Cancer in Africa

Epidemiology and Prevention

INTERNATIONAL AGENCY FOR RESEARCH ON CANCER

The International Agency for Research on Cancer (IARC) was established in 1965 by the World Health Assembly, as an independently financed organization within the framework of the World Health Organization. The headquarters of the Agency are at Lyon, France.

The Agency conducts a programme of research concentrating particularly on the epidemiology of cancer and the study of potential carcinogens in the human environment. Its field studies are supplemented by biological and chemical research carried out in the Agency's laboratories in Lyon, and, through collaborative research agreements, in national research institutions in many countries. The Agency also conducts a programme for the education and training of personnel for cancer research.

The publications of the Agency are intended to contribute to the dissemination of authoritative information on different aspects of cancer research. Information about IARC publications and how to order them, is available via the Internet at: **http://www.iarc.fr/**

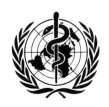

INTERNATIONAL AGENCY FOR RESEARCH ON CANCER
WORLD HEALTH ORGANIZATION

Cancer in Africa:

Epidemiology and Prevention

Edited by
**D.M. Parkin, J. Ferlay, M. Hamdi-Cherif,
F. Sitas, J. Thomas, H. Wabinga and S. L. Whelan**

IARC Scientific Publications No. 153

IARC*Press*
Lyon, France
2003

Published by the International Agency for Research on Cancer,
150 cours Albert Thomas, 69372 Lyon Cédex 08, France

Distributed by Oxford University Press, Walton Street, Oxford OX2 6DP, UK (fax: +44 1865 267782).
All IARC publications can also be ordered directly from IARC*Press* (fax: +33 04 72 73 83 02; E-mail: press@iarc.fr
or, in North America, tel. (toll-free) 877 WHO-IARC; fax 202-223-1776; E-mail iarcpress@who.int

IARC Library Cataloguing in Publication Data

Cancer in Africa : Epidemiology and prevention / editors, D.M. Parkin... [et al.]

(IARC scientific publication ; 153)

1. Epidemiology 2. Neoplasms – prevention 3. Africa   I.Parkin, D.M. II.Title III.Series

ISBN 92 832 2153 2   (NLM Classification W1)
ISSN 0300-5085

Printed in France

Contents

Foreword

Our knowledge of the geographic and ethnic patterns of cancer in the African continent is limited. There is an almost entire lack of valid mortality statistics by cause, and few registries have published incidence data in readily accessible sources – for example, the *Cancer Incidence in Five Continents* series. Yet the genetic diversity between populations living within the African continent is relatively large, and there are wide differences in environmental exposures, both external (climate, vegetation, micro-organisms) and social-cultural (e.g., diet, alcohol). Study of cancer risk in Africa, in relation to such factors, should therefore provide valuable clues to understanding the etiology of human cancer.

This book brings together all of the currently available data on the profile of cancer in the 52 countries of Africa, notably from cancer registries where data have not hitherto been published or have appeared only as journal articles or in local reports. The published literature on cancer patterns and trends in each country is reviewed. The book also provides a comprehensive review of the epidemiology and prevention of 20 major cancers, focusing on studies that have been performed in Africa, and the insights that these have provided. A special chapter deals with the impact of the AIDS epidemic on the burden of cancer on the continent.

The World Health Organization encourages all countries to plan their strategies for prevention, early diagnosis and care by means of a national cancer control programme. Appropriate decision-making depends on the availability of data on the burden and patterns of cancer, and it is hoped that this book will provide researchers and policy-makers with a comprehensive source of epidemiological information, as best it exists in Africa today.

Paul Kleihues, M.D.
Director, IARC

Contributors

Algeria, Algiers

D. Hammouda, Registre des tumeurs d'Alger, Institut National de Santé Publique, 4 chemin El Bakr, El Biar, Algiers
Tel: (213) 21-911140; Fax: (213) 21-912737
E-mail: dhammouda@sante.dz

Algeria, Batna

M.L. Bouhidel, Registre du Cancer de la Wilaya de Batna, Service d'Epidémiologie et de Médecine Préventive, CHU de Batna, Route de Tazoult, 03000 Batna
Tel: (213) 4-850000; Fax: (213) 4-856715

Algeria, Constantine

K. Mounia, Registre du Cancer de Constantine, Service d' Epidémiologie et de Médecine Préventive, C.H.U., Constantine 25000
Fax: (213) 4-697968

Algeria, Oran

L. Mokhtari, Registre du Cancer d'Oran, Service d'Epidémiologie et de Médecine Préventive, Centre Hospitalier et Universitaire d'Oran, Place Roux, 1 rue de Curie, Oran 31000
Tel/Fax: (213) 41-412246

Algeria, Sétif

M. Hamdi-Chérif, Registre du Cancer de Sétif, Service d'Epidémiologie, Hôpital Mère-Enfant, CHU de Sétif, Sétif 19000
Tel/Fax: (213) 36-911385
E-mail: hamdicherif@semepsetif.edu.dz

Algeria, Sidi-Bel-Abbès

A. Soulimane, Registre du Cancer de Sidi-Bel-Abbès, Service d'Epidémiologie et de Médecine Préventive, C.H.U. de Sidi-Bel-Abbès, 22000 Sidi-Bel-Abbès
Tel/Fax: (213) 7-549924

Burkina Faso, Ouagadougou

B. Sakande, Registre du Cancer de Burkina Faso/Ouagadougou, Centre Syfed, Ouagadougou, B.P. 4416, Ouagadougou 01
Tel: (226) 362264; Fax: (226) 31619

Cameroon, Yaoundé

A. Mbakop*, Service d'Anatomie Pathologique, Hôpital Général, B.P. 5408, Yaoundé (*Deceased)

Congo, Brazzaville

C. Gombe-Mbalawa, Registre du Cancer de Brazzaville, Service de Médecine et Cancérologie CHU, Université Marien Ngouabi, B.P. 69, 13 boulevard Maréchal Lyautey, Brazzaville
Tel: (242) 822365-68; Fax: (242) 828809 / 810411 / 810141
E-mail: unmgbuco@congonet.cg

Côte d'Ivoire, Abidjan

A. Echimane, Registre du Cancer d'Abidjan, Centre Hospitalier Universitaire de Treichville, 01 B.P. V.3, Abidjan 01
Tel: (225) 21-249122 / 258026; Fax: (225) 21-252852 / 350627
E-mail: echimane@ci.refer.org

The Gambia, Banjul

E. Bah, National Cancer Registry, The Gambia, c/o Gambia Hepatitis Intervention Study, MRC Laboratories, Fajara, P.O. Box 273, Banjul
Tel: (220) 495229; Fax: (220) 496117
E-mail: ebah@qanet.gm

Guinea, Conakry

M. Koulibaly, Guinean Tumour Registry, Centre National d'Anatomie Pathologique, Faculté de Médecine / Pharmacie, Université de Conakry, B.P. 4152, Conakry
Tel: (224) 228088; Fax: (224) 413990 / 455393

Kenya, Eldoret

N. Buziba, Eldoret Cancer Registry, Faculty of Health Sciences, Moi University, P.O. Box 4606, Eldoret
Tel: (254) 321-32781 / 2 / 3; Fax: (254) 321-33041
E-mail: mufhs@net2000ke.com

Malawi, Blantyre

C. Dzamalala & G. Liomba, Malawi National Cancer Registry, Queen Elizabeth Central Hospital, P.O. Box 95, Blantyre
Tel: (265) 630333, ext. 3029; Fax: (265) 631432
E-mail: dzamalala@hotmail.com

Mali, Bamako

S. Bayo, Registre du Cancer du Mali, Section des Maladies Néoplasiques, Institut National de Recherche en Santé Publique, Route de Koulikoro, B.P. 1771, Bamako
Tel: (223) 222-4231 / 222-0739; Fax: (223) 221-1999
E-mail: inrsp@spider.toolnet.org

Namibia, Windhoek

K. Johanesson & A. Zietsman, Cancer Association of Namibia, P.O. Box 30230, Windhoek
Tel: (264) 61-237740; Fax: (264) 61-237741
E-mail: kurtj@iafrica.com.na

Niger, Niamey

H. Nouhou, Registre du Cancer du Niger, Université de Niamey, Faculté des Sciences de la Santé, B.P. 10896, Niamey
Tel: (227) 734726 / 27, ext. 365; Fax: (227) 734731 / 733862
E-mail: hnouhou@yahoo.fr

Nigeria, Ibadan

J.O. Thomas, Ibadan Cancer Registry, Department of Pathology, University College Hospital, P.M.B. 5116, Ibadan
Tel: (234) 2-241-0088; Fax: (234) 2-241-0489
E-mail: dementia.uch@skannet.com.ng

France, La Réunion

J.Y. Vaillant, Registre des Cancers de l'île de la Réunion, CEPES (Cellule Epidémiologique, Prévention et Education pour la Santé), 12 rue Jean Chatel, 97400 St Denis
Tel: (262) 20.38.21 / 28.00.22; Fax: (262) 21.93.23
E-mail: cepes@cg974.fr

Rwanda, Butaré

Registre du Cancer de la Préfecture de Butaré, Faculté de Médecine, B.P. 30, Butaré
Tel/Fax: (250) 32012 / 3

South Africa, Cape Town

W. Gelderblom & W. Marasas, Programme on Mycotoxins and Experimental Carcinogenesis, Medical Research Council (MRC), P.O. Box 19070, Tygerberg Cape Town 7505
Tel: (27) 21-938-0286; Fax: (27) 21-938-0260
E-mail: wentzel.gelderblom@mrc.ac.za / wally.marasas@mrc.ac.za

South Africa, Elim

S. Lekhana, Elim Hospital, P.O. Box 12, Elim Hospital 0960, Limpopo
Tel: (27) 15-556-3201; Fax: (27) 15-556-3160
E-mail: chhaya@mweb.co.za

South Africa, National Pathology

F. Sitas & N. Mqoqi, National Cancer Registry, South African Institute for Medical Research, University of the Witwatersrand, P.O. Box 1038, Johannesburg 2000
Tel: (27) 11-489-9171; Fax: (27) 11-489-9152
E-mail:freddys@mail.saimr.wits.ac.za/
nokuzolam@mail.saimr.wits.ac.za

South Africa, Transkei, 4 Districts

N. Somdyala, PROMEC Cancer Registry, Medical Research Council, P.O. Box 19070, Tygerberg, Cape Town 7505
Tel: (27) 21-938-0290; Fax: (27) 21-938-0260
E-mail: ntuthu.somdyala@mrc.ac.za

South Africa, Transkei, Umtata

D. Mugwanya, Oesophageal Cancer Research Group, Department of Cardiothoracic and Vascular Surgery, Faculty of Health Sciences, UNITRA, Private Bag X1, Umtata, Transkei
Tel: (27) 47-502-2942 / 3; Fax: (27) 47-502-2946
E-mail: mugwanya@getafix.utr.ac.za

Swaziland, Manzini

S.L. Okonda, Swaziland National Cancer Registry, Central Public Health Laboratory, P.O. Box 54, Manzini
Tel: (268) 505-2126; Fax: (268) 505-6445

Tanzania, Dar es Salaam

J. Kitinya, Tanzania Cancer Registry, Department of Pathology, Muhimbili University College of Health Sciences, P.O. Box 65002, Dar es Salaam
Tel/Fax: (255) 51-151577
E-mail: jkitinya@muchs.ac.tz

Tanzania, Moshi

E. Moshi, Kilimanjaro Cancer Registry, Histopathology Department, Kilimanjaro Christian Medical Centre, P.O. Box 3010, Moshi
Tel : (255) 27-275-4377 / 83; Fax : (255) 27-275-4381
E-mail : kcmcadmin@kcmc.ac.tz

Tunisia, Centre

S. Korbi, Registre du Cancer de la Tunisie Centrale, Laboratoire d'Anatomie pathologique, C.H.U. F. Hached, Rue Dr Moro, 4002 Sousse
Tel/Fax: (216) 32-10355

Tunisia, North

M. Ben Abdallah, Registre des Cancers Nord-Tunisie, Service d'Epidémiologie, Biostatistique et Informatique, Institut Salah Azaiz, Boulevard du 9 Avril, Bab-Sâadoun, 1006 Tunis
Tel: (216) 1-577885; Fax: (216) 1-574725
E-mail: mansour.benabdallah@rns.tn

Tunisia, South

R. Jlidi, Registre des Cancers du Sud Tunisien, Laboratoire d'Anatomie et de Cytologie Pathologiques, Hôpital Universitaire Habib Bourguiba de Sfax, 3029 Sfax
Tel/Fax: (216) 4-240341
E-mail: rachid.jlidi@rns.tn

Uganda, Mbarara

F. Cruz Cordero, Department of Pathology, Mbarara University of Science and Technology, P.O. Box 1410, Mbarara
Fax: (256) 485-20782
E-mail: mustmed@infocom.co.ug

Uganda, Kyadondo

H. Wabinga, Kampala Cancer Registry, Department of Pathology, Makerere University Medical School, P.O. Box 7072, Kampala
Tel: (256) 41-531730 / 558731 / 17; Fax: (256) 41-530412 / 543895
E-mail: cancer-reg@infocom.co.ug

Zimbabwe, Harare

M. Bassett & E. Chokunonga, Zimbabwe National Cancer Registry, Parirenyatwa Hospital, P.O. Box A 449, Avondale, Harare
Tel: (263) 4-791631; Fax: (263) 4-794445
E-mail: cancer.registry@healthnet.zw

Acknowledgements

The editors would like to thank the following persons for their contributions to this volume:

Professor C. Wild (University of Leeds, UK), Dr S. Franceschi and Dr E. Šteliarová-Foucher (IARC) for their helpful comments on drafts of manuscripts; Mr E. Bah (Gambia Cancer Registry) and Dr D. Hammouda (Cancer Registry of Algiers) for preparing early drafts for certain chapters and Professor C. Ijsselmuiden (University of Pretoria, South Africa) for bibliographic research. Our thanks also to the following IARC staff: Ms Krittika Pitaksaringkarn for preparing the illustrations, Ms Chantal Déchaux for assistance with the manuscript and finally, Dr John Cheney for his invaluable work on the technical editing of the volume.

The cancer registries of Burkina Faso, Ouagadougou; Congo, Brazzaville; Côte d'Ivoire, Abidjan; Guinea, Conakry; Mali, Bamako and Niger, Niamey have been able to provide data for this publication through the generous support of the Association pour la Recherche Contre le Cancer (France).

1. Introduction

Africa was the birthplace of mankind. It is estimated that *Homo sapiens* and his ancestors were confined to the African continent for most of their evolutionary period before migration began to other areas of the world some 140 000 years ago. As a result of the long period of evolutionary history in Africa, there is more genetic diversity between populations living within the African continent than between Africans and the rest of mankind (Cavalli-Sforza, 1997). Not only do populations within Africa vary considerably with respect to their genes, but across the continent there is a very wide range of environments, in terms of climate, vegetation (12 of 16 vegetation zones defined by Matthews (1983) are represented) and zoology (including micro-organisms and human parasites). For all of these reasons, one might expect a wide diversity of cancer patterns, the study of which would be illuminating to our understanding of the causes of human cancer.

Alas, knowledge of cancer patterns in Africa is woefully inadequate, as anyone who has tried to obtain reasonably accurate estimates of cancer risk in different areas can attest. Until quite recently, knowledge of cancer patterns was based primarily on the work of pioneering clinicians and pathologists who described the composition of series of cancer patients encountered in their professional lives, in terms of age, sex, cancer site and histology. These clinical and pathological case series enriched the literature in the 1950s and 1960s, and were the subject of several reviews that drew together information on the relative frequency of different types of cancer in different areas, to piece together some sort of overall picture. Several of these reviews bear the title, like this book, of 'Cancer in Africa' (Oettlé, 1964; Clifford *et al*., 1968; Cook & Burkitt, 1971).

Unfortunately, comparisons based upon relative frequency of different cancers in case series can be very misleading. Almost all case series will be biased in terms of the probability that the different cancers occurring in the population will be included. Pathology series overrepresent those cancers that are readily biopsied and are correspondingly deficient in cancers such as liver, pancreas or brain, compared with the real incidence in the population. Hospital series are biased by the clinical facilities available (radiotherapy series always include, for example, many cancers of the head and neck and of the cervix, and few gastro-intestinal cancers). What is more, use of proportions (or percentages) of different cancers as the statistic for comparison introduces a further problem: since the total must always be 1 (or 100), so that if one cancer is 'common', all others in the series will appear to be rare, with respect to the comparison populations (see Boyle & Parkin, 1991).

The appropriate statistic for making comparisons of risk between populations is the incidence rate (although mortality rates may be used for the purpose for cancers with a high fatality or if incidence rates are not available). Incidence rates derive from population-based cancer registries, which aim to record information on *all* new cases of cancer which occur in a defined population (characterized, as a minimum, in terms of population size by age group and sex). The history of cancer registration in Africa, since the earliest registries set up in the 1950s, has, until fairly recently, been a sparse one. Cancer registration in economically under-

developed populations, such as all of the countries of northern and sub-Saharan Africa, is a difficult undertaking for a variety of reasons. The major problem is ensuring that every new case of cancer is identified. Cases can only be found when they come into contact with health services: hospitals, health centres, clinics and laboratories. When resources are restricted, the proportion of the population with access to such institutions may be limited, so that the statistics generated will not truly reflect the pattern of cancer. The ease with which the cases can be identified also depends on the extent of medical facilities available and the quality of statistical and record systems already in place (e.g., pathology request forms, hospital discharge abstracts, treatment records, etc.).

A further problem is to identify the 'usual' place of residence of the cancer patients so that, when incidence rates are calculated, the cases belonging to the population at risk can be selected. Place of residence is not an obvious concept in some African communities; especially in East and South Africa, individuals living and working in urban areas retain attachments to their home village, to which they may return intermittently, and permanently as they get older. On the other hand, persons normally living in rural areas frequently come to town to stay with a relative before visiting a hospital; the address given to the hospital will often be that of the city relative. Valid population estimates are also difficult to obtain. Censuses are infrequent (and also face problems of whom to include as residents of a particular area) and extensive, transient migrations make accurate intercensal and post-censal estimation problematic.

It is impossible to know, without an extensive population survey, what proportion of cancer cases never come into contact with modern diagnostic or treatment services, instead making use only of traditional healers or receiving no care at all. In the past, studies have suggested that some sections of the population may have been under-represented in hospital statistics, particularly older women or young men, who were more likely to return to their rural 'homes' to seek care (Flegg Mitchell, 1966). However, the consensus is that this is probably rather rare in contemporary urban Africa. Most cancer patients will, eventually, seek medical assistance, although very often at an advanced stage of disease. The situation in rural areas may be quite different. There have been few attempts to measure cancer incidence in rural populations, and certainly, when it has been tried, the recorded rates are low. For this reason, African cancer registries are almost all based on urban centres, where diagnostic and treatment facilities are situated. The main technical problem (as already noted) is then to exclude registration of 'temporary' residents, migrating into the urban area for treatment. From an epidemiological point of view, one must guess at how well the cancer profile from the urban areas reflects that in the country as a whole, given what is known of urban–rural differences in cancer patterns in other areas of the world (Nasca *et al*., 1980; Friis & Storm, 1993).

A further problem is the lack of trained personnel. There is very often a shortage not only of epidemiologists and statisticians to design and operate information systems, but also of suitably trained personnel to man the statistical infrastructure at all levels.

Health information systems—such as medical records departments—have been automated only very recently, if at all, and manual filing and processing leads to long delays, problems of quality control, lack of feedback and disillusionment of those responsible for collecting information.

Finally, it should be recalled that in most developing countries cancer has not been a priority for health ministries; nutritional, parasitic and infectious diseases have presented a greater and more immediate challenge. The level of interest in and development of cancer statistics may reflect the low priority that has been given to malignant disease in the past. Some of the problems in the collection and analysis of data on cancer cases have been reviewed (Olweny, 1985; Parkin & Sanghvi, 1991).

The development of registration can, to some extent, be gauged by the availability of incidence data through the *Cancer Incidence in Five Continents* series, which publishes data considered to be sufficiently complete and accurate to allow valid comparisons between geographical regions, ethnic groups, and over time. Table 1 shows the number of African cancer registries and different populations (a registry may provide rates on two or more ethnic groups, for example) in volumes I–VIII of this series.

Table 1. Cancer registries in *Cancer Incidence in Five Continents*

Volume	Period	Registries	Populations
I	1950s	4	4
II	1956–67	4*	7
III	1968–72	2*	2
IV	1973–77	1	1
V	1978–82	0	0
VI	1983–87	3	3
VII	1988–92	5	6
VIII	1993–97	6	6

* One updates the entry in previous volumes

The low point was reached in 1978–82 (Volume V) which might have been retitled as 'Cancer Incidence in Four Continents', since there was no contribution from Africa at all. Since then, as Table 1 shows, there has been a slow improvement with, in 1993–97, six cancer registries qualifying, although others might have done so, had reasonable data on populations at risk been available in what, for most countries, was a period during which no census had been carried out.

In this volume, we have included a description of all current cancer registration activity in Africa, as well as past activity. The tables showing incidence of cancer by site include data from the six cancer registries appearing in *Cancer Incidence in Five Continents*, Volume VIII (Parkin *et al.*, 2002), as well as from several others which provide data useful for comparison purposes. Some registries have been established only recently (their results will probably appear in *Cancer Incidence in Five Continents*, Volume IX) or use somewhat shaky population estimates. The results from other registries were considered to be too dependent upon histopathology data, or probably somewhat incomplete, although they provide useful 'lower bound' estimates of the true incidence for several cancer sites. Results from registries for which no realistic population at risk could be derived, or for which calculated rates were considered by the editors to be too misleading, are simply reproduced as tables showing numbers of cases, by age group and sex, with the percentage frequencies by site and sex.

These recent data are presented country by country, within the five 'areas' used by the United Nations Population Division in presenting demographic statistics (Northern, Western, Middle (Central), Eastern and Southern Africa). The countries comprising these 'areas' may be different from those in other regional groupings—for example, Zimbabwe (and Zambia) are grouped with Eastern Africa, although considered in many other contexts as part of Southern Africa. Within these country chapters, other available data on the cancer profile are also presented. These include cancer mortality rates, plus historical data from cancer registries or, when no incidence data are available, published case series which give some clue as to the likely cancer profile.

With respect to mortality data, the situation in Africa is even more dismal than for incidence. Death registration and medical certification of cause of death are neither feasible nor a statutory requirement in almost all countries, and deaths are generally registered only for a definite purpose, such as inheritance or insurance claims. Reasonably complete and accurate statistics on mortality by cause are available only for Mauritius and the French overseas department of Reunion. The background to death registration in South Africa is described in the chapter on that country. It has never been complete, particularly for the rural black population. Nevertheless, something could be made of the data, at least until the 'race' variable was removed from the death certificate for several years after the end of the apartheid regime in 1994.

To accompany the country-by-country description of cancer profiles, a little background material on each country is presented. The brief synopsis on climate, geography, natural resources etc. has been taken from the on-line version of the World Factbook of the United States Central Intelligence Agency (http://www.odci.gov/cia/publication/factbook/index.html), editing out that organization's economic and social nostrums. Here, we also present some summary statistical data on each of the 53 countries in Africa (Table 2). These have been taken from the UN Demographic Yearbook for 2000 (UN, 2002). Included in Table 2 are:
- Population size (by sex)
- Percentage of the population aged less than 15 (children), 15–24, and 65+ years
- Annual average percentage growth rate (1995–2000)
- Crude birth rate
- Fertility rate
- Crude death rate
- Infant mortality rate
- Expectation of life at birth (by sex)

In addition to the 'country profiles', this volume includes reviews of the epidemiology and prevention of 19 major cancers of importance on the African continent, together with chapters on cancer in children and cancers related to AIDS. These chapters bring together all the descriptive data from Part 1, notably in cancer-specific tables summarizing recent estimates of incidence and, for certain cancers, the proportions of different histological subtypes in the different registry series. Historic data on incidence (or mortality) of the cancer are reviewed (Table 3). In addition, we have carried out what we hope is an exhaustive review of the literature on the epidemiology and prevention of each of these cancers in the African context. This review omits published articles which are simply descriptions of case series in different clinical settings (unless such data are the only pertinent material relating to the epidemiology of the cancer), but we hope that very little else of significance has been missed. The authors of any papers that have been overlooked are asked for their indulgence in advance. These chapters also include a description of geographical patterns (and sometimes ethnic and temporal variation) and of etiological studies. Few reports have been identified related to research on cancer prevention in Africa (and, for that matter, not a single study that has investigated cancer survival in a representative (population-based) sample of cancer patients). This surely reflects the low priority

Table 2. Demographic statistics: 2000

Country	Country code	Population (2000) Both sexes All ages	Male All ages	Female All ages	% 0-14	% 15-24	% 65+	Average annual population growth rate (%) 1995-2000	Crude birth rate (per 1000 population) 1995-2000	Total fertility (children per woman) 1995-2000	Crude death rate (per 1000 population) 1995-2000	Infant mortality (deaths per 1000 live births) 1995-2000	Male expectation of life at birth (in years) 1995-2000	Female expectation of life at birth (in years) 1995-2000
AFRICA	**903**	**793,627**	**396,374**	**397,253**	**42.6%**	**20.3%**	**3.3%**	**2.41**	**38.7**	**5.3**	**14.1**	**91.2**	**50.3**	**52.4**
North Africa	**912**	**174,150**	**87,955**	**86,195**	**35.6%**	**20.7%**	**4.1%**	**1.86**	**27.6**	**3.6**	**7.5**	**57.7**	**63.0**	**66.1**
Algeria	12	30,291	15,346	14,945	34.8%	21.7%	4.1%	1.82	25.7	3.3	5.7	50.0	67.5	70.3
Egypt	818	67,884	34,364	33,521	35.4%	20.3%	4.1%	1.82	26.2	3.4	6.8	50.8	64.7	67.9
Libyan Arab Jamahiriya	434	5,290	2,741	2,549	33.9%	23.7%	3.4%	2.13	26.4	3.8	4.7	27.8	68.3	72.2
Morocco	504	29,878	14,964	14,914	34.7%	20.6%	4.1%	1.87	26.8	3.4	6.6	52.2	64.8	68.5
Sudan	736	31,095	15,639	15,457	40.1%	19.7%	3.4%	2.13	36.1	4.9	12.2	85.9	53.6	56.4
Tunisia	788	9,459	4,776	4,682	29.7%	21.1%	5.9%	1.12	18.7	2.3	6.7	30.3	68.4	70.7
West Africa	**914**	**224,189**	**112,388**	**111,801**	**44.8%**	**20.3%**	**3.0%**	**2.67**	**42.3**	**5.9**	**15.1**	**96.0**	**49.3**	**50.7**
Benin	204	6,272	3,092	3,180	46.4%	20.3%	2.7%	2.66	42.8	6.1	13.1	87.8	51.8	55.3
Burkina Faso	854	11,535	5,576	5,959	48.7%	20.8%	3.2%	2.32	46.7	6.9	17.9	99.1	44.2	46.2
Cape Verde	132	427	199	228	39.3%	21.6%	4.6%	2.30	31.8	3.6	6.4	55.6	65.5	71.3
Côte d'Ivoire	384	16,013	8,206	7,807	42.1%	21.5%	3.1%	2.14	36.0	5.1	15.4	89.0	47.4	48.1
Gambia	270	1,303	644	658	40.3%	17.9%	3.1%	3.11	40.4	5.2	18.5	125.3	44.0	46.8
Ghana	288	19,306	9,613	9,692	40.9%	21.4%	3.2%	2.20	34.0	4.6	10.8	68.6	55.0	57.6
Guinea	324	8,154	4,102	4,052	44.1%	20.1%	2.8%	2.13	45.7	6.3	18.2	124.2	46.0	47.0
Guinea-Bissau	624	1,199	591	608	43.5%	18.7%	3.6%	2.14	44.8	6.0	20.4	130.8	42.7	45.5
Liberia	430	2,913	1,465	1,448	42.7%	25.0%	2.9%	7.07	50.1	6.8	16.6	111.4	47.1	49.0
Mali	466	11,351	5,624	5,727	46.1%	19.7%	4.0%	2.68	49.9	7.0	18.5	130.3	49.8	51.8
Mauritania	478	2,665	1,321	1,344	44.1%	19.7%	3.2%	3.16	43.5	6.0	15.4	105.6	48.9	52.1
Niger	562	10,832	5,459	5,373	49.9%	19.5%	2.0%	3.46	55.4	8.0	20.7	136.1	43.9	44.5
Nigeria	566	113,862	57,383	56,479	45.1%	20.2%	3.0%	2.74	41.7	5.9	14.1	88.1	51.0	51.5
Senegal	686	9,421	4,697	4,723	44.3%	20.0%	2.5%	2.54	39.5	5.6	13.0	62.4	50.5	54.2
Sierra Leone	694	4,405	2,165	2,239	44.2%	19.2%	2.9%	1.53	49.5	6.5	26.4	165.4	36.0	38.6
Togo	768	4,527	2,248	2,279	44.3%	20.3%	3.1%	3.27	40.5	5.8	13.9	83.1	50.1	52.6
Central Africa	**911**	**95,404**	**47,240**	**48,164**	**47.2%**	**19.2%**	**3.1%**	**2.61**	**46.0**	**6.4**	**16.2**	**98.2**	**47.5**	**50.2**
Angola	24	13,134	6,499	6,635	48.2%	19.0%	2.8%	2.94	51.0	7.2	20.2	126.2	43.3	46.0
Cameroon	120	14,876	7,405	7,471	43.1%	20.6%	3.7%	2.28	37.6	5.1	14.8	87.3	49.1	50.8
Central African Republic	140	3,717	1,811	1,907	43.0%	19.8%	4.0%	2.10	39.6	5.3	19.1	101.2	42.7	46.0
Chad	148	7,885	3,900	3,985	46.5%	19.1%	3.1%	3.15	48.4	6.7	19.6	122.5	43.9	46.4
Congo	178	3,018	1,478	1,540	46.3%	19.2%	3.3%	2.96	44.5	6.3	14.7	72.1	48.8	53.1
Democratic Republic of the Congo	180	50,948	25,245	25,703	48.8%	18.9%	2.9%	2.56	47.7	6.7	15.0	90.6	49.2	51.9
Equatorial Guinea	226	457	225	231	43.7%	18.3%	3.9%	2.68	43.2	5.9	16.5	107.7	48.4	51.6
Gabon	266	1,230	609	621	40.2%	17.1%	5.8%	2.63	37.8	5.4	15.8	87.7	51.2	53.7

Table 2 (Contd). Demographic statistics: 2000

Country	Country code	Population (2000)						Average annual population growth rate (%) 1995–2000	Crude birth rate (per 1000 population) 1995–2000	Total fertility (children per woman) 1995–2000	Crude death rate (per 1000 population) 1995–2000	Infant mortality (deaths per 1000 live births) 1995–2000	Male expectation of life at birth (in years) 1995–2000	Female expectation of life at birth (in years) 1995–2000
		Both sexes All ages	Male All ages	Female All ages	% 0–14	% 15–24	% 65+							
East Africa	**910**	**250,318**	**124,381**	**125,938**	**45.3%**	**20.3%**	**2.9%**	**2.67**	**43.0**	**6.1**	**17.5**	**103.1**	**44.8**	**46.5**
Burundi	108	6,356	3,088	3,268	47.6%	20.5%	2.9%	0.89	43.1	6.8	21.3	120.0	39.6	41.5
Comoros	174	706	354	352	43.0%	21.5%	2.6%	2.95	38.9	5.4	9.5	76.3	57.4	60.2
Djibouti	262	632	297	335	43.2%	19.4%	3.2%	2.96	40.7	6.1	18.0	116.6	43.9	46.9
Eritrea	232	3,659	1,817	1,842	43.9%	19.2%	2.9%	2.75	40.9	5.7	14.0	89.3	50.1	53.0
Ethiopia	231	62,908	31,259	31,649	45.2%	19.1%	3.0%	2.55	44.6	6.8	19.0	114.8	43.6	45.4
Kenya	404	30,669	15,273	15,396	43.5%	22.7%	2.8%	2.32	35.4	4.6	12.1	64.7	51.2	53.2
Madagascar	450	15,970	7,943	8,028	44.7%	19.2%	3.0%	2.94	44.0	6.1	14.7	100.2	50.5	52.8
Malawi	454	11,308	5,617	5,692	46.3%	20.0%	2.9%	2.42	47.2	6.8	22.2	139.8	40.7	40.7
Mauritius	480	1,161	579	583	25.6%	18.2%	6.2%	0.83	17.1	2.0	6.7	18.5	66.9	74.8
Mozambique	508	18,292	9,042	9,251	43.9%	19.7%	3.2%	2.31	44.7	6.3	22.4	136.7	39.4	41.8
Réunion	638	721	352	369	28.1%	17.4%	6.7%	1.67	19.9	2.3	5.7	9.0	69.4	78.3
Rwanda	646	7,609	3,765	3,844	44.3%	22.2%	2.6%	8.48	42.4	6.2	21.7	121.9	38.7	40.2
Somalia	706	8,778	4,358	4,420	48.0%	19.3%	2.4%	3.56	52.3	7.3	18.5	122.3	45.4	48.5
Tanzania, United Republic of	834	35,119	17,422	17,697	45.0%	20.6%	2.4%	2.58	40.4	5.5	13.3	81.3	50.0	52.3
Uganda	800	23,300	11,625	11,676	49.2%	20.1%	2.5%	2.95	50.4	7.1	20.3	106.5	41.4	42.5
Zambia	894	10,421	5,236	5,185	46.5%	20.7%	2.9%	2.46	43.8	6.1	20.7	93.6	40.9	40.1
Zimbabwe	716	12,627	6,315	6,313	45.2%	21.8%	3.2%	1.91	37.4	5.0	18.0	65.0	43.2	42.7
Southern Africa	**913**	**49,567**	**24,411**	**25,156**	**35.0%**	**20.6%**	**3.6%**	**1.61**	**27.8**	**3.3**	**11.5**	**63.0**	**52.9**	**57.9**
Botswana	72	1,541	755	787	42.1%	22.5%	2.8%	1.61	33.6	4.4	17.0	73.9	43.8	44.7
Lesotho	426	2,035	1,009	1,026	39.3%	19.8%	4.2%	1.69	35.0	4.8	14.6	108.1	50.7	51.6
Namibia	516	1,757	868	889	43.7%	19.6%	3.8%	2.06	37.6	5.3	17.6	78.5	44.9	45.3
South Africa	710	43,309	21,323	21,986	34.0%	20.6%	3.6%	1.57	26.7	3.1	10.8	58.2	53.9	59.5
Swaziland	748	925	456	469	41.6%	20.5%	3.5%	2.04	35.6	4.8	14.0	86.9	49.3	52.2

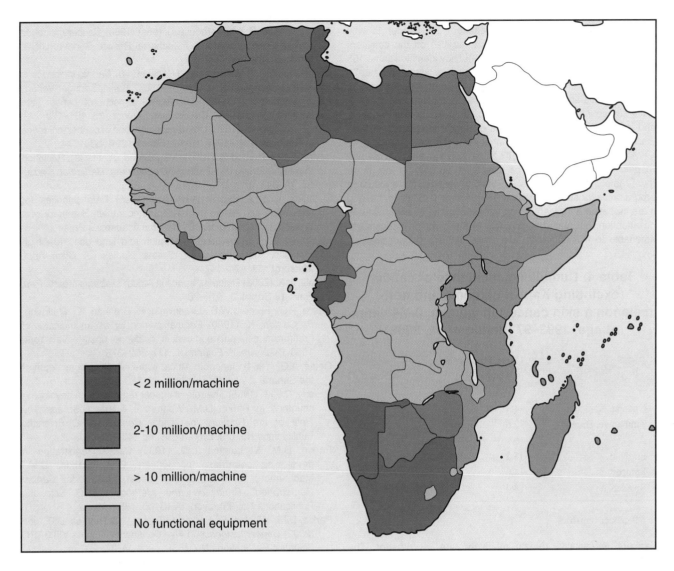

Figure 1. Radiotherapy services in Africa
From Levin *et al.* (1999)

which cancer has been accorded among the health and welfare problems facing African governments, and the international agencies involved in dealing with them.

In fact, a review of the policy documents published by the major agencies advising on (and financing) health care for the people of Africa shows no concern for the care of persons suffering from

Table 3. Sources of historic incidence data (1953–74) in Chapter 4

No.	Source
1	Doll *et al.*, 1966 (*Cancer Incidence in Five Continents* vol. I)
2	Doll *et al.*, 1970 (*Cancer Incidence in Five Continents* vol. II
3	Waterhouse *et al.*, 1976 (*Cancer Incidence in Five Continents* vol. III)
4	Waterhouse *et al.*, 1982 (*Cancer Incidence in Five Continents* vol. IV)
5	Wabinga *et al.*, 2000
6	Skinner *et al.*, 1993

cancer. The European Union's Directorate of Development (http://europa.eu.int/comm/development/sector/social/hap_policy_en.htm) gives priority to family planning, sexual and reproductive health and communicable disease (HIV/AIDS, malaria and tuberculosis). USAID (Malanick & Pebley, 1996) defines four strategic objectives—reduction of unintended pregnancies, maternal mortality, infant and child mortality, and sexually-transmitted disease (with a focus on HIV). The World Bank (1994) believes that better health in Africa will be achieved by reformed health care systems concentrating on basic health services delivered largely through local health centres and district hospitals.

From the purely objective point of view, concentration upon health problems in Africa that have been largely solved in the developed world (infant and child mortality, maternal mortality, infectious diseases) appears eminently reasonable. Unfortunately, these 'old' diseases co-exist in Africa with the emergence of new ones, most evidently AIDS, but also some of the non-communicable diseases, such as hypertension, diabetes and accidents/violence (Motala, 2002; Seedat, 2000; Reza *et al.*, 2001; Walker *et al.*, 2000) as well as cancer. Cancer is not a rare disease in Africa. Even ignoring the huge load of AIDS-related Kaposi sarcoma, the probability of developing a cancer by age 65 years in a woman living in present-day Kampala or Harare is only about 20% lower that of her sisters in western Europe (Table 4). Yet the facilities for providing treatment for cancer cases in most of Africa are minimal.

This paucity of specialized treatment for cancer is well illustrated by a survey of radiotherapy facilities on the continent undertaken in 1998 by Levin *et al.* (1999). They identified some 155 megavoltage machines (cobalt units or linear accelerators), but 79 of these (51%) were in just four countries of North Africa (Morocco, Algeria, Tunisia and Egypt) and 40 (26%) in the Republic of South Africa. 34 countries (out of 56) had no radiotherapy facilities at all, and in many others, provision was grossly inadequate, with less than one machine per 10 million inhabitants (Figure 1).

Although there are no data, it seems likely that the situation with respect to chemotherapy or specialist surgery is no more favourable. In turn, there is little incentive to encourage programmes for early detection of cancer when facilities for treating it are inadequate. Primary cancer prevention has received virtually no attention, not least because few of the common cancers are amenable to this approach, and those that are (tobacco-related

Table 4. Cumulative incidence of cancer (excluding Kaposi sarcoma and non-melanoma skin cancer) in women, 0–64 years of age, 1993–97 (Parkin *et al.*, 2002)

	Cumulative incidence (0–64 years) %
Uganda, Kampala	11.3
Zimbabwe, Harare	12.6
England	15.2
France*	14.0
Sweden	14.4

* 9 cancer registries

cancers, especially) remain relatively rare, at present. The exception is liver cancer, largely preventable by vaccination, as discussed in the relevant chapter, but where logistic problems and competing priorities have slowed implementation.

Hopefully, as the 21st century advances, cancer sufferers in Africa will receive more attention to their plight than has been evident in the past. The World Health Organization (2002) encourages all countries to implement a national cancer control programme within a comprehensive, systemic framework, comprising prevention, early diagnosis, screening, curative therapy, pain relief and palliative care. Appropriate decision-making can only be based upon the availability of epidemiological and programmatic data. It is hoped that this book will provide researchers and policy makers with this type of information, as best it exists in Africa today.

References

Boyle, P. & Parkin, D.M. (1991) Statistical methods for registries. In: Jensen, O.M., Parkin, D.M., MacLennan, R., Muir, C.S. & Skeet, R.G., eds, *Cancer Registration: Principles and Methods* (IARC Scientific Publications No. 95), IARC, Lyon, pp. 126–158

Cavalli-Sofrza, L.L. (1997) Genes, peoples and languages. *Proc. Natl Acad. Sci. USA*, **94**, 7719–7724

Clifford, P., Linsell, C.A. & Timms, G.L., eds, (1968) *Cancer in Africa*, Nairobi, East African Publishing House

Cook, P.J. & Burkitt, D.P. (1971) Cancer in Africa. *Br. Med. Bull.*, **27**, 14–20

Doll, R., Payne, P. & Waterhouse, J. (eds) (1966) *Cancer Incidence in Five Continents*, Vol. I. A Technical Report. Geneva, UICC; Berlin, Springer-Verlag

Doll, R., Muir, C. & Waterhouse, J. (eds) (1970) *Cancer Incidence in Five Continents*, Vol. II. Geneva, UICC; Berlin, Springer-Verlag

Flegg Mitchell, H. (1966) Sociological aspects of cancer rate surveys in Africa. *Natl Cancer Inst. Monogr.*, **25**, 151–170

Friis, S. & Storm H. (1993) Urban-rural variation in cancer incidence in Denmark 1943-1987. *Eur. J. Cancer*, **29A**, 538–544

Levin, C.V., el Gueddari, B. & Meghzifene, A. (1999) Radiation therapy in Africa; distribution and equipment. *Radiother. Oncol.*, **52**, 79–84

Malanick, C.E. & Pebley, A.R., eds (1996) Data priorities for population and health in developing countries. Summary of a Workshop. Washington DC, National Academies Press

Matthews, E. (1983) Global vegetation and land use: new high resolution data bases for climate studies. *J. Clim. Appl. Meteorol.*, **22**, 474–487

Motala, A.A. (2002) Diabetes trends in Africa. *Diabetes Metab. Res. Rev.*, **18 Suppl. 3**, S14–20

Nasca, P.C., Burnett, W.S., Greenwald, P., Brennan, K., Wolfgang, P., Carlton, K. (1980) Population density as an indicator of urban-rural differences in cancer incidence, upstate New York, 1968-1972. *Am. J. Epidemiol.*, **112**, 362–375

Oettlé, A.G. (1964) Cancer in Africa, especially in regions south of the Sahara. *J. Natl Cancer Inst.*, **33**, 383–439

Olweny, C.L.M. (1985) The role of cancer registration in developing countries. In: Parkin, D.M., Wagner, G. & Muir, C.S., eds, *The Role of the Registry in Cancer Control* (IARC Scientific Publications No. 66), Lyon, IARC, pp.143-152.

Parkin, D.M. & Sanghvi, L.D. (1991) Cancer registration in developing countries. In: Jensen, O.M., Parkin, D.M., MacLennan, R., Muir, C.S. & Skeet, R.G., eds, *Cancer Registration: Principles and Methods* (IARC Scientific Publications No. 95), Lyon, IARC, pp. 185–198

Parkin, D.M., Whelan, S., Ferlay, J., Teppo, L. & Thomas, D.B., eds (2002) *Cancer Incidence in Five Continents,* Volume VIII (IARC Scientific Publications No. 155) , Lyon, IARC

Reza, A., Mercy, J.A. & Krug, E. (2001) Epidemiology of violent deaths in the world. *Inj. Prev.*, **7**, 104–111

Seedat, Y.K. (2000) Hypertension in developing nations in sub-Saharan Africa. *J. Hum. Hypertens.*, **14**, 739–747

Skinner, M.E.G., Parkin, D.M., Vizcaino, A.P. & Ndhlovu, A. (1993) *Cancer in the African Population of Bulawayo, Zimbabwe, 1963–1977: Incidence, Time Trends and Risk Factors* (IARC Technical Report No. 15), Lyon, IARC

Wabinga, H.R., Parkin, D.M., Wabwire-Mangen, F. & Nambooze, S. (2000) Trends in incidence in Kyadondo County, Uganda, 1960–1997. *Br. J. Cancer*, **82**, 1585–1592

Walker, R.W., McLarty, D.G., Kitange, H.M., Whiting, D., Masuki, G., Mtasiwa, D.M., Machibya, H., Unwin, N. & Alberti, K.G. (2000) Stroke mortality in urban and rural Tanzania. Adult Morbidity and Mortality Project. *Lancet*, **355**, 1684–1687

Waterhouse, J.A.H., Muir, C.S., Correa, P. (eds) (1976) *Cancer Incidence in Five Continents*. Vol. III (IARC Scientific Publications No. 15.) Lyon, IARC

Waterhouse, J.A.H., Muir, C.S., Shanmugaratnam, K., Powell, J. (eds) (1982) *Cancer Incidence in Five Continents*. Vol. IV (IARC Scientific Publications No. 42.) Lyon, IARC

World Bank (1994) *Better Health in Africa*, Washington, World Bank

World Health Organization (2002) *National Cancer Control Programmes: Policies and Managerial Guidelines*, Geneva, WHO

2. Processing and presentation of the data

Processing of the data

The data used to create the tables presented in this book were generally submitted as listings of individual anonymous cases with the following variables (minimum):

1. a registration number which identifies the patient or the case
2. sex
3. ethnic group or race (optional)
4. age
5. date of incidence
6. site of the tumour
7. morphology of the tumour
8. behaviour of the tumour
9. basis of diagnosis

The processing of such data followed a regular procedure established in the Unit of Descriptive Epidemiology of IARC that is described in more detail in the *Cancer Incidence in Five Continents* series (Parkin *et al.*, 1997, 2002). When necessary, the data-sets were first converted into a full ICD-O-2 coding schema, then passed through the IARC-CHECK program (Parkin *et al.*, 1994) for verification. After validation, the records were converted to ICD-10 for presentation purposes. It should be noted that many cancer registries in Africa used the Canreg system, a software program developed at IARC and designed for population-based cancer registries. The data entry module of Canreg is based on the ICD-O-2 coding schema, and incorporates the same edits as those performed by the IARC-CHECK program, so that many data-sets had already been checked before submission. This simplified and speeded up the data validation process.

Presentation of the data

The largest set of tables in this book presents data on age-specific and age-standardized incidence, either by population (cancer registry) or as summary tables by cancer site.

Tables of incidence by registry

Population-at-risk: Whenever possible, registries were asked to provide data on population at risk by sex and age for as many years as possible, so that an accurate denominator corresponding to the period of the incident cases (person-years at risk) could be calculated. For those registries able to supply this information, the annual average population during the period covered appears at the foot of the table.

The age-specific incidence table: The numbers given in the body of the tables are the number of cancer cases registered during the corresponding period by sex, site and age-group. An example is given in Table 1. The column headings are defined as below:

SITE: A shortened version of the full ICD-10 title describing each site or site grouping.
ALL AGES: The total number of cases by site and for all sites.

AGE UNK: The number of cases of unknown age. They are included in the total number of cases and in the calculation of the crude rate. They are also taken into account in the computation of the world age-standardized and cumulative incidence rates.
MV (%): This is the proportion of cases known to be diagnosed by a microscopic method (either histology or cytology) and expressed as a percentage of all cases registered, including cases of unknown age or of unknown basis of diagnosis.
0-, 15-, , , 65+: The number of cancer cases registered by age-groups.
CRUDE RATE: The crude average annual incidence rate, calculated by dividing the total number of cases (including unknown age) by the corresponding population at risk (all males or all females) and expressed per 100 000 person-years.
%: The proportional frequency of each site to the total of all sites excluding C44 (other skin).
CR64: The cumulative incidence rate up to age 64 years. This is the sum over each year of age of the age-specific incidence rates, taken from birth to age 64. The cumulative rates are computed using five-year age-bands 0-, 5-, 10-,..., 64-, 65+, and have been adjusted to account for cases of unknown age (Parkin *et al.*, 1997).
ASR (W): The world age-standardized incidence rate. It is calculated by the direct method, using the world standard population and five-year age-bands 0-, 5-, 10-, ..., 64-, 65+, and has been adjusted to account for cases of unknown age (Parkin *et al.*, 1997). Note that the result would be slightly different if the ASR were calculated using the data presented in the table by 10-year age bands.
ICD-10: The ICD-10 code(s) corresponding to the site or group of sites given in the left-hand column.
Average annual population: If the user wishes to calculate the annual incidence rate per 100 000 for a particular age group, cancer site and sex, the number of cancer cases should be divided by the average annual population and the number of years for which the data are presented, then multiplied by 100 000.

For those registries that did not supply information on population at risk, a simplified version of the table, without summary rates, is presented.

Childhood table: Whenever possible (notably if sufficient cases were recorded), data on childhood cancer are presented by registry. The layout of the table follows that used in International Incidence of Childhood Cancer Vol. II (Parkin *et al.*, 1998) with a limited number of cancer types defined by the *International Classification of Childhood Cancer* (Kramarova *et al.*, 1996). The data are presented for the three age-group (0–4, 5–9, 10–14 years) and for both sexes combined only. An example is given in Table 2. The column headings are defined as below:

NUMBER OF CASES: The number of cases by age-group and the total age 0–14 years.
M/F: The ratio of the number of cases in males to that in females.
Overall REL. FREQ.(%): The percentage contribution of each cancer type (or group) to the total case series.

Table 1. Elsewhere (1995-1998)

NUMBER OF CASES BY AGE GROUP AND SUMMARY RATES OF INCIDENCE - MALE

SITE	ALL AGES	AGE UNK	MV (%)	0-	15-	25-	35-	45-	55-	65+	CRUDE RATE	%	CR 64	ASR (W)	ICD (10th)
Mouth	142	1	97	4	2	5	10	20	40	60	1.2	2.0	0.11	**1.9**	C00-06
Salivary gland	30	3	97	-	2	4	4	5	3	9	0.3	0.4	0.02	**0.4**	C07-08
Nasopharynx	416	6	97	15	73	67	62	81	69	43	3.5	5.9	0.35	**4.4**	C11
Other pharynx	111	1	95	1	1	3	9	16	40	40	0.9	1.6	0.11	**1.5**	C09-10,C12-14
Oesophagus	63	0	75	-	-	2	7	8	17	29	0.5	0.9	0.05	**0.8**	C15
Stomach	465	7	90	2	11	19	54	91	107	174	3.9	6.6	0.38	**6.1**	C16
Colon, rectum and anus	495	10	89	1	13	58	77	82	106	148	4.2	7.0	0.40	**6.2**	C18-21
Liver	65	2	55	3	-	1	5	4	18	32	0.6	0.9	0.05	**0.9**	C22
Gallbladder etc.	115	4	70	-	-	2	5	11	34	59	1.0	1.6	0.09	**1.6**	C23-24
Pancreas	76	0	54	-	-	1	9	10	16	39	0.6	1.1	0.05	**1.0**	C25
Larynx	332	9	94	2	1	3	17	59	99	142	2.8	4.7	0.28	**4.6**	C32
Trachea, bronchus and lung	1252	48	85	-	2	22	87	207	398	488	10.6	17.8	1.12	**17.3**	C33-34
Bone	162	2	85	34	48	16	20	4	18	20	1.4	2.3	0.09	**1.5**	C40-41
Melanoma of skin	34	2	100	-	1	3	4	6	8	9	0.3	0.5	0.03	**0.4**	C43
Other skin	504	19	98	6	8	14	46	67	117	227	4.3		0.36	**6.8**	C44
Mesothelioma	26	1	100	-	-	1	6	4	8	6	0.2	0.4	0.03	**0.3**	C45
Kaposi sarcoma	21	0	100	-	-	3	-	2	4	12	0.2	0.3	0.01	**0.3**	C46
Peripheral nerves	6	0	100	4	-	-	-	-	1	-	0.1	0.1	0.00	**0.1**	C47
Connective and soft tissue	101	1	90	21	11	10	16	8	17	17	0.9	1.4	0.07	**1.1**	C49
Breast	51	1	94	-	-	2	6	12	12	18	0.4	0.7	0.04	**0.7**	C50
Penis	1	0	100	-	-	-	-	-	-	1	0.0	0.0	0.00	**0.0**	C60
Prostate	385	31	92	1	-	2	5	16	70	260	3.3	5.5	0.17	**5.5**	C61
Testis	54	1	87	3	10	11	16	6	2	5	0.5	0.8	0.04	**0.5**	C62
Kidney	76	2	89	27	1	2	3	11	17	13	0.6	1.1	0.06	**0.9**	C64
Renal pelvis, ureter and other urinary	35	4	80	-	-	3	1	3	12	11	0.3	0.5	0.03	**0.5**	C65-66,C68
Bladder	649	56	87	3	6	18	32	71	185	278	5.5	9.2	0.51	**8.9**	C67
Eye	44	1	95	25	1	1	3	4	1	9	0.4	0.6	0.02	**0.5**	C69
Brain, nervous system	214	3	79	54	16	28	33	28	23	29	1.8	3.0	0.15	**2.2**	C70-72
Thyroid	77	1	92	1	9	9	15	12	12	18	0.7	1.1	0.06	**0.9**	C73
Hodgkin disease	163	2	100	39	33	35	19	16	11	8	1.4	2.3	0.10	**1.4**	C81
Non-Hodgkin lymphoma	422	5	100	85	44	41	60	47	76	64	3.6	6.0	0.32	**4.5**	C82-85,C96
Multiple myeloma	56	0	98	-	3	1	7	7	18	20	0.5	0.8	0.05	**0.7**	C90
Lymphoid leukaemia	153	1	96	75	9	5	10	9	17	27	1.3	2.2	0.08	**1.5**	C91
Myeloid leukaemia	97	1	99	22	8	11	16	13	7	19	0.8	1.4	0.06	**1.0**	C92-94
Leukaemia, unspecified	34	1	97	11	3	5	4	3	2	5	0.3	0.5	0.02	**0.3**	C95
Other and unspecified	622	21	79	55	34	51	64	97	133	167	5.3	8.8	0.50	**7.6**	O&U
All sites	7549	247	89	495	353	458	732	1040	1718	2506	63.9		5.82	**94.6**	ALL
All sites but C44	7045	228	88	489	345	444	686	973	1601	2279	59.7	100.0	5.45	**87.8**	ALLbC44
Average annual population				1036708	655833	489168	303293	201329	141181	123886					

Table 1. Elsewhere (1995-1998)

NUMBER OF CASES BY AGE GROUP AND SUMMARY RATES OF INCIDENCE - FEMALE

SITE	ALL AGES	AGE UNK	MV (%)	0-	15-	25-	35-	45-	55-	65+	CRUDE RATE	%	CR 64	ASR (W)	ICD (10th)
Mouth	64	0	97	1	1	1	10	12	14	25	0.5	0.8	0.05	0.8	*C00-06*
Salivary gland	24	1	88	-	-	2	5	7	2	5	0.2	0.3	0.02	0.3	*C07-08*
Nasopharynx	188	3	93	17	22	34	32	28	35	17	1.6	2.4	0.16	1.9	*C11*
Other pharynx	26	0	88	1	-	-	3	6	8	8	0.2	0.3	0.02	0.3	*C09-10,C12-14*
Oesophagus	33	0	79	1	1	1	4	2	7	18	0.3	0.4	0.02	0.4	*C15*
Stomach	284	4	87	1	4	28	46	50	70	81	2.4	3.7	0.24	3.4	*C16*
Colon, rectum and anus	463	20	92	1	20	46	81	69	100	126	3.9	6.0	0.37	5.4	*C18-21*
Liver	82	3	63	1	2	1	7	13	24	32	0.7	1.1	0.07	1.1	*C22*
Gallbladder etc.	491	6	84	1	1	9	60	98	148	168	4.2	6.4	0.44	6.3	*C23-24*
Pancreas	82	4	57	-	1	1	8	11	20	37	0.7	1.1	0.06	1.1	*C25*
Larynx	23	1	83	-	1	-	1	3	6	10	0.2	0.3	0.02	0.3	*C32*
Trachea, bronchus and lung	154	6	86	-	-	3	14	18	44	68	1.3	2.0	0.12	2.0	*C33-34*
Bone	125	3	88	32	34	10	16	9	10	11	1.1	1.6	0.07	1.1	*C40-41*
Melanoma of skin	38	1	100	2	1	2	3	8	8	13	0.3	0.5	0.03	0.5	*C43*
Other skin	270	10	95	5	12	15	18	40	53	117	2.3		0.18	3.3	*C44*
Mesothelioma	8	0	100	-	-	2	2	-	2	2	0.1	0.1	0.01	0.1	*C45*
Kaposi sarcoma	7	0	86	-	-	2	-	-	4	3	0.1	0.1	0.01	0.1	*C46*
Peripheral nerves	5	0	100	1	-	-	1	-	-	-	0.0	0.1	0.00	0.0	*C47*
Connective and soft tissue	87	2	94	8	16	20	12	9	6	14	0.7	1.1	0.05	0.8	*C49*
Breast	1995	35	96	-	7	199	600	540	360	254	17.0	25.9	1.90	23.1	*C50*
Vulva	12	0	83	-	-	-	2	3	4	3	0.1	0.2	0.01	0.2	*C51*
Vagina	18	0	89	1	-	2	1	4	6	4	0.2	0.2	0.02	0.2	*C52*
Cervix uteri	1146	26	96	-	4	46	220	336	321	193	9.8	14.9	1.19	14.2	*C53*
Uterus	213	7	96	-	3	7	29	42	61	64	1.8	2.8	0.19	2.7	*C54-55*
Ovary	200	5	95	3	12	27	36	49	38	30	1.7	2.6	0.18	2.3	*C56*
Placenta	0	0	-	-	-	-	-	-	-	-	0.0	0.0	0.00	0.0	*C58*
Kidney	79	2	91	39	-	3	8	7	12	8	0.7	1.0	0.05	0.8	*C64*
Renal pelvis, ureter and other urinary	40	1	78	-	4	4	5	7	10	9	0.3	0.5	0.03	0.5	*C65-66,C68*
Bladder	109	8	82	-	-	-	6	11	32	52	0.9	1.4	0.08	1.5	*C67*
Eye	37	1	92	20	1	-	1	2	5	7	0.3	0.5	0.02	0.4	*C69*
Brain, nervous system	118	3	86	25	14	17	16	17	18	8	1.0	1.5	0.09	1.2	*C70-72*
Thyroid	321	11	94	2	36	59	50	65	49	49	2.7	4.2	0.26	3.4	*C73*
Hodgkin disease	92	0	100	19	22	19	13	7	6	6	0.8	1.2	0.05	0.8	*C81*
Non-Hodgkin lymphoma	283	4	100	38	32	36	38	31	54	50	2.4	3.7	0.21	3.0	*C82-85,C96*
Multiple myeloma	49	0	100	-	1	2	8	7	9	22	0.4	0.6	0.03	0.6	*C90*
Lymphoid leukaemia	76	0	99	42	6	4	6	1	5	12	0.6	1.0	0.04	0.7	*C91*
Myeloid leukaemia	94	0	98	13	8	22	9	13	19	10	0.8	1.2	0.08	1.0	*C92-94*
Leukaemia, unspecified	25	0	96	8	1	2	1	3	6	4	0.2	0.3	0.02	0.3	*C95*
Other and unspecified	601	16	81	39	30	51	76	116	115	158	5.1	7.8	0.47	7.0	*O&U*
All sites	7962	183	92	320	299	679	1448	1644	1691	1698	67.8	100.0	6.86	93.0	*ALL*
All sites but C44	7692	173	92	315	287	664	1430	1604	1638	1581	65.5	100.0	6.68	89.6	*ALLbC44*
Average annual population				1002804	643707	482465	313292	214201	144816	132591					

RATES PER MILLION: The age-specific and crude incidence rates are calculated by dividing the number of cases of a specified age-group by the corresponding population at risk (both sexes combined) and expressed per million person-years. The ASR (see above) is the truncated age-standardized rate for the age range 0–14 years, again using the direct method and expressed per million person-years.

MV (%): See definition above.

Summary tables

Summary rates: The tables which appear in the section of the volume reviewing results for specific cancers present the summary incidence rates (crude, world age-standardized and cumulative), by sex and tumour type. There is a table for each site or grouping of sites presented in the age-specific tables. A summary table presents data for the African cancer registries that provided data on population at risk together with non-African populations extracted from *Cancer Incidence in Five Continents Vol. VIII* (Parkin *et al.*, 2002) for comparison purposes. The cancer registries are grouped by geographical area. Results from registries which are pathology-based are italicized, since they represent only minimum estimates of incidence.

Similar tables for childhood cancers accompany the chapter on childhood cancer. They present the crude and age-standardized rates by sex and for both sexes combined (expressed per million person-years), the total number of cases and the sex ratio (M/F).

For minor sites for which there is no chapter, data on summary rates are available on the CD-ROM (see below).

Percentage distribution of microscopically verified cases by histological type: These tables show the frequency of different histological subtypes within the total of microscopically verified (see the definition of MV (%) above) cases for nine tumour types. These tumour types and their associated histological sub-groups are fully described in *Cancer Incidence in Five Continents Vol. VII* (Parkin *et al.*, 1997). The information is presented for those African cancer registries that provided data originally coded to ICD-O, and for both sexes combined. The total number of registrations at the site is also printed to indicate the proportion of cases with microscopic verification.

CD-ROM

The CD-ROM that comes with this book contains a Windows™-based program called **CinA** to analyse the data contained in the present volume. With this software, users can examine the data with more flexibility and greater detail than in the printed tables. The data are stored in the traditional form of number of cases by sex and five-year age-groups (0-, 5-, ..., 64-, 65+). The standard three-digit ICD-10 anatomical sites used in the book have been replaced by a set of 80 categories based on a combination of ICD-10 three- or four-digit site codes and, for three tumours, of ICD-O-2

morphological subtypes (Table 3). Users can also create their own groupings, both of registry populations and of diagnostic units, which are then retained in the database. Only African registries that supplied data on population at risk are included in the database, together with some non-African populations extracted from *Cancer Incidence in Five Continents* Vol. VIII for comparison purposes.

There is considerable flexibility too in defining the indices to be calculated; thus the usual summary rates (crude, cumulative, world age-standardized) can be calculated over any chosen age range. The software also performs some elementary statistical tests, e.g. for homogeneity, trend and significance of ratio of age-specific rates in two populations. Finally, the software has inbuilt graphic capabilities for displaying age-specific rates as line graphs and the summary indices as bar charts; both may be exported as bitmap or JPEG files to a suitable software for reproduction.

System requirements:

- A PC running Microsoft Windows™ 95/98/Me/NT/2000/XP
- Microsoft Windows™ NT/2000/XP recommended
- 64 Mb of RAM recommended
- 10 Mb hard-disk space required

Installation:

1. Insert the disk in your CD-drive.
2. Double-click the e:\setup.exe file (e being the letter that identifies your CD-ROM drive: change if necessary).
3. Follow the instructions on the screen.

The installation procedure copies the program and all the necessary data files (the so-called 'database') in a specific binary file so that **CinA** can run without the CD-ROM.

References

Kramárová, E., Stiller, C.A., Ferlay, J., Parkin, D.M., Draper, G.J., Michaelis, J., Neglia, J. & Qureshi, S. (1996) *International Classification of Childhood Cancer* (IARC Technical Report No. 29), Lyon, IARC

Parkin, D.M., Chen, V.W., Ferlay, J., Galceran, J., Storm, H.H. & Whelan, S.L. (1994) *Comparability and Quality Control in Cancer Registration* (IARC Technical Report No. 19), Lyon, IARC

Parkin, D.M., Whelan, S.L., Ferlay, J., Raymond, L. & Young, J., eds (1997) *Cancer Incidence in Five Continents,* Vol. VII (IARC Scientific Publications No. 143), Lyon, IARC

Parkin, D.M., Kramárová, E., Draper, G.J., Masuyer, E., Michaelis, J., Neglia, J., Qureshi, S. & Stiller, C.A., eds (1998) *International Incidence of Childhood Cancer,* Vol. II (IARC Scientific Publications No. 144), Lyon, IARC

Parkin, D.M., Whelan, S.L., Ferlay, J., Teppo, L. & Thomas, D.B., eds (2002) *Cancer Incidence in Five Continents,* Vol. VIII (IARC Scientific Publications No. 155), Lyon, IARC

Table 2. Childhood cancer, Elsewhere (1995-1998)

| | NUMBER OF CASES | | | | | REL. FREQ.(%) | RATES PER MILLION | | | | | |
	0-4	5-9	10-14	All	M/F	Overall	0-4	5-9	10-14	Crude	ASR	%MV
Leukaemia	49	69	53	**171**	*1.7*	21.0	18.6	25.3	19.0	21.0	**20.9**	98.3
Acute lymphoid leukaemia	35	47	29	**111**	*1.8*	13.6	13.3	17.2	10.4	13.6	**13.7**	99.1
Lymphoma	49	75	57	**181**	*2.2*	22.2	18.6	27.5	20.4	22.2	**22.0**	100.0
Hodgkin Disease	9	29	20	**58**	*2.1*	7.1	3.4	10.6	7.2	7.1	**6.8**	100.0
Burkitt lymphoma	0	1	2	**3**	*2.0*	0.4	-	0.4	0.7	0.4	**0.3**	100.0
Central nervous system	13	28	24	**65**	*2.1*	8.0	4.9	10.3	8.6	8.0	**7.7**	83.1
Neuroblastoma	25	20	8	**53**	*2.5*	6.5	9.5	7.3	2.9	6.5	**6.9**	98.1
Retinoblastoma	29	10	1	**40**	*1.2*	4.9	11.0	3.7	0.4	4.9	**5.5**	100.0
Wilms tumour	35	20	8	**63**	*0.7*	7.7	13.3	7.3	2.9	7.7	**8.3**	96.8
Bone tumour	5	16	45	**66**	*1.1*	8.1	1.9	5.9	16.1	8.1	**7.3**	90.9
Connective tissue	7	10	12	**29**	*2.6*	3.6	2.7	3.7	4.3	3.6	**3.5**	86.2
Kaposi sarcoma	0	0	0	**0**	-	-	-	-	-	-	**-**	-
Germ cell tumours	9	2	2	**13**	*0.9*	1.6	3.4	0.7	0.7	1.6	**1.8**	100.0
Other	34	37	63	**134**	*1.2*	16.4	12.9	13.6	22.6	16.4	**15.9**	81.3
All	255	287	273	**815**	*1.5*	100.0	96.7	105.2	97.7	99.9	**99.7**	93.7

Table 3. List of cancers available in the *CinA* program

01	All sites (C00–97)	41	Corpus uteri (C54)
02	All sites but skin (C00–97 but C44)	42	Uterus unspecified (C55)
03	Oral cavity and pharynx (C00–14)	43	Ovary (C56)
04	Mouth (C00–06)	44	Placenta (C58)
05	Lip (C00)	45	Male genital organs (C60–63)
06	Salivary glands (C07–08)	46	Penis (C60)
07	Nasopharynx (C11)	47	Prostate (C61)
08	Other pharynx (C09–10,C12–14)	48	Testis (C62)
09	Digestive organs (C15–26)	49	Urinary tract (C64–68)
10	Oesophagus (C15)	50	Kidney (C64)
11	Stomach (C16)	51	Bladder (C67)
12	Colon (C18)	52	Squamous cell carcinoma
13	Rectum, rectosigmoid junction and anus (C19–21)	53	Transitional cell and adenocarcinoma
14	Liver (C22)	54	Other specified morphology
15	Gallbladder (C23)	55	Unspecified morphology
16	Pancreas (C25)	56	Other urinary organs (C65–66, C68)
17	Respiratory organs (C30–39)	57	Eye, brain and central nervous system (C69–72)
18	Larynx (C32)	58	Eye (C69)
19	Trachea, bronchus and lung (C33–34)	59	Retinoblastoma
20	Bone (C40–41)	60	Squamous cell carcinoma of the conjunctiva
21	Bone of limbs (C40)	61	Brain, central nervous system (C70–72)
22	Other bones (C41)	62	Meninges (C70)
23	Skin (C43–44)	63	Brain (C71)
24	Melanoma of skin (C43)	64	Thyroid and other endocrine glands (C73–75)
25	Other skin (C44)	65	Thyroid (C73)
26	Mesothelial and soft tissues (C45–49)	66	Adrenal gland (C74)
27	Mesothelioma (C45)	67	Lymphoid tissues (C81–96)
28	Kaposi sarcoma (C46)	68	Non-Hodgkin lymphoma (C82–85,C96)
29	Peripheral nerves (C47)	69	Burkitt lymphoma (C83.7)
30	Peritoneum and retroperitoneum (C48)	70	Mycosis fungoides (C84.0)
31	Connective and soft tissue (C49)	71	Hodgkin disease (C81)
32	Breast (C50)	72	Immunoproliferative disease (C88)
33	Female genital organs (C51–58)	73	Multiple myeloma (C90)
34	Vulva (C51)	74	Leukaemia (C91–95)
35	Vagina (C52)	75	Lymphoid leukaemia (C91)
36	Cervix uteri (C53)	76	Myeloid leukaemia (C92–94)
37	Squamous cell carcinoma	77	Chronic myeloid leukaemia (C92.1, C93.1, C94.1)
38	Adenocarcinoma	78	Leukaemia, cell unspecified (C95)
39	Other specified morphology	79	Other and unspecified cancers (C80, C97)
40	Unspecified morphology		

3. Cancer occurrence by country

3.1 North Africa

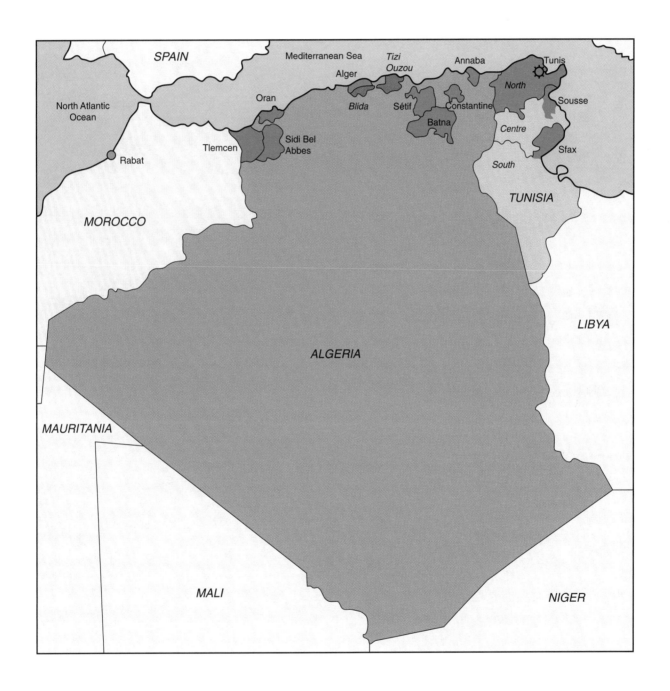

3.1.1 Algeria

Background

Climate: In the north, typically Mediterranean climate with hot, dry summers and mild, wet winters. Average temperatures 25°C in August and 12°C in January in Algiers. On the high plateaus and in the Sahara, low rainfall, with very large diurnal variations in temperature; occasional very violent sand storms.

Terrain: In the north, the Atlas chain of mountains and a narrow discontinuous coastal plain covering an area of 1000 km^2; in the south, the Sahara desert.

Ethnic groups: Largely Arabs (80%) with a strong Berber minority. Europeans less than 1%.

Religions: Sunni Muslim (state religion) 99%, Christian and Jewish 1%

Economy—overview: The hydrocarbons sector is the backbone of the economy, accounting for roughly 57% of government revenues, 25% of GDP and almost all export earnings. Algeria has the fifth largest reserves of natural gas in the world and is the second largest gas exporter; it ranks fourteenth for oil reserves.

Industries: Petroleum, natural gas, light industries, mining, electrical, petrochemical, food processing

Agriculture: Low wheat production has made it necessary to import food. Other products include barley, oats, grapes, olives, citrus, fruits; sheep, cattle

Cancer registration

There are eight cancer registries in Algeria (see map): the registries of Algiers in the capital, the registries of Sétif, Constantine, Annaba and Batna in the east of the country and the registries of Oran, Tlemcen, and Sidi-bel-Abbès in the west.

Cancer Registry of Algiers

The registry was established in 1991 in the National Institute of Public Health, with assistance from the WHO Regional Office for Africa. The registry began with a pilot year of retrospective data collection for the year 1990. Registration of new cases began in January 1993, covering at first the population of the city of Algiers (Alger). In 1997, registry coverage was increased to include the neighbouring wilayas (departments) of Blida and Tizi-Ouzu, increasing the population coverage from about 1.8 million (Algiers) to 4.3 million.

Data collection is active, in two specialized cancer hospitals (Algiers and Blida), 11 teaching hospitals, 9 specialist hospitals, 1 military hospital, 17 pathology laboratories (10 of which in the private sector), 5 private surgical clinics, the social security service financing overseas treatment. Death certificates are also consulted. There are six full-time data collectors with training in registration methods. A consulting pathologist assists with quality control of diagnosis.

Cancer Registry of Batna

The registry was established in 1995. Data collection is both active and passive. Information on cancer cases is collected primarily from the pathology laboratory of Batna University Hospital and a private laboratory, as well as chemotherapy clinics in Constantine and Anaba, the Sétif University Hospital, and private clinics in Batna wilaya. The registry receives bi-annual reports from hospitals in the wilaya on new cancer cases that have been treated.

Cancer Registry of Constantine

The registry was established in 1994, in the epidemiology service of the University Hospital (CHU) of Constantine. A retrospective survey of cancer cases for 1994–97 was followed by prospective registration from 1998. The principal sources of information are clinical services of the CHU (especially the departments of radiotherapy, oncology and nuclear medicine, paediatrics and haematology) and the department of pathology. Several private clinics and laboratories also contribute cases, Data collection is active by specially trained personnel. Death certificates are not used as a source of information. The registry has had problems because of insufficient personnel, with some periods of interrupted activity.

Cancer Registry of Oran

The cancer registry of Oran is part of the Epidemiology and Preventive Medicine Service of the University Hospital. It was established in 1993, following a retrospective survey of cancer cases in hospitals serving the wilaya. The registry is population-based and covers the wilaya of Oran (population 1.2 million in 1998). Oran is the second city of Algeria, and the University Hospital (CHU) includes a full range of treatment services for cancer, including radiotherapy.

The registry is operated by the professional (medical) personnel of the service. Data collection is carried out by postgraduate students (residents) in epidemiology. They identify cancer cases from clinical departments in the CHU, and from one large private hospital, and paediatric hospital. The pathology laboratories in these hospitals and private laboratories also contribute, as does the national service which funds overseas treatment for Algerian residents. Death certificates are not used as a source of information. Data management is by the CANREG-3 package (IARC). Annual reports have been published since 1992.

Cancer Registry of Sétif

The Sétif cancer registry was founded in January 1989 with the collaboration of the International Agency for Research on Cancer. It covers the population of the wilaya of Setif (population 1.3 million in 1998).The registry is attached to the Unit of Health Information and Biostatistics of the Department of Epidemiology and Public Health situated in the University Hospital (CHU) of Sétif. It is financed by the Ministry of Health and by the Ministry of Higher Education and Scientific Research.

Data are collected by active methods by the health technician of the Registry. Data sources include:
*   In the CHU of Sétif: the 'Admissions', the pathology laboratory, clinical chemistry laboratory, the central pharmacy and different hospital departments including the haematology service and its laboratory.
*   The health sectors of the dairas,
*   The Anti-cancer Centre of Constantine,
*   The Pierre et Marie Curie Centre in Algiers
*   Social security (insurance),
*   Municipal records for death certificates,
*   Physicians in the private sector.

Cancer Registry of Sidi-bel-Abbès

Registration began in 1994 with retrospective collection of data for the years 1991–93; registration has been prospective since 1995.

Cancer Registry of Tlemcen

A cancer registry for the wilaya of Tlemcen was set up in the Epidemiology Department of the medical school in 1994. It is part of a registration network in western Algeria (comprising Oran, Sidi bel Abbès and Tlemcen) using a common protocol. It relied entirely upon postgraduate students (residents) for case-finding in the services of the main teaching hospital (CHU) and several smaller private hospitals. At the CHU, there is a service of medical oncology (for day cases), but no other specialized cancer treatment facilities; patients are referred to Oran for radiotherapy. Pathologists have been asked to complete notification forms. Cases of cancer from Tlemcen identified by the Oran cancer registry are notified.

Cooperation with the various medical services has been uneven, and pathology notifications are inadequate (most pathology has devolved to the private sector), so that registration cannot be considered complete. A report was prepared based on the registrations for the years 1994–96 and a population estimated from the census of 1988, but has not been published.

Review of data
Algiers
Since 1993, the registry has published annual reports presenting results for the wilaya of Algiers. Since 1997, results from Blida and Tizi Ouzou have been included.

The results for 1993–97 are shown in Table 1. In men, the highest incidence rates are observed for tobacco-related cancers: lung (ASR 17.2 per 100 000) and bladder (10.8). Cancers of the gastrointestinal tract have shown steady increases in incidence, with colorectal cancers now third in frequency in both sexes (ASR 7.1 in men, 6.1 in women). Prostate cancer has also been increasing in incidence and is now fifth in frequency in men. The incidence of nasopharyngeal cancer in men is modest (ASR 2.7).

In women, breast cancer (ASR 21.2) and cervix cancer (ASR 12.6) are the dominant cancers. Of note is the relatively high incidence of gallbladder cancer in women (ASR 5.3; F:M sex ratio of 3.5:1).

Batna
The results for the four-year period 1995–98 are shown in Table 2. The calculated incidence rates are low, so that data are shown simply as relative frequency of different cancers.

Cancer of the stomach (10.3%) is the most frequent cancer of men; the frequency of cancer of the nasopharynx (10.7%) is rather higher than in the other series reported in this volume. In women, breast cancer (24.2% of the total) is dominant, with slightly more cases of gallbladder cancer (11.6%) than of cervix cancer (9.6%).

Constantine
The results for 1994–97 are shown in Table 3. The incidence for all cancers (excluding non-melanoma skin cancers) is low (ASR 79.0 per 100 000 in men and 90.4 per 100 000 in women) in comparison with the other major cities (Algiers, Oran) suggesting some under-registration. Nevertheless, the cancer profile is broadly similar, although in men bladder cancer incidence is rather low, being sixth in frequency following cancers of the lung (ASR 13.1), larynx (ASR 5.8), prostate (ASR 5.8), non-Hodgkin lymphoma (ASR 5.4) and nasopharynx (ASR 5.3).

The pattern of female cancer is similar to that elsewhere: breast (ASR 28.3), cervix (12.1) and gallbladder (ASR 6.3) are the principal sites.

Oran
The results for 1996–98 are presented in Table 4. Overall incidence rates are rather higher than for Algiers, despite a relatively high proportion of cases with morphological verification of diagnosis (93% in males, 95% in females). In men, the principal cancers (excluding non-melanoma skin cancers) are lung cancer (ASR 23.7), bladder cancer (ASR 13.6) and non-Hodgkin lymphoma (ASR 8.2); the rates for the latter are considerably higher than

recorded in the other Algerian registries. In women, breast cancer is the principal cancer (ASR 34.5), followed by cancer of the cervix (ASR 24.9), and gallbladder (ASR 6.6). The incidence of non-Hodgkin lymphoma is also high (ASR 6.2).

Sétif
The first results from the population-based cancer registry in Sétif for the years 1986–88 were published by Hamdi-Chérif et al. (1991). The standardized incidence rates for all sites (excluding non-melanoma skin cancer), were 70.1 per 100 000 for men and 59.9 per 100 000 for women. The most frequent cancers were lung, stomach and nasopharynx in men, and cervix, breast and gallbladder in women. These results represented the first detailed incidence data for all cancers in an Algerian population.

Data from Sétif were subsequently published in volumes VI (1986–89) and VII (1990–93) of Cancer Incidence in Five Continents and Volume II of International Incidence of Childhood Cancer.

In this volume, the results are presented for the five year period 1993–97 (Table 5). A total of 2865 new cases were registered. The standardized incidence rate for males is 78.5 per 100 000 and for females 74.8 per 100 000.

In men, lung cancer was the most frequent malignancy (ASR 15.5), followed by cancer of the stomach (ASR 7.8), nasopharyngeal carcinoma (ASR 6.3), large bowel (ASR 4.6) and non-Hodgkin lymphomas (ASR 3.6).

The most frequently reported cancers in women were breast (ASR 17.0); cervix (ASR 11.5); gallbladder (ASR 8.6); large bowel (colon and rectum) (ASR 4.3) and stomach (ASR 3.1).

Tlemcen
The results from 1994–96 are shown in Table 6. Cancer of the stomach (15.4% of cases) is the most common cancer of men, and is third in frequency (6.6%) in women. Breast cancer dominates the picture (29.4% of cases) in women.

Previous studies
A study was carried out on histological material from the anatomo-pathology laboratories in Algiers, Oran and Constantine from the years 1966–75 (Yaker, 1980, 1986). This involved retrospective extraction of data on cancer cases from the records of each of the laboratories onto edge-punched cards. Each register was extracted twice and the cards were verified after perforation. The cases included were limited to those coming from the three wilayate (prefectures), so that minimal rates of incidence were calculated. In males the most commonly recorded sites were larynx (9.2%), nasopharynx (5%) and buccal cavity (4.1%) and lymphomas (Table 6). Cervix cancer was the most common (30%) among female cancers; with an age-standardized rate of 24.1 per 100 000), it was almost three times more frequent than breast cancer.

In the years 1986–92, a population-based cancer registry for the wilaya of Algiers, confined to tumours of the gastrointestinal tract, was maintained in the department of surgery at Bologhine Hospital. Case-finding procedures were quite extensive, and similar to those later employed by the general population-based registry of Algiers (see above). A report for the three-year period 1987–89 has been published (Abid & Benabadji, 1999). 1143 cases were recorded (80% with histological verification of diagnosis), with an average of 1.9 notifications (sources) per case. The results are presented in Table 7. The incidence rates are somewhat similar to those in the general registry of Algiers in 1993–97, except for a rather higher incidence of stomach and colorectal cancers in men (ASR 17.5 and 15.2, respectively) in the digestive registry compared with the general registry (ASR 5.6 and 7.1, respectively). Most biliary tract malignancies were gallbladder cancers (94/120 in women, for example), and 75% of the latter had associated gallstones.

Summary

In all of the recent registry data, lung cancer is the major neoplasm of men, reflecting a high and increasing prevalence of smoking. Other tobacco-related cancers, notably bladder cancers and larynx cancers, are also common in most series. Lung cancer remains rare among women who, for the great majority, are non-smokers.

In the gastro-intestinal tract, cancers of the large bowel are generally the leading site, followed by stomach cancer. Cancer of the oesophagus is rare.

The incidence of cancers of the nasopharynx is moderately high, with rates between 3.9 per 100 000 and 7.6 per 100 000 in men, and 1.8–3.7 per 100 000 in women. As noted in earlier studies of populations in the Maghreb (see chapter on nasopharyngeal carcinoma), there is a bimodal incidence peak, with the first in adolescents (age 15–19 years) and the second in older adults (age 50+ years).

Cancer of the gallbladder is relatively common in women, with age-standardized rates in the range 6.3–8.9 per 100 000. It is much less common in men, with the sex ratio (F:M) generally around 4:1. This probably relates to the frequency of gallstones in the population.

In all of the recent series, breast cancer is the most common cancer, with incidence rates in some of the registries that are quite high (an ASR of 34.5 per 100 000 in Oran, for example). The registry reports often remark upon the low average age of the cases, but this almost certainly relates to the young age of the population at risk. Age-specific incidence rates appear to rise until around the menopause, and then are more or less constant.

In the early data from 1966–75, based on histopathology only, the incidence of cervix cancer was quite high (ASR 27.1). Incidence in more recent series is generally lower (ASR 12.1–29.3), although these rates are rather higher than those observed in Arab populations in western Asia.

Childhood cancer

Results from three registries are presented in Table 8 (Algiers, 1993–96), Table 9 (Oran, 1996–98) and Table 10 (Sétif, 1993–97). The data from these three series, plus 139 cases registered in Constantine in 1994–97 are pooled in Table 11.

In Algiers, childhood cancers comprise 4.5% of the total, and are more common in boys (218 cases versus 121 among girls). There is a slight preponderance of central nervous system tumours over lymphomas and leukaemias. The incidence of neuroblastoma (10.5 per million) is rather high.

Childhood cancers comprise 6.2% of the total in Oran (Table 9), with lymphomas (mainly non-Hodgkin lymphoma) the most commonly registered cancer. Wilms tumour (18.5 per million) and retinoblastoma (17.2 per million) have high incidence.

In Sétif, the overall childhood cancer incidence rate of 71.2 per million is relatively low compared with other registries (Table 10). Underdiagnosis of cases probably plays a role. Leukaemia and lymphomas are the most common malignancies in children, representing 62% of childhood cancer.

The pooled data-set (Table 11) includes 815 cases. Overall incidence is 99.7 per million. Lymphoma (ASR 22.0) is slightly more common than leukaemia (ASR 20.9), and Wilms tumour has a higher incidence rate than CNS tumours, although numerically less common.

References

Abid, L. & Benabadji, R. (1999) *Les cancers digestifs à Alger. Bilan de 3 années d'enregistrement prospectif*, Algiers, Service de Chirurgie, Hôpital Bologhine

Hamdi Chérif, M., Sekfali, N. & Coleman, M.P. (1991) Incidence du cancer dans la Wilaya de Sétif, Algérie. *Bull. Cancer*, **78**, 155–167

Meguenni (1998) Le registre du cancer à Tlemcen. Approche étiologique et perspectives. Thèse du doctorat, Institut des Sciences Médicales, Université Aboubekr Belkaid Tlemcen

Yaker, A. (1980) *Profil de la morbidité cancéreuse en Algérie 1966-1975*, Algiers, Société Nationale d'Edition et de Diffusion (SNED)

Yaker, A. (1986) Algeria. Histopathology Study, Algiers, Oran and Constantine, 1966-1975. In: Parkin, D.M., ed., *Cancer Occurrence in Developing Countries* (IARC Scientific Publications No. 75), Lyon, IARC, pp. 27–31

Table 1. Algeria, Algiers (1993-1997)

NUMBER OF CASES BY AGE GROUP AND SUMMARY RATES OF INCIDENCE - MALE

SITE	ALL AGES	AGE UNK	MV (%)	0-	15-	25-	35-	45-	55-	65+	CRUDE RATE	%	CR 64	ASR (W)	ICD (10th)
Mouth	49	1	100	2	1	3	5	6	15	16	0.9	1.4	0.08	1.3	C00-06
Salivary gland	18	3	94	-	-	3	3	2	3	3	0.3	0.5	0.03	0.4	C07-08
Nasopharynx	128	6	93	5	18	23	12	28	24	12	2.3	3.7	0.22	2.7	C11
Other pharynx	31	1	87	-	1	2	4	5	6	12	0.6	0.9	0.05	0.8	C09-10,C12-14
Oesophagus	34	0	74	-	-	1	4	4	11	14	0.6	1.0	0.06	0.9	C15
Stomach	211	7	89	1	4	5	18	35	61	80	3.8	6.2	0.35	5.6	C16
Colon, rectum and anus	284	10	88	-	6	29	44	39	56	100	5.2	8.3	0.41	7.1	C18-21
Liver	34	2	76	2	-	1	1	2	7	19	0.6	1.0	0.04	0.9	C22
Gallbladder etc.	53	4	83	-	1	-	4	5	15	28	1.0	1.5	0.07	1.5	C23-24
Pancreas	44	0	57	-	-	-	4	7	10	22	0.8	1.3	0.06	1.2	C25
Larynx	155	9	92	-	-	2	7	27	45	65	2.8	4.5	0.26	4.3	C32
Trachea, bronchus and lung	635	48	81	-	1	13	41	111	184	237	11.5	18.5	1.08	17.2	C33-34
Bone	94	2	80	25	22	13	8	3	9	12	1.7	2.7	0.11	1.8	C40-41
Melanoma of skin	22	2	100	1	-	-	3	4	5	7	0.4	0.6	0.03	0.6	C43
Other skin	292	19	98	2	5	4	26	41	73	122	5.3	8.5	0.44	7.8	C44
Mesothelioma	17	1	100	-	-	1	5	2	6	3	0.3	0.5	0.04	0.4	C45
Kaposi sarcoma	16	0	100	-	1	-	-	1	4	10	0.3	0.5	0.02	0.4	C46
Peripheral nerves	2	0	100	-	1	-	-	-	-	-	0.0	0.1	0.00	0.0	C47
Connective and soft tissue	51	1	84	10	3	4	11	3	11	8	0.9	1.5	0.08	1.1	C49
Breast	26	1	92	-	-	1	3	5	8	8	0.5	0.8	0.05	0.7	C50
Penis	0	0	-	-	-	-	-	-	-	-	0.0	0.0	0.00	0.0	C60
Prostate	194	31	89	1	-	2	5	4	35	116	3.5	5.7	0.18	5.4	C61
Testis	38	1	82	2	7	9	13	3	1	2	0.7	1.1	0.05	0.7	C62
Kidney	30	2	100	12	1	1	-	5	5	4	0.5	0.9	0.05	0.7	C64
Renal pelvis, ureter and other urinary	30	4	77	3	5	3	1	2	10	9	0.5	0.9	0.05	0.7	C65-66,C68
Bladder	402	56	85	3	5	12	22	43	103	158	7.3	11.7	0.61	10.8	C67
Eye	20	1	90	11	1	1	1	2	-	4	0.4	0.6	0.02	0.5	C69
Brain, nervous system	128	3	91	34	8	18	18	15	12	20	2.3	3.7	0.17	2.7	C70-72
Thyroid	52	1	92	1	6	4	8	8	10	14	0.9	1.5	0.08	1.2	C73
Hodgkin disease	33	2	100	4	6	11	6	3	7	-	0.6	1.0	0.04	0.5	C81
Non-Hodgkin lymphoma	161	5	100	23	11	16	26	16	42	22	2.9	4.7	0.28	3.6	C82-85,C96
Multiple myeloma	24	0	100	-	-	-	-	2	9	13	0.4	0.7	0.04	0.7	C90
Lymphoid leukaemia	56	1	100	27	2	2	2	5	7	10	1.0	1.6	0.07	1.2	C91
Myeloid leukaemia	37	1	100	11	2	4	9	4	2	4	0.7	1.1	0.05	0.8	C92-94
Leukaemia, unspecified	18	1	100	5	2	2	3	-	2	3	0.3	0.5	0.02	0.4	C95
Other and unspecified	299	21	73	36	15	17	36	41	56	77	5.4	8.7	0.45	7.2	O&U
All sites	3718	247	87	218	131	206	350	483	849	1234	67.6	100.0	5.65	93.8	ALL
All sites but C44	3426	228	86	216	126	202	324	442	776	1112	62.3	100.0	5.21	86.0	ALLbC44
Average annual population				334285	248972	205423	120263	81940	59187	49549					

Table 1. Algeria, Algiers (1993-1997)

NUMBER OF CASES BY AGE GROUP AND SUMMARY RATES OF INCIDENCE - FEMALE

SITE	ALL AGES	AGE UNK	MV (%)	0-	15-	25-	35-	45-	55-	65+	CRUDE RATE	%	CR 64	ASR (W)	ICD (10th)
Mouth	29	0	93	-	1	1	7	4	6	10	0.5	0.8	0.05	0.7	C00-06
Salivary gland	9	1	78	-	-	-	2	3	-	3	0.2	0.2	0.01	0.2	C07-08
Nasopharynx	61	3	97	5	9	10	10	10	8	6	1.1	1.7	0.09	1.2	C11
Other pharynx	10	0	70	-	-	-	3	3	1	3	0.2	0.3	0.02	0.2	C09-10,C12-14
Oesophagus	19	0	74	-	-	1	2	2	3	12	0.3	0.5	0.02	0.5	C15
Stomach	155	4	87	1	4	17	23	20	39	47	2.8	4.3	0.25	3.7	C16
Colon, rectum and anus	248	20	90	-	8	17	32	35	65	71	4.6	6.8	0.42	6.1	C18-21
Liver	34	3	68	-	1	1	2	2	6	19	0.6	0.9	0.03	0.9	C22
Gallbladder etc.	204	6	82	-	1	5	21	27	61	83	3.7	5.6	0.33	5.3	C23-24
Pancreas	36	4	58	-	1	-	4	5	8	14	0.7	1.0	0.05	0.9	C25
Larynx	11	1	73	-	-	2	1	1	2	6	0.2	0.3	0.01	0.3	C32
Trachea, bronchus and lung	73	6	81	-	1	5	5	7	22	30	1.3	2.0	0.12	1.9	C33-34
Bone	56	3	80	8	20	5	8	3	3	6	1.0	1.5	0.06	1.0	C40-41
Melanoma of skin	19	1	100	2	1	2	1	4	3	5	0.3	0.5	0.03	0.4	C43
Other skin	142	10	93	2	9	4	8	18	25	66	2.6	3.8	0.17	3.5	C44
Mesothelioma	5	0	100	-	-	1	2	-	-	2	0.1	0.1	0.00	0.1	C45
Kaposi sarcoma	3	0	100	-	-	-	-	-	-	1	0.1	0.1	0.01	0.1	C46
Peripheral nerves	2	0	100	-	-	2	-	-	-	-	0.0	0.1	0.00	0.0	C47
Connective and soft tissue	48	2	92	5	6	13	11	3	2	6	0.9	1.3	0.06	0.9	C49
Breast	906	35	95	-	3	82	259	239	169	119	16.6	25.0	1.73	21.2	C50
Vulva	3	0	33	-	-	-	1	1	1	1	0.1	0.1	0.00	0.1	C51
Vagina	3	0	100	-	-	-	-	1	-	1	0.1	0.1	0.01	0.1	C52
Cervix uteri	506	26	94	-	4	20	83	139	153	81	9.3	14.0	1.07	12.6	C53
Uterus	125	7	94	-	2	2	12	25	38	39	2.3	3.4	0.23	3.2	C54-55
Ovary	42	5	100	-	-	5	7	12	8	5	0.8	1.2	0.08	1.0	C56
Placenta	0	0	-	-	-	-	-	-	-	-	0.0	0.0	0.00	0.0	C58
Kidney	33	2	94	15	-	1	2	3	6	4	0.6	0.9	0.05	0.7	C64
Renal pelvis, ureter and other urinary	34	1	79	-	3	3	5	6	6	8	0.6	0.9	0.06	0.8	C65-66,C68
Bladder	86	8	84	-	-	-	5	7	24	42	1.6	2.4	0.12	2.3	C67
Eye	22	1	86	10	1	-	1	2	3	4	0.4	0.6	0.03	0.5	C69
Brain, nervous system	70	3	97	16	11	10	9	7	8	6	1.3	1.9	0.10	1.4	C70-72
Thyroid	192	11	93	-	24	23	31	45	31	27	3.5	5.3	0.33	4.2	C73
Hodgkin disease	27	0	100	7	9	8	-	1	1	1	0.5	0.7	0.03	0.5	C81
Non-Hodgkin lymphoma	109	4	100	7	11	16	17	12	19	23	2.0	3.0	0.16	2.4	C82-85,C96
Multiple myeloma	23	0	100	-	-	-	2	4	4	13	0.4	0.6	0.03	0.6	C90
Lymphoid leukaemia	29	0	100	16	1	1	3	-	3	5	0.5	0.8	0.03	0.7	C91
Myeloid leukaemia	26	0	100	4	3	-	4	5	3	2	0.5	0.7	0.04	0.5	C92-94
Leukaemia, unspecified	14	0	100	3	1	5	1	1	5	2	0.3	0.4	0.02	0.3	C95
Other and unspecified	353	16	80	20	14	34	48	66	64	91	6.5	9.7	0.54	8.3	O&U
All sites	3767	183	90	121	149	292	632	722	804	864	69.2		6.37	89.4	ALL
All sites but C44	3625	173	90	119	140	288	624	704	779	798	66.6	100.0	6.20	85.9	ALLbC44

| Average annual population | | | | 326543 | 243710 | 199869 | 120925 | 86448 | 58799 | 52034 | | | | | |

Table 2. Algeria, Batna (1995-1999)

NUMBER OF CASES BY AGE GROUP - MALE

SITE	ALL AGES	AGE UNK	MV (%)	0-	15-	25-	35-	45-	55-	65+	%	ICD (10th)
Mouth	20	0	100	-	-	2	-	1	8	9	3.1	C00-06
Salivary gland	0	0	-	-	-	-	-	-	-	-	0.0	C07-08
Nasopharynx	70	0	100	8	10	6	13	15	11	7	10.7	C11
Other pharynx	11	0	100	-	-	-	-	2	2	7	1.7	C09-10,C12-14
Oesophagus	5	0	100	-	-	-	-	1	-	4	0.8	C15
Stomach	67	0	88	-	-	-	6	11	15	35	10.3	C16
Colon, rectum and anus	45	0	87	-	1	7	5	10	9	13	6.9	C18-21
Liver	12	0	8	-	1	-	-	1	3	7	1.8	C22
Gallbladder etc.	20	0	70	-	-	-	1	2	6	11	3.1	C23-24
Pancreas	13	0	23	-	-	-	1	1	3	8	2.0	C25
Larynx	24	0	92	-	-	-	2	6	8	8	3.7	C32
Trachea, bronchus and lung	65	0	77	-	-	-	5	11	31	18	10.0	C33-34
Bone	22	0	77	9	4	2	2	-	1	4	3.4	C40-41
Melanoma of skin	2	0	100	-	-	-	-	-	-	2	0.3	C43
Other skin	127	0	94	1	1	4	10	8	26	77	-	C44
Mesothelioma	1	0	100	-	-	-	-	-	-	1	0.2	C45
Kaposi sarcoma	0	0	-	-	-	-	-	-	-	-	0.0	C46
Peripheral nerves	0	0	-	-	-	-	-	-	-	-	0.0	C47
Connective and soft tissue	15	0	93	1	3	2	4	1	2	2	2.3	C49
Breast	12	0	100	-	-	-	-	-	4	8	1.8	C50
Penis	0	0	-	-	-	-	-	-	-	-	0.0	C60
Prostate	25	0	84	-	-	-	2	1	3	19	3.8	C61
Testis	6	0	83	-	-	2	2	-	2	-	0.9	C62
Kidney	16	0	75	3	-	-	-	3	3	7	2.5	C64
Renal pelvis, ureter and other urinary	1	0	100	-	-	-	-	-	-	1	0.2	C65-66,C68
Bladder	18	0	67	-	-	1	1	2	4	10	2.8	C67
Eye	3	0	67	-	2	-	-	-	-	1	0.5	C69
Brain, nervous system	36	0	22	6	4	4	10	3	2	7	5.5	C70-72
Thyroid	9	0	100	-	1	-	3	1	1	3	1.4	C73
Hodgkin disease	12	0	83	5	3	3	1	-	-	-	1.8	C81
Non-Hodgkin lymphoma	30	0	100	6	5	3	3	3	1	9	4.6	C82-85,C96
Multiple myeloma	3	0	0	-	-	-	-	-	-	3	0.5	C90
Lymphoid leukaemia	24	0	8	10	3	-	-	4	4	3	3.7	C91
Myeloid leukaemia	28	0	7	4	5	2	6	1	5	5	4.3	C92-94
Leukaemia, unspecified	2	0	0	1	-	-	-	1	-	-	0.3	C95
Other and unspecified	35	0	54	8	4	3	3	4	3	10	5.4	O&U
All sites	779	0	76	62	47	42	76	96	157	299	100.0	ALL
All sites but C44	652	0	73	61	46	38	66	88	131	222		ALLbC44

Table 2. Algeria, Batna (1995-1999)

NUMBER OF CASES BY AGE GROUP - FEMALE

SITE	ICD (10th)	ALL AGES	AGE UNK	MV (%)	0-	15-	25-	35-	45-	55-	65+	%
Mouth	C00-06	5	0	100	-	-	-	-	1	1	3	0.7
Salivary gland	C07-08	0	0	-	-	-	-	-	-	-	-	0.0
Nasopharynx	C11	22	0	100	1	4	3	5	2	3	4	2.9
Other pharynx	C09-10,C12-14	4	0	100	-	-	-	1	-	1	2	0.5
Oesophagus	C15	9	0	89	-	-	-	1	1	2	5	1.2
Stomach	C16	34	0	85	-	-	-	2	10	8	14	4.5
Colon, rectum and anus	C18-21	47	0	81	-	-	7	4	8	15	13	6.2
Liver	C22	21	0	24	1	-	-	2	6	5	7	2.8
Gallbladder etc.	C23-24	87	0	76	-	-	-	7	23	28	29	11.6
Pancreas	C25	9	0	44	-	-	-	-	1	4	4	1.2
Larynx	C32	3	0	67	-	-	1	1	-	1	1	0.4
Trachea, bronchus and lung	C33-34	11	0	100	-	-	1	1	4	4	1	1.5
Bone	C40-41	15	0	73	3	3	1	1	3	1	3	2.0
Melanoma of skin	C43	2	0	100	-	-	-	-	-	2	-	0.3
Other skin	C44	92	0	90	1	3	4	4	14	13	53	
Mesothelioma	C45	2	0	100	-	-	-	-	-	-	2	0.3
Kaposi sarcoma	C46	0	0	-	-	-	-	-	-	-	-	0.0
Peripheral nerves	C47	0	0	-	-	-	-	-	-	-	-	0.0
Connective and soft tissue	C49	10	0	100	1	1	1	2	2	2	1	1.3
Breast	C50	182	0	99	-	-	20	64	47	26	25	24.2
Vulva	C51	5	0	100	-	-	-	-	4	1	-	0.7
Vagina	C52	3	0	100	-	-	-	2	-	1	-	0.4
Cervix uteri	C53	72	0	100	-	1	2	6	20	20	23	9.6
Uterus	C54-55	22	0	100	-	-	-	5	6	3	8	2.9
Ovary	C56	29	0	97	-	2	3	7	8	3	6	3.9
Placenta	C58	1	0	100	-	-	-	1	-	-	-	0.1
Kidney	C64	8	0	75	2	1	-	-	2	3	-	1.1
Renal pelvis, ureter and other urinary	C65-66,C68	0	0	-	-	-	-	-	-	-	-	0.0
Bladder	C67	1	0	100	-	-	-	-	-	-	1	0.1
Eye	C69	0	0	-	-	-	-	-	-	-	-	0.0
Brain, nervous system	C70-72	27	0	19	5	3	4	3	4	2	6	3.6
Thyroid	C73	22	0	86	-	1	3	2	7	6	3	2.9
Hodgkin disease	C81	9	0	89	1	4	2	2	-	-	-	1.2
Non-Hodgkin lymphoma	C82-85,C96	19	0	95	1	3	2	2	3	1	7	2.5
Multiple myeloma	C90	3	0	33	-	-	-	-	2	-	1	0.4
Lymphoid leukaemia	C91	14	0	14	10	-	-	-	1	3	-	1.9
Myeloid leukaemia	C92-94	24	0	13	7	3	6	-	4	3	1	3.2
Leukaemia, unspecified	C95	2	0	0	-	1	1	-	-	-	-	0.3
Other and unspecified	O&U	29	0	66	3	2	2	1	4	10	7	3.9
All sites	ALL	845	0	82	36	32	61	127	187	172	230	
All sites but C44	ALLbC44	753	0	81	35	29	57	123	173	159	177	100.0

Table 3. Algeria, Constantine (1994-1997)

NUMBER OF CASES BY AGE GROUP AND SUMMARY RATES OF INCIDENCE - MALE

SITE	ALL AGES	AGE UNK	0-	15-	25-	35-	45-	55-	65+	CRUDE RATE	%	CR 64	ASR (W)	ICD (10th)
Mouth	21	0	-	1	-	2	3	7	8	1.4	3.0	0.16	**2.5**	C00-06
Salivary gland	2	0	-	-	-	1	1	-	-	0.1	0.3	0.02	**0.2**	C07-08
Nasopharynx	51	0	2	4	3	7	9	14	12	3.3	7.3	0.38	**5.3**	C11
Other pharynx	7	0	-	-	-	1	2	2	2	0.5	1.0	0.06	**0.8**	C09-10,C12-14
Oesophagus	3	0	-	-	-	-	1	-	2	0.2	0.4	0.01	**0.4**	C15
Stomach	32	0	-	1	4	6	-	7	12	2.1	4.6	0.20	**3.6**	C16
Colon, rectum and anus	42	0	-	3	9	7	8	6	9	2.7	6.0	0.28	**4.1**	C18-21
Liver	6	0	1	-	-	1	1	2	1	0.4	0.9	0.05	**0.6**	C22
Gallbladder etc.	15	0	-	-	1	3	1	4	9	1.0	2.1	0.08	**1.8**	C23-24
Pancreas	13	0	-	-	-	3	-	-	7	0.8	1.8	0.06	**1.5**	C25
Larynx	49	0	-	-	1	4	9	16	19	3.2	7.0	0.37	**5.8**	C32
Trachea, bronchus and lung	108	0	-	-	2	7	16	47	36	7.0	15.4	0.96	**13.1**	C33-34
Bone	16	0	1	5	2	3	1	3	1	1.0	2.3	0.10	**1.3**	C40-41
Melanoma of skin	3	0	-	-	-	-	1	-	1	0.2	0.4	0.02	**0.3**	C43
Other skin	27	0	1	1	1	3	3	6	13	1.7	0.9	0.15	**3.2**	C44
Mesothelioma	6	0	-	-	-	1	1	1	3	0.4	0.9	0.03	**0.7**	C45
Kaposi sarcoma	2	0	-	-	-	-	-	-	2	0.1	0.3	0.00	**0.3**	C46
Peripheral nerves	0	0	-	-	-	-	-	-	-	0.0	0.0	0.00	**0.0**	C47
Connective and soft tissue	5	0	1	-	1	-	-	2	-	0.3	0.7	0.04	**0.4**	C49
Breast	6	0	-	-	-	-	1	-	5	0.4	0.9	0.01	**0.7**	C50
Penis	0	0	-	-	-	-	-	-	-	0.0	0.0	0.00	**0.0**	C60
Prostate	46	0	-	-	-	-	3	7	36	3.0	6.5	0.15	**5.8**	C61
Testis	4	0	1	-	2	1	-	-	-	0.3	0.6	0.02	**0.2**	C62
Kidney	10	0	3	-	-	2	2	3	-	0.6	1.4	0.09	**0.9**	C64
Renal pelvis, ureter and other urinary	0	0	-	-	-	-	-	-	-	0.0	0.0	0.00	**0.0**	C65-66,C68
Bladder	37	0	-	-	-	2	-	13	20	2.4	5.3	0.23	**4.6**	C67
Eye	2	0	-	-	-	-	1	-	1	0.1	0.3	0.01	**0.2**	C69
Brain, nervous system	13	0	3	1	1	3	2	3	1	0.8	1.8	0.09	**1.1**	C70-72
Thyroid	11	0	-	-	3	1	2	1	2	0.7	1.6	0.07	**1.1**	C73
Hodgkin disease	19	0	2	5	3	2	5	2	2	1.2	2.7	0.10	**1.5**	C81
Non-Hodgkin lymphoma	57	0	7	6	7	10	6	7	14	3.7	8.1	0.32	**5.4**	C82-85,C96
Multiple myeloma	13	0	-	3	1	3	2	2	2	0.8	1.8	0.08	**1.2**	C90
Lymphoid leukaemia	29	0	7	2	2	4	3	4	8	1.9	4.1	0.15	**2.7**	C91
Myeloid leukaemia	25	0	5	-	3	2	6	2	7	1.6	3.6	0.13	**2.4**	C92-94
Leukaemia, unspecified	2	0	1	-	-	1	-	-	-	0.1	0.3	0.01	**0.2**	C95
Other and unspecified	48	0	4	3	3	4	11	13	10	3.1	6.8	0.38	**5.1**	O&U
All sites	730	0	39	38	49	81	104	174	245	47.3	100.0	4.82	**79.0**	ALL
All sites but C44	703	0	38	38	48	78	101	168	232	45.5		4.66	**75.9**	ALLbC44

	MV (%)
Mouth	90
Salivary gland	100
Nasopharynx	100
Other pharynx	100
Oesophagus	33
Stomach	84
Colon, rectum and anus	93
Liver	83
Gallbladder etc.	53
Pancreas	46
Larynx	92
Trachea, bronchus and lung	74
Bone	100
Melanoma of skin	100
Other skin	100
Mesothelioma	100
Kaposi sarcoma	100
Peripheral nerves	-
Connective and soft tissue	100
Breast	83
Penis	-
Prostate	93
Testis	100
Kidney	100
Renal pelvis, ureter and other urinary	-
Bladder	76
Eye	100
Brain, nervous system	62
Thyroid	100
Hodgkin disease	100
Non-Hodgkin lymphoma	98
Multiple myeloma	92
Lymphoid leukaemia	90
Myeloid leukaemia	96
Leukaemia, unspecified	100
Other and unspecified	71
All sites	87
All sites but C44	86

Average annual population

0-	15-	25-	35-	45-	55-	65+
155198	84204	59284	31858	24629	17086	13725

Table 3. Algeria, Constantine (1994-1997)

NUMBER OF CASES BY AGE GROUP AND SUMMARY RATES OF INCIDENCE - FEMALE

SITE	ALL AGES	AGE UNK	MV (%)	0-	15-	25-	35-	45-	55-	65+	CRUDE RATE	%	CR 64	ASR (W)	ICD (10th)
Mouth	9	0	100	-	-	-	1	2	1	5	0.6	1.0	0.04	1.0	C00-06
Salivary gland	2	0	100	1	-	-	-	-	-	1	0.1	0.2	0.00	0.2	C07-08
Nasopharynx	26	0	100	-	1	4	6	6	7	2	1.7	2.8	0.22	2.5	C11
Other pharynx	1	0	100	-	-	-	-	-	1	-	0.1	0.1	0.02	0.1	C09-10,C12-14
Oesophagus	1	0	100	-	-	-	-	-	1	-	0.1	0.1	0.02	0.1	C15
Stomach	21	0	71	-	-	1	3	4	7	6	1.4	2.3	0.16	2.2	C16
Colon, rectum and anus	43	0	98	-	3	7	4	7	7	15	2.8	4.7	0.24	4.2	C18-21
Liver	6	0	67	-	-	1	-	3	1	1	0.4	0.7	0.04	0.6	C22
Gallbladder etc.	58	0	81	-	-	1	8	13	15	21	3.8	6.4	0.40	6.3	C23-24
Pancreas	14	0	50	-	-	1	-	2	4	7	0.9	1.5	0.08	1.5	C25
Larynx	8	0	88	-	-	-	-	2	4	2	0.5	0.9	0.06	0.8	C32
Trachea, bronchus and lung	20	0	85	-	-	-	2	3	6	9	1.3	2.2	0.12	2.2	C33-34
Bone	13	0	92	6	2	-	1	4	-	-	0.9	1.4	0.07	0.9	C40-41
Melanoma of skin	3	0	100	-	-	-	-	-	1	2	0.2	0.3	0.02	0.4	C43
Other skin	15	0	93	-	-	1	3	1	5	5	1.0		0.10	1.5	C44
Mesothelioma	2	0	100	-	-	-	-	-	1	1	0.1	0.2	0.02	0.2	C45
Kaposi sarcoma	2	0	50	-	-	-	-	-	1	1	0.1	0.2	0.02	0.3	C46
Peripheral nerves	0	0	-	-	-	-	-	-	-	-	0.0	0.0	0.00	0.0	C47
Connective and soft tissue	8	0	100	-	3	-	1	-	1	3	0.5	0.9	0.03	0.7	C49
Breast	291	0	95	-	-	32	103	74	45	37	19.1	31.9	2.25	28.3	C50
Vulva	2	0	100	-	-	-	-	-	1	1	0.1	0.2	0.01	0.2	C51
Vagina	2	0	100	-	-	-	1	-	-	1	0.1	0.2	0.00	0.2	C52
Cervix uteri	113	0	99	-	-	3	16	32	32	30	7.4	12.4	0.89	12.1	C53
Uterus	23	0	100	-	-	1	8	3	3	8	1.5	2.5	0.18	2.6	C54-55
Ovary	43	0	93	1	4	7	8	9	7	7	2.8	4.7	0.28	3.8	C56
Placenta	0	0	-	-	-	-	-	-	-	-	0.0	0.0	0.00	0.0	C58
Kidney	12	0	75	8	-	2	1	-	-	1	0.8	1.3	0.04	0.8	C64
Renal pelvis, ureter and other urinary	1	0	0	-	-	1	-	-	-	-	0.1	0.1	0.01	0.1	C65-66,C68
Bladder	6	0	83	-	-	-	-	2	2	2	0.4	0.7	0.05	0.7	C67
Eye	2	0	100	-	-	-	-	-	1	1	0.1	0.2	0.03	0.2	C69
Brain, nervous system	12	0	67	3	1	1	2	3	2	-	0.8	1.3	0.07	0.9	C70-72
Thyroid	31	0	97	-	1	8	7	3	6	6	2.0	3.4	0.20	2.8	C73
Hodgkin disease	16	0	100	4	3	2	5	2	-	-	1.1	1.8	0.08	1.1	C81
Non-Hodgkin lymphoma	36	0	97	3	6	7	4	2	9	5	2.4	3.9	0.24	3.1	C82-85,C96
Multiple myeloma	7	0	100	-	-	-	-	1	1	5	0.5	0.8	0.01	0.8	C90
Lymphoid leukaemia	13	0	92	3	2	2	2	-	1	3	0.9	1.4	0.05	1.1	C91
Myeloid leukaemia	24	0	92	2	1	7	3	5	4	2	1.6	2.6	0.16	2.0	C92-94
Leukaemia, unspecified	0	0	-	-	-	-	-	-	-	-	0.0	0.0	0.00	0.0	C95
Other and unspecified	42	0	88	7	3	2	4	11	5	10	2.8	4.6	0.24	3.9	O&U
All sites	928	0	92	38	30	92	188	195	186	199	61.0	100.0	6.44	90.4	ALL
All sites but C44	913	0	92	38	30	91	185	194	181	194	60.0		6.34	88.8	ALLbC44
Average annual population				148012	81398	56096	34737	27460	18256	14654					

Table 4. Algeria, Oran (1996-1998)

NUMBER OF CASES BY AGE GROUP AND SUMMARY RATES OF INCIDENCE - MALE

SITE	ALL AGES	AGE UNK	MV (%)	0-	15-	25-	35-	45-	55-	65+	CRUDE RATE	%	CR 64	ASR (W)	ICD (10th)
Mouth	26	0	96	1	-	1	2	5	7	10	1.5	1.7	0.14	2.3	C00-06
Salivary gland	3	0	100	-	-	-	-	-	-	3	0.2	0.2	0.00	0.3	C07-08
Nasopharynx	103	0	99	5	16	18	26	18	11	9	5.8	6.6	0.50	6.6	C11
Other pharynx	15	0	93	-	-	-	3	-	7	5	0.8	1.0	0.10	1.3	C09-10,C12-14
Oesophagus	17	0	76	-	-	1	2	3	4	7	1.0	1.1	0.08	1.5	C15
Stomach	91	0	98	-	2	4	16	16	18	35	5.1	5.9	0.42	7.6	C16
Colon, rectum and anus	87	0	91	-	-	8	15	15	26	23	4.9	5.6	0.51	7.2	C18-21
Liver	2	0	0	-	-	-	1	-	1	1	0.1	0.1	0.01	0.2	C22
Gallbladder etc.	18	0	50	-	-	-	1	2	7	8	1.0	1.2	0.11	1.7	C23-24
Pancreas	16	0	56	-	-	-	1	2	4	9	0.9	1.0	0.06	1.5	C25
Larynx	91	0	100	2	1	-	3	20	24	41	5.1	5.9	0.46	8.3	C32
Trachea, bronchus and lung	263	0	90	-	-	5	25	42	86	105	14.8	16.9	1.48	23.7	C33-34
Bone	29	0	83	4	15	-	4	-	2	4	1.6	1.9	0.09	1.7	C40-41
Melanoma of skin	9	0	100	1	-	2	-	2	2	1	0.5	0.6	0.05	0.6	C43
Other skin	130	0	98	1	2	2	11	18	28	68	7.3	8.4	0.53	11.7	C44
Mesothelioma	3	0	100	-	-	1	-	1	1	-	0.2	0.2	0.02	0.2	C45
Kaposi sarcoma	3	0	100	-	-	2	-	1	-	-	0.2	0.2	0.02	0.2	C46
Peripheral nerves	0	0	-	-	-	-	-	-	-	-	0.0	0.0	0.00	0.0	C47
Connective and soft tissue	29	0	93	9	3	2	2	4	3	6	1.6	1.9	0.12	2.1	C49
Breast	11	0	100	-	-	1	2	3	1	4	0.6	0.7	0.05	0.9	C50
Penis	0	0	-	-	-	-	-	-	-	-	0.0	0.0	0.00	0.0	C60
Prostate	74	0	96	-	-	-	-	5	13	56	4.2	4.8	0.20	7.2	C61
Testis	8	0	100	-	3	-	1	3	-	1	0.5	0.5	0.03	0.5	C62
Kidney	22	0	77	8	-	1	-	1	6	6	1.2	1.4	0.10	1.7	C64
Renal pelvis, ureter and other urinary	5	0	100	-	-	-	-	1	2	2	0.3	0.3	0.03	0.5	C65-66,C68
Bladder	148	0	93	-	1	5	5	18	44	75	8.4	9.5	0.70	13.6	C67
Eye	18	0	100	12	-	-	2	-	-	4	1.0	1.2	0.04	1.2	C69
Brain, nervous system	42	0	64	11	3	5	8	6	6	3	2.4	2.7	0.21	2.8	C70-72
Thyroid	7	0	86	-	-	2	3	1	1	-	0.4	0.5	0.04	0.4	C73
Hodgkin disease	56	0	100	19	14	9	6	3	4	1	3.2	3.6	0.22	3.1	C81
Non-Hodgkin lymphoma	125	0	99	34	20	9	14	18	15	15	7.1	8.0	0.54	8.2	C82-85,C96
Multiple myeloma	13	0	100	-	-	-	-	3	7	3	0.7	0.8	0.11	1.2	C90
Lymphoid leukaemia	25	0	88	16	1	1	2	1	3	3	1.4	1.6	0.09	1.5	C91
Myeloid leukaemia	13	0	100	2	1	2	2	-	2	3	0.7	0.8	0.05	0.9	C92-94
Leukaemia, unspecified	5	0	80	1	-	2	-	-	-	1	0.3	0.3	0.01	0.3	C95
Other and unspecified	178	0	96	8	12	21	17	31	39	50	10.0	11.4	0.92	14.2	O&U
All sites	1685	0	93	133	97	104	172	243	374	562	95.1		8.04	136.9	ALL
All sites but C44	1555	0	93	132	95	102	161	225	346	494	87.8	100.0	7.51	125.2	ALLbC44
Average annual population				191541	127986	102891	70736	44279	29493	23673					

Table 4. Algeria, Oran (1996-1998)

NUMBER OF CASES BY AGE GROUP AND SUMMARY RATES OF INCIDENCE - FEMALE

SITE	ALL AGES	AGE UNK	MV (%)	0-	15-	25-	35-	45-	55-	65+	CRUDE RATE	%	CR 64	ASR (W)	ICD (10th)
Mouth	10	0	100	-	-	-	-	4	3	3	0.6	0.6	0.07	0.9	C00-06
Salivary gland	5	0	80	-	-	-	3	1	-	1	0.3	0.3	0.02	0.3	C07-08
Nasopharynx	50	0	94	4	4	10	12	7	10	3	2.8	2.9	0.28	3.3	C11
Other pharynx	6	0	100	1	-	-	-	2	2	1	0.3	0.3	0.04	0.5	C09-10,C12-14
Oesophagus	8	0	88	-	1	-	-	-	1	5	0.5	0.5	0.02	0.6	C15
Stomach	52	0	88	-	-	8	5	12	9	18	3.0	3.0	0.24	4.0	C16
Colon, rectum and anus	83	0	92	-	5	6	22	11	15	24	4.7	4.8	0.39	6.1	C18-21
Liver	10	0	100	-	-	1	-	3	5	2	0.6	0.6	0.08	0.9	C22
Gallbladder etc.	77	0	82	-	-	-	3	18	29	26	4.4	4.5	0.49	6.6	C23-24
Pancreas	22	0	55	-	-	-	2	3	6	11	1.2	1.3	0.10	1.8	C25
Larynx	2	0	100	-	-	1	-	-	-	1	0.1	0.1	0.00	0.1	C32
Trachea, bronchus and lung	30	0	87	-	-	1	5	7	9	8	1.7	1.7	0.18	2.4	C33-34
Bone	25	0	92	11	4	2	3	-	3	2	1.4	1.4	0.09	1.5	C40-41
Melanoma of skin	15	0	100	-	-	-	2	4	4	5	0.9	0.9	0.08	1.2	C43
Other skin	89	0	98	3	2	7	4	18	19	36	5.1	5.1	0.41	7.1	C44
Mesothelioma	1	0	100	-	-	-	-	-	1	-	0.1	0.1	0.01	0.1	C45
Kaposi sarcoma	1	0	100	-	-	-	-	-	1	-	0.1	0.1	0.01	0.1	C46
Peripheral nerves	2	0	100	1	-	-	1	-	-	-	0.1	0.1	0.01	0.1	C47
Connective and soft tissue	20	0	100	3	4	3	-	3	2	4	1.1	1.2	0.08	1.3	C49
Breast	481	0	98	-	3	54	158	137	73	56	27.3	27.8	2.83	34.5	C50
Vulva	2	0	100	-	-	-	-	-	-	1	0.1	0.1	0.01	0.2	C51
Vagina	9	0	78	-	-	1	-	3	2	-	0.5	0.5	0.05	0.7	C52
Cervix uteri	324	0	98	-	-	18	81	117	70	38	18.4	18.7	2.14	24.9	C53
Uterus	48	0	98	-	-	4	14	11	9	9	2.7	2.8	0.27	3.5	C54-55
Ovary	50	0	96	1	1	7	7	14	11	9	2.8	2.9	0.29	3.7	C56
Placenta	0	0	-	-	-	-	-	-	-	-	0.0	0.0	0.00	0.0	C58
Kidney	28	0	93	13	-	-	4	2	6	3	1.6	1.6	0.14	1.9	C64
Renal pelvis, ureter and other urinary	4	0	100	-	-	-	-	-	2	1	0.2	0.2	0.03	0.3	C65-66,C68
Bladder	15	0	73	-	-	-	1	2	4	8	0.9	0.9	0.07	1.3	C67
Eye	8	0	100	6	-	-	-	-	-	2	0.5	0.5	0.02	0.6	C69
Brain, nervous system	19	0	68	5	1	2	1	3	6	1	1.1	1.1	0.12	1.3	C70-72
Thyroid	62	0	97	1	5	20	9	10	7	10	3.5	3.6	0.28	4.0	C73
Hodgkin disease	20	0	100	3	5	1	4	-	3	4	1.1	1.2	0.08	1.3	C81
Non-Hodgkin lymphoma	88	0	100	16	10	6	10	10	20	16	5.0	5.1	0.44	6.2	C82-85,C96
Multiple myeloma	16	0	100	-	1	2	4	1	4	4	0.9	0.9	0.08	1.2	C90
Lymphoid leukaemia	12	0	100	7	1	-	1	-	-	2	0.7	0.7	0.03	0.8	C91
Myeloid leukaemia	10	0	100	1	1	3	1	2	2	-	0.6	0.6	0.06	0.6	C92-94
Leukaemia, unspecified	0	0	-	-	-	-	-	-	-	-	0.0	0.0	0.00	0.0	C95
Other and unspecified	114	0	97	8	7	7	12	22	25	33	6.5	6.6	0.59	8.7	O&U
All sites	1818	0	95	85	56	165	370	431	363	348	103.2	100.0	10.14	134.4	ALL
All sites but C44	1729	0	95	82	54	158	366	413	344	312	98.1		9.73	127.3	ALLbC44

Average annual population: 186009 | 126289 | 102612 | 70593 | 44430 | 29832 | 27584

Table 5. Algeria, Setif (1993-1997)

NUMBER OF CASES BY AGE GROUP AND SUMMARY RATES OF INCIDENCE - MALE

SITE	ALL AGES	AGE UNK	MV (%)	0-	15-	25-	35-	45-	55-	65+	CRUDE RATE	%	CR 64	ASR (W)	ICD (10th)
Mouth	46	0	98	1	-	1	1	6	11	26	1.5	3.4	0.14	2.8	C00-06
Salivary gland	7	0	100	-	1	-	-	2	-	3	0.2	0.5	0.01	0.4	C07-08
Nasopharynx	134	0	98	3	35	23	17	26	20	10	4.5	9.8	0.52	6.3	C11
Other pharynx	58	0	100	1	-	1	-	9	25	21	1.9	4.3	0.30	3.8	C09-10,C12-14
Oesophagus	9	0	89	1	-	-	1	-	2	6	0.3	0.7	0.02	0.5	C15
Stomach	131	0	89	1	4	6	14	38	21	47	4.4	9.6	0.51	7.8	C16
Colon, rectum and anus	82	0	90	1	4	12	11	20	18	16	2.7	6.0	0.36	4.6	C18-21
Liver	23	0	22	-	-	-	3	1	8	11	0.8	1.7	0.09	1.4	C22
Gallbladder etc.	29	0	69	-	-	1	3	3	8	14	1.0	2.1	0.11	1.8	C23-24
Pancreas	3	0	33	-	-	-	-	-	1	1	0.1	0.2	0.01	0.2	C25
Larynx	37	0	89	-	1	2	3	3	14	17	1.2	2.7	0.16	2.3	C32
Trachea, bronchus and lung	246	0	91	-	-	-	14	38	81	110	8.2	18.1	1.04	15.5	C33-34
Bone	23	0	96	4	6	1	5	-	4	3	0.8	1.7	0.07	1.0	C40-41
Melanoma of skin	0	0	-	-	-	-	-	-	-	-	0.0	0.0	0.00	0.0	C43
Other skin	55	0	100	2	1	7	6	5	10	24	1.8		0.17	3.0	C44
Mesothelioma	0	0	-	-	-	-	-	-	-	-	0.0	0.0	0.00	0.0	C45
Kaposi sarcoma	0	0	-	-	-	-	-	-	-	-	0.0	0.0	0.00	0.0	C46
Peripheral nerves	4	0	100	4	-	-	-	-	-	-	0.1	0.3	0.00	0.1	C47
Connective and soft tissue	16	0	100	1	4	3	3	1	1	3	0.5	1.2	0.04	0.7	C49
Breast	8	0	100	-	-	-	1	3	3	1	0.3	0.6	0.05	0.5	C50
Penis	1	0	100	-	-	-	-	-	-	1	0.0	0.1	0.00	0.1	C60
Prostate	71	0	94	-	-	-	1	4	15	52	2.4	5.2	0.16	4.3	C61
Testis	4	0	100	-	1	-	1	-	1	2	0.1	0.3	0.01	0.2	C62
Kidney	14	0	79	4	-	-	1	3	3	3	0.5	1.0	0.06	0.8	C64
Renal pelvis, ureter and other urinary	0	0	-	-	-	-	-	-	-	-	0.0	0.0	0.00	0.0	C65-66,C68
Bladder	62	0	87	-	-	1	3	8	25	25	2.1	4.6	0.29	4.0	C67
Eye	4	0	100	2	2	-	-	-	1	-	0.1	0.3	0.02	0.2	C69
Brain, nervous system	31	0	58	6	2	4	6	6	2	5	1.0	2.3	0.10	1.4	C70-72
Thyroid	7	0	86	-	2	-	1	1	-	2	0.2	0.5	0.02	0.3	C73
Hodgkin disease	55	0	100	14	8	12	5	5	6	5	1.8	4.0	0.16	2.3	C81
Non-Hodgkin lymphoma	79	0	100	21	7	9	10	7	12	13	2.6	5.8	0.25	3.6	C82-85,C96
Multiple myeloma	6	0	100	-	-	-	4	-	-	2	0.2	0.4	0.01	0.3	C90
Lymphoid leukaemia	43	0	100	25	4	1	4	-	3	6	1.4	3.2	0.08	1.5	C91
Myeloid leukaemia	22	0	100	4	4	2	3	3	1	5	0.7	1.6	0.06	1.0	C92-94
Leukaemia, unspecified	9	0	100	4	-	1	3	3	-	1	0.3	0.7	0.03	0.4	C95
Other and unspecified	97	0	74	7	4	10	7	14	25	30	3.2	7.1	0.38	5.4	O&U
All sites	1416	0	90	105	87	99	129	210	321	465	47.3	100.0	5.25	78.5	ALL
All sites but C44	1361	0	90	103	86	92	123	205	311	441	45.5		5.08	75.5	ALLbC44
Average annual population				255997	131540	76749	54443	32852	22393	24376					

Table 5. Algeria, Setif (1993-1997)

NUMBER OF CASES BY AGE GROUP AND SUMMARY RATES OF INCIDENCE - FEMALE

SITE	ALL AGES	AGE UNK	MV (%)	0-	15-	25-	35-	45-	55-	65+	CRUDE RATE	%	CR 64	ASR (W)	ICD (10th)
Mouth	16	0	100	1	-	-	2	2	4	7	0.5	1.1	0.05	0.9	C00-06
Salivary gland	8	0	100	-	-	2	-	3	2	1	0.3	0.6	0.04	0.4	C07-08
Nasopharynx	51	0	84	8	8	10	4	5	10	6	1.7	3.6	0.17	2.2	C11
Other pharynx	9	0	100	-	-	-	-	1	4	4	0.3	0.6	0.04	0.5	C09-10,C12-14
Oesophagus	5	0	80	-	-	-	2	-	2	1	0.2	0.4	0.02	0.3	C15
Stomach	56	0	89	-	-	2	15	14	15	10	1.9	3.9	0.26	3.1	C16
Colon, rectum and anus	89	0	93	1	4	16	23	16	13	16	3.0	6.2	0.32	4.3	C18-21
Liver	32	0	47	1	-	-	4	5	12	10	1.1	2.2	0.15	1.9	C22
Gallbladder etc.	152	0	90	-	-	2	28	40	43	39	5.1	10.7	0.69	8.6	C23-24
Pancreas	10	0	70	-	-	-	2	1	2	5	0.3	0.7	0.03	0.6	C25
Larynx	2	0	100	-	-	-	-	1	-	1	0.1	0.1	0.00	0.1	C32
Trachea, bronchus and lung	31	0	97	-	-	1	2	2	7	21	1.0	2.2	0.07	1.7	C33-34
Bone	31	0	97	7	8	3	4	2	4	3	1.0	2.2	0.09	1.2	C40-41
Melanoma of skin	1	0	100	-	-	-	-	-	1	-	0.0	0.1	0.00	0.1	C43
Other skin	24	0	100	-	1	3	3	3	4	10	0.8	1.7	0.07	1.3	C44
Mesothelioma	0	0	-	-	-	-	-	-	-	-	0.0	0.0	0.00	0.0	C45
Kaposi sarcoma	1	0	100	-	-	-	-	-	-	1	0.0	0.1	0.00	0.1	C46
Peripheral nerves	1	0	100	-	1	-	-	-	-	-	0.0	0.1	0.00	0.0	C47
Connective and soft tissue	11	0	91	1	3	2	2	2	1	1	0.4	0.8	0.03	0.5	C49
Breast	317	0	96	-	1	31	80	90	73	42	10.5	22.2	1.47	17.0	C50
Vulva	5	0	100	-	-	-	1	1	3	1	0.2	0.4	0.04	0.3	C51
Vagina	4	0	100	-	-	-	-	-	3	1	0.1	0.3	0.03	0.3	C52
Cervix uteri	203	0	96	-	-	5	40	48	66	44	6.7	14.2	0.96	11.5	C53
Uterus	17	0	94	-	-	-	-	3	6	8	0.6	1.2	0.07	1.0	C54-55
Ovary	65	0	91	1	7	8	14	14	12	9	2.2	4.6	0.26	3.2	C56
Placenta	0	0	-	-	-	-	-	-	-	-	0.0	0.0	0.00	0.0	C58
Kidney	6	0	100	3	1	-	1	1	-	-	0.2	0.4	0.02	0.3	C64
Renal pelvis, ureter and other urinary	1	0	0	-	-	-	1	-	-	-	0.0	0.1	0.00	0.0	C65-66,C68
Bladder	2	0	50	-	-	-	-	-	2	-	0.1	0.1	0.02	0.1	C67
Eye	5	0	100	4	1	-	-	-	-	1	0.2	0.4	0.00	0.2	C69
Brain, nervous system	17	0	71	1	1	4	4	4	3	-	0.6	1.2	0.07	0.8	C70-72
Thyroid	36	0	94	1	6	8	3	7	5	6	1.2	2.5	0.12	1.7	C73
Hodgkin disease	29	0	100	-	5	8	7	4	2	1	1.0	2.0	0.09	1.1	C81
Non-Hodgkin lymphoma	50	0	100	5	5	8	7	7	6	6	1.7	3.5	0.15	2.1	C82-85,C96
Multiple myeloma	3	0	100	-	-	-	1	-	-	-	0.1	0.2	0.02	0.2	C90
Lymphoid leukaemia	22	0	100	16	2	-	1	1	1	2	0.7	1.5	0.03	0.7	C91
Myeloid leukaemia	34	0	100	6	3	7	7	2	10	6	1.1	2.4	0.12	1.6	C92-94
Leukaemia, unspecified	11	0	91	5	-	1	1	2	-	2	0.4	0.8	0.05	0.5	C95
Other and unspecified	92	0	64	4	6	8	12	17	21	24	3.1	6.5	0.34	4.8	O&U
All sites	1449	0	91	76	64	130	258	296	338	287	48.1	100.0	5.88	74.8	ALL
All sites but C44	1425	0	91	76	63	127	255	293	334	277	47.4		5.81	73.5	ALLbC44

	0-	15-	25-	35-	45-	55-	65+
Average annual population	245685	130365	79658	59563	36286	24550	25765

Table 6. Algeria: case series

Site	Histopathology series: Algiers, Oran, Constantine. 1966–75 (Yaker, 1980, 1986)					Tlemcen, 1994–96 (Meguenni, 1998)				
	Male		Female		%HV	Male		Female		%HV
	No.	%	No.	%		No.	%	No.	%	
Oral cavity[1]	402	4.1%	136	1.4%	100	10	2.9%	10	2.1%	
Nasopharynx	497*	5.0%	222*	2.2%	100	25	7.3%	10	2.1%	
Other pharynx						2	0.6%	1	0.2%	
Oesophagus	56	0.6%	30	0.3%	100	6	1.7%	7	1.5%	
Stomach	436	4.4%	174	1.7%	100	53	15.4%	31	6.6%	
Colon/rectum	398	4.0%	266	2.7%	100	16	4.7%	24	5.1%	
Liver	189	1.9%	180	1.8%	100	16	4.7%	20	4.3%	
Pancreas	33	0.3%	21	0.2%	100	13	3.8%	12	2.6%	
Larynx	907	9.2%	82	0.8%	100	29	8.4%	1	0.2%	
Lung	309	3.1%	50	0.5%	100	19	5.5%	4	0.9%	
Melanoma	111	1.1%	82	0.8%	100	4	1.2%	0	0.0%	
Other skin	2449	24.8%	1267	12.7%	100	13	3.8%	9	1.9%	
Kaposi sarcoma										
Breast	53	0.5%	1147	11.5%	100	1	0.3%	138	29.4%	
Cervix uteri			3002	30.1%	100			26	5.5%	
Corpus uteri			502	5.0%	100			5	1.1%	
Ovary etc.			241	2.4%	100			32	6.8%	
Prostate	138	1.4%			100	3	0.9%			
Penis	47	0.5%			100	0	0.0%			
Bladder	314	3.2%	48	0.5%	100	3	0.9%	0	0.0%	
Kidney etc.	121	1.2%	88	0.9%	100	1	0.3%	0	0.0%	
Eye	154	1.6%	126	1.3%	100	0	0.0%	1	0.2%	
Brain, nervous system	112	1.1%	81	0.8%	100	1	0.3%	3	0.6%	
Thyroid	83	0.8%	183	1.8%	100	1	0.3%	6	1.3%	
Non-Hodgkin lymphoma	788	8.0%	412	4.1%	100	7	2.0%	5	1.1%	
Hodgkin disease	383	3.9%	112	1.1%	100	17	4.9%	14	3.0%	
Myeloma	12	0.1%	9	0.1%	100	9	2.6%	7	1.5%	
Leukaemia	431	4.4%	300	3.0%	100	27	7.8%	30	6.4%	
ALL SITES	9867	100.0%	9957	100.0%	100	344	100.0%	470	100.0%	

[1] Includes salivary gland tumours

* Includes oropharynx

Table 7. Registry of digestive tract cancer, Algiers, 1987–89 (Abid & Benabadji, 1999)

Male		0–14	15–24	25–34	35–44	45–54	55–64	65+	Total	%	Crude rate	ASR (world)
Oesophagus	C15	0	0	0	0	6	8	9	25	3.8%	1.0	2.1
Stomach	C16	0	5	17	30	43	43	84	241	36.9%	9.2	17.5
Colon/rectum	C18–21	4	12	18	26	44	40	66	215	32.9%	8.2	15.2
Liver	C22	1	0	1	4	9	5	14	34	5.2%	1.3	2.5
Gallbladder etc.	C23–24	0	0	0	1	6	12	14	33	5.1%	1.3	2.6
Pancreas	C25	0	0	0	1	6	15	13	36	5.5%	1.4	2.9
All sites	C15–C26	22	26	41	64	117	131	220	653	100.0%	24.9	46.6
Population (1988)		413372	177571	114135	57793	49674	30468	30989	874005			

Female		0–14	15–24	25–34	35–44	45–54	55–64	65+	Total	%	Crude rate	ASR (world)
Oesophagus	C15	0	0	0	0	4	4	3	11	2.2%	0.4	0.8
Stomach	C16	3	0	13	23	24	28	29	126	25.7%	4.8	7.7
Colon/rectum	C18–21	1	4	10	22	25	29	40	136	27.8%	5.2	8.4
Liver	C22	0	0	3	3	7	9	8	30	6.1%	1.1	2.0
Gallbladder etc.	C23–24	0	0	3	10	32	31	43	120	24.5%	4.6	7.8
Pancreas	C25	0	0	0	0	3	6	6	15	3.1%	0.6	1.0
All sites	C15–C26	13	5	31	60	98	122	146	490	100.0%	18.7	30.8
Population (1988)		393171	168923	111122	66589	58070	36068	37329	871272			

Table 8. Childhood cancer, Algeria, Algiers (1993-1997)

	NUMBER OF CASES					REL. FREQ.(%)	RATES PER MILLION					
	0-4	5-9	10-14	All	M/F	Overall	0-4	5-9	10-14	Crude	ASR	%MV
Leukaemia	25	22	19	66	1.9	19.5	24.6	20.0	15.9	20.0	20.6	100.0
Acute lymphoid leukaemia	16	15	9	40	1.7	11.8	15.8	13.7	7.5	12.1	12.7	100.0
Lymphoma	10	17	14	41	1.9	12.1	9.9	15.5	11.7	12.4	12.2	100.0
Hodgkin disease	3	3	5	11	0.6	3.2	3.0	2.7	4.2	3.3	3.2	100.0
Burkitt lymphoma	0	0	0	0	-	-	-	-	-	-	-	-
Brain and spinal neoplasms	7	22	15	44	1.9	13.0	6.9	20.0	12.6	13.3	12.8	93.2
Neuroblastoma	12	16	5	33	3.1	9.7	11.8	14.6	4.2	10.0	10.5	100.0
Retinoblastoma	14	4	1	19	0.9	5.6	13.8	3.6	0.8	5.8	6.8	100.0
Wilms tumour	15	8	4	27	0.8	8.0	14.8	7.3	3.4	8.2	9.0	96.3
Bone tumours	1	7	25	33	3.1	9.7	1.0	6.4	21.0	10.0	8.5	87.9
Soft tissue sarcomas	4	5	6	15	2.0	4.4	3.9	4.6	5.0	4.5	4.5	80.0
Kaposi sarcoma	0	0	0	0	-	-	-	-	-	-	-	-
Germ cell tumours	9	0	2	11	0.8	3.2	8.9	-	1.7	3.3	3.9	100.0
Other	14	14	22	50	1.9	14.7	13.8	12.8	18.5	15.1	14.8	76.0
All	111	115	113	339	1.8	100.0	109.4	104.8	94.8	102.6	103.7	93.2

Table 9. Childhood cancer, Algeria, Oran (1996-1998)

	NUMBER OF CASES					REL. FREQ.(%)	RATES PER MILLION					
	0-4	5-9	10-14	All	M/F	Overall	0-4	5-9	10-14	Crude	ASR	%MV
Leukaemia	3	11	13	**27**	2.4	12.4	8.5	29.3	32.3	23.8	**22.1**	100.0
Acute lymphoid leukaemia	3	8	9	**20**	2.3	9.2	8.5	21.3	22.4	17.7	**16.6**	95.0
Lymphoma	19	34	19	**72**	2.8	33.0	53.6	90.5	47.2	63.6	**63.6**	100.0
Hodgkin disease	2	12	8	**22**	6.3	10.1	5.6	31.9	19.9	19.4	**18.3**	100.0
Burkitt lymphoma	0	0	0	**0**	-	-	-	-	-	-	**-**	-
Brain and spinal neoplasms	2	3	3	**8**	3.0	3.7	5.6	8.0	7.5	7.1	**6.9**	50.0
Neuroblastoma	6	3	1	**10**	1.5	4.6	16.9	8.0	2.5	8.8	**9.8**	90.0
Retinoblastoma	11	6	0	**17**	2.4	7.8	31.0	16.0	-	15.0	**17.2**	100.0
Wilms tumour	8	8	4	**20**	0.7	9.2	22.6	21.3	9.9	17.7	**18.5**	100.0
Bone tumours	3	2	10	**15**	0.4	6.9	8.5	5.3	24.8	13.2	**12.2**	93.3
Soft tissue sarcomas	3	5	4	**12**	3.0	5.5	8.5	13.3	9.9	10.6	**10.5**	91.7
Kaposi sarcoma	0	0	0	**0**	-	-	-	-	-	-	**-**	-
Germ cell tumours	0	0	0	**0**	-	-	-	-	-	-	**-**	-
Other	9	10	18	**37**	0.8	17.0	25.4	26.6	44.7	32.7	**31.4**	97.3
All	64	82	72	**218**	1.6	100.0	180.6	218.3	178.9	192.5	**192.2**	95.9

Table 10. Childhood cancer, Algeria, Setif (1993-1997)

	NUMBER OF CASES					REL. FREQ.(%)	RATES PER MILLION					
	0-4	5-9	10-14	All	M/F	Overall	0-4	5-9	10-14	Crude	ASR	%MV
Leukaemia	16	28	16	**60**	1.2	33.1	19.4	32.9	19.2	23.9	**23.7**	94.7
Acute lymphoid leukaemia	13	19	9	**41**	1.6	22.7	15.7	22.3	10.8	16.3	**16.4**	100.0
Lymphoma	15	17	20	**52**	2.1	28.7	18.1	20.0	24.1	20.7	**20.5**	100.0
Hodgkin disease	3	10	6	**19**	2.8	10.5	3.6	11.8	7.2	7.6	**7.3**	100.0
Burkitt lymphoma	0	1	2	**3**	2.0	1.7	-	1.2	2.4	1.2	**1.1**	100.0
Brain and spinal neoplasms	1	3	3	**7**	6.0	3.9	1.2	3.5	3.6	2.8	**2.7**	85.7
Neuroblastoma	5	1	0	**6**	-	3.3	6.0	1.2	-	2.4	**2.7**	100.0
Retinoblastoma	4	0	0	**4**	0.3	2.2	4.8	-	-	1.6	**1.9**	100.0
Wilms tumour	4	2	0	**6**	1.0	3.3	4.8	2.4	-	2.4	**2.6**	100.0
Bone tumours	0	5	6	**11**	0.6	6.1	-	5.9	7.2	4.4	**4.0**	90.9
Soft tissue sarcomas	0	0	1	**1**	-	0.6	-	-	1.2	0.4	**0.3**	100.0
Kaposi sarcoma	0	0	0	**0**	-	-	-	-	-	-	**-**	-
Germ cell tumours	0	0	0	**0**	-	-	-	-	-	-	**-**	-
Other	6	9	19	**34**	0.9	18.8	7.3	10.6	22.9	13.6	**12.9**	67.6
All	51	65	65	**181**	1.4	100.0	61.7	76.4	78.2	72.2	**71.2**	92.3

Table 11. Childhood cancer, Algeria, 4 Registries

	NUMBER OF CASES					REL. FREQ.(%)	RATES PER MILLION					
	0-4	5-9	10-14	All	M/F	Overall	0-4	5-9	10-14	Crude	ASR	%MV
Leukaemia	49	69	53	171	1.7	21.0	18.6	25.3	19.0	21.0	20.9	98.3
Acute lymphoid leukaemia	35	47	29	111	1.8	13.6	13.3	17.2	10.4	13.6	13.7	99.1
Lymphoma	49	75	57	181	2.2	22.2	18.6	27.5	20.4	22.2	22.0	100.0
Hodgkin disease	9	29	20	58	2.1	7.1	3.4	10.6	7.2	7.1	6.8	100.0
Burkitt lymphoma	0	1	2	3	2.0	0.4	-	0.4	0.7	0.4	0.3	100.0
Brain and spinal neoplasms	13	28	24	65	2.1	8.0	4.9	10.3	8.6	8.0	7.7	83.1
Neuroblastoma	25	20	8	53	2.5	6.5	9.5	7.3	2.9	6.5	6.9	98.1
Retinoblastoma	29	10	1	40	1.2	4.9	11.0	3.7	0.4	4.9	5.5	100.0
Wilms tumour	35	20	8	63	0.7	7.7	13.3	7.3	2.9	7.7	8.3	96.8
Bone tumours	5	16	45	66	1.1	8.1	1.9	5.9	16.1	8.1	7.3	90.9
Soft tissue sarcomas	7	10	12	29	2.6	3.6	2.7	3.7	4.3	3.6	3.5	86.2
Kaposi sarcoma	0	0	0	0	-	-	-	-	-	-	-	-
Germ cell tumours	9	2	2	13	0.9	1.6	3.4	0.7	0.7	1.6	1.8	100.0
Other	34	37	63	134	1.2	16.4	12.9	13.6	22.6	16.4	15.9	81.3
All	255	287	273	815	1.5	100.0	96.7	105.2	97.7	99.9	99.7	93.7

3.1.2 Egypt

Background
Climate: Desert; hot dry summers with moderate winters.

Terrain: Vast desert plateau interrupted by Nile valley and delta.

Ethnic groups: Eastern Hamitic stock (Egyptians, Bedouins and Berbers) 99%, Greek, Nubian, Armenian, other European (primarily Italian and French) 1%.

Religions: Muslim (mostly Sunni) 94% (official estimate), Coptic Christian and other 6% (official estimate).

Economy—overview: At the end of the 1980s, Egypt faced problems of low productivity and a poor economy with excessive population growth, high inflation and urban overcrowding. Substantial progress has been made in improving macroeconomic performance, with moves towards a more decentralized, market-oriented economy. Foreign investment has been increasing but since 1997 there has been a sharp downturn in tourism.

Industries: Textiles, food processing, tourism, chemicals, petroleum, construction, cement, metals.

Agriculture—products: Cotton, rice, corn, wheat, beans, fruits, vegetables; cattle, water buffalo, sheep, goats. The annual fish catch is about 140 000 metric tons.

Cancer registration
Cancer Registry of Alexandria
Alexandria is the second largest governorate in Egypt, situated on the Mediterranean coast, with an estimated population of over three million. The Alexandria Regional Cancer Registry was initiated by the Alexandria Faculty of Medicine in 1960. In its early phase, it was a hospital registry covering only university hospitals. In 1963, the registry headquarters was transferred to the Department of Medical Statistics at the Medical Research Institute and the registry became a central hospital-based registry, covering 18 hospitals all over Alexandria (university, health insurance, medical organization, school health, and Ministry of Health hospitals).

Data are collected actively on standardized registration forms. Cases are ascertained from a variety of sources (medical and surgical departments, radiology, pathology and medical records). The data collected are revised and coded centrally. An index system is used to allow rapid manual retrieval of information and to avoid duplicate registration. Tumour diagnoses are classified according to the ninth revision of the ICD and to the ICD-O coding systems.

Cairo Metropolitan Cancer Registry
The cancer registry of the metropolitan Cairo area (CMCR) was started in 1973 and has published several reports. The registry was a multi-hospital register of patients with cancer attending nine hospitals belonging to the Universities of Cairo, Azhar and Ain Shams and six Ministry of Health hospitals in the metropolitan Cairo area. Hospitals in the private sector were not included, but these provided only a small percentage of hospital care for cancer at that time. Cases were also contributed from Assiut University hospital, located 350 km to the south of Cairo. Data on cancer cases were recorded on reporting forms from inpatient departments, outpatient clinics and pathology and haematology departments and sent to the central registry, which maintains an alphabetical index in order to avoid duplicate registrations. At the time, the estimated population

of the Greater Cairo Area was 8.6 million and that of Assiut Governorate 1.8 million.

Registry of the National Cancer Institute, Cairo
The Registry of the National Cancer Institute (NCI) in Cairo has recorded details of all patients hospitalized at the Institute since 1970. At least until 1988, registration was restricted to inpatients. A card system with different indices was in use at least until 1987 (Sherif & Ibrahim, 1987).

The NCI has a wide catchment area, covering the entire country. Although this might in theory allow a fairly good estimate of the relative frequencies of different types of cancer in Egypt, there is undoubtedly some selection of the type of patients referred and admitted to the Institute, related to the facilities and expertise available.

Pathology Registry of Cairo
This registry was established in 1969 at the National Cancer Institute. It has published frequencies for the five years 1985–89 (see below).

Population-based cancer registration
In 2000, a national Cancer Registry project was launched by the Ministry of Health and Population. A coordinating centre in Cairo was charged with the tasks of coordinating the work of eight regional cancer registries, located in Aswan, Damanhour, Elsalem, Menya, Tanta, Sohag, Domiatt and Nasser Institute Hospital (Cairo). Some of the registries had been established for some time, including the registries in Aswan (1988) and Tanta, Gharbia Governorate (1997). Detailed results are not so far available (2002).

Review of data
Alexandria cancer registry
Frequency data have been published for the period 1972–91, together with estimated incidence rates, based on the estimated average population at risk during this period (Table 1). Out of a total of 43 496 cases, 21 792 were men and 21 604 women. In men, bladder cancer occupies the first place (15.9%), followed by brain and central nervous system cancers (11%), non-Hodgkin lymphomas (10.8%) and lung (7.9%) and larynx (6.2%) cancers. Breast cancer is the commonest cancer in women (32.7%), followed by central nervous system cancers (7.2%), non-Hodgkin lymphomas (6.3%), cervix cancer (4.5%) and cancers of the colon and rectum (4.2%).

The estimated incidence rates must be considered approximations. They suggest a relatively high incidence of breast cancer in women (ASR 35.6 per 100 000), bladder cancer in men (ASR 19.2) and non-Hodgkin lymphoma in both sexes (ASR 10.1 in men and 6.4 in women). The rather high relative frequency of 'brain cancer' presumably represents mis-diagnosis or misrecording of metastatic cancers.

Cairo Metropolitan Cancer Registry
The data presented in Table 2 are for 1978 and 1979, from Aboul Nasr *et al.* (1986). The most striking feature is the very high frequency of bladder cancer, which comprises 28.8% of cancers in males and 11.7% of cancers in females. This elevated frequency has often been reported (Ibrahim & Elsebai, 1983) and is related to the prevalence of schistosomiasis in Egypt. The frequency in this series is somewhat higher than in the general population, since the National Cancer Institute (one of the hospitals reporting to the

Registry) has a particular interest and expertise in the management of this cancer; 31.8% of cases registered at the Institute in 1976–77 were bladder cancer (Ibrahim, 1982).

In females, breast cancer is the dominant tumour (23.3% of cases); it is considerably more common than cervical cancer (8.8%).

The relatively high frequencies of lymphomas in people of each sex are of note, and are partly related to the young age structure of the population.

Registry of the National Cancer Institute, Cairo
The results for 1970–85 (Sherif & Ibrahim, 1987) are shown in Table 2. The frequency of bladder cancers (40.6% of cancers in men, 14.3% in women) and of female breast cancer (33.9% of female cancers) are more extreme than those in the CMCR, presumably reflecting the special treatment services provided by this hospital.

Pathology Registry of Cairo
This has published frequencies for the five years 1985 to 1989, out of a total of 23 567 biopsies, 26.3% were cancer of the bladder, 12.2% lymphomas, 11.3% breast, 7.6% oral cavity and pharynx, 6.7% leukaemias and 3.5% cervix cancer.

Cancer mortality rates in Egypt
Soliman et al. (1999) have published cancer mortality rates, based on the mandatory and routinely available mortality records of Menofeia province in the Nile Delta region of Egypt (Table 3). They compared the results with data from the Surveillance Epidemiology, and End Results (SEER) mortality rates of the United States.

Bladder and liver cancers are the two most common causes of cancer mortality in Menofeia province. The high frequency and age-adjusted mortality rates of bladder and liver cancer revealed by this study may be explained by the fact that Menofeia is a rural region exposed to schistosomal infections.

Childhood cancer
Data on childhood cancer from the Alexandria cancer registry (Bedwani, 1992; Bedwani et al., 1998) and from the register of tumour pathology in the National Cancer Institute (Mokhtar, 1991) are summarized in Table 4.

References

Aboul Nasr, A.L., Boutros, S.G. & Husein, M.H. (1986) Cairo Metropolitan cancer registry, 1978–1979. In: Parkin, D.M., ed., *Cancer Occurrence in Developing Countries* (IARC Scientific Publications No. 75), Lyon, IARC

Bedwani, R. (1992) *Alexandria Cancer Registry 1972-1991.* Alexandria, Medical Statistic and Clinical Epidemiology Unit, Alexandria University Medical Research Institute

Bedwani, R.N., Zaki A., Abuseif, H.H., Khewesky, F.S., El-Shazly, M., Abdel-Fattah, M. & Bassili, A. (1998) Egypt: Alexandria Regional Cancer Registry, 1980–1989. In: Parkin, D.M., Kramárová, E., Draper, G.J., Masuyer, E., Michaelis, J., Neglia, J, Qureshi, S. & Stiller, C.A., eds, *International Incidence of Childhood Cancer,* vol. II (IARC Scientific Publications No. 144), Lyon, IARC, pp. 27–29

Ibrahim, A.S. (1982) *The Registry of the Cairo Cancer Institute 1970-77.* In: Aoki, K., Tominaga, S., Hirayama, T. & Hirota, Y., eds, *Cancer Prevention in Developing Countries*, Nagoya, University of Nagoya Press, pp. 173–182

Ibrahim, A.S. & Elsebai, I. (1983) *Epidemiology of Bladder Cancer.* In: Elsebai, I., ed., *Bladder Cancer, Vol. I*, Boca Raton, FL, CRC Press, pp. 17–38

Mokhtar, N. (1991) *Cancer Pathology Registry 1985-1989.* Cairo, Department of Pathology, National Cancer Institute, Cairo University

Sherif, M. & Ibrahim, A.S. (1987) NCI, Cairo, 1970-1985. In: *The Profile of Cancer in Egypt*, Cairo, National Cancer Institute

Soliman, A.S., Bondy, M.L., Raouf, A.A., Makram, M.A., Jonston, D.A. & Levin, B. (1999) Cancer mortality in Menofeia, Egypt: comparison with US mortality rates. *Cancer Causes Control,* **10**, 349–354

Table 1. Alexandria Cancer Registry: 1972–91

Site		Male				Female			
		Total	%	Crude rate	ASR (world)	Total	%	Crude rate	ASR (world)
Mouth	C00–08	669	3.1%	2.6	3.2	333	1.5%	1.4	2
Nasopharynx	C11	328	1.5%	1.3	1.5	163	0.8%	0.7	0.6
Other pharynx	C09–10,C12–14	719	3.3%	2.8	2.1	309	1.4%	1.3	0.8
Oesophagus	C15	729	3.3%	2.8	2.9	1062	4.9%	4.3	1.1
Stomach	C16	399	1.8%	1.5	2.0	346	1.6%	1.4	1.5
Colon/rectum	C18–21	937	4.3%	3.6	4.4	914	4.2%	3.7	1.9
Liver	C22	60	0.3%	0.2	0.6	568	2.6%	2.3	1.8
Pancreas	C25	299	1.4%	1.2	2.0	180	0.8%	0.7	0.5
Larynx	C32	1346	6.2%	5.2	7.4	146	0.7%	0.6	0.9
Lung	C33–34	1726	7.9%	6.6	9.5	368	1.7%	1.5	1.8
Melanoma of skin	C43	0	0.0%			0	0.0%		
Other skin	C44	1420	6.5%	5.5	6.9	568	2.6%	2.3	2.9
Kaposi sarcoma	C46	0	0.0%			0	0.0%		
Breast	C50					7068	32.7%	27.9	35.6
Cervix	C53					970	4.5%	3.9	5.5
Corpus	C54					625	2.9%	2.5	3.8
Ovary etc.	C56–57					526	2.4%	2.1	2.4
Prostate	C61	442	2.0%	1.7	2.6				
Testis	C62	115	0.5%	0.4	0.6				
Bladder	C67	3466	15.9%	13.3	19.2	675	3.1%	2.7	3.6
Kidney etc.	C64–66	263	1.2%	1.0	1.1	230	1.1%	0.9	1.0
Brain	C71–72	2398	11.0%	9.2	10.2	1561	7.2%	6.3	6.1
Thyroid	C73	294	1.4%	1.1	1.4	568	2.6%	2.3	2.9
Non-Hodgkin lymphoma	C82–85,C96	2349	10.8%	9.0	10.1	1369	6.3%	5.5	6.4
Hodgkin disease	C81	656	3.0%	2.5	2.6	378	1.7%	1.5	1.5
Myeloma	C90	198	0.9%	0.8	1.0	131	0.6%	0.5	0.7
Leukaemia	C91–95	1065	4.9%	4.1	4.0	776	3.6%	3.1	3.4
Other sites	Other	1591	7.3%	6.1	6.8	1517	7.0%	6.1	7.0
All sites	ALL	21792	100.0%	82.4	102.0	21604	100.0%	85.6	95.6

Source: Alexandria Cancer Registry 1972–1991. Alexandria University Medical Research Institute, The Medical Statistics and Clinical Epidemiology Unit, 1992

Table 2. Egypt: frequency data

Site	Cairo Metropolitan Cancer Registry 1978–79 (Aboul Nasr et al., 1986)					National Cancer Institute (NCI), 1970–85 (Sherif & Ibrahim, 1987)				
	Male		Female		%HV	Male		Female		%HV
	No.	%	No.	%		No.	%	No.	%	
Oral cavity[1]	194	4.6%	95	3.5%		815	4.2%	565	4.5%	
Nasopharynx	49	1.2%	16	0.6%		136	0.7%	67	0.5%	
Other pharynx	142	3.3%	53	1.9%		548	2.8%	376	3.0%	
Oesophagus	68	1.6%	16	0.6%		710	3.6%	211	1.7%	
Stomach	42	1.0%	27	1.0%		252	1.3%	87	0.7%	
Colon/rectum	199	4.7%	108	4.0%		783	4.0%	243	1.9%	
Liver	104	2.4%	47	1.7%		33	0.2%	13	0.1%	
Pancreas	10	0.2%	11	0.4%		113	0.6%	33	0.3%	
Lung	121	2.8%	18	0.7%		440	2.2%	74	0.6%	
Melanoma	234	5.5%	241	8.8%		1002	5.1%	529	4.2%	
Other skin										
Kaposi sarcoma										
Breast	52	1.2%	635	23.3%		228	1.2%	4305	33.9%	
Cervix uteri			241	8.8%				579	4.6%	
Corpus uteri			40	1.5%				267	2.1%	
Ovary etc.			94	3.4%				357	2.8%	
Prostate						103	0.5%		0.0%	
Penis						28	0.1%		0.0%	
Bladder	1225	28.8%	319	11.7%		7953	40.6%	1820	14.3%	
Kidney etc.	31	0.7%	14	0.5%						
Eye	72	1.7%	40	1.5%		122	0.6%	71	0.6%	
Brain, nervous system	78	1.8%	45	1.6%		28	0.1%	13	0.1%	
Thyroid	47	1.1%	65	2.4%		183	0.9%	320	2.5%	
Non-Hodgkin lymphoma	224	5.3%	106	3.9%		1024	5.2%	446	3.5%	
Hodgkin disease	142	3.3%	62	2.3%		861	4.4%	244	1.9%	
Myeloma	15	0.4%	8	0.3%		37	0.2%	29	0.2%	
Leukaemia	157	3.7%	105	3.8%		931	4.7%	363	2.9%	
ALL SITES	4252	100.0%	2729	100.0%		19610	100.0%	12695	100.0%	

[1] Includes salivary gland tumours

Table 3. Menofeia, Egypt: age-adjusted mortality rates (per 100 000) (1992–96) (Soliman et al., 1999)

Site (ICD)	Total	Male	Female
Urinary bladder	9.5	15.6	3.9
Liver	8.4	10.5	4.4
Leukaemia	4.0	5.0	3.5
Breast	4.8	0.4	8.9
Colorectum	3.5	4.4	2.7
Lung	3.3	5.4	0.9
Brain	1.8	2.2	1.5
Stomach	1.8	2.2	1.5
Non-Hodgkin lymphoma	1.2	1.6	0.9

Table 4. Egypt: Childhood cancer

Cancer	Cancer Pathology Register National Cancer Institute 1985–89 (Mokhtar, 1991)[a]		Alexandria Cancer Registry 1972–1991 (Bedwani, 1992)		1980–89 (Bedwani *et al.*, 1998)	
	No.	%	No.	%	No.	%
Leukaemia	409	25.9%	1023	24.5%	259	19.7%
Acute lymphocytic leukaemia					81	6.2%
Lymphoma	512	32.5%	1102	26.4%	400	30.4%
Burkitt lymphoma					1	0.1%
Hodgkin disease					126	9.6%
Brain and spinal neoplasms	10	0.6%	1064	25.4%	244	18.6%
Neuroblastoma			142	3.4%	66	5.0%
Retinoblastoma			43	1.0%	8	0.6%
Wilms tumour	44	2.8%	335	8.0%	50	3.8%
Bone tumour	124	7.9%	335	8.0%	83	6.3%
Soft-tissue sarcomas	151	9.6%	66	1.6%	62	4.7%
Kaposi sarcoma					0	0.0%
Other	327	20.7%	71		143	10.9%
Total	1577	100.0%	4181	100.0%	1315	100.0%

[a] Cases aged <20 years

3.1.3 Libya

Background

Climate: Mediterranean along coast; dry, extreme desert interior.

Terrain: mostly barren, flat to undulating plains, plateaux, depressions.

Ethnic groups: Berber and Arab 97%; remainder Greek, Maltese, Italian, Egyptian, Pakistani, Turkish, Indian and Tunisian.

Religions: Sunni Muslim 97%.

Economy—overview: The economy depends primarily upon revenues from the oil sector, which contributes practically all export earnings and about one-third of GDP. The non-oil manufacturing and construction sectors, which account for about 20% of GDP, have expanded from processing mostly agricultural products to include production of petrochemicals, iron, steel, and aluminium. Although agriculture accounts for only 5% of GDP, it employs 18% of the labour force. Climatic conditions and poor soils severely limit farm output and Libya imports about 75% of its food requirements.

Industries: petroleum, food processing, textiles, handicrafts, cement.

Agriculture—products: wheat, barley, olives, dates, citrus, vegetables, peanuts; meat, eggs.

Cancer registration

There has been no cancer registration in Libya.

Review of data

A study on 1124 histologically-diagnosed cases (664 males and 460 females), seen at the oncology clinic of the central Hospital, Tripoli, from 1981 to 1985 was reported by Akhtar *et al.* (1993). In males, lung cancer was the most common cancer (22.4%), followed by non-Hodgkin lymphoma (10.4%), Hodgkin disease (9.0%), larynx caner (4.7%) and stomach cancer (4.7%). In females, breast cancer was in the first position (29.8%), followed by ovary (7.8%), non-Hodgkin lymphoma (7.6%) and Hodgkin disease (3.7%).

Reference

Akhtar, S.S., Abu Bakr, M.A., Dawi, S.A. & Huq, I.U. (1993) Cancer in Libya – a retrospective study 1981-1985. *Afr. J. Med.Sci.,* **22**, 17–24

3.1.4 Morocco

Background

Climate: Mediterranean, becoming more extreme in the interior

Terrain: Northern coast and interior are mountainous with large areas of bordering plateaux, intermontane valleys, and rich coastal plains

Ethnic groups: Arab-Berber 99.1%, other 0.7%, Jewish 0.2%

Religions: Muslim 98.7%, Christian 1.1%, Jewish 0.2%

Economy—overview: Morocco is essentially an agricultural country, although only 19% of the total land is cultivated

Industries: Phosphate rock mining and processing, food processing, leather goods, textiles, construction, tourism

Agriculture—products: Barley, wheat, citrus, wine, vegetables, olives; livestock

Cancer registration

A hospital-based registry was set up in the newly founded National Institute of Oncology in 1986. This registry expanded its activities to cover the province of Rabat-Salé in October 1990.

Review of data

Data from the hospital registry of the National Institute of Oncology (Table 1) were published for 1986 to 1987 on the basis of 5148 cases (Chaoki & Gueddari, 1991). In women, cervix cancer accounts for 35% of all cancers, followed by breast cancer (22.3%). In men, cancer of the nasopharynx came first at 12.3%, followed by lymphomas 10.1%, larynx 8.2%, and lung cancers 6.5%.

Childhood cancer

Table 2 shows details of a series of 444 cases of childhood cancer admitted to the Hospital for Children in Rabat over a three-year period, 1983–85 (Msefer Alaoui, 1988). It excludes children requiring neurosurgery, who were not treated in this hospital. The most commonly recorded childhood cancers were lymphomas (32.6% of the total), of which about 20% were Burkitt lymphoma, leukaemias (22.7% of cases) and Wilms tumour (10%).

References

Chaouki, N. & El Gueddari, B. (1991) Epidemiological descriptive approach of cancer in Morocco through the activity of the National Institute of Oncology 1986-1987. *Bull. Cancer (Paris)*, **78**, 603–609

Msefer Alaoui, F. (1988) Rabat: Hospital for Children, 1983–1985. In: Parkin, D.M., Stiller, C.A., Draper, G.J., Bieber, C.A., Terracini, B. & Young, J.L., eds, *International Incidence of Childhood Cancer* (IARC Scientific Publications No. 87), Lyon, IARC, pp. 33–35

Table 1. Morocco: case series

| Site | National Oncology Institute,1986–87 (Chaouki & Gueddari, 1991) | | | | %HV |
| | Male | | Female | | |
	No.	%	No.	%	
Oral cavity[1]	73	4.5%	25	1.2%	
Nasopharynx	200	12.3%	107	5.3%	
Other pharynx					
Oesophagus	37	2.3%	22	1.1%	
Stomach	25	1.5%	8	0.4%	
Colon/rectum					
Liver					
Pancreas					
Lung	106	6.5%		0.0%	
Melanoma					
Other skin	82	5.1%		0.0%	
Kaposi sarcoma					
Breast	21	1.3%	453	22.3%	
Cervix uteri			710	34.9%	
Corpus uteri			47	2.3%	
Ovary etc.			60	2.9%	
Prostate	39	2.4%			
Penis		0.0%			
Bladder	25	1.5%	5	0.2%	
Kidney etc.					
Eye					
Brain, nervous system	67	4.1%		0.0%	
Thyroid					
Non-Hodgkin lymphoma	103	6.4%	56	2.8%	
Hodgkin's disease	61	3.8%	23	1.1%	
Myeloma					
Leukaemia					
ALL SITES	1620	100.0%	2034	100.0%	

[1]Lip and tongue

Table 2. Morocco: childhood case series

| Cancer | Rabat, Hospital for Children, 1983–85 (Msefer Alaoui, 1988) | |
	No.	%
Leukaemia	101	22.7%
Acute lymphocytic leukaemia	75	16.9%
Lymphoma	145	32.7%
Burkitt lymphoma	30	6.8%
Hodgkin disease	49	11.0%
Brain and spinal neoplasms	15	3.4%
Neuroblastoma	39	8.8%
Retinoblastoma	21	4.7%
Wilms tumour	44	9.9%
Bone tumours	16	3.6%
Soft-tissue sarcomas	20	4.5%
Kaposi sarcoma	0	0.0%
Other	43	9.7%
Total	444	100.0%

3.1.5 Sudan

Background

Climate: Tropical in south; arid desert in north; rainy season (April to October)

Terrain: Generally flat, featureless plain; mountains in east and west

Ethnic groups: Black 52%, Arab 39%, Beja 6%, foreigners 2%, other 1%

Religions: Sunni Muslim 70% (in north), indigenous beliefs 25%, Christian 5% (mostly in south and Khartoum)

Economy—overview: Sudan is very poor. The income per inhabitant is $250 a year and inflation is high. The private sector's main areas of activity are agriculture and trading, with most private industrial investment predating 1980. Agriculture employs 80% of the work force. Industry mainly processes agricultural items. There are potentially lucrative oilfields in south-central Sudan

Industries: Cotton ginning, textiles, cement, edible oils, sugar, soap distilling, shoes, petroleum refining

Agriculture—products: Cotton, groundnuts, sorghum, millet, wheat, gum arabic, sesame; sheep

Cancer registration

There has been no population-based cancer registry in Sudan. Registration activity has been confined to a hospital-based registry, based on records of patients attending the only oncological hospital, the Radiation and Isotope Centre, Khartoum (the only facility offering specialized treatment for cancer in the country), and the Sudan Cancer Registry, based on histopathologically confirmed cases dianosed in the National Health Laboratories in Khartoum.

Review of data

Early reports presented data on histopathologically confirmed cases. Hickey (1959) described 1335 malignant epithelial neoplasms collected from the Stack Medical Research Laboratories during the period 1935–54. Lynch *et al.* (1963) published a report on 2234 malignant tumours collected from the same source and from the Department of Pathology, University of Khartoum, for the period 1954–61. This series was reproduced by Daoud *et al.* (1968) and compared with 1578 malignant tumours from Khartoum district examined at the Department of Pathology in 1957–65.

Data from the pathology-based Sudan Cancer Registry for 1978 were published by Mukhtar (1986) (Table 1). Breast cancer was the dominant tumour (26% of tumours in females). Other cancers of particular interest in this series were nasopharyngeal cancer, the relative importance of which, especially in males, was described previously (Hidayatalla *et al.*, 1983), eye tumours, which are mainly epithelial tumours of the conjunctiva (Malik *et al.*, 1974), and oral cancer.

Hidayatalla and Rahman (1986) published a series of 10 410 cases seen in the Radiation and Isotope Centre for the years 1967–84 (Table 1). The distribution of cases is on the whole similar to that at the Sudan Cancer Registry, with some bias towards the more radiosensitive tumours (of the breast and nasopharynx) and against surgically treated and radioresistant cancers (of the skin and digestive tract). The commonest cancers in males are those of the nasopharynx, which is most frequent among the southern and Sudanic tribes (Hidayatalla *et al.*, 1983), non-Hodgkin lymphoma

(Malik *et al.*, 1974), cancer of the mouth, especially the gingiva (Lynch *et al.*, 1963), and of the bladder. Kaposi sarcoma, which comprises 1.2% of tumours in males, is commoner in patients from the four provinces in the south and west, as noted previously by Wasfi *et al.* (1967); in that area, it comprises 7.2% of cancers in males. In females, the commonest cancers are of the breast (Hidayatalla, 1969), cervix, ovary and mouth.

Childhood cancer

A series of 775 childhood cancer cases from the Registry of the Radiation and Isotope Centre, Khartoum, in the period 1967–84 was published by Hidayatalla (1988). The series was divided into two broad ethnic groupings—Arabs (including Arabs, Mowalad, Nubians and Bejas) and Sudanics (including Nilotic and Sudanic tribes, and Beggara). However, it was emphasized that there is no clear demarcation between the two; there is, in fact, considerable sharing of characteristics between them.

Table 2 shows the results. For the two groups taken together, and for the Arab subgroup, the commonest diagnostic category was the lymphomas, with 23% of all cases. For Hodgkin disease, the relative frequencies were similar for Arabs and Sudanics, while Burkitt lymphoma had a higher relative frequency among Sudanics. Leukaemia was uncommon in both groups, but particularly in the Sudanics. An exceptionally high proportion (29%) of all leukaemias were classified as chronic myeloid. The next largest category is retinoblastoma (15% of the total); however, among the Sudanic subgroup this tumour accounted for 23% of all cases and was more common than the lymphomas. The proportion of brain tumours, neuroblastoma and Ewing sarcoma was low in both ethnic groups.

Although not shown in the table, nasopharyngeal cancers were common in both groups: 8.2% of cancers in Arab children and 14.8% in the Sudanic

A previous report (Abdel Rahman & Hidayatalla, 1969) described the 63 childhood cancer cases seen at the Centre in its first two years.

References

Abdel Rahman, S. & Hidayatalla. A. (1969) The pattern of malignant disease in children seen at the Radiation and Isotope Centre, Khartoum. *Sudan Med. J.*, **7**, 7–12

Daoud, E.H., Hassan, A.M., Zak, F. & Zakova, N. (1968) *Aspects of Malignant Disease in the Sudan.* In: Clifford, P., Linsell, C.A. & Timms, G.L., eds, *Cancer in Africa*, Nairobi, East African Publishing House, pp. 43–50

Hickey, B.B. (1959) Malignant epithelial tumours in the Sudanese. *Ann. R. Coll. Surg.*, **24**, 303–322

Hidayatalla, A. (1969) Carcinoma of the breast in Sudan. I. Epidemiological survey. *Sudan Med. J.*, **1**, 43–49

Hidayatalla, A. (1988) Registry of the Radiation and Isotope Centre, Khartoum, 1967–1984. In: Parkin, D.M., Stiller, C.A., Draper, G.J., Bieber, C.A., Terracini, B. & Young, J.L., eds, *International Incidence of Childhood Cancer* (IARC Scientific Publications No. 87), Lyon, IARC, pp. 43–47

Hidayatalla, A., Malik, M.O.A., El Hadai, A.E., Osman, A.A. & Hutt, M.S.R. (1983) Studies on nasopharyngeal carcinoma in the Sudan — I. Epidemiology and aetiology. *Eur. J. Cancer*, **6**, 705–710

Hidayatalla, A. & Rahman, E.A. (1986) The Radiation and Isotope Centre, Khartoum, 1967-1984. In: Parkin, D.M., ed., *Cancer Occurrence in Developing Countries* (IARC Scientific Publications No. 75), Lyon, IARC, pp. 82–87

Lynch, J.B., Hassan, A.M. & Omar, A. (1963) Cancer in the Sudan. *Sudan Med. J.*, **2**, 29–37

Malik, M.O.A., Hidayatalla, A., Daoud, E.H. & El Hassan, H.M. (1974) Superficial cancer in the Sudan. A study of 1,225 primary malignant superficial tumours. *Br. J. Cancer*, **30**, 355–364

Mukhtar, B.I. (1986) The Sudan Cancer registry, 1978. In: Parkin, D.M., ed., *Cancer Occurrence in Developing Countries* (IARC Scientific Publications No. 75), Lyon, IARC, pp. 81–85

Wasfi, A., El Hassan, A. & Zak, F. (1967) Kaposi's sarcoma in the Sudan. *Sudan Med. J.*, **5**, 213–222

Table 1. Sudan: case series

Site	Sudan Cancer Registry, 1978 (Mukhtar, 1986)				%HV	Radiation and Isotope Centre, Khartoum, 1967–84 (Hidayatalla & Rahman, 1986)				%HV
	Male		Female			Male		Female		
	No.	%	No.	%		No.	%	No.	%	
Oral cavity[1]	33	6.7%	22	4.0%	100	471	10.0%	350	6.2%	
Nasopharynx	22	4.5%	8	1.5%	100	560	11.9%	166	2.9%	
Other pharynx	7	1.4%	1	0.2%	100	102	2.2%	83	1.5%	
Oesophagus	16	3.3%	21	3.8%	100	159	3.4%	188	3.3%	
Stomach	13	2.7%	8	1.5%	100	26	0.6%	18	0.3%	
Colon/rectum	22	4.5%	19	3.5%	100	154	3.3%	69	1.2%	
Liver	25	5.1%	14	2.6%	100	43	0.9%	19	0.3%	
Pancreas						6	0.1%	7	0.1%	
Lung	4	0.8%	4	0.7%	100	89	1.9%	26	0.5%	
Melanoma	14	2.9%	10	1.8%	100	39	0.8%	16	0.3%	
Other skin	53	10.8%	30	5.5%	100	311	6.6%			
Kaposi sarcoma						59	1.2%	3	0.1%	
Breast	7	1.4%	142	26.0%	100	122	2.6%	1962	34.5%	
Cervix uteri			82	15.0%	100			812	14.3%	
Corpus uteri			21	3.8%	100			144	2.5%	
Ovary etc			38	6.9%	100			206	3.6%	
Prostate	19	3.9%			100	40	0.8%			
Penis										
Bladder	20	4.1%	4	0.7%	100	224	4.7%	68	1.2%	
Kidney etc.	7	1.4%	7	1.3%	100	101	2.1%	78	1.4%	
Eye	27	5.5%	6	1.1%	100	156	3.3%	110	1.9%	
Brain, nervous system	2	0.4%	1	0.2%	100	99	2.1%	79	1.4%	
Thyroid	6	1.2%	10	1.8%	100	73	1.5%	136	2.4%	
Non-Hodgkin lymphoma	36	7.4%	16	2.9%	100	472	10.0%	180	3.2%	
Hodgkin disease	16	3.3%	3	0.5%	100	215	4.6%	89	1.6%	
Myeloma										
Leukaemia	22	4.5%	10	1.8%	100	246	5.2%	189	3.3%	
ALL SITES	489	100.0%	547	100.0%	100	4721	100.0%	5689	100.0%	

[1] Includes salivary gland tumours

Table 2. Sudan: childhood cancer

Cancer	Radiation and Isotope Centre, Khartoum, 1967–84 (Hidayatalla, 1988)			
	Arab		Sudanic	
	No.	%	No.	%
Leukaemia	63	11.3%	10	4.6%
Acute lymphocytic leukaemia	37	6.6%	4	1.8%
Lymphoma	129	23.1%	46	21.2%
Burkitt lymphoma	16	2.9%	15	6.9%
Hodgkin disease	52	9.3%	19	8.8%
Brain and spinal neoplasms	25	4.5%	5	2.3%
Neuroblastoma	12	2.2%	4	1.8%
Retinoblastoma	72	12.9%	49	22.6%
Wilms tumour	47	8.4%	15	6.9%
Bone tumours	40	7.1%	9	4.1%
Soft-tissue sarcomas	46	8.2%	15	6.9%
Kaposi sarcoma	1	0.2%	1	0.5%
Other	124	22.2%	64	29.5%
Total	558	100.0%	217	100.0%

3.1.6 Tunisia

Background

Climate: Mediterranean climate, with temperatures averaging 10.6°C in January and 26.1°C in July. Mild rainy winters in the north. Going south, the climate becomes progressively hotter and dryer.

Terrain: The low Atlas mountain range crosses the north of the country from south-west to north-east, with valleys and fertile plains between the mountains. To the south, a plateau descends progressively to a succession of salty depressions known as 'sebkhas' on the border of the Sahara desert, which constitutes nearly 40% of the Tunisian land surface.

Ethnic groups: Arab 98%, European 1%, Jewish and other 1%

Religions: Muslim 98%, Christian 1%, Jewish and other 1%

Economy—overview: The economy is diverse, with important agricultural, mining, energy, tourism and manufacturing sectors. Government control of economic affairs has gradually lessened over the past decade with increasing privatization of trade and commerce. Both tourism and trade have markedly increased in recent years.

Industries: Tunisia possesses many large oil deposits, concentrated in the south, that easily cover the needs of the country. The reserves of phosphate in the south-west are the greatest in the world. Other mineral resources are iron, lead and zinc.

Agriculture—products: Olives, dates, oranges, almonds, grain, sugar beet, grapes, poultry, beef, dairy products

Cancer registration

Until fairly recently, the only information available on cancer patterns in Tunisia was derived from the hospital registry of the Institut Salah Azaiz, the main cancer treatment centre in the country. However, there are now three regional population-based cancer registries, covering the entire national population. These are, in the northern region, the Cancer Registry of Tunis, in the centre, the Cancer Registry of Sousse, and in the south, the Cancer Registry of Sfax.

Cancer Registry of Tunis

The registry was established in 1997 and covers the populations of the 10 governorates of the northern region of the country (4.3 million inhabitants in 1994). It is located in the Institut Salah Azaiz in Tunis, the only specialized public cancer hospital in the country. The registry depends upon active case-finding by physicians attached temporarily to the registry, during their training in public health. The hospital cancer registry of Institut Salah Azaiz is an important source of cancer cases (40% of registrations), but there are many other public and private hospitals in Tunis (including fifteen teaching hospitals, and two private radiotherapy centres), and nine regional hospitals in the governorates. Private practice in surgery and medical oncology is common. Information on cancers diagnosed in 15 pathology laboratories is an important source of information, but can be used only if the hospital admission can be traced, as the demographic data available, notably the address, are otherwise too sparse. Death certification is unreliable and incomplete, and this source is not used for case-finding. For 1994 (see below), there were an average of 1.3 sources per case registered, with 87% of cases having a single source of information.

Cancer Registry of Sousse

The registry was established in 1987 with the support of the Ministry of Health, and is located in the pathology laboratory of the University Hospital Farhat Hached, the principal hospital of the city of Sousse. The registry aims to cover the population of the central region of Tunisia, comprising six governorates, with a population estimated (mid-1996) at 2.5 million. Initially, however, the registry has restricted registration to the governorate of Sousse, with a population of 455 000 (mid-1996).

Information is collected on cancer cases diagnosed in the pathology department and in the services of haematology, medical oncology and radiotherapy of Farhat Hached hospital, as well as from private pathology laboratories, and other hospitals. Registration is largely limited to cases with a diagnosis based upon histology or cytology.

Cancer Registry of Sfax

The registry was established in 1997, and covers the wilaya (district) of Sfax (population 771 000 in 1997), in the southern region of the country. It is located in the pathology department of the Habib Bourgiba University Hospital. The registry depends on active case-finding by physicians (two public health specialists, two part-time) in hospitals (including two university hospitals and two regional hospitals, as well as smaller local hospitals), laboratories (one public, one private) and departments of haematology and radiotherapy (one public service, one private), plus private practitioners. Death certificates are not used as a source of information.

Review of data

Cancer Registry of Tunis

Data from the first year of registration (1994) are presented (Table 1). There were 2085 cases in males (ASR 122 per 100 000) and 1601 cases in females (ASR 94.7 per 100 000). The principal cancers in men are cancers of lung (ASR 26.6) and bladder (12.3). In women, breast is the leading cancer site (24.1). The incidence of nasopharyngeal cancer appears to be rather lower than in northern Algeria.

There is a relatively high proportion of cases with morphological verification of diagnosis (89% in men, 92% in women).

Cancer Registry of Sousse

2039 cases were registered in the period 1993–97 among the residents of Sousse (Table 2). Almost all cases were morphologically verified (the registry is essentially pathology-based). The age-standardized incidence rates are 138.7 per 100 000 in men and 91.4 per 100 000 in women. The principal cancers in men are lung (ASR 30.6), bladder (ASR 17.4), skin (ASR 12.4), prostate (ASR 9.3) and non-Hodgkin lymphoma (ASR 8.2). The principal cancers among women were breast (ASR 22.7), non-melanoma skin cancers (ASR 8.9) and cervix cancer (ASR 7.9); this latter rate is a little higher than in the other Tunisian data.

The registry has published its results in reports for an earlier period (1987–93) as well as for 1993–97.

Cancer Registry of Sfax

Data for 1997 are presented (Table 3). The recorded incidence (ASR 140.5 per 100 000 in men, 99.1 per 100 000 in women) is rather higher than in the northern region, in part due to the relatively large numbers of skin cancers recorded (13.4% of the total cases). The majority of cases (96%) have a morphological validation of diagnosis, suggesting that the pathology department where the registry is located is the major source of cases. The principal sites in men are cancers of the lung (ASR 24.2), bladder (ASR 14.9) and prostate (ASR 12.4), and in women, cancer of the breast (ASR 22.7).

Other data

Before the establishment of cancer registration in Tunisia, information on the cancer profile was obtainable from published case series. For example, Chadli *et al.* (1976) reported on 7959 cancers diagnosed histologically in 1960–69 in the Institut Pasteur laboratory in Tunis; at that time, this was the only histopathology laboratory in the country (Table 4). The data from the hospital cancer registry of the National Cancer Institute (Institut Salah Azaiz) have also been published (Mourali, 1986; Ben Abdallah, 1997). Table 4 shows the results for the 17-year period 1969–85 (Ben Abdallah, 1997). There are some similarities between them. Breast cancer (especially in the hospital series) and cervix cancer are the dominant malignancies, and there are raised frequencies of skin cancers, respiratory cancer in men (in the hospital series), and nasopharyngeal cancer and non-Hodgkin lymphoma.

Childhood cancer

Table 5 shows the distribution by type of 1637 childhood cancers recorded in the hospital cancer registry of the Institut Salah Azaiz in the 17-year period 1969–85 (Ben Abdallah, 1997). Lymphomas were the most common cancers (28.2%) with 12% leukaemias (mainly acute lymphocytic).

The population-based data are in Table 6. They represent a pooled data-set from the three registries, with 112 cases contributed from the Northern Region (Tunis) for 1994, 68 from Sousse (Centre) for 1993–97 and 28 cases from Sfax in 1997. Leukaemias are the most common childhood cancers (ASR 27.8 per million), of which the majority (72%) are acute lymphocytic. Lymphomas comprise 17% of childhood cancers, with an ASR of 14.7 per million. Few cases of Burkitt lymphoma are recorded, although this may be due to differences in diagnostic practice: in Tunis, five cases were recorded among the 16 childhood non-Hodgkin lymphomas, in Sousse none among 4 non-Hodgkin lymphomas. Among the 'other' category were seven cancers of the nasopharynx and six skin cancers.

References

Ben Abdallah, M. (1997) *Cancer in Tunisia*, Tunis, Institut Salah Azaiz

Chadli,A., Rethers, L., Landreat, A. & Habanec, B. (1976) La physiognomie du cancer en Tunisie. Etude de 7959 cancers primitifs. *Arch. Inst. Pasteur Tunis*, **4,** 317–423

Mourali, N. (1986) Institut Salah-Azaiz, Tunis, 1976–1980. In: Parkin, D.M., ed., *Cancer Occurrence in Developing Countries* (IARC Scientific Publications No. 75), Lyon, IARC, pp. 93–96

Table 1. Tunisia, North, Tunis (1994)

NUMBER OF CASES BY AGE GROUP AND SUMMARY RATES OF INCIDENCE - MALE

SITE	ALL AGES	AGE UNK	MV (%)	0-	15-	25-	35-	45-	55-	65+	CRUDE RATE	%	CR 64	ASR (W)	ICD (10th)
Mouth	48	0	98	-	-	3	3	6	22	14	2.2	2.5	0.23	2.8	C00-06
Salivary gland	3	0	100	-	-	-	-	-	1	2	0.1	0.2	0.01	0.2	C07-08
Nasopharynx	67	0	99	1	2	8	13	7	28	8	3.1	3.4	0.34	3.7	C11
Other pharynx	16	0	88	-	1	-	3	3	7	2	0.7	0.8	0.09	0.9	C09-10,C12-14
Oesophagus	19	1	89	-	-	-	-	2	9	7	0.9	1.0	0.09	1.2	C15
Stomach	102	2	91	-	-	2	13	13	29	43	4.7	5.2	0.37	6.1	C16
Colon, rectum and anus	109	4	94	-	1	6	20	13	29	36	5.0	5.6	0.41	6.2	C18-21
Liver	49	0	65	3	1	1	3	8	7	26	2.3	2.5	0.13	2.9	C22
Gallbladder etc.	29	0	59	-	-	-	2	4	10	17	1.3	1.5	0.08	1.7	C23-24
Pancreas	39	1	33	-	-	-	-	4	8	26	1.8	2.0	0.09	2.4	C25
Larynx	103	7	99	-	1	-	6	18	31	48	4.8	5.3	0.38	6.3	C32
Trachea, bronchus and lung	437	7	86	-	1	2	26	65	160	176	20.2	22.4	1.78	26.6	C33-34
Bone	15	0	93	3	8	-	1	-	2	1	0.7	0.8	0.04	0.7	C40-41
Melanoma of skin	8	0	100	-	1	-	-	1	2	4	0.4	0.4	0.02	0.5	C43
Other skin	138	1	100	1	3	4	13	19	32	65	6.4		0.44	8.1	C44
Mesothelioma	4	1	100	-	-	-	1	1	-	2	0.2	0.2	0.01	0.2	C45
Kaposi sarcoma	2	0	100	-	-	-	-	-	-	2	0.1	0.1	0.00	0.1	C46
Peripheral nerves	1	0	100	-	-	-	-	1	-	-	0.0	0.1	0.01	0.1	C47
Connective and soft tissue	30	0	100	1	2	6	3	2	8	8	1.4	1.5	0.11	1.6	C49
Breast	6	0	100	-	-	1	-	1	-	3	0.3	0.3	0.02	0.3	C50
Penis	1	0	100	-	-	-	1	-	1	-	0.0	0.1	0.01	0.1	C60
Prostate	132	4	89	-	-	-	-	2	20	105	6.1	6.8	0.18	7.9	C61
Testis	12	0	92	-	1	4	2	3	-	2	0.6	0.6	0.04	0.6	C62
Kidney	24	0	92	3	1	1	4	2	6	7	1.1	1.2	0.09	1.4	C64
Renal pelvis, ureter and other urinary	5	0	100	-	-	2	-	1	2	2	0.2	0.3	0.02	0.3	C65-66,C68
Bladder	204	2	99	1	-	2	8	15	65	111	9.4	10.5	0.64	12.3	C67
Eye	9	0	78	2	-	4	-	1	2	3	0.4	0.5	0.03	0.5	C69
Brain, nervous system	48	1	88	9	6	3	3	7	12	6	2.2	2.5	0.19	2.6	C70-72
Thyroid	12	0	100	-	-	3	3	2	2	-	0.6	0.6	0.05	0.6	C73
Hodgkin disease	33	2	100	4	7	4	6	5	5	2	1.5	1.7	0.13	1.6	C81
Non-Hodgkin lymphoma	97	2	99	9	6	9	6	13	22	30	4.5	5.0	0.34	5.4	C82-85,C96
Multiple myeloma	30	0	90	-	-	-	4	4	11	11	1.4	1.5	0.13	1.8	C90
Lymphoid leukaemia	42	0	100	9	4	4	6	3	5	11	1.9	2.2	0.12	2.2	C91
Myeloid leukaemia	37	0	100	2	9	6	3	3	3	11	1.7	1.9	0.10	1.9	C92-94
Leukaemia, unspecified	3	0	100	-	-	-	-	-	-	2	0.1	0.2	0.00	0.2	C95
Other and unspecified	171	3	68	5	6	3	13	22	39	80	7.9	8.8	0.53	10.1	O&U
All sites	2085	28	89	54	61	74	166	247	581	874	96.5		7.24	122.0	ALL
All sites but C44	1947	27	88	53	58	70	153	228	549	809	90.1	100.0	6.80	113.9	ALLbC44
Average annual population				702684	425829	359013	269655	153026	133480	117433					

Table 1. Tunisia, North, Tunis (1994)

NUMBER OF CASES BY AGE GROUP AND SUMMARY RATES OF INCIDENCE - FEMALE

SITE	ALL AGES	AGE UNK	MV (%)	0-	15-	25-	35-	45-	55-	65+	CRUDE RATE	%	CR 64	ASR (W)	ICD (10th)
Mouth	16	0	100	-	-	-	2	-	5	9	0.8	1.1	0.05	1.0	C00-06
Salivary gland	5	0	100	-	-	-	-	-	2	3	0.2	0.3	0.02	0.3	C07-08
Nasopharynx	33	0	100	-	5	3	8	7	7	3	1.6	2.2	0.15	1.8	C11
Other pharynx	6	0	100	-	-	2	-	2	1	1	0.3	0.4	0.03	0.3	C09-10,C12-14
Oesophagus	16	0	94	-	-	-	2	1	6	7	0.8	1.1	0.06	1.0	C15
Stomach	61	1	92	-	1	10	8	5	20	17	2.9	4.0	0.25	3.5	C16
Colon, rectum and anus	113	9	95	-	1	3	12	16	23	49	5.4	7.5	0.37	7.0	C18-21
Liver	29	0	62	1	-	-	2	4	8	14	1.4	1.9	0.10	1.8	C22
Gallbladder etc.	71	0	65	-	-	3	5	8	21	34	3.4	4.7	0.24	4.4	C23-24
Pancreas	26	1	46	-	-	-	1	1	9	14	1.2	1.7	0.09	1.7	C25
Larynx	4	0	100	-	-	-	-	1	2	1	0.2	0.3	0.02	0.3	C32
Trachea, bronchus and lung	37	2	95	-	2	-	7	6	10	12	1.8	2.5	0.16	2.3	C33-34
Bone	8	0	100	3	2	2	1	-	-	-	0.4	0.5	0.02	0.3	C40-41
Melanoma of skin	12	0	100	1	2	-	-	1	3	4	0.6	0.8	0.04	0.7	C43
Other skin	91	3	100	-	2	3	8	17	17	41	4.3	5.7	0.30	5.7	C44
Mesothelioma	0	0	-	-	-	-	-	-	-	-	0.0	0.0	0.00	0.0	C45
Kaposi sarcoma	2	1	100	-	-	-	-	1	-	-	0.1	0.1	0.01	0.1	C46
Peripheral nerves	5	0	100	-	1	1	1	-	-	3	0.2	0.3	0.01	0.3	C47
Connective and soft tissue	17	1	94	2	1	5	1	3	3	3	0.8	1.1	0.07	0.9	C49
Breast	409	0	98	-	-	40	107	113	74	75	19.4	27.1	1.85	24.1	C50
Vulva	14	0	100	-	-	-	1	4	3	6	0.7	0.9	0.05	0.9	C51
Vagina	5	0	100	-	-	-	1	2	1	1	0.2	0.3	0.02	0.3	C52
Cervix uteri	103	0	99	-	2	6	28	23	28	16	4.9	6.8	0.51	6.1	C53
Uterus	37	0	100	-	-	-	2	6	18	11	1.8	2.5	0.19	2.4	C54-55
Ovary	50	0	98	2	2	4	10	10	12	10	2.4	3.3	0.23	2.9	C56
Placenta	3	0	67	-	1	-	2	-	-	-	0.1	0.2	0.01	0.1	C58
Kidney	19	0	74	4	-	1	-	5	3	6	0.9	1.3	0.07	1.2	C64
Renal pelvis, ureter and other urinary	1	0	100	-	-	-	-	-	-	1	0.0	0.1	0.00	0.1	C65-66,C68
Bladder	15	0	100	-	-	-	-	3	4	8	0.7	1.0	0.05	1.0	C67
Eye	6	0	100	1	-	-	2	1	1	1	0.3	0.4	0.02	0.4	C69
Brain, nervous system	27	0	93	9	4	6	4	3	1	-	1.3	1.8	0.09	1.3	C70-72
Thyroid	55	0	100	-	4	11	18	5	4	13	2.6	3.6	0.18	2.9	C73
Hodgkin disease	18	0	100	1	4	6	2	3	1	1	0.9	1.2	0.06	0.9	C81
Non-Hodgkin lymphoma	60	1	100	7	2	6	6	6	8	24	2.9	4.0	0.17	3.5	C82-85,C96
Multiple myeloma	25	0	96	-	-	-	1	1	13	10	1.2	1.7	0.11	1.6	C90
Lymphoid leukaemia	32	0	100	10	6	-	-	3	9	3	1.5	2.1	0.13	1.7	C91
Myeloid leukaemia	47	1	100	7	1	5	8	7	12	6	2.2	3.1	0.21	2.6	C92-94
Leukaemia, unspecified	3	0	100	2	-	-	1	-	-	-	0.1	0.2	0.01	0.1	C95
Other and unspecified	120	3	73	8	-	6	13	18	28	44	5.7	7.9	0.44	7.3	O&U
All sites	1601	23	93	58	38	125	265	286	357	449	76.1		6.41	94.7	ALL
All sites but C44	1510	20	92	58	36	122	257	269	340	408	71.8	100.0	6.11	89.1	ALLbC44
Average annual population				673698	415596	362546	260562	152397	129125	109870					

Table 2. Tunisia, Centre, Sousse (1993-1997)

NUMBER OF CASES BY AGE GROUP AND SUMMARY RATES OF INCIDENCE - MALE

SITE	ALL AGES	AGE UNK	MV (%)	0-	15-	25-	35-	45-	55-	65+	CRUDE RATE	%	CR 64	ASR (W)	ICD (10th)
Mouth	31	0	100	-	-	-	3	4	7	17	2.7	2.8	0.19	3.7	C00-06
Salivary gland	3	0	100	-	-	1	-	-	-	2	0.3	0.3	0.01	0.3	C07-08
Nasopharynx	46	0	100	1	4	7	9	8	8	9	4.0	4.2	0.36	4.9	C11
Other pharynx	6	0	100	-	-	-	-	2	2	2	0.5	0.6	0.06	0.8	C09-10,C12-14
Oesophagus	3	0	100	-	-	-	-	1	-	2	0.3	0.3	0.01	0.4	C15
Stomach	42	0	100	-	-	-	4	5	10	23	3.6	3.9	0.26	5.0	C16
Colon. rectum and anus	65	0	100	1	2	2	6	10	15	29	5.6	6.0	0.45	7.7	C18-21
Liver	11	0	100	1	-	-	2	2	3	3	1.0	1.0	0.10	1.3	C22
Gallbladder etc.	6	0	100	-	-	-	2	-	2	4	0.5	0.6	0.03	0.7	C23-24
Pancreas	19	0	100	-	-	-	2	3	6	8	1.6	1.7	0.15	2.3	C25
Larynx	51	0	100	-	-	2	5	5	20	21	4.4	4.7	0.43	6.2	C32
Trachea, bronchus and lung	255	0	99	-	-	2	20	26	73	134	22.1	23.4	1.70	30.6	C33-34
Bone	10	0	100	2	2	3	2	1	-	-	0.9	0.9	0.06	0.8	C40-41
Melanoma of skin	4	0	100	-	-	-	-	-	2	2	0.3	0.4	0.03	0.5	C43
Other skin	109	0	100	2	1	5	19	20	16	46	9.4		0.70	12.4	C44
Mesothelioma	0	0	-	-	-	-	1	-	-	-	0.0	0.0	0.00	0.0	C45
Kaposi sarcoma	11	0	100	-	-	3	1	1	1	5	1.0	1.0	0.05	1.2	C46
Peripheral nerves	1	0	100	1	-	-	-	-	-	-	0.1	0.1	0.00	0.1	C47
Connective and soft tissue	15	0	100	2	2	1	3	3	1	3	1.3	1.4	0.10	1.5	C49
Breast	5	0	100	-	-	1	-	-	2	2	0.4	0.5	0.04	0.6	C50
Penis	1	0	100	-	-	-	-	-	-	1	0.1	0.1	0.00	0.1	C60
Prostate	79	0	99	-	-	-	-	2	5	72	6.8	7.2	0.11	9.3	C61
Testis	7	0	100	1	2	1	3	-	-	-	0.6	0.6	0.04	0.6	C62
Kidney	19	0	100	3	-	-	1	4	7	4	1.6	1.7	0.18	2.3	C64
Renal pelvis, ureter and other urinary	9	0	100	-	-	-	-	3	-	6	0.8	0.8	0.04	1.1	C65-66,C68
Bladder	146	0	99	-	-	4	3	11	40	88	12.7	13.4	0.83	17.4	C67
Eye	5	0	100	2	-	-	1	-	2	-	0.4	0.5	0.04	0.5	C69
Brain, nervous system	15	0	93	-	2	3	4	2	1	3	1.3	1.4	0.10	1.5	C70-72
Thyroid	7	0	100	-	1	-	1	1	1	3	0.6	0.6	0.04	0.8	C73
Hodgkin disease	20	0	100	3	1	1	1	6	2	3	1.7	1.8	0.16	2.2	C81
Non-Hodgkin lymphoma	76	0	100	3	5	8	14	4	21	21	6.6	7.0	0.57	8.2	C82-85,C96
Multiple myeloma	4	0	100	-	-	-	-	3	-	1	0.3	0.4	0.04	0.6	C90
Lymphoid leukaemia	25	0	100	12	-	2	-	5	1	4	2.2	2.3	0.14	2.5	C91
Myeloid leukaemia	21	1	100	1	4	2	5	3	-	6	1.8	1.9	0.11	2.1	C92-94
Leukaemia, unspecified	1	0	100	-	-	-	-	1	-	-	0.1	0.1	0.01	0.1	C95
Other and unspecified	71	0	97	3	2	4	4	10	21	27	6.2	6.5	0.54	8.3	O&U
All sites	1199	0	99	38	29	50	116	146	269	551	103.9	100.0	7.73	138.7	ALL
All sites but C44	1090	0	99	36	28	45	97	126	253	505	94.5		7.03	126.2	ALLbC44
Average annual population				78380	47180	37480	27820	15320	12460	12160					

Table 2. Tunisia, Centre, Sousse (1993-1997)

NUMBER OF CASES BY AGE GROUP AND SUMMARY RATES OF INCIDENCE - FEMALE

SITE	ALL AGES	AGE UNK	MV (%)	0-	15-	25-	35-	45-	55-	65+	CRUDE RATE	%	CR 64	ASR (W)	ICD (10th)
Mouth	8	0	100	-	-	-	1	1	4	2	0.7	1.1	0.08	1.0	C00-06
Salivary gland	4	0	100	-	2	-	-	-	-	2	0.4	0.5	0.01	0.4	C07-08
Nasopharynx	16	0	100	1	2	3	6	2	1	1	1.4	2.1	0.12	1.5	C11
Other pharynx	2	0	100	-	-	-	-	1	-	-	0.2	0.3	0.02	0.2	C09-10,C12-14
Oesophagus	3	0	100	-	1	-	-	-	2	1	0.3	0.4	0.03	0.4	C15
Stomach	24	0	100	-	1	2	3	4	4	10	2.1	3.2	0.15	2.7	C16
Colon, rectum and anus	77	0	100	-	1	3	9	14	20	30	6.8	10.2	0.58	8.8	C18-21
Liver	6	0	100	-	-	-	1	1	1	2	0.5	0.8	0.04	0.7	C22
Gallbladder etc.	19	0	100	-	-	-	-	1	4	13	1.7	2.5	0.09	2.2	C23-24
Pancreas	7	0	100	-	-	-	-	1	1	5	0.6	0.9	0.03	0.8	C25
Larynx	1	0	100	-	-	-	1	-	-	-	0.1	0.1	0.01	0.1	C32
Trachea, bronchus and lung	16	0	100	-	1	-	1	3	2	9	1.4	2.1	0.08	1.8	C33-34
Bone	5	0	100	2	-	1	1	-	-	-	0.4	0.7	0.03	0.4	C40-41
Melanoma of skin	9	0	100	-	-	-	1	6	1	6	0.8	1.2	0.03	1.0	C43
Other skin	82	0	100	3	3	3	10	6	8	49	7.3		0.32	8.9	C44
Mesothelioma	0	0		-	-	-	-	-	-	-	0.0	0.0	0.00	0.0	C45
Kaposi sarcoma	3	0	100	-	-	-	-	-	-	2	0.3	0.4	0.00	0.3	C46
Peripheral nerves	0	0		-	-	-	-	-	-	-	0.0	0.0	0.00	0.0	C47
Connective and soft tissue	15	0	100	1	2	-	2	2	3	5	1.3	2.0	0.10	1.6	C49
Breast	209	0	100	-	-	20	60	47	36	46	18.6	27.6	1.71	22.7	C50
Vulva	1	0	100	-	1	-	-	-	-	-	0.1	0.1	0.00	0.1	C51
Vagina	2	0	100	-	-	1	-	-	-	-	0.2	0.3	0.01	0.1	C52
Cervix uteri	70	0	100	-	-	4	18	20	13	15	6.2	9.2	0.61	7.9	C53
Uterus	20	0	95	-	-	-	1	-	12	7	1.8	2.6	0.20	2.4	C54-55
Ovary	24	0	96	-	-	2	-	3	11	8	2.1	3.2	0.22	2.8	C56
Placenta	0	0		-	-	-	-	-	-	-	0.0	0.0	0.00	0.0	C58
Kidney	14	0	100	3	1	-	1	1	2	6	1.2	1.8	0.07	1.5	C64
Renal pelvis, ureter and other urinary	3	0	100	-	-	-	-	1	-	1	0.3	0.4	0.02	0.3	C65-66,C68
Bladder	12	0	100	-	-	1	-	1	2	8	1.1	1.6	0.05	1.4	C67
Eye	5	0	100	2	-	-	-	-	-	2	0.4	0.7	0.02	0.5	C69
Brain, nervous system	13	0	92	4	-	1	2	2	4	-	1.2	1.7	0.12	1.3	C70-72
Thyroid	27	0	100	-	4	6	8	2	2	5	2.4	3.6	0.16	2.5	C73
Hodgkin disease	15	0	100	3	7	2	2	-	-	1	1.3	2.0	0.07	1.2	C81
Non-Hodgkin lymphoma	47	0	100	1	7	4	7	8	11	15	4.2	6.2	0.35	5.1	C82-85,C96
Multiple myeloma	10	0	100	-	-	-	2	2	3	3	0.9	1.3	0.09	1.2	C90
Lymphoid leukaemia	13	0	100	7	1	-	1	1	2	3	1.2	1.7	0.07	1.3	C91
Myeloid leukaemia	12	0	100	1	2	-	1	-	3	4	1.1	1.6	0.08	1.3	C92-94
Leukaemia, unspecified	1	0	0	-	-	-	-	-	-	1	0.1	0.1	0.00	0.1	C95
Other and unspecified	45	0	96	2	1	4	3	3	12	20	4.0	5.9	0.28	5.0	O&U
All sites	840	0	99	30	34	59	142	128	165	282	74.7	100.0	5.85	91.4	ALL
All sites but C44	758	0	99	27	31	56	132	122	157	233	67.4		5.54	82.5	ALLbC44
Average annual population				74740	44160	36780	27500	16200	13040	12600					

Table 3. Tunisia, Sfax (1997)

NUMBER OF CASES BY AGE GROUP AND SUMMARY RATES OF INCIDENCE - MALE

SITE	ALL AGES	AGE UNK	MV (%)	0-	15-	25-	35-	45-	55-	65+	CRUDE RATE	%	CR 64	ASR (W)	ICD (10th)
Mouth	13	0	100	-	-	1	-	2	4	6	3.3	3.3	0.26	4.2	C00-06
Salivary gland	1	0	100	-	-	-	1	-	2	-	0.3	0.3	0.02	0.3	C07-08
Nasopharynx	12	0	100	-	-	-	4	3	2	3	3.1	3.1	0.27	3.7	C11
Other pharynx	4	0	100	-	-	-	-	-	2	2	1.0	1.0	0.09	1.3	C09-10,C12-14
Oesophagus	2	0	50	-	-	-	-	-	-	2	0.5	0.5	0.00	0.6	C15
Stomach	10	0	100	-	-	-	2	-	3	5	2.5	2.6	0.18	3.1	C16
Colon, rectum and anus	28	0	100	-	1	-	-	3	6	18	7.1	7.2	0.38	8.9	C18-21
Liver	5	0	100	-	-	1	-	-	-	4	1.3	1.3	0.02	1.4	C22
Gallbladder etc.	4	0	100	-	-	-	-	-	2	2	1.0	1.0	0.09	1.3	C23-24
Pancreas	2	0	50	-	-	-	-	-	1	1	0.5	0.5	0.04	0.7	C25
Larynx	18	0	100	-	-	-	-	3	10	5	4.6	4.6	0.56	6.2	C32
Trachea, bronchus and lung	76	0	92	-	-	-	4	6	23	43	19.3	19.5	1.32	24.2	C33-34
Bone	1	0	100	-	-	1	-	-	-	-	0.3	0.3	0.02	0.2	C40-41
Melanoma of skin	2	0	100	-	-	1	-	-	-	1	0.5	0.5	0.02	0.6	C43
Other skin	65	0	100	-	-	2	10	8	9	36	16.5		0.95	20.2	C44
Mesothelioma	0	0	-	-	-	-	-	-	-	-	0.0	0.0	0.00	0.0	C45
Kaposi sarcoma	1	0	100	-	-	-	-	-	-	1	0.3	0.3	0.00	0.3	C46
Peripheral nerves	0	0	-	-	-	-	-	-	-	-	0.0	0.0	0.00	0.0	C47
Connective and soft tissue	5	0	100	-	-	-	1	1	2	1	1.3	1.3	0.14	1.6	C49
Breast	4	0	100	-	-	-	-	-	1	3	1.0	1.0	0.04	1.2	C50
Penis	0	0	-	-	-	-	-	-	-	-	0.0	0.0	0.00	0.0	C60
Prostate	41	0	98	-	-	-	-	-	5	36	10.4	10.5	0.22	12.4	C61
Testis	2	0	100	-	1	-	1	-	-	-	0.5	0.5	0.03	0.5	C62
Kidney	4	0	75	1	-	-	-	1	-	2	1.0	1.0	0.05	1.3	C64
Renal pelvis, ureter and other urinary	6	0	83	-	-	-	-	1	2	3	1.5	1.5	0.12	2.0	C65-66,C68
Bladder	47	0	98	-	-	2	4	4	14	23	12.0	12.1	0.89	14.9	C67
Eye	2	0	100	1	-	1	-	-	-	-	0.5	0.5	0.03	0.5	C69
Brain, nervous system	11	0	64	3	3	-	1	-	3	1	2.8	2.8	0.22	2.9	C70-72
Thyroid	1	0	100	-	-	1	-	-	-	-	0.3	0.3	0.02	0.3	C73
Hodgkin disease	10	0	100	2	3	-	1	1	2	-	2.5	2.6	0.23	2.8	C81
Non-Hodgkin lymphoma	17	0	100	2	2	-	3	2	2	6	4.3	4.4	0.27	4.9	C82-85,C96
Multiple myeloma	3	0	100	1	-	-	-	-	-	2	0.8	0.8	0.01	0.8	C90
Lymphoid leukaemia	19	0	100	5	2	-	2	1	-	9	4.8	4.9	0.19	5.3	C91
Myeloid leukaemia	13	0	100	2	1	2	-	-	1	6	3.3	3.3	0.17	3.8	C92-94
Leukaemia, unspecified	1	0	100	-	-	-	-	-	-	1	0.3	0.3	0.00	0.3	C95
Other and unspecified	24	0	92	1	-	-	-	4	5	14	6.1	6.2	0.38	7.8	O&U
All sites	454	0	96	18	13	12	34	40	101	236	115.5	100.0	7.24	140.5	ALL
All sites but C44	389	0	95	18	13	10	24	32	92	200	98.9		6.29	120.3	ALLbC44

Average annual population

	0-	15-	25-	35-	45-	55-	65+
	128200	78400	64400	48400	27400	22800	23600

Table 3. Tunisia, Sfax (1997)

NUMBER OF CASES BY AGE GROUP AND SUMMARY RATES OF INCIDENCE - FEMALE

SITE	ALL AGES	AGE UNK	MV (%)	0-	15-	25-	35-	45-	55-	65+	CRUDE RATE	%	CR 64	ASR (W)	ICD (10th)
Mouth	2	0	100	-	-	-	-	-	1	1	0.5	0.7	0.06	**0.6**	*C00-06*
Salivary gland	0	0	-	-	-	-	-	-	-	-	0.0	0.0	0.00	**0.0**	*C07-08*
Nasopharynx	3	0	100	-	1	-	-	1	-	1	0.8	1.1	0.05	**0.9**	*C11*
Other pharynx	4	0	100	-	-	-	-	2	-	2	1.1	1.4	0.06	**1.4**	*C09-10,C12-14*
Oesophagus	2	0	100	-	-	-	1	1	-	-	0.5	0.7	0.04	**0.7**	*C15*
Stomach	9	0	100	-	-	1	-	-	4	4	2.4	3.2	0.19	**2.9**	*C16*
Colon, rectum and anus	31	0	100	-	-	3	7	3	5	13	8.2	11.2	0.54	**9.6**	*C18-21*
Liver	1	0	100	-	-	-	1	-	-	-	0.3	0.4	0.01	**0.3**	*C22*
Gallbladder etc.	8	0	100	-	-	1	1	1	3	2	2.1	2.9	0.19	**2.6**	*C23-24*
Pancreas	3	0	33	-	-	-	-	-	1	2	0.8	1.1	0.04	**1.0**	*C25*
Larynx	1	0	100	-	-	-	-	-	-	1	0.3	0.4	0.00	**0.3**	*C32*
Trachea, bronchus and lung	7	0	100	-	-	-	1	-	3	3	1.9	2.5	0.15	**2.2**	*C33-34*
Bone	5	0	80	-	3	-	-	1	-	1	1.3	1.8	0.09	**1.4**	*C40-41*
Melanoma of skin	1	0	100	-	-	-	-	1	-	-	0.3	0.4	0.01	**0.2**	*C43*
Other skin	38	0	100	1	3	1	4	8	5	16	10.1		0.66	**12.0**	*C44*
Mesothelioma	0	0	-	-	-	-	-	-	-	-	0.0	0.0	0.04	**0.0**	*C45*
Kaposi sarcoma	1	0	100	1	-	-	-	-	-	-	0.3	0.4	0.04	**0.3**	*C46*
Peripheral nerves	0	0	-	-	-	-	-	-	-	-	0.0	0.0	0.00	**0.0**	*C47*
Connective and soft tissue	6	0	100	1	2	2	-	-	-	1	1.6	2.2	0.09	**1.4**	*C49*
Breast	73	0	100	-	-	7	24	14	15	13	19.3	26.4	1.81	**22.7**	*C50*
Vulva	0	0	-	-	-	-	-	-	-	-	0.0	0.0	0.00	**0.0**	*C51*
Vagina	0	0	-	-	-	-	-	-	-	-	0.0	0.0	0.00	**0.0**	*C52*
Cervix uteri	10	0	100	-	-	-	2	3	4	1	2.6	3.6	0.32	**3.4**	*C53*
Uterus	13	0	100	-	-	3	1	3	5	1	3.4	4.7	0.35	**4.5**	*C54-55*
Ovary	9	0	100	-	-	-	1	2	2	4	2.4	3.2	0.17	**3.0**	*C56*
Placenta	1	0	100	-	-	1	-	-	-	-	0.3	0.4	0.01	**0.2**	*C58*
Kidney	2	0	100	-	-	-	-	-	-	2	0.5	0.7	0.00	**0.6**	*C64*
Renal pelvis, ureter and other urinary	5	0	100	-	-	-	-	1	-	4	1.3	1.8	0.03	**1.6**	*C65-66,C68*
Bladder	13	0	100	-	-	-	-	3	7	3	3.4	4.7	0.41	**4.6**	*C67*
Eye	1	0	100	1	-	-	-	-	-	-	0.3	0.4	0.02	**0.2**	*C69*
Brain, nervous system	5	0	40	-	1	2	-	2	-	-	1.3	1.8	0.11	**1.4**	*C70-72*
Thyroid	7	0	100	-	1	1	-	1	1	3	1.9	2.5	0.11	**2.1**	*C73*
Hodgkin disease	4	0	100	-	-	-	2	-	-	2	1.1	1.4	0.03	**1.0**	*C81*
Non-Hodgkin lymphoma	11	0	91	-	1	1	3	2	-	4	2.9	4.0	0.26	**3.6**	*C82-85,C96*
Multiple myeloma	3	0	100	-	-	-	-	1	1	1	0.8	1.1	0.07	**1.0**	*C90*
Lymphoid leukaemia	11	0	100	4	1	1	-	1	2	2	2.9	4.0	0.15	**3.2**	*C91*
Myeloid leukaemia	4	0	100	1	-	-	-	-	1	2	1.1	1.4	0.06	**1.2**	*C92-94*
Leukaemia, unspecified	2	0	50	1	-	-	-	-	-	1	0.5	0.7	0.01	**0.5**	*C95*
Other and unspecified	19	0	89	-	1	1	1	2	6	7	5.0	6.9	0.40	**6.0**	*O&U*
All sites	315	0	97	10	16	21	44	50	72	102	83.4		6.57	**99.1**	*ALL*
All sites but C44	277	0	96	9	13	20	40	42	67	86	73.3	100.0	5.91	**87.1**	*ALLbC44*
Average annual population				120000	73400	63700	46600	28600	23000	22400					

Table 4. Tunisia: case series

Site	Institut Pasteur,Tunis: 1960–69 (Chadli *et al.*, 1976)					Institut Salah Azaiz,Tunis: 1969–85 (Ben Abdallah, 1997)				
	Male		Female		%HV	Male		Female		%HV
	No.	%	No.	%		No.	%	No.	%	
Oral cavity[1]	297	7.0%	107	2.9%	100	1027	8.2%	466	4.0%	
Nasopharynx	236	5.6%	101	2.7%	100	1324	10.5%	570	4.9%	
Other pharynx	49	1.2%	27	0.7%	100	224	1.8%	144	1.2%	
Oesophagus	31	0.7%	15	0.4%	100	121	1.0%	81	0.7%	
Stomach	138	3.3%	61	1.6%	100	241	1.9%	139	1.2%	
Colon/rectum	299	7.1%	157	4.2%	100	418	3.3%	312	2.7%	
Liver	65	1.5%	24	0.6%	100	64	0.5%	33	0.3%	
Pancreas	43	1.0%	15	0.4%	100	21	0.2%	8	0.1%	
Lung	167	4.0%	14	0.4%	100	1425	11.3%	87	0.7%	
Melanoma	56	1.3%	33	0.9%	100	103	0.8%	79	0.7%	
Other skin	631	14.9%	381	10.2%	100	1645	13.1%	993	8.5%	
Kaposi sarcoma	24	0.6%	6	0.2%	100					
Breast	20	0.5%	799	21.4%	100	108	0.9%	3429	29.2%	
Cervix uteri			758	20.3%	100			1872	15.9%	
Corpus uteri			122	3.3%	100			194	1.7%	
Ovary etc.			102	2.7%	100			376	3.2%	
Prostate	155	3.7%			100	150	1.2%			
Penis					100	23	0.2%			
Bladder	168	4.0%	22	0.6%	100	300	2.4%	38	0.3%	
Kidney etc.	60	1.4%	41	1.1%	100	135	1.1%	111	0.9%	
Eye	70	1.7%	35	0.9%	100	85	0.7%	69	0.6%	
Brain, nervous system	71	1.7%	23	0.6%	100	167	1.3%	103	0.9%	
Thyroid	36	0.9%	101	2.7%	100	129	1.0%	401	3.4%	
Non-Hodgkin lymphoma	369	8.7%	171	4.6%	100	976	7.8%	500	4.3%	
Hodgkin disease	195	4.6%	64	1.7%	100	460	3.7%	181	1.5%	
Myeloma	13	0.3%	8	0.2%	100	74	0.6%	33	0.3%	
Leukaemia	18	0.4%	5	0.1%	100	316	2.5%	122	1.0%	
ALL SITES	4222	100.0%	3737	100.0%	100	12571	100.0%	11747	100.0%	

[1] Includes salivary gland tumours

Table 5. Institut Salah Azaiz: childhood case series, 1969–85 (Ben Abdallah, 1997)

Cancer	Institute Salah Azaiz, Tunis: 1969–85 (Ben Abdallah, 1997)	
	No.	%
Leukaemia	198	12.1%
Acute lymphocytic leukaemia	149	9.1%
Lymphoma	462	28.2%
Burkitt lymphoma	86	5.3%
Hodgkin disease	176	10.8%
Brain and spinal neoplasms	73	4.5%
Neuroblastoma	54	3.3%
Retinoblastoma	77	4.7%
Wilms tumour	118	7.2%
Bone tumours	117	7.1%
Soft-tissue sarcomas	126	7.7%
Kaposi sarcoma		
Other*	412	25.2%
Total	1637	100.0%

*Includes nasopharynx (90; 5.5%) and skin (96; 5.9%)

Table 6. Childhood cancer, Tunisia, 3 Registries

	NUMBER OF CASES					REL. FREQ.(%)	RATES PER MILLION					
	0-4	5-9	10-14	All	M/F	Overall	0-4	5-9	10-14	Crude	ASR	%MV
Leukaemia	24	24	17	65	1.0	31.3	31.7	29.3	20.9	27.2	27.8	100.0
Acute lymphoid leukaemia	18	20	9	47	1.2	22.6	23.8	24.4	11.0	19.7	20.3	100.0
Lymphoma	8	16	12	36	2.0	17.3	10.6	19.5	14.7	15.1	14.7	100.0
Hodgkin disease	1	8	4	13	2.3	6.3	1.3	9.8	4.9	5.4	5.1	100.0
Burkitt lymphoma	3	2	1	6	1.0	2.9	4.0	2.4	1.2	2.5	2.7	83.3
Brain and spinal neoplasms	9	11	3	23	0.9	11.1	11.9	13.4	3.7	9.6	10.0	91.3
Neuroblastoma	19	1	0	20	0.8	9.6	25.1	1.2	-	8.4	10.1	85.0
Retinoblastoma	5	1	0	6	1.0	2.9	6.6	1.2	-	2.5	3.0	100.0
Wilms tumour	11	1	0	12	1.4	5.8	14.5	1.2	-	5.0	6.0	91.7
Bone tumours	0	1	9	10	1.0	4.8	-	1.2	11.0	4.2	3.6	100.0
Soft tissue sarcomas	4	0	3	7	0.8	3.4	5.3	-	3.7	2.9	3.1	100.0
Kaposi sarcoma	0	0	0	0	-	-	-	-	-	-	-	-
Germ cell tumours	1	0	3	4	1.0	1.9	1.3	-	3.7	1.7	1.6	100.0
Other	10	5	10	25	1.3	12.0	13.2	6.1	12.3	10.5	10.6	84.0
All	91	60	57	208	1.1	100.0	120.2	73.3	70.0	87.0	90.5	94.7

3.2 West Africa

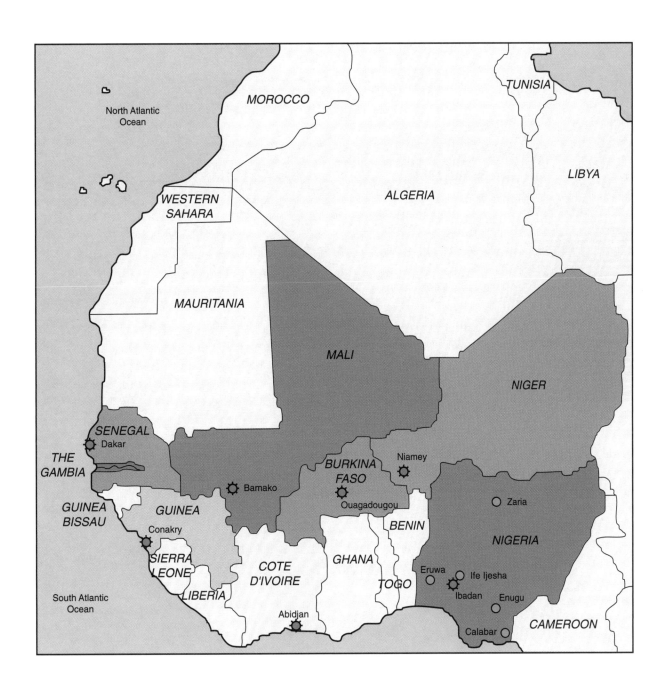

3.2.1 Benin

Background

Climate: Tropical; hot, humid in south; semiarid in north

Terrain: Mostly flat to undulating plain; some hills and low mountains

Ethnic groups: African 99% (42 ethnic groups, most important being Fon, Adja, Yoruba, Bariba), Europeans 5500

Religions: Indigenous beliefs 70%, Muslim 15%, Christian 15%

Economy—overview: The economy of Benin remains underdeveloped and dependent on subsistence agriculture, cotton production and regional trade. Commercial and transport activities, which make up a large part of the GDP, are extremely vulnerable to developments in Nigeria, particularly fuel shortages.

Industries: Textiles, cigarettes; beverages, food; construction materials, petroleum

Agriculture—products: Corn, sorghum, cassava (tapioca), yams, beans, rice, cotton, palm oil, peanuts; poultry, livestock

Cancer registration

There has been no cancer registry in Benin.

Review of data

There is no published material on the cancer profile in the country.

3.2.2 Burkina Faso

Background

Climate: Tropical; warm, dry winters; hot, wet summers

Terrain: Mostly flat to dissected, undulating plains; hills in west and southeast

Ethnic groups: Mossi about 24%, Gurunsi, Senufo, Lobi, Bobo, Mande, Fulani

Religions: Indigenous beliefs 40%, Muslim 50%, Christian (mainly Roman Catholic) 10%

Economy—overview: One of the poorest countries in the world, landlocked Burkina Faso has a high population density, few natural resources and a fragile soil. Over 80% of the population is engaged in subsistence agriculture, which is highly vulnerable to variations in rainfall. Industry remains undeveloped.

Industries: Cotton lint, beverages, agricultural processing, soap, cigarettes, textiles, gold

Agriculture—products: Peanuts, shea nuts, sesame, cotton, sorghum, millet, corn, rice; livestock

Cancer registration

A population-based cancer registry was established in 1997, in the Department of Anatomical Pathology, in the main teaching hospital of the capital, Ouagadougou. The objective was to record all cases of cancer among residents of the city, but cases in non-residents, from hospital or laboratory sources, were also registered. Registration was principally by active case finding through visits to the various clinical services in the National Hospital Yalgado Ouedraogo (the only major tertiary care facility) and to several smaller private clinics. All pathology reports mentioning cancer are obtained from the laboratory in the hospital, and from laboratories in three private clinics.

The registration process is carried out with a microcomputer using the CANREG software.

Review of data

The results are presented in Table 1 for the first complete year of registration (1998). 407 cases were registered, 51% of which had microscopically verified diagnosis.

In males, liver cancer is the most commonly registered tumour (25.9%) with 14% microscopic verification, followed by prostate (16.2%) and bladder cancers (9.1%). In women, breast cancer (28.6%) is registered more frequently than cervix cancer (20.6%), with liver cancer (7.5%) in third rank.

We are not aware of any other published data of the cancer profile in Burkina Faso.

Table 1. Burkina Faso, Ouagadougou (1998)

NUMBER OF CASES BY AGE GROUP - MALE

SITE	ICD (10th)	ALL AGES	AGE UNK	MV (%)	0-	15-	25-	35-	45-	55-	65+	%
Mouth	C00-06	5	0	40	1	-	-	1	1	1	1	2.5
Salivary gland	C07-08	1	0	0	-	-	-	-	-	1	-	0.5
Nasopharynx	C11	0	0	-	-	-	-	-	-	-	-	0.0
Other pharynx	C09-10,C12-14	4	0	50	-	-	-	-	-	2	2	2.0
Oesophagus	C15	5	0	60	-	-	-	-	-	3	2	2.5
Stomach	C16	5	0	20	-	-	-	1	-	2	2	2.5
Colon, rectum and anus	C18-21	8	0	88	-	1	-	-	2	1	4	4.1
Liver	C22	51	0	14	1	1	7	15	13	6	8	25.9
Gallbladder etc.	C23-24	1	0	100	-	-	-	-	-	-	1	0.5
Pancreas	C25	0	0	-	-	-	-	-	-	-	-	0.0
Larynx	C32	0	0	-	-	-	-	-	-	-	-	0.0
Trachea, bronchus and lung	C33-34	9	0	100	-	-	-	-	1	4	4	4.6
Bone	C40-41	9	0	33	1	2	2	1	-	2	1	4.6
Melanoma of skin	C43	0	0	-	-	-	-	-	-	-	-	0.0
Other skin	C44	4	0	25	2	-	-	-	-	1	1	-
Mesothelioma	C45	1	0	100	-	-	-	-	-	1	-	0.5
Kaposi sarcoma	C46	3	0	100	-	-	1	2	-	-	-	1.5
Peripheral nerves	C47	0	0	-	-	-	-	-	-	-	-	0.0
Connective and soft tissue	C49	6	0	67	1	-	1	1	1	-	2	3.0
Breast	C50	2	0	100	-	-	-	-	-	2	-	1.0
Penis	C60	0	0	-	-	-	-	-	-	-	-	0.0
Prostate	C61	32	0	31	-	-	-	-	-	6	26	16.2
Testis	C62	1	0	100	-	-	-	1	-	-	-	0.5
Kidney	C64	1	0	0	-	-	-	-	-	1	-	0.5
Renal pelvis, ureter and other urinary	C65-66,C68	0	0	-	-	-	-	-	-	-	-	0.0
Bladder	C67	18	0	17	1	1	-	2	5	2	6	9.1
Eye	C69	9	0	44	7	-	-	-	2	-	-	4.6
Brain, nervous system	C70-72	0	0	-	-	-	-	-	-	-	-	0.0
Thyroid	C73	0	0	-	-	-	-	-	-	-	-	0.0
Hodgkin disease	C81	3	0	100	2	-	-	1	-	-	-	1.5
Non-Hodgkin lymphoma	C82-85,C96	7	0	100	2	-	1	2	-	-	2	3.6
Multiple myeloma	C90	0	0	-	-	-	-	-	-	-	-	0.0
Lymphoid leukaemia	C91	2	0	100	-	-	-	-	-	2	-	1.0
Myeloid leukaemia	C92-94	2	0	100	1	1	-	-	-	-	-	1.0
Leukaemia, unspecified	C95	1	0	100	1	-	-	-	-	-	-	0.5
Other and unspecified	O&U	11	0	55	1	-	1	1	1	3	4	5.6
All sites	ALL	201	0	42	22	6	14	26	27	40	66	100.0
All sites but C44	ALLbC44	197	0	43	20	6	14	26	27	39	65	

Table 1. Burkina Faso, Ouagadougou (1998)

NUMBER OF CASES BY AGE GROUP - FEMALE

SITE	ICD (10th)	ALL AGES	AGE UNK	MV (%)	0-	15-	25-	35-	45-	55-	65+	%
Mouth	C00-06	1	0	100	-	-	-	-	-	-	1	0.5
Salivary gland	C07-08	1	0	100	-	-	-	-	1	-	-	0.5
Nasopharynx	C11	0	0	0	-	-	-	-	-	-	-	0.0
Other pharynx	C09-10,C12-14	1	0	0	-	-	1	-	-	-	-	0.5
Oesophagus	C15	4	0	50	-	-	-	-	4	-	-	2.0
Stomach	C16	5	0	80	1	-	-	-	1	2	1	2.5
Colon, rectum and anus	C18-21	2	0	50	-	-	-	-	1	-	1	1.0
Liver	C22	15	0	13	-	1	3	4	1	5	1	7.5
Gallbladder etc.	C23-24	0	0	-	-	-	-	-	-	-	-	0.0
Pancreas	C25	2	0	0	-	-	-	2	-	-	-	1.0
Larynx	C32	0	0	-	-	-	-	-	-	-	-	0.0
Trachea, bronchus and lung	C33-34	3	0	100	-	-	1	-	-	1	1	1.5
Bone	C40-41	4	0	50	1	1	-	-	1	1	-	2.0
Melanoma of skin	C43	1	0	100	-	-	-	-	-	-	1	0.5
Other skin	C44	7	0	43	-	-	3	2	1	1	-	0.0
Mesothelioma	C45	0	0	-	-	-	-	-	-	-	-	0.0
Kaposi sarcoma	C46	0	0	-	-	-	-	-	-	-	-	0.0
Peripheral nerves	C47	0	0	-	-	-	-	-	-	-	-	0.0
Connective and soft tissue	C49	0	0	-	-	-	-	-	-	-	-	0.0
Breast	C50	57	0	63	-	5	13	14	9	10	6	28.6
Vulva	C51	0	0	-	-	-	-	-	-	-	-	0.0
Vagina	C52	0	0	-	-	-	-	-	-	-	-	0.0
Cervix uteri	C53	41	0	73	1	1	12	9	11	5	2	20.6
Uterus	C54-55	15	0	87	-	2	5	4	2	1	1	7.5
Ovary	C56	4	0	100	-	-	1	1	1	1	-	2.0
Placenta	C58	0	0	-	-	-	-	-	-	-	-	0.0
Kidney	C64	1	0	0	1	-	-	-	-	-	-	0.5
Renal pelvis, ureter and other urinary	C65-66,C68	0	0	-	-	-	-	-	-	-	-	0.0
Bladder	C67	5	0	40	-	-	2	2	-	1	-	2.5
Eye	C69	7	0	43	5	-	1	-	1	-	-	3.5
Brain, nervous system	C70-72	0	0	-	-	-	-	-	-	-	-	0.0
Thyroid	C73	1	0	100	-	-	-	-	-	-	1	0.5
Hodgkin disease	C81	0	0	-	-	-	-	-	-	-	-	0.0
Non-Hodgkin lymphoma	C82-85,C96	5	0	60	1	1	1	-	2	-	-	2.5
Multiple myeloma	C90	0	0	-	-	-	-	-	-	-	-	0.0
Lymphoid leukaemia	C91	2	0	50	1	-	-	1	-	-	-	1.0
Myeloid leukaemia	C92-94	2	0	50	2	-	-	-	-	-	-	1.0
Leukaemia, unspecified	C95	1	0	100	-	-	-	-	1	-	-	0.5
Other and unspecified	O&U	19	0	47	2	-	3	2	4	3	5	9.5
All sites	ALL	206	0	60	15	11	47	40	40	32	21	100.0
All sites but C44	ALLbC44	199	0	61	15	11	44	38	40	31	20	

3.2.3 Cape Verde

Background

Climate: Temperate; warm, dry summer; precipitation meager and very erratic

Terrain: Steep, rugged, rocky, volcanic

Ethnic groups: Creole (mulatto) 71%, African 28%, European 1%

Religions: Roman Catholicism fused with indigenous beliefs

Economy—overview: Cape Verde's low per capita GDP reflects a poor natural resource base, serious water shortages exacerbated by cycles of long-term drought, and a high birth rate. The economy is service-oriented, with commerce, transport and public services accounting for almost 70% of GDP. Although nearly 70% of the population lives in rural areas, the share of agriculture in the GDP in 1995 was only 8%, of which fishing accounted for 1.5%. About 90% of food must be imported. The fishing potential, mostly lobster and tuna, is not fully exploited.

Industries: Food and beverages, fish processing, shoes and garments, salt mining, ship repair

Agriculture—products: Bananas, corn, beans, sweet potatoes, sugarcane, coffee, peanuts; fish

Cancer registration

There has been no cancer registration in the country to date

Review of data

There are no published data on cancer incidence, or on clinical/pathological case series.

Mysteriously, some mortality data for 1980 were published in the World Health Statistics Annual of WHO (1983) for a limited series of sites (Table 1). No such data have appeared since. The rates are low and suggest under-registration of deaths. But some interesting features emerge, such as the frequency of stomach cancer as a cause of death (the leading cause of cancer death in both sexes).

Reference

WHO (1983) *World Health Statistics Annual, 1983*, Geneva

Table 1. Cape Verde: 1980 (source: WHO, 1983)

Site	ICD 8	Males			Females		
		Deaths	Rate	ASR(W)	Deaths	Rate	ASR(W)
Buccal cavity and pharynx	A045	1	0.7	0.6	2	1.3	0.8
Oesophagus	A046	6	4.4	3.3	6	3.8	3.1
Stomach	A047	21	15.3	12.1	20	12.6	9.2
Rectum, rectosigmoid junction, anus	A049	1	0.7	0.3	1	0.6	0.5
Larynx	A050	2	1.5	1.3	0	0	0
Trachea, bronchus and lung	A051	6	4.4	3.4	4	2.5	1.5
Bone	A052	1	0.7	0.6	1	0.6	0.4
Breast	A054				6	3.8	2.8
Cervix uteri	A055				12	7.5	5.6
Prostate	A057	4	2.9	2.3			
Leukaemia	A059	1	0.7	0.6	1	0.6	0.3
Other and unspecified sites	A058	15	10.9	7.1	16	10.1	8.0
ALL MALIGNANT NEOPLASMS		62	45.2	33.4	80	50.3	37.9

Male population: 137 100
Female population: 159 000
Rate: Crude rate per 100 000
ASR(W): Age-standardized rate (World population) per 100 000

3.2.4 Côte d'Ivoire

Background

Climate: Tropical along coast, semi-arid in far north; three seasons—warm and dry (November to March), hot and dry (March to May), hot and wet (June to October)

Terrain: Mostly flat to undulating plains; mountains in north-west

Ethnic groups: Baoule 23%, Bete 18%, Senoufou 15%, Malinke 11%, Agni, foreign Africans (mostly Burkinabe and Malians, about 3 million), non-Africans 130 000 to 330 000

Religions: Muslim 60%, Christian 12%, indigenous beliefs 25% (some overlap with the Christians and Muslims)

Economy—overview: Côte d'Ivoire is among the world's largest producers and exporters of coffee, cocoa beans, and palm oil. Consequently, the economy is highly sensitive to fluctuations in international prices for these products and to weather conditions. Despite attempts by the government to diversify the economy, it is still largely dependent on agriculture and related activities, which engage roughly 85% of the population.

Industries: Foodstuffs, beverages; wood products, oil refining, automobile assembly, textiles, fertilizer, construction materials, electricity

Agriculture—products: Coffee, cocoa beans, bananas, palm kernels, corn, rice, cassava (tapioca), sweet potatoes, sugar; cotton, rubber; timber

Cancer registration

The Abidjan cancer registry was founded in 1994, under the auspices of the Ministry of Public Health. It is located in the Department of Oncology at the University Hospital of Treichville. This department is a referral centre for cancer treatment in the capital. The registry was, from its inception, designed to be population-based with complete recording of all cancer cases diagnosed among the population of the city of Abidjan. The city comprises 10 administrative subdivisions and in 1996 the population was estimated to be almost 3 million.

Case finding is carried out by a cancer registrar and two full-time clerks, by active search for cases in all of the hospital services in the city where cancer might be diagnosed. Weekly visits are made to the major services (surgery, urology, medicine, gynaecology, paediatrics etc.) in the three major teaching hospitals (Treichville, Cocody and Yopougon), as well as less frequent visits to government, private hospitals, health centres and private clinics. Cases of cancer in residents of Abidjan who are admitted to the mission hospital in Dabou 50 km from Abidjan are notified to the registry by medical staff. In addition, cancer cases are identified from various case series (haematological malignancies, lymphomas, Kaposi sarcomas, etc.) collected by clinicians.

An important source of information is the two university departments of pathology which provide histopathology and cytology services for the whole of the south of the country. Two private laboratories are also used as sources of data. Death certificates are not used as a source of information, because of the difficulty in retrieving them from the different administrative offices where they are stored, and because the primary sources (hospitals, pathology laboratories) were already covered by the case-finding system.

Care is taken to distinguish residents of Abidjan from temporary visitors (the latter are generally individuals domiciled with their extended family for the purpose of receiving treatment). The definition of 'usual resident' is a person who has lived in Abidjan for at least six months. The registration process is carried out with a microcomputer using the CANREG software.

Results for the three-year period 1995–97 have been published (Echimane *et al.*, 2000) and are reproduced in Table 1. The incidence rates calculated based on the estimated resident population are a little low, suggesting that some cases are not being found. In addition, the level of diagnostic confirmation by histology or cytology is relatively high (81.8%) compared with that in other registries in West Africa. Although this partly reflects the failure to detect a proportion of cases diagnosed without histology, it is quite likely that the proportion of cancer cases receiving a biopsy is higher in Abidjan, where there are numerous laboratories and pathologists, than elsewhere in the region. Suspected cases of liver cancer are frequently examined by aspiration cytology to confirm the diagnosis.

Review of data

Cancer Registry

The ranking of the different cancers differs depending on whether they are considered in terms of numbers of cases or ASRs. In men, prostate (15.3% cancers, ASR 31.4 per 100 000) and liver cancer (14.6 % of cases, ASR 10.0 per 100 000) rank first and second by both indices, but while the next most frequent in terms of numbers are non-Hodgkin lymphoma (10%), Kaposi sarcoma (7.5%) and lung cancer (5.1%), in terms of ASR, they are lung (6.2 per 100 000), stomach (3.3 per 100 000) and non-Hodgkin lymphoma (3.0 per 100 000).

In women, the most important sites are breast (25.2%), cervix uteri (23.6%), non-Hodgkin lymphoma (7.2%), ovary (4.8%) and liver (4.2%). Because of the different age distributions, the age-standardized incidence for cervix cancer (26.8 per 100 000) is rather higher than that for breast cancer (21.4 per 100 000); liver cancer has the third highest incidence (5.6 per 100 000), followed by stomach cancer (4.5 per 100 000). Of the 215 cases of cervix cancer with a histological diagnosis, 92.5% were squamous-cell carcinomas and 3.3% adenocarcinomas.

Among the non-Hodgkin lymphomas, 70 cases (44%) were recorded as Burkitt lymphoma; the proportion of non-Hodgkin lymphoma considered to be Burkitt lymphoma fell with age from 49/55 cases (89%) at 0–14 years to 20/74 (27%) at 15–44 years.

Previous studies

In an analysis of 5758 cancers histologically diagnosed in the laboratory of the University Hospital of Treichville between 1974 and 1983, Diomande *et al.* (1988) found cervix cancer to be almost three times more frequent (29.1% of female cancers) than breast cancer (10.5%). In the modern registry data, cervix cancer is slightly less common, despite similar rates of histological verification.

The high incidence of cervix cancer is presumably related to a high prevalence of infection with oncogenic subtypes of human papillomavirus, now accepted as the major causative agent for cervical cancer. In a study of women attending gynaecology clinics in Abidjan, La Ruche *et al.* (1998) found that 23.2% of women with no cytological abnormality of the cervix were infected with this virus.

Childhood cancer

Table 2 presents the neoplasms occurring in the childhood population (age 0–14 years) of Abidjan. There were a total of 137 cases, but because 21% had no histological diagnosis, 29 cases (21% of the total) fell into the 'other unspecified' category. The most frequent childhood cancer was lymphoma (58 cases, 42.3% of the total), of which 49 (84.5%) were Burkitt lymphoma, followed by leukaemias (12 cases, 8.8%) and brain tumour (9 cases, 6.6 %). The peak incidence for Burkitt lymphoma cases was in the 10–14-year age group. Some underdiagnosis of childhood cancers is likely, as witnessed by the low rates, absence of any cases in infants less than one year old, and the few cases of leukaemias and brain tumours recorded.

In a series of childhood cancers, collected over 10 years in the paediatric service of Treichville Hospital, Essoh et al. (1988) found that 50.5% of cancer cases admitted were non-Hodgkin lymphomas, of which Burkitt lymphoma comprised 96%.

References

Diomande, I., D'Horpock, A.F., Heroin, P., Ette, M., Dago, A., Battesti, F., Honde, M. & Beaumel, A. (1988) Evolution des cancers en Côte d'Ivoire. Rev. Méd. Côte d'Ivoire, 75, 81–84

Echimane, A.K., Ahnoux, A.A., Adoubi, I., Hien, S., M'Bra, K., D'Horpock, A., Diomande, M., Anongba, D., Mensah-Adoh, I. & Parkin, D.M. (2000) Cancer incidence in Abidjan, Ivory Coast: first results from the cancer registry, 1995-1997. Cancer, 89, 653–663

Essoh, N., Andoh, J., Tea, D., Mobiot, L., et al. (1988) Panorama de l'oncologie pédiatrique. A propos de 495 cas observés dans la service de pédiatrie de CHU de Treichville. Rev. Méd. Côte d'Ivoire, 75, 81–84

La Ruche, G., You, B., Mensah-Ado, I., Bergeron, C., Montcho, C., Ramon, R., Touré-Coulibaly, K., Welffens-Ekra, C., Dabis, F. & Orth, G. (1998) Human papillomavirus and human immunodeficiency virus infections: relation with cervical dysplasia-neoplasia in African women. Int J. Cancer, 76, 480–486

Table 1. Abidjan Cancer Registry, Côte d'Ivoire, 1995–97 (Echimane et al., 2000)

Site		Male				Female				HV%
		Total	%	Crude rate	ASR (world)	Total	%	Crude rate	ASR (world)	
Mouth	C00–08	18	2.1%	0.3	2.4	15	1.5%	0.3	2.4	97.0
Nasopharynx	C11	7	0.8%	0.2	0.5	2	0.2%	0.0	0.1	55.6
Other pharynx	C09–10, C12–14	10	1.1%	0.2	0.7	4	0.4%	0.1	0.7	85.7
Oesophagus	C15	9	1.0%	0.2	0.7	1	0.1%	0.0	0.2	90.0
Stomach	C16	37	4.3%	0.8	3.3	23	2.3%	0.5	4.5	90.0
Colon/rectum	C18–21	37	4.3%	0.8	2.4	23	2.3%	0.6	2.5	80.0
Liver	C22	125	14.6%	2.7	10.0	43	4.2%	1.0	5.6	50.6
Pancreas	C25	11	1.3%	0.2	1.0	6	0.6%	0.1	0.9	47.1
Lung	C33–34	44	5.1%	1.0	6.2	9	0.9%	0.2	1.2	90.6
Melanoma of skin	C43	5	0.6%	0.1	0.7	5	0.5%	0.1	1.4	100
Other skin	C44	28	3.3%	0.6	2.2	17	1.7%	0.4	2.3	82.2
Kaposi sarcoma	C46	64	7.5%	1.4	2.2	19	1.9%	0.4	1.4	100
Breast	C50	9	1.0%	0.2	0.9	255	25.2%	5.9	21.4	89.0
Cervix	C53					239	23.6%	5.5	26.8	90.0
Corpus	C54					11	1.1%	0.3	2.3	75.0
Ovary etc.	C56–57					49	4.8%	1.1	4.0	65.3
Prostate	C61	131	15.3%	2.8	31.4					76.3
Penis	C60	3	0.3%	0.1	0.2					100
Bladder	C67	24	2.8%	0.5	2.2	9	0.9%	0.2	1.8	63.6
Kidney etc.	C64–66, C68	16	1.9%	0.3	1.0	10	1.0%	0.2	0.7	70.8
Eye	C69	3	0.3%	0.1	0.0	9	0.9%	0.3	0.9	58.3
Brain, nervous system	C71–72	9	1.0%	0.2	0.3	13	1.3%	0.3	0.9	63.6
Thyroid	C73	3	0.3%	0.1	0.1	17	1.7%	0.4	1.5	90.0
Non-Hodgkin lymphoma	C82–85, C96	86	10.0%	1.9	3.0	73	7.2%	1.7	2.9	98.1
Hodgkin disease	C81	21	2.4%	0.5	0.8	13	1.3%	0.3	0.7	100
Myeloma	C90	8	0.9%	0.2	1.8	5	0.5%	0.1	0.5	100
Leukaemia	C91–95	30	3.5%	0.7	1.0	28	2.8%	0.7	2.7	98.6
All sites	ALL	859	100.0%	18.7	83.7	1012	100.0%	23.3	98.6	100

Table 2. Côte d'Ivoire: childhood cancer

Cancer	Abidjan Cancer Registry, 1995–97 (Echimane *et al.*, 2000)		
	No.	%	ASR
Leukaemia	12	8.8%	3.3
Acute lymphocytic leukaemia	6	4.4%	1.6
Lymphoma	58	42.3%	16.8
Burkitt lymphoma	49	35.8%	13.5
Hodgkin disease	3	2.2%	0.8
Brain and spinal neoplasms	9	6.6%	2.5
Neuroblastoma	1	0.7%	0.3
Retinoblastoma	4	2.9%	1
Wilms tumour	7	5.1%	1.8
Bone tumours	8	5.8%	2.3
Soft-tissue sarcomas	4	2.9%	1.1
Kaposi sarcoma	2	1.5%	0.5
Other	34	24.8%	8.5
Total	137	100.0%	37.6

3.2.5 The Gambia

Background

Climate: Tropical; hot rainy season (June to November); cooler dry season (November to May)

Terrain: Flood plain of the Gambia River flanked by some low hills

Ethnic groups: African 99% (Mandinka 42%, Fula 18%, Wolof 16%, Jola 10%, Serahuli 9%, other 4%), non-African 1%

Religions: Muslim 90%, Christian 9%, indigenous beliefs 1%

Economy—overview: The Gambia has no important mineral or other natural resources and has a limited agricultural base. About 75% of the population depends on crops and livestock for its livelihood. Small-scale manufacturing activity features the processing of peanuts, fish and hides. Reexport trade constituted a major segment of economic activity, but the 50% devaluation of the CFA franc in January 1994 made Senegalese goods more competitive and hurt the reexport trade. The Gambia also has an important tourism industry.

Industries: Processing peanuts, fish and hides; tourism; beverages; agricultural machinery assembly, wood-working, metalworking; clothing

Agriculture—products: Peanuts, millet, sorghum, rice, corn, cassava (tapioca), palm kernels; cattle, sheep, goats; forest and fishing resources are not fully exploited

Cancer registration

The Gambian National Cancer Registry was started in July 1986 as part of the Gambia Hepatitis Intervention Study (GHIS). This collaborative project, involving the IARC, the Government of The Gambia and the UK Medical Research Council (MRC), was supported by the Government of Italy through its Ministry of Foreign Affairs and the Swedish Medical Research Council. It was designed as a community-based randomized controlled trial to evaluate the protective efficacy of infant hepatitis B immunization in preventing chronic liver disease, particularly primary liver cancer, in adult life. The registry is the first population-based one with nationwide coverage in Africa, and thus covers both rural and urban populations.

Since the inception of the GHIS, improvements have been made in the diagnosis of chronic liver disease, especially primary liver cell carcinoma, by use of alpha-fetoprotein estimation, abdominal ultrasound examination and blood testing for hepatitis B surface antigen (HBsAg). In addition, a local histopathology service was revived during the middle phase of the project so as to improve histological diagnosis of all cancers. The registry receives copies of all histology reports from the National Health Laboratory Services located in the capital city of Banjul. Until recently, the Gambia had three tertiary care hospitals, two of which are government-owned, namely the Royal Victoria Hospital (RVH) in Banjul and Bansang Hospital (BSG) located in the eastern region of the country and serving mainly a rural population. These hospitals are the major referral centres for the various government dispensaries and health centres, which are evenly located around the country. They provide general medical and laboratory services. The MRC ward hospital in Fajara is another major referral centre, with four out-reach stations in rural areas; this institution has a broad-based laboratory research facility. In addition, there are various private clinics and hospitals located mainly in and around Banjul and a few mission clinics in the peri-urban and rural areas that offer general medical care.

Data collection is an active process. Initially, this was done by regular visits (their frequency determined by the yield of cancer cases) to the hospitals, collaborating private clinics, mission clinics and seven of the major health centres manned by medical doctors. Since 1997, a registry clerk has been posted in each of the three tertiary care facilities, with responsibility to work closely with the clinical, nursing and medical records staff. All possible sources (medical records, log books, ward/admission books, histology report books, specific biochemistry request books, surgical operation lists, nursing report books, death certificate stubs) are scanned for diagnosis of cancer. Cases found during admission or consultation are interviewed personally by the registry staff.

Data entry and management are performed with the IARC CANREG-3 programme. Site and histology are coded according to ICD-O second edition.

Quality control checks, which involve re-abstracting tumour and patient details from the sources of information, are undertaken by the supervisor at regular intervals.

The population denominators for calculation of incidence rates are based on annual estimates using 1983 and 1993 census figures.

Review of data

Registry data

After the change in registration methodology in 1999, there was a noticeable increase in the annual number of registrations, from and average of 280 per year in 1988–96 to 463 per year in 1997–99. Table 1 therefore shows the incidence rates for the period 1997–98. Data for the 10-year period 1988–97 have been published (Bah *et al.*, 2001), as well as the results from the first two years of activity (Bah *et al.*, 1990).

During the period under review (1997–98), 926 malignant tumours (448 in males and 478 in females) were registered among residents of The Gambia (Table 1).

The most common cancer in male Gambians is liver cancer, which constitutes 58% of all malignancies. Cancers of the lung and prostate are next in importance. Among female Gambians, cervix cancer dominates (36.5% of cases), with an age-standardized incidence rate of 29.6 per 100 000 person-years, while cancer of the liver (19.5%) and breast (9%) rank second and third, respectively.

Table 1 shows that, of the 926 cancer cases, 22.7% were based on microscopic examination. The percentage is lowest for liver cancer (3.5%), mainly due to the wide use of alpha-fetoprotein estimation and ultrasound examination in the confirmation of suspected liver disease in this population. On average, 40% of the diagnoses of liver cancer were based on suggestive ultrasonography, while positive alpha-foetoprotein estimation accounted for an additional 30%.

Childhood cancer

Table 2 shows an analysis of childhood cancer cases registered in a 11-year period, 1988–98 There were 162 cases. The overall incidence is low (ASR 34.7 per million). Lymphomas are the most commonly recorded cancer type, with 44.8% of lymphoma cases diagnosed as Burkitt lymphoma (corresponding to an ASR of 6.1 per million). The paucity of CNS tumours probably reflects the absence of diagnostic facilities.

References

Bah, E., Hall, A.J. & Inskip, H.M. (1990) The first two years of the Gambia National Cancer Registry. *Br. J. Cancer*, **62**, 647–650

Bah, E., Parkin, D.M., Hall, A.J., Jack, A.D. & Whittle, H. (2001) Cancer in The Gambia: 1988–97. *Br. J. Cancer*, **84**, 1207–1214

Table 1. The Gambia (1997-1998)

NUMBER OF CASES BY AGE GROUP AND SUMMARY RATES OF INCIDENCE - MALE

SITE	ALL AGES	AGE UNK	MV (%)	0-	15-	25-	35-	45-	55-	65+	CRUDE RATE	%	CR 64	ASR (W)	ICD (10th)
Mouth	4	0	75	-	-	-	-	2	1	1	0.4	0.9	0.07	0.9	C00-06
Salivary gland	2	0	100	2	-	-	-	-	-	-	0.2	0.5	0.01	0.1	C07-08
Nasopharynx	1	1	100	-	-	-	-	-	-	-	0.1	0.2	0.00	0.0	C11
Other pharynx	0	0	-	-	-	-	-	-	-	-	0.0	0.0	0.00	0.0	C09-10,C12-14
Oesophagus	7	1	0	-	-	1	1	3	1	1	0.7	1.6	0.10	1.4	C15
Stomach	11	1	27	-	-	2	2	2	2	5	1.1	2.5	0.12	2.5	C16
Colon, rectum and anus	8	0	13	-	-	-	-	-	-	-	0.8	1.8	0.10	1.5	C18-21
Liver	257	17	4	1	13	43	52	55	45	31	26.0	58.1	3.92	48.9	C22
Gallbladder etc.	0	0	-	-	-	-	-	-	-	-	0.0	0.0	0.00	0.0	C23-24
Pancreas	9	1	0	-	-	1	2	2	2	1	0.9	2.0	0.16	1.8	C25
Larynx	1	0	100	-	-	-	1	-	-	-	0.1	0.2	0.02	0.2	C32
Trachea, bronchus and lung	22	1	14	-	-	-	-	2	6	12	2.2	5.0	0.25	5.1	C33-34
Bone	7	0	0	2	1	-	-	-	2	-	0.7	1.6	0.08	1.0	C40-41
Melanoma of skin	2	0	50	1	-	-	1	1	-	1	0.2	0.5	0.02	0.3	C43
Other skin	6	2	100	-	1	-	-	-	-	-	0.6		0.05	1.0	C44
Mesothelioma	0	0	-	-	-	-	-	-	-	-	0.0	0.0	0.00	0.0	C45
Kaposi sarcoma	4	2	0	-	-	-	-	-	-	-	0.4	0.9	0.04	0.6	C46
Peripheral nerves	1	0	100	1	-	-	-	-	-	-	0.1	0.2	0.00	0.1	C47
Connective and soft tissue	7	1	0	-	-	-	-	-	2	2	0.7	1.6	0.10	1.5	C49
Breast	0	0	-	-	-	-	-	-	-	-	0.0	0.0	0.00	0.0	C50
Penis	4	0	25	-	-	2	-	1	-	-	0.4	0.9	0.04	0.7	C60
Prostate	20	2	20	-	-	-	-	1	3	15	2.0	4.5	0.10	4.7	C61
Testis	2	0	50	1	-	-	-	-	-	1	0.2	0.5	0.00	0.3	C62
Kidney	3	0	0	1	1	-	-	-	-	-	0.3	0.7	0.01	0.4	C64
Renal pelvis, ureter and other urinary	0	0	-	-	-	-	-	-	-	1	0.0	0.0	0.00	0.0	C65-66,C68
Bladder	6	0	50	-	-	-	2	2	1	-	0.6	1.4	0.09	1.2	C67
Eye	6	0	67	1	-	-	2	1	-	-	0.6	1.4	0.06	1.0	C69
Brain, nervous system	1	0	0	1	-	-	-	-	-	-	0.1	0.2	0.00	0.1	C70-72
Thyroid	0	0	-	-	-	-	-	-	-	-	0.0	0.0	0.00	0.0	C73
Hodgkin disease	6	2	67	3	-	-	-	-	-	-	0.6	1.4	0.03	0.5	C81
Non-Hodgkin lymphoma	19	0	53	10	-	1	3	2	-	2	1.9	4.3	0.16	2.4	C82-85,C96
Multiple myeloma	0	0	-	-	-	-	-	-	-	-	0.0	0.0	0.00	0.0	C90
Lymphoid leukaemia	1	0	0	-	-	1	-	-	-	-	0.1	0.2	0.01	0.1	C91
Myeloid leukaemia	0	0	-	-	-	-	-	-	-	-	0.0	0.0	0.00	0.0	C92-94
Leukaemia, unspecified	3	0	0	3	-	-	-	-	-	-	0.3	0.7	0.01	0.2	C95
Other and unspecified	28	4	36	-	1	2	5	4	7	5	2.8	6.3	0.46	5.8	O&U
All sites	448	35	15	27	18	57	75	81	72	83	45.4		6.05	84.3	ALL
All sites but C44	442	33	14	27	17	57	74	80	72	82	44.8	100.0	5.99	83.2	ALLbC44
Average annual population				250517	97019	53467	35224	25671	16280	15177					

Table 1. The Gambia (1997-1998)

NUMBER OF CASES BY AGE GROUP AND SUMMARY RATES OF INCIDENCE - FEMALE

SITE	ALL AGES	AGE UNK	MV (%)	0-	15-	25-	35-	45-	55-	65+	CRUDE RATE	%	CR 64	ASR (W)	ICD (10th)
Mouth	7	1	57	1	1	-	1	2	-	1	0.7	1.5	0.07	1.2	C00-06
Salivary gland	2	2	100	-	-	-	-	-	-	-	0.2	0.4	0.00	0.0	C07-08
Nasopharynx	0	0	-	-	-	-	-	-	-	-	0.0	0.0	0.00	0.0	C11
Other pharynx	0	0	-	-	-	-	-	-	-	-	0.0	0.0	0.00	0.0	C09-10,C12-14
Oesophagus	5	2	20	-	-	-	-	2	-	2	0.5	1.1	0.05	1.1	C15
Stomach	8	0	25	-	-	-	-	2	4	2	0.8	1.7	0.19	2.1	C16
Colon, rectum and anus	14	0	14	-	-	5	1	4	1	3	1.4	3.0	0.16	2.5	C18-21
Liver	91	8	2	1	1	17	19	16	17	13	8.9	19.5	1.45	17.6	C22
Gallbladder etc.	0	0	-	-	-	-	-	-	-	-	0.0	0.0	0.00	0.0	C23-24
Pancreas	7	0	57	-	-	-	1	1	3	2	0.7	1.5	0.17	1.9	C25
Larynx	1	0	100	-	1	-	-	-	-	-	0.1	0.2	0.02	0.2	C32
Trachea, bronchus and lung	3	0	67	-	1	-	-	1	1	-	0.3	0.6	0.04	0.5	C33-34
Bone	4	0	25	2	-	-	-	1	-	-	0.4	0.9	0.03	0.5	C40-41
Melanoma of skin	1	0	0	-	-	-	1	-	-	-	0.1	0.2	0.01	0.1	C43
Other skin	12	4	83	2	-	-	-	2	1	3	1.2		0.14	2.4	C44
Mesothelioma	0	0	-	-	-	-	-	-	-	-	0.0	0.0	0.00	0.0	C45
Kaposi sarcoma	4	1	100	-	-	2	-	-	-	-	0.4	0.9	0.03	0.4	C46
Peripheral nerves	0	0	-	-	-	-	-	-	-	-	0.0	0.0	0.00	0.0	C47
Connective and soft tissue	6	1	83	2	-	-	-	1	-	-	0.6	1.3	0.05	0.7	C49
Breast	41	10	51	-	3	4	11	8	-	5	4.0	8.8	0.47	7.0	C50
Vulva	1	0	0	-	-	-	-	-	-	-	0.1	0.2	0.03	0.2	C51
Vagina	2	0	0	-	1	1	-	-	-	-	0.2	0.4	0.01	0.2	C52
Cervix uteri	170	14	27	-	3	37	53	31	20	12	16.6	36.5	2.53	29.6	C53
Uterus	20	1	45	-	1	3	6	6	2	2	2.0	4.3	0.31	3.6	C54-55
Ovary	13	1	31	-	3	1	5	2	1	-	1.3	2.8	0.17	2.0	C56
Placenta	1	0	0	-	-	-	1	-	-	-	0.1	0.2	0.01	0.1	C58
Kidney	6	0	17	3	-	1	1	1	-	-	0.6	1.3	0.11	1.0	C64
Renal pelvis, ureter and other urinary	0	0	-	-	-	-	-	-	-	-	0.0	0.0	0.00	0.0	C65-66,C68
Bladder	3	0	0	-	-	-	-	-	2	2	0.3	0.6	0.01	0.5	C67
Eye	5	0	40	2	1	1	1	-	-	-	0.5	1.1	0.05	0.6	C69
Brain, nervous system	1	0	100	-	1	-	-	-	-	-	0.1	0.2	0.03	0.2	C70-72
Thyroid	4	2	50	-	-	-	-	1	1	-	0.4	0.9	0.12	1.0	C73
Hodgkin disease	3	1	100	1	1	-	-	-	-	-	0.3	0.6	0.00	0.4	C81
Non-Hodgkin lymphoma	13	3	69	8	-	-	-	1	-	1	1.3	2.8	0.04	1.0	C82-85,C96
Multiple myeloma	0	0	-	-	-	-	-	-	-	-	0.0	0.0	0.00	0.0	C90
Lymphoid leukaemia	0	0	-	-	-	-	-	-	-	-	0.0	0.0	0.00	0.0	C91
Myeloid leukaemia	0	0	-	-	-	-	-	-	-	-	0.0	0.0	0.00	0.0	C92-94
Leukaemia, unspecified	3	0	0	2	-	-	1	-	-	-	0.3	0.6	0.04	0.4	C95
Other and unspecified	27	3	26	4	3	2	2	5	2	6	2.6	5.8	0.28	4.6	O&U
All sites	478	53	30	27	21	74	104	83	60	56	46.7	100.0	6.71	84.5	ALL
All sites but C44	466	49	29	25	21	74	104	81	59	53	45.5	100.0	6.57	82.1	ALLbC44
Average annual population				246741	96651	73334	42577	23105	13728	15848					

Table 2. Childhood cancer, The Gambia (1988-1998)

	NUMBER OF CASES					REL. FREQ.(%)	RATES PER MILLION					
	0-4	5-9	10-14	**All**	*M/F*	Overall	0-4	5-9	10-14	Crude	**ASR**	%MV
Leukaemia	4	6	3	**13**	*1.6*	8.0	2.3	3.5	2.4	2.8	**2.7**	25.0
Acute lymphoid leukaemia	2	2	1	**5**	*1.5*	3.1	1.1	1.2	0.8	1.1	**1.1**	40.0
Lymphoma	14	29	22	**65**	*1.6*	40.1	8.0	17.1	17.6	13.8	**13.7**	59.3
Hodgkin disease	2	4	3	**9**	*3.5*	5.6	1.1	2.4	2.4	1.9	**1.9**	66.7
Burkitt lymphoma	5	13	11	**29**	*1.1*	17.9	2.9	7.7	8.8	6.2	**6.1**	44.8
Brain and spinal neoplasms	0	1	0	**1**	-	0.6	-	0.6	-	0.2	**0.2**	-
Neuroblastoma	1	0	1	**2**	*1.0*	1.2	0.6	-	0.8	0.4	**0.5**	50.0
Retinoblastoma	11	2	0	**13**	*0.9*	8.0	6.3	1.2	-	2.8	**2.8**	76.9
Wilms tumour	10	6	1	**17**	*1.4*	10.5	5.7	3.5	0.8	3.6	**3.6**	41.2
Bone tumours	0	0	8	**8**	*0.6*	4.9	-	-	6.4	1.7	**1.9**	12.5
Soft tissue sarcomas	3	2	0	**5**	*0.3*	3.1	1.7	1.2	-	1.1	**1.0**	100.0
Kaposi sarcoma	1	1	0	**2**	*1.0*	1.2	0.6	0.6	-	0.4	**0.4**	100.0
Germ cell tumours	1	0	0	**1**	-	0.6	0.6	-	-	0.2	**0.2**	100.0
Other	12	8	17	**37**	*0.9*	22.8	6.8	4.7	13.6	7.9	**8.1**	43.2
All	56	54	52	**162**	*1.2*	100.0	31.9	31.8	41.5	34.4	**34.7**	49.4

3.2.6 Ghana

Background

Climate: Tropical; warm and comparatively dry along the south-east coast; hot and humid in south-west; hot and dry in north

Terrain: Mostly low plains with dissected plateau in south-central area

Ethnic groups: Black African 99.8% (major tribes—Akan 44%, Moshi-Dagomba 16%, Ewe 13%, Ga 8%), European and other 0.2%

Religions: Indigenous beliefs 38%, Muslim 30%, Christian 24%, other 8%

Economy—overview: Well endowed with natural resources, Ghana has a much higher per capita output than many countries in West Africa, although it remains heavily dependent on international financial and technical assistance. Gold, timber and cocoa are major sources of foreign exchange. The domestic economy continues to revolve around subsistence agriculture, which accounts for 41% of GDP and employs 60% of the work force, mainly small landholders.

Industries: Mining, lumbering, light manufacturing, aluminium smelting, food processing

Agriculture—products: Cocoa, rice, coffee, cassava (tapioca), peanuts, corn, shea nuts, bananas; timber

Cancer registration

In 1972, with the aid of a grant from IARC, a cancer registry was established in the Korle Bu Teaching Hospital and later extended to cover all three major hospitals in Accra (Foli & Christian, 1976). There does not appear to be any comprehensive report of the results of this registry

Review of data

The only comprehensive review of the cancer profile in Ghana is the publication by Edington (1956), which presented data from histologically diagnosed cases from the Medical Research Institute, Accra, from 1942 to 1955 and autopsy cases from 1923 to 1955 (Table 1). Liver cancer accounted for 7.6% of cancers. Foli and Christian (1976), reporting cancer registry data, which included cases diagnosed using alpha-foetoprotein, pointed out that this was probably an underestimate; they found relative frequencies of 21.3% in men and 6.5% in women (overall, 14.5%).

Childhood cancer

Welbeck and Hesse (1998) reported the frequency of different cancers among children treated in the children's department of Korle Bu Teaching Hospital in 1992 to 1995 (Table 2). By far the most common malignant tumour was Burkitt lymphoma (60% of the total). The relatively high incidence of this tumour in Ghana had prompted the establishment of the Burkitt's Tumor Project at Korle Bu Hospital in 1965, and several publications have described epidemiological and clinical features of Burkitt lymphoma in Ghana (Biggar & Nkrumah, 1979; Biggar *et al.*, 1981).

References

Biggar, R.J, Nkrumah, F.K., Neequaye J. & Levine P.H. (1981) Changes in the presenting tumour site of Burkitt's lymphoma in Ghana, West Africa, 1965-1978. *Br. J. Cancer*, **43**, 632–636

Biggar, R.J. & Nkrumah, F.K. (1979) Burkitt's lymphoma in Ghana: urban-rural distribution, time-space clustering and seasonality. *Int. J. Cancer*, **23**, 330–336

Edington, G.M. (1956) Malignant disease in the Gold Coast. *Br. J. Cancer*, **10**, 595–608

Foli, A.K. & Christian, E.C. (1976) Primary liver-cell carcinoma in Accra [letter]. *Lancet*, **ii**, 696–697

Welbeck, J.E. & Hesse, A.A.J. (1998) Pattern of childhood malignancy in Korle Bu Teaching Hospital, Ghana. *W. Afr. J. Med.*, **17**, 81–84

Table 1. Ghana: case series

Site	Medical Research Institute, Accra, 1942–55 (Edington, 1956)						%HV
	Male		Female		Both sexes		
	No.	%	No.	%	No.	%	
Oral cavity[1]	13	3.3%	7	2.1%	53	4.4%	100
Nasopharynx	2	0.5%	2	0.6%	14	1.2%	93
Other pharynx	0	0.0%	0	0.0%	0	0.0%	
Oesophagus	1	0.3%	0	0.0%	1	0.1%	0
Stomach	23	5.9%	14	4.2%	43	3.6%	72
Colon/rectum	9	2.3%	2	0.6%	20	1.7%	90
Liver	67	17.1%	9	2.7%	91	7.6%	34
Pancreas	10	2.6%	0	0.0%	11	0.9%	18
Lung	2	0.5%	2	0.6%	4	0.3%	0
Melanoma					63	5.3%	95
Other skin[2]	38	9.7%	36	10.7%	153	12.8%	99
Kaposi sarcoma					10	0.8%	100
Breast	2	0.5%	42	12.5%	64	5.4%	97
Uterus (cervix & corpus)			71	21.1%	71	6.0%	99
Ovary etc.			33	9.8%	33	2.8%	88
Prostate	25	6.4%			25	2.1%	88
Penis	16	4.1%			16	1.3%	100
Bladder	20	5.1%	2	0.6%	30	2.5%	53
Kidney etc.	3	0.8%	1	0.3%	14	1.2%	79
Eye			1	0.3%	19	1.6%	100
Brain, nervous system					6	0.5%	100
Thyroid	5	1.3%	1	0.3%	13	1.1%	100
Non-Hodgkin lymphoma[3]					77	6.5%	100
Hodgkin's disease					30	2.5%	100
Myeloma					7	0.6%	100
Leukaemia (non-lymph.)					12	1.0%	100
ALL SITES	392	100.0%	337	100.0%	1192	100.0%	84

[1] Includes salivary gland tumours
[2] Distribution between males and females estimated from subtotals
[3] Includes lymphocytic leukaemia

Table 2. Ghana: childhood cancer

Cancer	Korle Bu Hospital, Accra, 1992–95 (Welbeck & Hesse, 1998)	
	No.	%
Leukaemia	21	8.1%
Acute lymphocytic leukaemia		0.0%
Lymphoma	179	69.4%
Burkitt lymphoma	153	59.3%
Hodgkin disease	6	2.3%
Brain and spinal neoplasms	2	0.8%
Neuroblastoma	3	1.2%
Retinoblastoma	22	8.5%
Wilms tumour	20	7.8%
Bone tumours		0.0%
Soft-tissue sarcomas		0.0%
Kaposi sarcoma		0.0%
Other	7*	2.7%
Total	254	100.0%

* 5 cases of hepatoma

3.2.7 Guinea

Background

Climate: Varies between regions, but generally hot and humid; monsoonal-type rainy season (June to November) with south-westerly winds; dry season (December to May) with north-easterly harmattan winds

Terrain: Generally flat coastal plain, hilly to mountainous interior, with savannah forest in some areas.

Ethnic groups: Peuhl, Malinke, Soussou and other smaller tribal groups.

Religions: Muslim 85%, Christian 8%, indigenous beliefs 7%

Economy—overview: Although possessing major mineral, hydropower and agricultural resources, Guinea remains one of the poorest countries in the world. The agricultural sector employs 80% of the work force. Guinea possesses over 25% of the world's bauxite reserves and is the second largest bauxite producer. The mining sector accounted for about 75% of exports in 1995.

Industries: Bauxite, gold, diamonds; alumina refining; light manufacturing and agricultural processing industries

Agriculture—products: Rice, coffee, pineapples, palm kernels, cassava (tapioca), bananas, sweet potatoes; cattle, sheep, goats; poultry; timber

Cancer registration

The cancer registry of Guinea is population-based, covering the capital city of Conakry. It was established in 1990 and is located in the Department of Pathology at the University Hospital of Donka, Conakry. There were approximately one million inhabitants in the city according to 1993 estimates. However, over the last decade Guinea has experienced a massive influx of refugees to the capital city and the forest region from neighbouring countries at war. Since 1990, refugees from Liberia, then Sierra Leone and Guinea Bissau have entered the country.

Case-finding is mainly active. Personnel from the registry search for cases from all hospitals that provide services to patients with cancer. These include two hospitals within the city, namely the university hospital (CHU) de Donka and Hôpital Ignace Deen, where major services, including surgery, urology, general medicine and gynaecology, are provided. Regular visits are made to these two hospitals, with visits to health centres and private clinics less frequently. The registry also relies on notifications received from medical officers in selected hospitals in Kindia, Kamsar and Fria, where some patients from Conakry receive treatment.

Copies of all reports of cancer cases diagnosed by histopathology, ultrasonography or specific biochemical assays (human chorionic gonadotrophin (HCG), alpha-foetoprotein) are received by the registry. For cultural and religious reasons, autopsies are not routinely performed in Guinea except for medico-legal purposes.

A six-month duration of stay is used as the criterion to distinguish cancer patients who are usual residents of the city from temporary visitors (cases domiciled with their families for the purpose of receiving medical care). There is no system of death registration in Guinea, although deaths occurring in hospital are certified. Death certificates are not used as a source of information.

The cancer registry of Guinea was computerized from its inception, using the CANREG software of IARC.

Review of data

Cancer registry

The first results from the cancer registry, for the period 1992–95, were published by Koulibaly *et al.* (1997).

For the four-year period under review (1996–99), 1161 males and 1486 females were registered with cancer among residents of Conakry. Table 1 shows the distribution of cancers by sex, site and age group, as well as percentage frequency, crude and age-standardized rates (ASR). The population at risk has been estimated from the 1993 census.

Liver cancer ranks as the most common cancer in males (40.4%, ASR 37.6 per 100 000) followed by lung cancer (9%, ASR 8.2), prostate cancer (5.5%, ASR 9.7) and stomach cancer (5.3%, ASR 6.1).

In females, cervix cancer (45.4%, ASR 49.6 per 100 000) ranks first, followed by cancers of the breast (12.9%, ASR 15.5) and liver (9.9%, ASR 12.1).

43% of cancers in men and 59% in women had a diagnosis based on histology. Only 15% of liver cancers were diagnosed on the basis of microscopic examination of tissue. Liver cancer is three times more common in males than in females, in contrast to stomach cancer, for which the male/female ratio is 1.5.

The incidence of cervix cancer in Guinea is one of the highest recorded in the world.

Age-specific rates of liver cancer show a rapid increase in early age to reach a peak at ages 45–49 years among the male population. In contrast, a less dramatic increase in rates is observed in females. In this population, the incidence of liver cancer reaches a plateau at age 50 years. In both sexes, most liver cancers occur before the age of 55 years; as in most data-sets from sub-Saharan Africa.

Childhood cancer

Table 2 presents the neoplasms occurring in the childhood population (age 0–14 years) of Conakry. There were a total of 193 cases, with 60.6% having a histological diagnosis. The most frequent childhood cancer was lymphoma (64 cases, 33.2% of the total), of which 34 (17.6%) were Burkitt lymphoma, with an age-standardized incidence of 11.9 per million. Retinoblastoma comprised 16.1% of cancers (ASR 8.6 per million). Some underdiagnosis of childhood cancers is likely, in view of the low rates recorded and the few cases of leukaemias and brain tumours.

Reference

Koulibaly, M., Kabba, I.S., Cisse, A., Diallo, S.B., Diallo, M.B., Keita, N., Camara, N.D., Diallo, M.S., Sylla, B.S. & Parkin, D.M. (1997) Cancer incidence in Conakry, Guinea: first results from the Cancer Registry 1992-1995. *Int. J. Cancer,* **70**, 39–45

Table 1. Guinea, Conakry (1996-1999)

NUMBER OF CASES BY AGE GROUP AND SUMMARY RATES OF INCIDENCE - MALE

SITE	ALL AGES	AGE UNK	MV (%)	0-	15-	25-	35-	45-	55-	65+	CRUDE RATE	%	CR 64	ASR (W)	ICD (10th)
Mouth	33	0	67	-	1	2	11	12	4	3	1.4	2.9	0.21	2.9	C00-06
Salivary gland	3	0	67	1	-	-	1	1	-	-	0.1	0.3	0.01	0.2	C07-08
Nasopharynx	5	0	60	-	-	1	1	1	2	-	0.2	0.4	0.05	0.5	C11
Other pharynx	18	0	39	-	-	2	5	7	2	2	0.8	1.6	0.11	1.6	C09-10,C12-14
Oesophagus	13	0	62	-	-	4	2	6	1	-	0.6	1.2	0.08	0.9	C15
Stomach	59	0	58	-	1	2	17	18	11	10	2.6	5.3	0.38	6.1	C16
Colon, rectum and anus	35	0	57	-	-	3	12	8	8	4	1.5	3.1	0.23	3.2	C18-21
Liver	453	0	15	5	-	28	166	143	81	29	19.8	40.4	3.02	37.6	C22
Gallbladder etc.	1	0	100	-	-	-	-	-	1	-	0.0	0.1	0.02	0.1	C23-24
Pancreas	8	0	25	-	-	-	3	5	-	-	0.3	0.7	0.08	0.8	C25
Larynx	7	0	57	-	-	-	3	2	1	1	0.3	0.6	0.04	0.7	C32
Trachea, bronchus and lung	101	0	27	-	-	6	43	34	11	7	4.4	9.0	0.61	8.2	C33-34
Bone	22	0	91	9	3	1	1	5	3	-	1.0	2.0	0.10	1.3	C40-41
Melanoma of skin	18	0	100	-	-	1	2	9	6	-	0.8	1.6	0.16	1.6	C43
Other skin	40	0	55	-	-	3	11	13	9	4	1.7	3.4	0.30	3.8	C44
Mesothelioma	0	0	-	-	-	-	-	-	-	-	0.0	0.0	0.00	0.0	C45
Kaposi sarcoma	2	0	100	-	-	-	-	2	-	-	0.1	0.2	0.02	0.2	C46
Peripheral nerves	5	0	100	2	2	1	-	-	-	-	0.2	0.4	0.01	0.2	C47
Connective and soft tissue	26	0	81	2	2	1	5	11	3	2	1.1	2.3	0.16	2.2	C49
Breast	0	0	-	-	-	-	-	-	-	-	0.0	0.0	0.00	0.0	C50
Penis	0	0	-	-	-	-	-	-	-	-	0.0	0.0	0.00	0.0	C60
Prostate	62	0	45	-	-	-	-	10	26	26	2.7	5.5	0.46	9.7	C61
Testis	6	0	67	1	-	-	1	2	2	-	0.3	0.5	0.03	0.3	C62
Kidney	26	0	54	16	-	-	2	6	1	1	1.1	2.3	0.09	1.5	C64
Renal pelvis, ureter and other urinary	0	0	-	-	-	-	-	-	-	-	0.0	0.0	0.00	0.0	C65-66,C68
Bladder	12	0	58	-	-	1	-	2	6	3	0.5	1.1	0.10	1.5	C67
Eye	31	0	10	15	2	4	4	2	3	1	1.4	2.8	0.11	1.7	C69
Brain, nervous system	2	0	50	-	-	1	-	1	-	-	0.1	0.2	0.01	0.1	C70-72
Thyroid	6	0	67	-	2	-	1	2	-	1	0.3	0.5	0.02	0.5	C73
Hodgkin disease	27	0	100	6	4	4	9	1	1	2	1.2	2.4	0.09	1.6	C81
Non-Hodgkin lymphoma	61	0	95	17	6	7	10	11	7	3	2.7	5.4	0.29	3.9	C82-85,C96
Multiple myeloma	0	0	-	-	-	-	-	-	-	-	0.0	0.0	0.00	0.0	C90
Lymphoid leukaemia	12	0	100	3	3	-	4	1	1	-	0.5	1.1	0.05	0.6	C91
Myeloid leukaemia	14	0	100	-	3	1	6	2	1	1	0.6	1.2	0.06	0.9	C92-94
Leukaemia, unspecified	2	0	100	-	-	-	1	1	-	-	0.1	0.2	0.01	0.1	C95
Other and unspecified	51	0	69	1	-	3	10	22	6	9	2.2	4.5	0.32	5.4	O&U
All sites	1161	0	43	78	29	77	331	340	197	109	50.7	100.0	7.24	99.8	ALL
All sites but C44	1121	0	42	78	29	74	320	327	188	105	49.0		6.94	96.0	ALLbC44
Average annual population				250782	109336	93152	62963	30064	18015	7810					

Table 1. Guinea, Conakry (1996-1999)

NUMBER OF CASES BY AGE GROUP AND SUMMARY RATES OF INCIDENCE - FEMALE

SITE	ALL AGES	AGE UNK	MV (%)	0-	15-	25-	35-	45-	55-	65+	CRUDE RATE	%	CR 64	ASR (W)	ICD (10th)
Mouth	14	0	79	-	1	2	5	2	3	1	0.6	1.0	0.10	1.3	C00-06
Salivary gland	4	0	75	-	-	1	1	2	-	-	0.2	0.3	0.02	0.3	C07-08
Nasopharynx	1	0	100	-	-	1	1	-	-	-	0.0	0.1	0.00	0.1	C11
Other pharynx	5	0	20	-	1	1	3	1	-	-	0.2	0.3	0.02	0.3	C09-10,C12-14
Oesophagus	5	0	40	-	-	-	1	3	1	-	0.2	0.3	0.05	0.5	C15
Stomach	34	0	56	-	-	3	7	13	7	4	1.5	2.3	0.26	3.6	C16
Colon, rectum and anus	30	0	87	-	1	8	5	5	5	6	1.4	2.1	0.16	3.2	C18-21
Liver	144	0	15	3	2	11	58	36	27	7	6.5	9.9	1.02	12.1	C22
Gallbladder etc.	1	0	100	-	-	-	1	-	-	-	0.0	0.1	0.00	0.1	C23-24
Pancreas	5	0	60	-	-	-	1	4	-	-	0.2	0.3	0.04	0.4	C25
Larynx	1	0	0	-	-	-	-	1	-	-	0.0	0.1	0.01	0.1	C32
Trachea, bronchus and lung	20	0	20	-	-	1	10	5	3	1	0.9	1.4	0.14	1.7	C33-34
Bone	10	0	80	2	1	2	1	1	2	1	0.5	0.7	0.05	0.8	C40-41
Melanoma of skin	14	0	100	-	-	-	5	6	1	2	0.6	1.0	0.09	1.5	C43
Other skin	33	0	70	-	1	3	11	7	8	3	1.5	2.3	0.26	3.2	C44
Mesothelioma	0	0	-	-	-	-	-	-	-	-	0.0	0.0	0.00	0.0	C45
Kaposi sarcoma	1	0	100	-	-	1	-	-	-	-	0.0	0.1	0.00	0.0	C46
Peripheral nerves	2	0	100	-	-	-	-	-	-	1	0.1	0.1	0.03	0.3	C47
Connective and soft tissue	11	0	82	2	1	1	1	3	2	1	0.5	0.8	0.08	1.0	C49
Breast	188	0	74	-	5	21	69	51	34	8	8.5	12.9	1.33	15.5	C50
Vulva	8	0	88	-	-	-	2	1	2	3	0.4	0.6	0.04	1.2	C51
Vagina	9	0	100	-	2	-	3	3	3	-	0.4	0.6	0.10	0.9	C52
Cervix uteri	659	0	54	-	3	103	265	202	62	24	29.7	45.4	4.03	49.6	C53
Uterus	44	0	36	-	-	2	14	12	12	4	2.0	3.0	0.36	4.5	C54-55
Ovary	51	0	88	-	8	8	10	13	7	4	2.3	3.5	0.32	4.4	C56
Placenta	9	0	100	-	5	4	-	-	-	-	0.4	0.6	0.02	0.4	C58
Kidney	14	0	43	7	1	2	1	1	-	-	0.6	1.0	0.08	0.8	C64
Renal pelvis, ureter and other urinary	1	0	100	-	-	-	1	-	-	-	0.0	0.1	0.00	0.0	C65-66,C68
Bladder	13	0	38	-	-	1	1	3	6	3	0.6	0.9	0.13	1.9	C67
Eye	10	0	10	6	2	1	1	1	-	-	0.5	0.7	0.02	0.4	C69
Brain, nervous system	0	0	-	-	-	-	-	-	-	-	0.0	0.0	0.00	0.0	C70-72
Thyroid	17	0	47	-	-	3	5	5	4	-	0.8	1.2	0.13	1.3	C73
Hodgkin disease	10	0	100	2	1	1	5	1	-	-	0.5	0.7	0.03	0.4	C81
Non-Hodgkin lymphoma	44	0	100	17	4	9	6	5	2	1	2.0	3.0	0.17	2.4	C82-85,C96
Multiple myeloma	0	0	-	-	-	-	-	-	-	-	0.0	0.0	0.00	0.0	C90
Lymphoid leukaemia	10	0	100	1	1	1	3	2	-	2	0.5	0.7	0.03	1.0	C91
Myeloid leukaemia	11	0	100	-	3	3	2	3	-	-	0.5	0.8	0.05	0.6	C92-94
Leukaemia, unspecified	3	0	100	-	-	-	-	1	1	-	0.1	0.2	0.04	0.3	C95
Other and unspecified	50	0	80	1	3	5	15	14	4	8	2.3	3.4	0.26	5.0	O&U
All sites	1486	0	59	42	45	197	510	409	200	83	67.0	100.0	9.49	121.0	ALL
All sites but C44	1453	0	58	42	44	194	499	402	192	80	65.5	100.0	9.23	117.7	ALLbC44
Average annual population				245143	106017	88641	62420	31151	14583	6635					

Table 2. Childhood cancer, Guinea, Conakry (1993-1999)

	NUMBER OF CASES					REL. FREQ.(%)	RATES PER MILLION					
	0-4	5-9	10-14	**All**	*M/F*	Overall	0-4	5-9	10-14	Crude	**ASR**	%MV
Leukaemia	5	3	3	**11**	*1.8*	5.7	3.5	2.8	4.2	3.4	**3.5**	80.0
Acute lymphoid leukaemia	4	1	1	**6**	*1.0*	3.1	2.8	0.9	1.4	1.9	**1.8**	100.0
Lymphoma	9	24	31	**64**	*1.1*	33.2	6.4	22.4	43.4	20.0	**22.3**	87.5
Hodgkin disease	1	6	7	**14**	*3.7*	7.3	0.7	5.6	9.8	4.4	**4.9**	100.0
Burkitt lymphoma	6	11	17	**34**	*0.9*	17.6	4.2	10.3	23.8	10.6	**11.9**	100.0
Brain and spinal neoplasms	0	0	1	**1**	-	0.5	-	-	1.4	0.3	**0.4**	100.0
Neuroblastoma	0	0	0	**0**	-	-	-	-	-	-	**-**	-
Retinoblastoma	25	6	0	**31**	*2.1*	16.1	17.7	5.6	-	9.7	**8.6**	-
Wilms tumour	6	6	7	**19**	*2.8*	9.8	4.2	5.6	9.8	5.9	**6.3**	68.4
Bone tumours	3	3	8	**14**	*3.7*	7.3	2.1	2.8	11.2	4.4	**5.0**	85.7
Soft tissue sarcomas	1	2	5	**8**	*3.0*	4.1	0.7	1.9	7.0	2.5	**2.9**	50.0
Kaposi sarcoma	0	0	0	**0**	-	-	-	-	-	-	**-**	-
Germ cell tumours	2	0	0	**2**	*1.0*	1.0	1.4	-	-	0.6	**0.5**	100.0
Other	12	13	18	**43**	*1.4*	22.3	8.5	12.1	25.2	13.4	**14.5**	30.2
All	63	57	73	**193**	*1.6*	100.0	44.5	53.2	102.1	60.3	**64.0**	60.6

3.2.8 Guinea-Bissau

Background

Climate: Tropical; generally hot and humid; monsoonal-type rainy season (June to November) with southwesterly winds; dry season (December to May) with northeasterly harmattan winds

Terrain: Mostly low coastal plain rising to savanna in east

Ethnic groups: African 99% (Balanta 30%, Fula 20%, Manjaca 14%, Mandinga 13%, Papel 7%), European and mulatto less than 1%

Religions: Indigenous beliefs 50%, Muslim 45%, Christian 5%

Economy—overview: Guinea-Bissau depends mainly on farming and fishing. The country ranks sixth in cashew production. Guinea-Bissau exports fish and seafood along with small amounts of peanuts, palm kernels, and timber. Rice is the major crop and staple food.

Industries: Agricultural products processing, beer, soft drinks

Agriculture—products: Rice, corn, beans, cassava (tapioca), cashew nuts, peanuts, palm kernels, cotton; fishing and forest potential not fully exploited

Cancer registration

There has been no cancer registry in Guinea-Bissau.

Review of data

There is no published material on the cancer profile in the country.

3.2.9 Liberia

Background

Climate: Tropical; hot, humid; dry winters with hot days and cool to cold nights; wet, cloudy summers with frequent heavy showers

Terrain: Mostly flat to rolling coastal plains rising to rolling plateau and low mountains in north-east

Ethnic groups: Indigenous African tribes 95% (including Kpelle, Bassa, Gio, Kru, Grebo, Mano, Krahn, Gola, Gbandi, Loma, Kissi, Vai, and Bella), Americo-Liberians 2.5% (descendants of immigrants from the United States who had been slaves)

Religions: Traditional 70%, Muslim 20%, Christian 10%

Economy—overview: Civil war since 1990 has destroyed much of Liberia's economy, especially the infrastructure in and around Monrovia. Many businessmen have fled the country, taking capital and expertise with them, although some have returned. Richly endowed with water, mineral resources, forests, and a climate favourable to agriculture, Liberia used to be a producer and exporter of basic products, while local manufacturing, mainly foreign owned, was small in scope.

Industries: Rubber processing, food processing, construction materials, furniture, palm-oil processing, iron ore, diamonds

Agriculture—products: Rubber, coffee, cocoa, rice, cassava (tapioca), palm oil, sugar-cane, bananas; sheep, goats; timber

Cancer registration

There is no active cancer registration in the country.

Review of data

A cancer registry functioned in Liberia for around 10 years, from 1973–82. It was located in the Department of Radiotherapy of the J.F. Kennedy Memorial Hospital in the capital, Monrovia. The registry attempted national cancer registration, achieved by personal visits of the Director to all 34 hospitals throughout the country. The only pathology service in the country (in the J.F. Kennedy Memorial Hospital) was another important source of information (although a few biopsies, especially from 'concession' hospitals belonging to private companies, were sent overseas). Registration was believed to be relatively complete for cancer cases from whom a biopsy was taken or receiving hospital inpatient care. However, these must have been a minority of cases, since the crude incidence rates were very low (15.6 per 100 000 for males and 21.2 per 100 000 for females in 1976–80).

The registry produced two reports, and the results for 1973–77 were published by Sobo (1982) and for 1976–80 by Sobo (1986). Although the periods overlap, the two sets of results are shown in Table 1. During these two periods, an average 300 cases of cancer were recorded by the registry each year.

In 1973–77, liver (16.2 %) and prostate (11.0 %) cancers were the most common in men. Bladder cancers constituted 7.7% of all male cancers, about the same frequency as Burkitt lymphoma and Hodgkin disease. The ranking was somewhat different in the period 1976–80, when non-Hodgkin lymphomas (14.9%) and prostate (11.3 %) and liver (10.9 %) cancers were the commonest.

In females, cervix (28.2%), breast (11.1%) and ovary (10.4%) cancers were the most common malignancies in 1973–77. The ranking was similar in 1976–80, with these three sites accounting for 30.0%, 15.0% and 8.9% of cancers, respectively.

The fluctuations in proportions probably relate to variations in diagnosis, rather than any change in incidence. Thus, it was noted that in 1973–77, 63.7% of two cancers had a histological diagnosis; this is a very high proportion and implies that liver cancers were almost certainly under-diagnosed or under-registered. Several studies have confirmed a high rate of infection with hepatitis B virus in the Liberian population (Frentzel-Beyme *et al.*, 1977; Skinhoj, 1979; Prince *et al.*, 1981). The relatively high frequency of bladder cancer and the high percentage among them of squamous-cell carcinomas (75% of histologically diagnosed cases) are consistent with the presence of endemic schistosomiasis (Sobo, 1982).

No data are available on the frequency of Kaposi sarcoma in these time periods. Wendler *et al.* (1986) found no antibody to HIV in 935 serum samples obtained in Liberia between 1976 and 1984.

Childhood cancer

Burkitt lymphoma was by far the most common cancer of children, accounting for 49.6% of cancers in boys and 59.2% of cancers in girls in 1973–77, and 44% of cancers in boys and 41.9% of cancers in girls in 1976–80. Hodgkin disease also appears to be relatively frequent in childhood.

References

Frentzel-Beyme, R.R., Traavik, T., Ulstrup, J. & Tonjum, A.M. (1977).The prevalence of HB-Ag (Australia antigen) in the population of Liberia. *Soc. Sci. Med.*, **11**, 749–756

Prince, A.M., White, T., Pollock, N., Riddle, J., Brotman, B. & Richardson, L. (1981) Epidemiology of hepatitis B infection in Liberian infants *Infect. Immun.*, **32**, 675–680

Skinhoj, P. (1979) Hepatitis B virus infection in children. A sero-epidemiological study in three endemic areas.*Trans. R. Soc. Trop. Med. Hyg.*, **73**, 549–552

Sobo, A.O. (1982). A review of cases registered from Liberia Cancer Registry 1973-1977. *Cancer*, **49**, 1945–1950

Sobo, A.O. (1986) Liberia Cancer Registry, 1976–80. In: Parkin D.M., ed., *Cancer Occurrence in Developing Countries* (IARC Scientific Publications No. 75), Lyon, IARC, pp. 55–58

Wendler, I., Schneider, J., Gras, B., Fleming, A.F., Hunsmann, G. & Schmitz, H. (1986) Seroepidemiology of human immunodeficiency virus in Africa. *Br. Med. J. (Clin. Res. Ed.)*, **27**, 782–785

Table 1. Liberia: case series

| Site | Liberia 1973–77 (Sobo, 1982) | | | | | Liberia 1976–80 (Sobo, 1986) | | | | |
| | Male | | Female | | %HV | Male | | Female | | %HV |
	No.	%	No.	%		No.	%	No.	%	
Oral cavity						30	4.5%	17	1.9%	
Nasopharynx	29	3.8%	15	1.7%		0	0.0%	1	0.1%	
Other pharynx						4	0.6%	0	0.0%	
Oesophagus	10	1.3%	1	0.1%		7	1.1%	0	0.0%	
Stomach	14	1.8%	9	1.0%		23	3.5%	12	1.3%	
Colon/rectum	21	2.7%	23	2.7%		26	3.9%	22	2.5%	
Liver[a]	125	16.2%	47	5.4%	63.7	72	10.9%	35	3.9%	
Pancreas[b]	9	1.2%	8	0.9%		4	0.6%	7	0.8%	
Lung	30	3.9%	11	1.3%		10	1.5%	5	0.6%	
Melanoma	25	3.3%	26	3.0%		15	2.3%	24	2.7%	
Other skin	30	3.9%	22	2.5%		20	3.0%	11	1.2%	
Kaposi sarcoma										
Breast			96	11.1%	68.8	4	0.6%	133	15.0%	
Cervix uteri			244	28.2%	75.8			267	30.0%	
Corpus uteri			22	2.5%				37	4.2%	
Ovary etc.			90	10.4%	82.2			79	8.9%	
Prostate	84	11.0%			82.1	75	11.3%			
Penis	9	1.2%				10	1.5%			
Bladder	59	7.7%	18	2.1%	100	35	5.3%	23	2.6%	
Kidney etc.	18	2.3%	9	1.0%		7	1.1%	8	0.9%	
Eye	3	0.4%	6	0.7%		5	0.8%	7	0.8%	
Brain, nervous system	7	0.9%	1	0.1%		3	0.5%	2	0.2%	
Thyroid	12	1.6%	18	2.1%		15	2.3%	18	2.0%	
Non-Hodgkin lymphoma	80	10.4%	46	5.3%	86.3	99	14.9%	45	5.1%	
Hodgkin disease	65	8.5%	16	1.8%	73.8[c]	43	6.5%	22	2.5%	
Myeloma						4	0.6%	1	0.1%	
Leukaemia	26	3.4%	16	1.8%		11	1.7%	8	0.9%	
ALL SITES	766	100.0%	866	100.0%		663	100.0%	889	100.0%	

[a] Includes gallbladder

[b] Includes retroperitoneum

[c] Males only

3.2.10 Mali

Background

Climate: Subtropical to arid; hot and dry March to June; rainy, humid and mild June to November; cool and dry November to February

Terrain: Mostly flat to rolling northern plains covered by sand; savanna in south, rugged hills in north-east

Ethnic groups: Mande 50% (Bambara, Malinke, Sarakole), Peul 17%, Mowsi 12%, Songhvi 6%, Tuareg and Moor 10%, other 5%

Religions: Muslim 90%, indigenous beliefs 9%, Christian 1%

Economy—overview: 65% of the land area of Mali is desert or semi-desert. Economic activity is largely confined to the riverine area irrigated by the Niger. About 10% of the population is nomadic and some 80% of the labour force is engaged in farming and fishing. Industrial activity is concentrated on processing farm commodities. Mali is heavily dependent on foreign aid and vulnerable to fluctuations in world prices for cotton and gold, its main export.

Industries: Minor local consumer goods production and food processing; construction; phosphate and gold mining

Agriculture—products: Cotton, millet, rice, corn, vegetables, peanuts; cattle, sheep, goats

Cancer registration

The Cancer Registry of Mali started operations in 1986. It is located in the Department of Pathology of the National Institute of Public Health Research in the capital city, Bamako. This department provides the basic source of information for the registry, and is the only histopathology service in the country.

The registry was from the start conceived as population-based covering the District of Bamako, which includes the population of the capital city and its immediate surroundings. In 1987, the population was 646 163. As in most developing countries, the health care system in Mali is far from adequate. Hospitals, clinics and other health facilities are concentrated in the capital city of Bamako. Two major hospitals provide tertiary care services: Hôpital Gabriel Touré, and Hôpital de Point G.

Active case-finding is carried out by a cancer registrar who regularly visits these two public hospitals and Kati hospital, 15 km distant. Visits are also made to two specialized institutes (dermatology and ophthalmology) and to two centres of maternal and child health staffed by gynaecologists. In each service, there is a contact person for the registry, usually the head nurse who, under the supervision of the consulting physician, records information on all cancer diagnoses using a form provided by the registry. During his regular visits, the technician checks these forms for completeness and verifies the information contained from other sources (e.g., ward books, operation lists), as well as with the medical and nursing staff. The frequency of visits is determined by the number of the cases detected.

Death registration is incomplete in Mali and covers only the city of Bamako, where a death certificate is required in order to obtain a burial permit. Copies of death certificates are obtained and the death register is scanned by the registry as a source of information.

Registration is confined to 'usual residents', defined as having lived for at least six months in Bamako or having the intention to stay for six months. For data management, the registry uses the CANREG software.

Review of data

Cancer Registry

The results from the cancer registry have been published for 1988–82 (Parkin *et al.*, 1997) and for 1993–97 (Parkin *et al.*, 2002). An error was present in the population at risk data in the former, and for this reason, both sets of data are published together here, which allows a comparison between them. In the "Summary Tables" that accompany the site-specific chapters, the data are presented for the full ten-year period 1988–97.

In the more recent period (Table 2), the most common cancers of men are liver (ASR 33.4 per 100 000; 36.2 %), stomach (ASR 17.3; 15.8%) and bladder (ASR 9.6; 9.6%). Only 3% of the liver malignancies in men were confirmed by histology. In females, cervix (ASR 32.0 per 100 000; 27.1%), breast (ASR 17.2, 15.2%), stomach (ASR 16.6; 13.1%) and liver (ASR 15.1; 12.0%) are the most frequent cancer sites. Age-specific incidence for cervix cancer rises rapidly after age 15 years, reaching a peak after age 45. Over 60% of the malignancies occurring in the cervix uteri were based on histology.

Comparison with the earlier data for 1988–1992 (Table 1) suggests some decline in the incidence of liver cancer (–23% in men and –20% in women) and an increase in the incidence of prostate cancer (+81%), and breast cancer (+38%). The incidence of stomach cancer and cervix cancer is much the same. Kaposi sarcoma remains quite rare (2–3% of cancers in men, 0.5–1% cancers in women) with little change in the incidence.

An interesting feature of these data is the moderately high incidence of stomach cancer in both sexes, which is in contrast with series from neighbouring countries. Whether this is artificial (inclusion of non-residents, increasing availability of gastroscopy) or related to local diets rich in nitrosamines as suggested in an earlier review (see Bayo *et al.*, 1990) remains to be investigated further.

Childhood cancer

Table 3 presents the neoplasms occurring in the childhood population (age 0–14 years) of Bamako. Out of a total of 133 cases, 67.7% had a histological diagnosis. The most frequent childhood cancers were lymphomas (32 cases, 24.1% of the total, of which only three were were Burkitt lymphoma), and retinoblastoma (19.5% of the total, corresponding to an ASR of 7.7 per million). Some underdiagnosis of childhood cancers is likely, as witnessed by the low rates, the absence of any central nervous system tumours, and small number of leukaemia cases (of which none was diagnosed as acute lymphocytic).

References

Bayo, S., Parkin, D.M., Koumare, A.K., Diallo, A.N., Ba, T., Soumare, S. & Sangare, S. (1990) Cancer in Mali, 1987-1988. *Int. J. Cancer*, **45**, 679–684

Parkin, D.M., Muir, C.S., Whelan, S.L., Gao, Y.-T., Ferlay, J. & Powell, J. (1992) *Cancer Incidence in Five Continents*, Vol. VI (IARC Scientific Publications No. 120), Lyon, IARC

Parkin, D.M., Whelan, S.L., Ferlay, J., Raymond, L. & Young, J., eds (1997) *Cancer Incidence in Five Continents*, Vol. VII (IARC Scientific Publications No. 143), Lyon, IARC

Parkin, D.M., Whelan, S.L., Ferlay, J., Teppo, L. and Thomas, D.B. eds (2002) *Cancer Incidence in Five Continents*, Vol. VIII (IARC Scientific Publications No. 155), Lyon, IARC

Table 1. Mali, Bamako (1988-1992)

NUMBER OF CASES BY AGE GROUP AND SUMMARY RATES OF INCIDENCE - MALE

SITE	ALL AGES	AGE UNK	MV (%)	0-	15-	25-	35-	45-	55-	65+	CRUDE RATE	%	CR 64	ASR (W)	ICD (10th)
Mouth	10	0	70	-	-	1	2	1	5	1	0.6	1.0	0.11	1.2	C00-06
Salivary gland	0	0	-	-	-	-	-	-	-	-	0.0	0.0	0.00	0.0	C07-08
Nasopharynx	1	0	0	-	-	-	-	1	-	-	0.1	0.1	0.01	0.1	C11
Other pharynx	6	0	33	-	-	-	3	2	-	1	0.3	0.6	0.03	0.6	C09-10,C12-14
Oesophagus	12	0	42	-	-	-	2	5	3	2	0.7	1.2	0.12	1.5	C15
Stomach	143	0	50	1	3	10	20	47	31	31	7.9	14.5	1.22	17.3	C16
Colon, rectum and anus	48	0	40	-	3	6	14	6	10	9	2.6	4.9	0.37	5.3	C18-21
Liver	416	0	3	2	22	61	97	95	79	60	22.9	42.1	3.26	43.5	C22
Gallbladder etc.	1	0	100	-	-	-	-	-	-	1	0.1	0.1	0.00	0.2	C23-24
Pancreas	17	0	35	-	-	1	2	5	4	5	0.9	1.7	0.13	2.2	C25
Larynx	15	0	0	-	1	-	1	4	5	4	0.8	1.5	0.16	2.1	C32
Trachea, bronchus and lung	38	0	18	-	-	3	6	12	9	8	2.1	3.8	0.33	4.6	C33-34
Bone	8	0	88	2	3	-	1	-	1	1	0.4	0.8	0.04	0.7	C40-41
Melanoma of skin	5	0	100	-	1	2	-	-	1	1	0.3	0.5	0.03	0.4	C43
Other skin	36	0	78	1	1	1	8	8	8	9	2.0		0.29	4.5	C44
Mesothelioma	0	0	-	-	-	-	-	-	-	-	0.0	0.0	0.00	0.0	C45
Kaposi sarcoma	19	0	100	-	2	7	1	6	-	3	1.0	1.9	0.11	1.7	C46
Peripheral nerves	0	0	-	-	-	-	-	-	-	-	0.0	0.0	0.00	0.0	C47
Connective and soft tissue	4	0	75	-	2	-	1	1	-	-	0.2	0.4	0.02	0.3	C49
Breast	3	0	33	-	-	-	1	1	1	-	0.2	0.3	0.03	0.5	C50
Penis	2	0	50	-	-	-	-	1	-	1	0.1	0.2	0.01	0.3	C60
Prostate	33	0	21	-	-	-	-	5	7	21	1.8	3.3	0.17	5.3	C61
Testis	4	0	25	-	-	2	1	1	-	-	0.2	0.4	0.03	0.3	C62
Kidney	17	0	29	8	1	1	1	3	2	1	0.9	1.7	0.09	1.2	C64
Renal pelvis, ureter and other urinary	2	0	100	2	-	-	-	-	-	-	0.1	0.2	0.00	0.1	C65-66,C68
Bladder	71	0	8	-	3	4	10	14	15	25	3.9	7.2	0.51	9.5	C67
Eye	16	0	50	9	2	-	1	2	1	1	0.9	1.6	0.06	1.1	C69
Brain, nervous system	3	0	0	1	1	-	1	-	-	-	0.2	0.3	0.03	0.3	C70-72
Thyroid	3	0	100	-	1	1	1	-	-	-	0.2	0.3	0.01	0.1	C73
Hodgkin disease	19	0	95	7	7	4	1	-	-	-	1.0	1.9	0.05	0.8	C81
Non-Hodgkin lymphoma	24	0	100	3	3	6	3	1	3	5	1.3	2.4	0.12	2.2	C82-85,C96
Multiple myeloma	0	0	-	-	-	-	-	-	-	-	0.0	0.0	0.00	0.0	C90
Lymphoid leukaemia	0	0	-	-	-	-	-	-	-	-	0.0	0.0	0.00	0.0	C91
Myeloid leukaemia	2	0	100	1	-	1	-	-	-	-	0.1	0.2	0.01	0.1	C92-94
Leukaemia, unspecified	9	0	44	-	2	1	4	1	1	-	0.5	0.9	0.04	0.5	C95
Other and unspecified	38	0	37	1	5	1	7	4	8	12	2.1	3.8	0.26	4.7	O&U
All sites	1025	0	28	38	62	117	188	221	196	203	56.4	100.0	7.68	113.2	ALL
All sites but C44	989	0	26	37	61	116	180	213	188	194	54.4		7.38	108.7	ALLbC44
Average annual population				153211	74059	59718	36556	21415	10737	7662					

Table 1. Mali, Bamako (1988-1992)

NUMBER OF CASES BY AGE GROUP AND SUMMARY RATES OF INCIDENCE - FEMALE

SITE	ICD (10th)	ASR (W)	CR 64	%	CRUDE RATE	0-	15-	25-	35-	45-	55-	65+	MV (%)	AGE UNK	ALL AGES
Mouth	C00-06	0.9	0.03	0.9	0.5	-	1	2	2	-	-	3	63	0	8
Salivary gland	C07-08	0.4	0.02	0.3	0.2	-	-	-	1	1	-	1	100	0	3
Nasopharynx	C11	0.0	0.00	0.1	0.0	-	-	-	-	-	-	-	-	0	0
Other pharynx	C09-10,C12-14	0.1	0.01	0.1	0.1	-	-	-	1	-	-	-	0	0	1
Oesophagus	C15	0.7	0.03	0.8	0.4	-	-	2	3	-	-	2	86	0	7
Stomach	C16	12.5	1.01	9.8	5.1	-	2	6	12	24	26	17	45	0	87
Colon, rectum and anus	C18-21	2.5	0.17	2.4	1.2	-	2	5	2	5	3	4	38	0	21
Liver	C22	20.7	1.51	18.6	9.6	2	10	22	35	32	33	31	4	0	165
Gallbladder etc.	C23-24	0.0	0.00	0.0	0.0	-	-	-	-	-	-	-	-	0	0
Pancreas	C25	1.0	0.06	0.7	0.3	-	-	-	-	3	1	2	50	0	6
Larynx	C32	0.7	0.01	0.6	0.3	-	-	1	1	1	-	2	0	0	5
Trachea, bronchus and lung	C33-34	1.8	0.18	1.5	0.8	-	-	-	1	3	6	3	15	0	13
Bone	C40-41	1.2	0.13	1.1	0.6	2	1	2	1	-	4	-	30	0	10
Melanoma of skin	C43	1.2	0.14	0.9	0.5	1	-	-	-	2	5	-	100	0	8
Other skin	C44	3.0	0.24		1.2	-	-	4	2	4	7	4	90	0	21
Mesothelioma	C45	0.0	0.00	0.0	0.0	-	-	-	-	-	-	-	-	0	0
Kaposi sarcoma	C46	0.4	0.04	0.4	0.2	-	-	1	1	1	1	-	100	0	4
Peripheral nerves	C47	0.0	0.00	0.0	0.0	-	-	-	-	-	-	-	-	0	0
Connective and soft tissue	C49	0.5	0.05	0.3	0.2	-	1	-	-	-	2	-	67	0	3
Breast	C50	12.5	0.99	11.2	5.8	-	1	16	28	20	21	14	48	0	100
Vulva	C51	0.5	0.04	0.6	0.3	-	-	-	3	2	-	-	80	0	5
Vagina	C52	0.3	0.02	0.4	0.2	-	-	3	1	-	-	-	75	0	4
Cervix uteri	C53	29.5	2.38	28.1	14.6	-	-	47	79	60	38	26	64	0	250
Uterus	C54-55	4.0	0.34	3.7	1.9	-	2	3	8	13	4	3	36	0	33
Ovary	C56	0.9	0.08	1.1	0.6	1	-	1	5	3	-	-	70	0	10
Placenta	C58	0.3	0.02	0.4	0.2	-	1	1	2	-	-	-	100	0	4
Kidney	C64	1.9	0.20	2.1	1.1	5	2	2	1	2	7	-	26	0	19
Renal pelvis, ureter and other urinary	C65-66,C68	0.0	0.00	0.0	0.0	-	-	-	-	-	-	-	-	0	0
Bladder	C67	3.0	0.26	2.9	1.5	-	2	1	13	4	5	1	12	0	26
Eye	C69	1.2	0.08	1.5	0.8	5	1	1	3	3	-	-	38	0	13
Brain, nervous system	C70-72	0.2	0.02	0.4	0.2	1	1	1	1	-	-	-	0	0	4
Thyroid	C73	2.1	0.12	2.0	1.0	-	1	1	9	3	1	4	56	0	18
Hodgkin disease	C81	0.4	0.01	0.6	0.3	1	2	-	1	-	-	1	100	0	5
Non-Hodgkin lymphoma	C82-85,C96	0.9	0.05	1.0	0.5	-	2	3	-	1	1	2	100	0	9
Multiple myeloma	C90	0.0	0.00	0.0	0.0	-	-	-	-	-	-	-	-	0	0
Lymphoid leukaemia	C91	0.0	0.00	0.0	0.0	-	-	-	-	-	-	-	-	0	0
Myeloid leukaemia	C92-94	1.4	0.10	1.2	0.6	-	-	3	1	3	2	2	82	0	11
Leukaemia, unspecified	C95	0.9	0.05	1.2	0.6	5	1	-	1	3	-	1	55	0	11
Other and unspecified	O&U	3.5	0.19	2.9	1.5	1	-	4	4	5	3	9	15	0	26
All sites	ALL	111.0	8.59	100.0	53.0	24	33	135	220	196	170	132	44	0	910
All sites but C44	ALLbC44	108.1	8.35		51.8	24	33	131	218	192	163	128	43	0	889
Average annual population						163114	75709	43852	27171	16504	9206	7711			

Table 2. Mali, Bamako (1993-1997)

NUMBER OF CASES BY AGE GROUP AND SUMMARY RATES OF INCIDENCE - MALE

SITE	ALL AGES	AGE UNK	MV (%)	0-	15-	25-	35-	45-	55-	65+	CRUDE RATE	%	CR 64	ASR (W)	ICD (10th)
Mouth	4	0	75	-	1	-	-	-	1	2	0.2	0.4	0.02	0.5	C00-06
Salivary gland	0	0	-	-	-	-	-	-	-	-	0.0	0.0	0.00	0.0	C07-08
Nasopharynx	0	0	-	-	-	-	-	-	-	-	0.0	0.0	0.00	0.0	C11
Other pharynx	4	0	75	-	-	1	-	-	1	2	0.2	0.4	0.02	0.5	C09-10,C12-14
Oesophagus	22	0	55	-	1	1	1	10	8	1	1.1	2.4	0.24	2.4	C15
Stomach	147	0	49	-	3	9	13	44	44	34	7.1	15.8	1.29	17.3	C16
Colon, rectum and anus	49	0	43	-	2	7	11	9	9	11	2.4	5.3	0.31	4.8	C18-21
Liver	336	0	3	1	6	40	77	83	71	58	16.3	36.2	2.48	33.4	C22
Gallbladder etc.	2	0	50	-	-	-	1	1	-	-	0.1	0.2	0.03	0.2	C23-24
Pancreas	12	0	8	-	-	-	-	1	5	6	0.6	1.3	0.09	1.7	C25
Larynx	6	0	50	-	-	1	-	2	2	1	0.3	0.6	0.05	0.8	C32
Trachea, bronchus and lung	22	0	32	-	-	-	1	2	12	7	1.1	2.4	0.22	2.9	C33-34
Bone	6	0	100	1	4	-	-	-	-	1	0.3	0.6	0.01	0.4	C40-41
Melanoma of skin	4	0	100	-	-	-	-	1	3	-	0.2	0.4	0.05	0.4	C43
Other skin	27	0	93	-	1	4	6	7	9	-	1.3	2.8	0.24	2.3	C44
Mesothelioma	0	0	-	-	-	-	-	-	-	-	0.0	0.0	0.00	0.0	C45
Kaposi sarcoma	27	0	100	-	3	9	8	3	-	4	1.3	2.9	0.10	1.8	C46
Peripheral nerves	1	0	100	-	-	-	1	-	-	-	0.0	0.1	0.02	0.2	C47
Connective and soft tissue	10	0	100	1	-	2	1	4	1	1	0.5	1.1	0.04	0.9	C49
Breast	7	0	43	-	-	1	1	2	2	1	0.3	0.8	0.04	0.6	C50
Penis	1	0	100	-	-	-	1	-	-	-	0.0	0.1	0.00	0.0	C60
Prostate	40	0	45	-	-	-	-	4	11	25	1.9	4.3	0.27	6.2	C61
Testis	4	0	0	-	1	1	1	1	-	-	0.2	0.4	0.02	0.4	C62
Kidney	16	0	63	12	-	-	1	1	2	-	0.8	1.7	0.07	0.9	C64
Renal pelvis, ureter and other urinary	0	0	-	-	-	-	-	-	-	-	0.0	0.0	0.00	0.0	C65-66,C68
Bladder	89	0	16	-	5	9	9	23	20	23	4.3	9.6	0.63	9.6	C67
Eye	12	0	67	4	1	2	1	1	1	2	0.6	1.3	0.04	0.8	C69
Brain, nervous system	0	0	-	-	-	-	-	-	-	-	0.0	0.0	0.00	0.0	C70-72
Thyroid	1	0	100	-	-	1	-	-	-	-	0.0	0.1	0.01	0.1	C73
Hodgkin disease	14	0	93	4	3	3	2	2	-	-	0.7	1.5	0.05	0.7	C81
Non-Hodgkin lymphoma	27	0	100	8	3	5	5	4	-	2	1.3	2.9	0.09	1.6	C82-85,C96
Multiple myeloma	0	0	-	-	-	-	-	-	-	-	0.0	0.0	0.00	0.0	C90
Lymphoid leukaemia	1	0	100	-	1	-	-	-	-	-	0.0	0.1	0.00	0.0	C91
Myeloid leukaemia	28	0	89	-	1	12	7	5	2	1	1.4	3.0	0.15	1.8	C92-94
Leukaemia, unspecified	0	0	-	-	-	-	-	-	-	-	0.0	0.0	0.00	0.0	C95
Other and unspecified	36	0	33	5	6	6	5	9	2	3	1.7	3.9	0.17	2.5	O&U
All sites	955	0	36	36	42	114	152	216	206	189	46.3	100.0	6.76	95.9	ALL
All sites but C44	928	0	34	36	41	110	146	209	197	189	45.0		6.51	93.5	ALLbC44
Average annual population				172458	87026	66594	42156	24341	11482	8817					

Table 2. Mali, Bamako (1993-1997)

NUMBER OF CASES BY AGE GROUP AND SUMMARY RATES OF INCIDENCE - FEMALE

SITE	ICD (10th)	ALL AGES	AGE UNK	MV (%)	0-	15-	25-	35-	45-	55-	65+	CRUDE RATE	%	CR 64	ASR (W)
Mouth	C00-06	3	0	100	1	-	-	-	1	-	1	0.2	0.3	0.01	0.3
Salivary gland	C07-08	0	0	-	-	-	-	-	-	-	-	0.0	0.0	0.00	0.0
Nasopharynx	C11	1	0	100	-	1	-	-	-	-	-	0.1	0.1	0.00	0.0
Other pharynx	C09-10,C12-14	1	0	100	-	-	1	-	-	-	-	0.1	0.1	0.01	0.1
Oesophagus	C15	10	0	50	-	-	-	4	5	1	-	0.5	1.0	0.10	1.1
Stomach	C16	129	0	52	-	3	12	25	29	35	25	6.8	13.1	1.31	16.6
Colon, rectum and anus	C18-21	38	0	45	-	1	6	6	15	5	5	2.0	3.9	0.36	4.5
Liver	C22	118	0	3	1	2	17	19	25	23	31	6.2	12.0	1.02	15.1
Gallbladder etc.	C23-24	2	0	50	-	-	-	-	-	2	-	0.1	0.2	0.05	0.4
Pancreas	C25	5	0	0	-	-	-	2	1	1	1	0.3	0.5	0.05	0.6
Larynx	C32	0	0	-	-	-	-	-	-	-	-	0.0	0.0	0.00	0.0
Trachea, bronchus and lung	C33-34	1	0	0	-	-	-	1	-	-	-	0.1	0.1	0.01	0.1
Bone	C40-41	4	0	100	1	3	-	-	-	-	-	0.2	0.4	0.01	0.1
Melanoma of skin	C43	8	0	100	-	-	2	2	2	1	1	0.4	0.8	0.11	1.2
Other skin	C44	21	0	100	2	-	2	4	5	3	5	1.1	2.1	0.17	2.5
Mesothelioma	C45	0	0	-	-	-	-	-	-	-	-	0.0	0.0	0.00	0.0
Kaposi sarcoma	C46	12	0	100	-	3	5	1	3	-	-	0.6	1.2	0.08	0.9
Peripheral nerves	C47	0	0	-	-	-	-	-	-	-	-	0.0	0.0	0.00	0.0
Connective and soft tissue	C49	8	0	75	2	-	2	1	2	-	1	0.4	0.8	0.05	0.6
Breast	C50	149	0	42	1	8	21	41	34	29	15	7.8	15.2	1.46	17.2
Vulva	C51	2	0	0	1	-	-	-	1	-	-	0.1	0.2	0.01	0.2
Vagina	C52	3	0	67	-	-	-	1	1	-	1	0.2	0.3	0.02	0.2
Cervix uteri	C53	266	0	64	-	12	32	64	65	57	36	14.0	27.1	2.62	32.0
Uterus	C54-55	31	0	61	-	1	4	4	10	6	6	1.6	3.2	0.30	3.9
Ovary	C56	26	0	62	2	3	4	3	8	2	4	1.4	2.6	0.21	2.8
Placenta	C58	7	0	100	-	1	2	3	1	-	-	0.4	0.7	0.05	0.6
Kidney	C64	13	0	38	5	1	-	2	1	2	2	0.7	1.3	0.08	1.2
Renal pelvis, ureter and other urinary	C65-66,C68	1	0	100	-	-	-	-	1	-	-	0.1	0.1	0.01	0.1
Bladder	C67	35	0	23	-	2	2	6	8	10	7	1.8	3.6	0.35	4.5
Eye	C69	12	0	83	8	-	-	-	-	-	4	0.6	1.2	0.01	0.9
Brain, nervous system	C70-72	2	0	0	1	-	1	-	-	-	-	0.1	0.2	0.01	0.1
Thyroid	C73	10	0	70	-	2	3	3	-	2	-	0.5	1.0	0.08	0.9
Hodgkin disease	C81	11	0	91	2	3	-	2	1	3	-	0.6	1.1	0.09	0.9
Non-Hodgkin lymphoma	C82-85,C96	30	0	100	7	8	4	2	5	4	-	1.6	3.1	0.20	2.3
Multiple myeloma	C90	0	0	-	-	-	-	-	-	-	-	0.0	0.0	0.00	0.0
Lymphoid leukaemia	C91	2	0	100	-	-	1	-	-	-	1	0.1	0.2	0.00	0.2
Myeloid leukaemia	C92-94	13	0	92	-	-	1	3	5	4	-	0.7	1.3	0.17	1.7
Leukaemia, unspecified	C95	0	0	-	-	-	-	-	-	-	-	0.0	0.0	0.00	0.0
Other and unspecified	O&U	30	0	37	-	3	4	5	6	5	7	1.6	3.1	0.24	3.6
All sites	ALL	1004	0	52	35	58	123	203	236	198	151	52.7	100.0	9.23	117.6
All sites but C44	ALLbC44	983	0	51	33	58	121	199	231	195	146	51.6	100.0	9.06	115.0
Average annual population					188820	87445	42056	26528	17430	9789	8710				

Table 3. Childhood cancer, Mali, Bamako (1988-1997)

	NUMBER OF CASES					REL. FREQ.(%)	RATES PER MILLION					
	0-4	5-9	10-14	All	M/F	Overall	0-4	5-9	10-14	Crude	ASR	%MV
Leukaemia	2	2	2	6	0.2	4.5	1.5	1.9	1.9	1.8	1.8	33.3
Acute lymphoid leukaemia	0	0	0	0	-	-	-	-	-	-	-	-
Lymphoma	4	16	12	32	2.2	24.1	3.0	15.3	11.7	9.4	9.5	100.0
Hodgkin disease	1	7	6	14	3.7	10.5	0.8	6.7	5.8	4.1	4.1	100.0
Burkitt lymphoma	0	2	1	3	2.0	2.3	-	1.9	1.0	0.9	0.9	100.0
Brain and spinal neoplasms	0	2	0	2	-	1.5	-	1.9	-	0.6	0.6	-
Neuroblastoma	0	0	0	0	-	-	-	-	-	-	-	-
Retinoblastoma	20	5	1	26	1.0	19.5	15.2	4.8	1.0	7.7	7.7	80.8
Wilms tumour	8	4	2	14	2.5	10.5	6.1	3.8	1.9	4.1	4.2	100.0
Bone tumours	1	2	3	6	1.0	4.5	0.8	1.9	2.9	1.8	1.8	66.7
Soft tissue sarcomas	2	1	0	3	0.5	2.3	1.5	1.0	-	0.9	0.9	100.0
Kaposi sarcoma	0	0	0	0	-	-	-	-	-	-	-	-
Germ cell tumours	0	0	0	0	-	-	-	-	-	-	-	-
Other	13	15	16	44	1.2	33.1	9.9	14.4	15.5	13.0	13.0	31.8
All	50	47	36	133	1.3	100.0	38.0	45.0	35.0	39.3	39.4	67.7

3.2.11 Mauritania

Background

Climate: Desert; constantly hot, dry, dusty

Terrain: Mostly barren, flat plains of the Sahara; some central hills

Ethnic groups: Mixed Maur/black 40%, Maur 30%, black 30%

Religions: Muslim 100%

Economy—overview: A majority of the population still depends on agriculture and livestock for a livelihood, even though most of the nomads and many subsistence farmers were forced into the cities by recurrent droughts in the 1970s and 1980s. Mauritania has extensive deposits of iron ore, which account for almost 50% of total exports. The decline in world demand for this ore, however, has led to cutbacks in production. The coastal waters are among the richest fishing areas in the world, but overexploitation by foreigners threatens this key resource. The country's first deep-water port opened near Nouakchott in 1986.

Industries: Fish processing, mining of iron ore and gypsum

Agriculture—products: Dates, millet, sorghum, root crops; cattle, sheep; fish products

Cancer registration

There has been no cancer registration in the country

Review of data

There has been no publication on the cancer profile of the country.

3.2.12 Niger

Background
Climate: Desert; mostly hot, dry, dusty; tropical in extreme south

Terrain: Predominantly desert plains and sand dunes; flat or rolling plains in south; hills in north

Ethnic groups: Hausa 56%, Djerma 22%, Fula 8.5%, Tuareg 8%, Beri Beri (Kanouri) 4.3%, Arab, Toubou, and Gourmantche 1.2%, about 1200 French expatriates

Religions: Muslim 90%, remainder indigenous beliefs and Christians

Economy—overview: Niger is a poor, landlocked sub-Saharan nation, whose economy centres on subsistence agriculture, animal husbandry, re-export trade, and decreasingly on uranium, its major export since the 1970s, of which prices have fallen dramatically. Other exports, primarily to Nigeria, to the south, include livestock, onions and the products of Niger's small cotton industry.

Industries: Cement, brick, textiles, food processing, chemicals, slaughterhouses, and a few other small light industries; uranium mining, gold mining. A search for petroleum in the north is promising.

Agriculture—products: Cowpeas, cotton, peanuts, millet, sorghum, cassava (tapioca), rice; cattle, sheep, goats, camels, donkeys, horses, poultry

Cancer registration
The Cancer Registry of Niger was founded in 1992, in the Faculté des Sciences de la Santé of the University of Niamey. It is located in the Department of Pathology at the University Hospital. This department is a referral centre for pathology services for the whole country. Nevertheless, the registry was designed to be population-based with complete recording of all cancer cases diagnosed among the population of the capital city, Niamey. Niger comprises eight administrative subdivisions, three in the capital city. In 1995 the population of Niamey was estimated to be 521 000.

Case finding was carried out by a cancer registry clerk during the first six years of operation and later by medical students as well, through active searching for cases in the hospital services in the city where cancer might be diagnosed. These include, especially, the National Hospital, the University Hospital and the main maternity hospital. Visits are made to the major services (surgery, urology, medicine, gynaecology, paediatrics and biology laboratory) once every two weeks, and the charge nurses are encouraged to make a note of cancer cases admitted, which can be collected by the registrar. Otherwise, the clerk examines sources such as the ward admission books, consultation registers, medical records in the departments (though information is often missing from this source) to obtain details of cancer cases, their diagnosis and place of residence. Other clinics visited include maternal and child health clinics and occasionally some private clinics with clinicians to collect biopsies.

An important source of information is the department of pathology, which provides histopathology and cytology services for the whole country. Although some specimens are sent out of the country, the registry receives copies of reports of all cancer cases diagnosed by the pathology services in the city, including biochemical tests such as human chorionic gonadotrophin (HCG), prostate-specific antigen (PSA) and alpha-foetoprotein.

Since no cause of death is recorded on death certificates in Niger, they cannot be used for cancer registration.

The definition of 'usual resident' of Niamey is six months' residence in the city. The registration process is carried out with a microcomputer using the CANREG software.

Review of data
Cancer Registry
For the seven-year period considered (1993–99), a total of 1527 cases were registered among residents of Niamey. Table 1 shows the numbers of cases by sex, site and age group, as well as the percentage frequencies and crude and age-standardized rates (ASRs).

The incidence rates, as calculated based on the estimated resident population, are a little low, and in any case must be considered approximate, because of the uncertainty of the estimate of the population at risk based on the 1988 census.

In men, liver cancer (22.5% of cases, ASR 16.9 per 100 000) ranks first, followed by non-Hodgkin lymphoma (7.5%).

In women, the most important cancers are breast (19.9%), cervix (19.0%), liver (7.4%), ovary (5.7%), other uterus (5.2%) and non-Hodgkin lymphoma (4.3%).

Table 1 also shows the percentage of cases with a morphological diagnosis. 49% had been diagnosed on the basis of microscopic examination of tissue. The percentage is lowest for liver (7%) and highest for the leukaemias (> 80%).

Previous studies
A three-year study (1989–91) of the relative frequency of cancer in Niger using records of the Faculté des Sciences de la Santé in Niamey showed that primary carcinoma of the liver (15.5%), skin cancer (14.2%), non-Hodgkin lymphoma (10.0%) and cancer of the prostate (7.3%) were the most common cancers in males. In females, cancers of the cervix (20.2%), breast (13.9%), liver (9.6%) and skin (7.7%) were most common (Nouhou *et al.*, 1994).

Childhood cancer
119 cases of childhood cancers were recorded by the registry in 1993–99 (Table 2). The overall incidence is low (ASR 71.7 per million). Lymphomas were the most commonly recorded tumour; one third of the cases were Burkitt lymphoma.

References
Nouhou, H., Mahamadou, O., Ramatou & Adehossi, E. (1994) Cancer au Niger: Etude de fréquence relative sur une période de 3 ans (1989-1991). *Médecine d'Afrique Noire*, **41**, 171–178

Table 1. Niger, Niamey (1993-1999)

NUMBER OF CASES BY AGE GROUP AND SUMMARY RATES OF INCIDENCE - MALE

SITE	ALL AGES	AGE UNK	MV (%)	0-	15-	25-	35-	45-	55-	65+	CRUDE RATE	%	CR 64	ASR (W)	ICD (10th)
Mouth	10	0	90	-	1	2	-	2	2	3	0.5	1.7	0.09	**1.8**	C00-06
Salivary gland	5	0	60	1	-	-	1	1	1	1	0.3	0.8	0.04	**0.7**	C07-08
Nasopharynx	1	0	0	-	-	-	-	-	-	-	0.1	0.2	0.00	**0.3**	C11
Other pharynx	7	0	57	-	1	-	1	4	-	1	0.4	1.2	0.05	**0.9**	C09-10,C12-14
Oesophagus	7	0	43	-	-	-	-	4	3	-	0.4	1.2	0.12	**1.0**	C15
Stomach	13	1	62	-	-	-	-	4	7	1	0.7	2.2	0.28	**2.7**	C16
Colon, rectum and anus	37	0	78	2	1	5	10	6	8	5	2.0	6.2	0.35	**4.8**	C18-21
Liver	135	1	7	-	2	14	39	42	24	13	7.3	22.5	1.30	**16.9**	C22
Gallbladder etc.	0	0	-	-	-	-	-	-	-	-	0.0	0.0	0.00	**0.0**	C23-24
Pancreas	7	0	29	-	-	-	1	1	3	2	0.4	1.2	0.10	**1.5**	C25
Larynx	11	1	18	-	-	-	3	3	4	-	0.6	1.8	0.17	**1.6**	C32
Trachea, bronchus and lung	23	2	17	-	-	1	3	3	5	9	1.2	3.8	0.22	**4.9**	C33-34
Bone	37	1	59	10	6	8	6	2	3	1	2.0	6.2	0.20	**2.7**	C40-41
Melanoma of skin	3	0	100	-	-	-	-	-	-	2	0.2	0.5	0.01	**0.7**	C43
Other skin	30	0	57	-	5	3	4	5	10	3	1.6	5.0	0.38	**4.4**	C44
Mesothelioma	0	0	-	-	-	-	-	-	-	-	0.0	0.0	0.00	**0.0**	C45
Kaposi sarcoma	5	0	100	-	-	1	3	1	-	-	0.3	0.8	0.03	**0.3**	C46
Peripheral nerves	0	0	-	-	-	-	-	-	-	-	0.0	0.0	0.00	**0.0**	C47
Connective and soft tissue	20	0	70	3	6	4	1	2	1	3	1.1	3.3	0.09	**2.1**	C49
Breast	7	0	86	-	-	-	1	3	3	-	0.4	1.2	0.13	**1.1**	C50
Penis	0	0	-	-	-	-	-	-	-	-	0.0	0.0	0.00	**0.0**	C60
Prostate	41	0	34	-	-	-	-	2	12	27	2.2	6.8	0.33	**10.8**	C61
Testis	1	0	0	-	-	-	-	-	-	-	0.1	0.2	0.02	**0.2**	C62
Kidney	14	0	29	3	1	3	2	1	4	-	0.8	2.3	0.17	**1.6**	C64
Renal pelvis, ureter and other urinary	1	0	100	-	-	-	-	-	-	-	0.1	0.2	0.00	**0.1**	C65-66,C68
Bladder	30	0	23	-	-	2	5	10	8	5	1.6	5.0	0.35	**4.8**	C67
Eye	15	0	47	7	-	1	2	-	4	-	0.8	2.5	0.11	**1.1**	C69
Brain, nervous system	5	0	80	2	3	1	-	-	1	-	0.3	0.8	0.03	**0.3**	C70-72
Thyroid	3	0	33	-	-	-	-	-	1	-	0.2	0.5	0.03	**0.3**	C73
Hodgkin disease	10	0	70	4	3	-	1	2	-	-	0.5	1.7	0.04	**0.6**	C81
Non-Hodgkin lymphoma	45	0	98	16	5	8	5	6	3	2	2.4	7.5	0.27	**3.7**	C82-85,C96
Multiple myeloma	3	0	100	-	-	1	1	1	-	-	0.2	0.5	0.02	**0.2**	C90
Lymphoid leukaemia	18	2	100	4	4	1	3	2	1	1	1.0	3.0	0.11	**1.6**	C91
Myeloid leukaemia	10	1	100	-	1	2	3	3	-	-	0.5	1.7	0.07	**0.8**	C92-94
Leukaemia, unspecified	0	0	-	-	-	-	-	-	-	-	0.0	0.0	0.00	**0.0**	C95
Other and unspecified	75	1	55	9	8	10	13	17	7	10	4.1	12.5	0.53	**8.8**	O&U
All sites	629	10	48	61	46	68	109	129	116	90	34.1	100.0	5.63	**83.2**	ALL
All sites but C44	599	10	47	61	41	65	105	124	106	87	32.5		5.25	**78.8**	ALLbC44

| Average annual population | | | | 122454 | 50066 | 39128 | 26064 | 13737 | 5730 | 3316 | | | | | |

Table 1. Niger, Niamey (1993-1999)

NUMBER OF CASES BY AGE GROUP AND SUMMARY RATES OF INCIDENCE - FEMALE

SITE	ICD (10th)	ALL AGES	AGE UNK	MV (%)	0-	15-	25-	35-	45-	55-	65+	CRUDE RATE	%	CR 64	ASR (W)
Mouth	C00-06	9	0	67	2	-	2	3	2	-	-	0.5	1.0	0.07	0.8
Salivary gland	C07-08	3	0	33	1	1	-	-	1	-	-	0.2	0.3	0.02	0.3
Nasopharynx	C11	0	0	-	-	-	-	-	-	-	-	0.0	0.0	0.00	0.0
Other pharynx	C09-10,C12-14	2	0	50	1	-	-	-	1	-	-	0.1	0.2	0.02	0.2
Oesophagus	C15	7	0	86	-	-	1	1	2	2	1	0.4	0.8	0.11	1.3
Stomach	C16	15	0	73	-	-	1	1	2	9	2	0.8	1.7	0.34	3.3
Colon, rectum and anus	C18-21	24	0	67	-	4	4	3	5	3	5	1.3	2.7	0.23	3.6
Liver	C22	65	0	8	2	6	8	21	8	10	10	3.6	7.4	0.67	9.3
Gallbladder etc.	C23-24	1	0	0	-	-	-	-	-	1	-	0.1	0.1	0.04	0.3
Pancreas	C25	7	0	14	-	-	1	1	3	-	2	0.4	0.8	0.06	1.2
Larynx	C32	3	0	0	-	-	-	1	-	1	1	0.2	0.3	0.04	0.6
Trachea, bronchus and lung	C33-34	2	0	0	-	-	1	-	-	1	-	0.1	0.2	0.05	0.4
Bone	C40-41	23	2	52	5	10	1	1	2	2	-	1.3	2.6	0.17	1.9
Melanoma of skin	C43	4	0	100	-	-	-	1	1	2	-	0.2	0.5	0.09	0.8
Other skin	C44	24	0	79	-	-	5	2	7	8	2	1.3	2.7	0.42	4.4
Mesothelioma	C45	0	0	-	-	-	-	-	-	-	-	0.0	0.0	0.00	0.0
Kaposi sarcoma	C46	4	0	100	-	1	3	-	-	-	-	0.2	0.5	0.02	0.2
Peripheral nerves	C47	0	0	-	-	-	-	-	-	-	-	0.0	0.0	0.00	0.0
Connective and soft tissue	C49	24	0	96	1	4	4	3	8	1	3	1.3	2.7	0.21	3.1
Breast	C50	175	0	48	1	8	31	48	48	24	15	9.7	19.9	2.05	25.0
Vulva	C51	8	0	63	-	1	2	3	-	2	-	0.4	0.9	0.10	0.9
Vagina	C52	6	0	83	-	-	1	1	3	1	-	0.3	0.7	0.09	0.9
Cervix uteri	C53	167	0	47	-	1	37	71	42	9	7	9.3	19.0	1.60	19.6
Uterus	C54-55	46	1	63	1	3	5	7	13	11	5	2.6	5.2	0.69	7.8
Ovary	C56	50	0	50	2	5	8	15	7	11	2	2.8	5.7	0.64	6.7
Placenta	C58	4	0	25	-	2	-	1	1	-	-	0.2	0.5	0.03	0.3
Kidney	C64	10	0	20	3	-	4	1	-	2	-	0.6	1.1	0.10	0.9
Renal pelvis, ureter and other urinary	C65-66,C68	1	0	100	-	-	-	-	1	-	-	0.1	0.1	0.03	0.2
Bladder	C67	25	0	24	-	1	6	5	6	2	5	1.4	2.8	0.23	3.7
Eye	C69	7	0	71	4	-	1	-	1	-	1	0.4	0.8	0.03	0.6
Brain, nervous system	C70-72	3	0	0	1	-	1	-	-	1	-	0.2	0.3	0.01	0.1
Thyroid	C73	13	0	69	-	2	4	3	2	1	1	0.7	1.5	0.10	1.4
Hodgkin disease	C81	1	0	100	-	1	-	-	-	-	-	0.1	0.1	0.01	0.1
Non-Hodgkin lymphoma	C82-85,C96	38	1	89	12	4	9	4	4	2	2	2.1	4.3	0.24	3.3
Multiple myeloma	C90	1	0	100	-	-	-	1	-	-	-	0.1	0.1	0.01	0.1
Lymphoid leukaemia	C91	16	1	75	2	1	2	3	4	1	2	0.9	1.8	0.15	2.1
Myeloid leukaemia	C92-94	15	0	87	2	-	6	4	2	-	1	0.8	1.7	0.09	1.4
Leukaemia, unspecified	C95	3	0	100	2	-	1	-	-	-	-	0.2	0.3	0.01	0.1
Other and unspecified	O&U	97	0	24	16	11	12	18	15	18	7	5.4	11.0	1.06	12.4
All sites	ALL	903	6	49	58	66	161	223	191	124	74	50.2	100.0	9.82	119.9
All sites but C44	ALLbC44	879	6	49	58	66	156	221	184	116	72	48.8	100.0	9.39	115.5
Average annual population					126763	52684	38584	19866	9043	4395	3832				

85

Table 2. Childhood cancer, Niger, Niamey (1993-1999)

	NUMBER OF CASES					REL. FREQ.(%)	RATES PER MILLION					
	0-4	5-9	10-14	All	M/F	Overall	0-4	5-9	10-14	Crude	ASR	%MV
Leukaemia	3	3	4	10	0.7	8.4	4.1	4.9	9.8	5.7	6.0	100.0
Acute lymphoid leukaemia	2	1	3	6	2.0	5.0	2.7	1.6	7.4	3.4	3.7	100.0
Lymphoma	4	11	17	32	1.7	26.9	5.5	18.1	41.7	18.3	20.1	100.0
Hodgkin disease	0	0	4	4	-	3.4	-	-	9.8	2.3	2.8	50.0
Burkitt lymphoma	1	6	4	11	1.2	9.2	1.4	9.9	9.8	6.3	6.6	81.8
Brain and spinal neoplasms	1	1	1	3	2.0	2.5	1.4	1.6	2.5	1.7	1.8	66.7
Neuroblastoma	1	0	1	2	-	1.7	1.4	-	2.5	1.1	1.2	50.0
Retinoblastoma	6	4	0	10	1.5	8.4	8.2	6.6	-	5.7	5.3	30.0
Wilms tumour	1	1	0	2	-	1.7	1.4	1.6	-	1.1	1.1	50.0
Bone tumours	2	6	6	14	1.8	11.8	2.7	9.9	14.7	8.0	8.5	64.3
Soft tissue sarcomas	1	1	2	4	3.0	3.4	1.4	1.6	4.9	2.3	2.5	75.0
Kaposi sarcoma	0	0	0	0	-	-	-	-	-	-	-	-
Germ cell tumours	1	0	0	1	-	0.8	1.4	-	-	0.6	0.5	100.0
Other	9	16	16	41	0.5	34.5	12.4	26.3	39.2	23.5	24.7	17.1
All	29	43	47	119	1.1	100.0	39.8	70.7	115.2	68.2	71.7	54.6

3.2.13 Nigeria

Background
Climate: Equatorial tropical to the south with dry savannah grassland to the north

Terrain: Southern lowlands merge into central hills and plateaux; plains in north

Ethnic groups: Hausa, Fulani, Yoruba, Ibo, Kanuri, Ibibio, Tiv, Ijaw

Religions: Muslim 50%, Christian 40%, indigenous beliefs 10%

Economy: Political instability, corruption and poor management have hobbled the oil-rich Nigerian economy. The oil sector provides 30% of GDP, 95% of foreign exchange earnings and about 80% of budgetary revenues. The largely subsistence agricultural sector has failed to keep up with rapid population growth, so that Nigeria, once a large net exporter of food, now must import food.

Industries: Crude oil, coal, tin, columbite, palm oil, peanuts, cotton, rubber, wood, hides and skins, textiles, cement and other construction materials, food products, footwear, chemicals, fertilizer, printing, ceramics, steel

Agriculture—products: Cocoa, peanuts, palm oil, corn, rice, sorghum, millet, cassava, yams, rubber; cattle, sheep, goats, pigs; fishing and forest resources extensively exploited

Cancer registration
There are several hospital-based cancer registries operating in Nigeria, but the only population-based registry has been, and remains, the one in Ibadan.

Ibadan Cancer Registry
One of the earliest population-based cancer registries in Africa, the Ibadan Cancer Registry was established in 1960 within the Pathology Department of the University College Hospital (UCH), Ibadan. Since its inception, the aim of the registry has been to monitor the incidence of cancer in the population of Ibadan and its environs, and to provide baseline data for use by health planners, physicians and research workers. For many years, it was the only active registry in Nigeria. It was population-based until 1994, when, as a result of staff shortage, data collection was limited to within the UCH. However, since 1997 the registry has been reactivated with assistance from IARC and data are actively collected from the population. The registry's defined population is the residents of the 70 km² area of the city of Ibadan, comprising five local government areas of Oyo state, with a total population of 1.22 million in 1991. Residents are defined as persons who have been living in the relevant area for at least one year.

The University College Hospital (UCH) is the major tertiary care facility serving the registry population, and it includes specialist cancer treatment services, including radiotherapy. In addition, there are two government state hospitals (Adeoyo Hospital and Ring Road Hospital) and several private and mission hospitals that provide general medical, gynaecological and paediatric services. Three pathology departments are present in the registry area, including the Pathology Department at UCH, which provides the bulk of the histology services and is a major source of information for the registry. The Haematology Department provides copies of reports of haematological malignancies for registration.

Case-finding is effected mainly through a schedule of regular visits by registry staff to the sources of data. Most of the registry's data is collected from UCH, Adeoyo and Ring Road Hospitals where the search for cancer cases is conducted through scrutiny of clinics, wards, surgical pathology records, surgical operation lists and autopsy reports. Case-finding visits are also made to selected large mission and private clinics (about ten in total) that care for cancer cases. Registration of non-hospital deaths is very limited in Ibadan, and the quality of cause-of-death information is very poor; this source of data has not been used until very recently. Autopsy reports from the mortuaries at UCH and Ring Road Hospital allow detection of deaths due to cancer which may have escaped the registration process.

The CANREG computer system has been used for data recording and management since 1997; previously, registration of cases and analysis of the registry database was carried out manually, using an alphabetic name and site card index system.

National Headquarters for Cancer Registries in Nigeria (NHCRN)
In 1990, the NHCRN was established by the Federal Ministry of Health and located in the UCH, with the main objective of coordinating the establishment and development of cancer registries in Nigeria, and as part of its activities to organize training programmes in cancer registration, as well as programmes for cancer prevention and control. Within the last decade, this has led to increased awareness of the importance of cancer registration and to the development of cancer registries nationwide. Many hospital-based cancer registries have been established in teaching hospitals with the assistance and support of the NCHRN. Through its workshops and conferences, the NHCRN has created awareness and provided an avenue for sharing ideas, reviewing the problems of establishing registries in Nigeria and comparing data generated.

Ife-Ijesha Cancer Registry
Ife-Ijesha Cancer Registry was established in 1989 in the Department of Morbid Anatomy of the Obafemi Awolowo University Teaching Hospital (OAUTH). The registry was designed as a population-based cancer registry covering the Ife-Ijesha zone of Osun State in south-western Nigeria. This zone consists of about seven local government areas—Atakumosa, Ife-Central, Ife-North, Ife-South, Ilesa, Obokun and Oriade. The population of this area was 782 000 in 1991.

A registry clerk carries out active case-finding in OAUTH. This hospital is the major source of information, especially its outreach stations at Ile-Ife and Ilesa, which are the main tertiary care facilities in Ife-Ijesha zone. The registry clerk searches for records of possible cancer patients in the various wards, haematology, radiology and consultant outpatient departments. All histology, cytology and surgical pathology reports that are generated by the Department of Morbid Anatomy of OAUTH are checked for cancer diagnoses on a routine basis. There is a system of death registration at OAUTH, and all death certificates issued at the hospital are searched for deaths due to neoplasms, in addition to scrutiny of autopsy reports (routine hospital and coroner).

In addition to OAUTH, a total of nine hospitals (public and private) are visited fortnightly or monthly, depending upon the number of cancer patients treated. Admission books, clinic registers and hospital case records constitute the main sources of information. In addition, a few medical practitioners in the registry area complete and forward notification cards supplied by the registry.

Just nine 'essential' variables are collected on each case; site and histology are coded using ICD-O, and the CANREG system is used for data entry and management.

Zaria Cancer Registry

The Registry is based in the Department of Pathology, Ahmadu Bello University Hospital, Zaria, in northern Nigeria, and serves the university hospitals complex in Zaria and the nearby larger town of Kaduna. The registry started recording cases prospectively in 1982, but the data from a retrospective survey of cases recorded in the Department of Pathology for the years 1976–78 were published by Cederquist and Attah (1986).

Calabar Cancer Registry

This hospital-based registry was established in 1983, based in the Department of Pathology, University of Calabar Teaching Hospital, Calabar, in south-eastern Nigeria. The hospital provides services for the inhabitants of Cross River and Akwa Ibom states as well as neighbouring Abia State and the Republic of Cameroon. The Department of Pathology provides diagnostic services. Cancer cases were retrospectively recorded from 1979.

Review of data

Cancer registries

Ibadan Cancer Registry

During the 40 years of its existence, various studies on the frequency and incidence of cancers have been published. The earliest publication from Ibadan was the report of a cancer rate survey for 1960–63 by Edington and MacLean (1965). Subsequently, cancer incidence data from the registry were published for the periods 1960–62, 1960–65 and 1960–69 in the first three volumes of *Cancer Incidence in Five Continents*. However problems in obtaining adequate denominator population data prevented subsequent results from appearing in later volumes. During the period 1960–69, 2420 cancer cases were registered (1206 males and 1214 females) among the residents of Ibadan and environs (Table 1). The age-standardized incidence (world) rates (ASR) for cancers at all sites were 78.0 and 105.1 per 100 000 for males and females respectively. Non-Hodgkin lymphoma (19.1%, ASR 9.8) and liver cancer (14.4%, ASR 10.0) were the commonest tumours among males. Prostate cancer (5.2%, ASR 9.5) showed high rates in the elderly population. In females, cancers of the cervix (15.6%, ASR 20.9) and breast (12.9%, ASR 14.4) were commonest.

Abioye (1981) and others subsequently reviewed cancer patterns derived from series of cases registered between 1970 and 1997. The profile remained broadly similar to that in 1960–69, with, in males, high frequencies of liver cancer and non-Hodgkin lymphoma, but with prostate cancer emerging as the third most common cancer. In females, cervix cancer remained the most common malignancy throughout the period, although its relative frequency declined. A comparison of the relative frequencies of the common cancer sites during two time periods (1960–80 and 1981–95) over the four decades of the existence of the Ibadan Cancer Registry is shown in Table 2. Breast cancer frequency increased two-fold, with only a minimal rise (1.2%) in cancer of the cervix. The percentage frequency of non-Hodgkin lymphoma including Burkitt lymphoma halved, but these cancers remained the most common malignancy in males. The frequency of prostate cancer increased 1.7 times, while that of choriocarcinoma decreased four-fold (from 8.5% to 2.8%). The frequency of colorectal, liver and lung cancers remained more or less unchanged.

Current data: Table 3 shows data from a recent two-year period, since the reactivation of the registry, with 496 and 652 cancers among males and females, respectively. The estimated age-adjusted incidence for all cancers is a little lower than in 1960–69 (63.9 per 100 000 in males, 74.5 per 100 000 in females). In men, the most common cancers are prostate (ASR 19.8; 23.8%), liver (ASR 7.7; 11.6%) and non-Hodgkin lymphoma (ASR 4.9; 10.3%). Only 32% of the liver malignancies in men were confirmed by histology. In females, breast (ASR 25.3; 35.3%), cervix (ASR 19.9; 24.4%) and ovary (ASR 3.2; 4.7%) are the three most common sites of cancer. The age-specific incidence for breast cancer rises gradually after age 25 years to a peak at age 50. 80% of the malignancies occurring in the breast were verified by histology or cytology.

In spite of the epidemic of HIV/AIDS (with an estimated prevalence of infection of 5.1% in Nigeria at the end of 1999 (UNAIDS, 2000)), current data from Ibadan do not show similar marked increases in incidence of some HIV/AIDS-associated cancers to those reported from parts of eastern and southern Africa.

The registry has always been faced with the problem of case-finding and ascertainment, with suggestion of a reduction in recent years compared with the 1960s. Coverage may indeed have been better in the earlier years, because health care was virtually free and accessible to all, with free treatment of cancer cases. The UCH was the major referral centre in the region, providing most of the specialty services. In addition there was economic and political stability with little or no disruption in the provision of social services and hospital care. The cost of treatment and services is now borne by the patients, who are often unable to cope with the expense of cancer care and management. As a result many are lost to conventional medical care, seeking less expensive alternative traditional care.

Trends in incidence, 1960–99:

Breast cancer was the second commonest female cancer recorded in the earlier years (1960–69) but it is now the commonest female cancer, and in fact the commonest cancer among both sexes. The increase may be related in part to increasing awareness and campaigns about breast cancer, as well as the availability of fine-needle aspiration facilities for quick and easy diagnosis in the hospital. Nevertheless, about 80–85% of these cancers still present in advanced stages, with attendant poor outcome.

Uterine cancer. Cancer of the cervix used to be the commonest gynaecological cancer, but it has recently been overtaken by breast cancer. The incidence rates show little change (ASR 20.9 in 1960–69 and 19.9 in 1998–99) and a recent study of gynaecological malignancies over a period of two decades (1976–95) based on registry data revealed a steady increase in the frequency of new cases (Babarinsa *et al.*, 1998). This reflects the poor development of screening facilities and the lack of a national screening programme. A decline has occurred in the frequency of choriocarcinoma. Endometrial cancer remains uncommon.

Prostate cancer has become the most common cancer among males in Ibadan. Current data (ASR 19.8) indicate a doubling of the incidence rate since 1960–69 (ASR 9.5). The median age of occurrence is 67.5 years and the mean age 71.4 years. The explanation for the rising trend of prostate cancer is uncertain, but may be partly related to improvements in diagnosis and a greater awareness of the importance of this cancer in an increasing elderly population.

Colorectal cancer is considered uncommon in Africa, and this has been related to consumption of high-fibre diet. The early data (1960–69) showed that cancers of the colon and rectum were not frequent, but the results for the period 1998–99 suggest an increase in rectal cancer in males, although there has been no significant change in the ASR for colon cancers in either males or females. An analysis of relative frequencies of these cancers reported a statistically significant 81% increase in frequency of colorectal neoplasms over a 20-year period (Iliyasu *et al.*, 1996), attributed to changing dietary habits, increasing cancer awareness and possibly increased access to health-care facilities.

Liver cancer has shown little change in incidence over the last four decades, with a male: female ratio of 3–4:1. Exposure to the risk factors, particularly hepatitis B virus and aflatoxins, remains widespread.

Table 1. Nigeria, Ibadan (1960-1969)

NUMBER OF CASES BY AGE GROUP AND SUMMARY RATES OF INCIDENCE - MALE

SITE	ALL AGES	AGE UNK	0-	15-	25-	35-	45-	55-	65+	CRUDE RATE	%	ASR (W)	ICD (10th)
Mouth	51	3	1	2	10	8	10	13	4	1.4	4.2	4.0	C00-C08
Nasopharynx	11	0	-	1	1	4	3	2	-	0.3	0.9	0.7	C11
Other pharynx	1	0	-	-	-	-	-	1	-	0.0	0.1	0.1	C09-C10,C12-C14
Oesophagus	11	1	-	-	-	1	1	7	1	0.3	0.9	1.4	C15
Stomach	85	5	-	1	10	21	21	19	8	2.4	7.0	7.0	C16
Colon, rectum and anus	36	0	1	2	7	8	9	8	1	1.0	3.0	2.4	C18-C21
Liver	174	6	5	11	29	61	31	26	5	4.9	14.4	10.0	C22
Pancreas	25	0	-	1	3	6	10	5	-	0.7	2.1	1.7	C25
Larynx	13	0	-	-	-	2	5	5	1	0.4	1.1	1.3	C32
Trachea, bronchus and lung	13	1	-	1	-	3	7	1	-	0.4	1.1	0.8	C33-C34
Melanoma of skin	10	1	1	-	2	2	1	3	1	0.3	0.8	0.9	C43
Other skin	22	6	1	3	3	3	3	2	1	0.6	1.8	1.3	C44
Kaposi sarcoma	1	0	-	-	-	-	-	-	1	0.0	0.1	0.2	C46
Breast	1	0	-	-	-	-	1	-	-	0.0	0.1		C50
Penis	2	1	-	-	-	-	-	-	1	0.1	0.2	0.1	C60
Prostate	63	4	-	-	-	-	9	23	27	1.8	5.2	9.5	C61
Kidney etc.	23	0	17	1	-	2	2	1	-	0.6	1.9	1.1	C64-C66,C68
Bladder	34	1	1	1	1	5	5	13	7	0.9	2.8	3.8	C67
Eye	8	0	4	2	-	2	-	-	-	0.3	0.7	0.3	C69
Brain, nervous system	20	0	11	3	-	3	1	-	2	0.6	1.7	1.0	C70-C72
Thyroid	12	1	-	2	1	5	1	-	2	0.3	1.0	0.7	C73
Hodgkin disease	71	0	11	13	14	12	10	8	3	2.0	5.9	3.6	C81
Non-Hodgkin lymphoma	230	3	120	23	18	29	21	10	6	6.4	19.1	9.8	C82-C85,C96
Multiple myeloma	14	0	1	1	3	3	3	2	1	0.4	1.2	0.9	C90
Leukaemia	82	0	20	11	16	15	8	11	1	2.3	6.8	3.9	C91-C95
Other and unspecified	193	12	19	22	33	40	26	25	16	5.4	16.0	11.9	O&U
All sites	1206	45	213	100	151	235	188	185	89	33.7	100.0	78.0	ALL
All sites but C44	1184	39	212	97	148	232	185	183	88	33.0	98.2	76.7	ALLbC44
Average annual population			92370	109708	95147	36716	14924	5628	3820				

Source: Cancer Incidence in Five Continents volume 3

Table 1. Nigeria, Ibadan (1960-1969)

NUMBER OF CASES BY AGE GROUP AND SUMMARY RATES OF INCIDENCE - FEMALE

SITE	ALL AGES	AGE UNK	0-	15-	25-	35-	45-	55-	65+	CRUDE RATE	%	ASR (W)	ICD (10th)
Mouth	33	4	1	1	4	9	6	7	1	1.2	2.7	3.0	C00-C08
Nasopharynx	3	0	-	1	-	1	-	1	-	0.1	0.2	0.2	C11
Other pharynx	1	0	-	-	-	-	1	1	-	0.0	0.1	0.2	C09-C10,C12-C14
Oesophagus	8	1	-	-	7	3	1	1	2	0.3	0.7	1.0	C15
Stomach	56	5	-	-	7	6	21	14	3	2.1	4.6	6.2	C16
Colon, rectum and anus	32	0	-	-	5	8	11	5	3	1.2	2.6	3.1	C18-C21
Liver	43	2	2	1	8	6	17	6	1	1.6	3.5	3.7	C22
Pancreas	12	1	-	-	1	1	2	6	1	0.4	1.0	1.7	C25
Larynx	3	0	-	-	-	1	1	-	-	0.1	0.2	0.5	C32
Trachea, bronchus and lung	11	0	-	-	2	5	2	2	-	0.4	0.9	0.8	C33-C34
Melanoma of skin	18	3	-	2	1	-	7	3	2	0.7	1.5	2.1	C43
Other skin	17	2	-	2	2	4	4	1	2	0.6		1.5	C44
Kaposi sarcoma													C46
Breast	157	9	-	2	27	44	39	21	15	5.8	12.9	14.4	C50
Cervix uteri	189	6	-	-	10	48	66	43	16	7.0	15.6	20.9	C53
Uterus	14	0	-	1	-	4	5	3	1	0.5	1.2	1.5	C54-C55
Ovary etc.	82	3	2	4	15	21	20	15	2	3.0	6.8	6.9	C56-C57
Kidney etc.	11	1	5	1	2	1	-	-	1	0.4	0.9	0.5	C64-C66,C68
Bladder	19	0	1	1	2	3	4	6	2	0.7	1.6	2.1	C67
Eye	14	1	11	-	-	2	-	-	-	0.5	1.2	0.5	C69
Brain, nervous system	13	0	6	1	2	3	1	1	1	0.5	1.1	0.7	C70-C72
Thyroid	26	4	2	1	6	6	6	-	-	1.0	2.1	1.6	C73
Hodgkin disease	23	1	2	2	5	2	4	7	-	0.9	1.9	2.1	C81
Non-Hodgkin lymphoma	132	1	55	13	14	16	20	12	1	4.9	10.9	7.7	C82-C85,C96
Multiple myeloma	7	0	-	-	1	1	2	3	-	0.3	0.6	0.8	C90
Leukaemia	46	0	5	3	12	4	11	9	2	1.7	3.8	3.8	C91-C95
Other and unspecified	244	10	14	32	59	47	36	35	11	9.1	20.1	17.7	O&U
All sites	1214	54	106	67	185	245	286	204	67	45.1	100.0	105.1	ALL
All sites but C44	1197	52	106	65	183	241	282	203	65	44.5	98.6	103.7	ALLbC44
Average annual population			89214	68953	67858	24450	10669	4550	3372				

Source: Cancer Incidence in Five Continents volume 3

Lung cancer rates in Nigeria remain low (ASR 0.8 in both sexes in 1960–69; 0.7 in men in 1998–99). The prevalence of cigarette smoking, the major risk factor, does not seem to have significantly increased among the general population—it is likely that the dwindling economic resources and purchasing power of individuals have not favoured the habit.

Ife-Ijesha cancer registry

During the three-year period 1993–95 since active registration began in the zone, a total of 400 resident cases, 187 males and 213 females, were registered (Table 4). The overall crude incidence rates of 15.7 per 100 000 (ASR 29.3) in males and 17.3 per 100 000 (ASR 25.7) in females are low, indicating a significant degree of under-reporting of cancer cases. Among males, prostate cancer (25.7%), non-Hodgkin lymphoma (17.1%) and liver cancer (7.0%) were the commonest malignancies, as elsewhere in the region. In females, cancers of the breast (28.2%), cervix (13.6%) and non-Hodgkin lymphoma (7.0%) were commonest.

Zaria Cancer registry

A series from the Department of Pathology, Ahmadu Bello University Hospital, Zaria was published by Cederquist and Attah (1986). The cases represent cancers diagnosed in 1976–78 by histology, cytology or bone marrow examination (the latter information coming from the haematology department) (Table 5). The most frequently recorded tumours in this series were non-Hodgkin lymphomas (22.9% of tumours in males, 10.4 in females). About half the cases occurred in children aged under 15 years, the great majority of which were Burkitt lymphoma, but there were also a considerable number of adult cases. In females, the importance of carcinomas of the cervix, breast and ovary was similar to that seen elsewhere in West Africa. In males, liver was the most common site (excluding skin and lymphomas), with a cancer frequency (8.4%) similar to that in Ibadan. The cases of prostate cancer were noted to be young (only 12% were aged 55 years or more).

More recent data, for 1991–92, were reported by Afolayan (1992). Frequencies of liver, breast and prostate cancers were higher than in the earlier series (Table 5).

Calabar cancer registry

The review of frequency series of data from Calabar (1979–88) (Table 4) showed cervical cancer to be the commonest cancer (37.0% of cancers in females), followed by breast (29.8%). Among males, prostate cancer is the commonest (28.6%), followed by liver (16.5%).

Other registries: Eruwa and Enugu

Though data available are essentially hospital-based, similar interesting patterns have emerged (Table 4). Prostate and liver cancers are the commonest among males in both centres. Cancer data from Eruwa, a more rural community, indicate that cervical cancer is still the commonest cancer in females (cervix 25%, breast 18%), while Enugu's report shows that breast cancer was more common (breast 44.5%, cervix 23%). Enugu Cancer Registry is located in a hospital that caters for an urban population.

Childhood cancer

An analysis of the relative frequencies of the principal types of childhood cancer during 1960–72 was published by Williams (1975). These relative frequencies were compared by Olisa *et al.* (1975) with those observed in a series of black children in the United States and with registry data from the United Kingdom and Uganda. Akang (1996) also compared the early series with the relative frequencies observed in 1973–90 and noted increased frequencies of intracranial neoplasms, leukaemias, renal neoplasms and retinoblastomas, with a relative decline in the frequencies of bone neoplasms and Burkitt lymphoma. The rising frequencies of retinoblastomas, renal and intracranial tumours were ascribed to the increased number of qualified physicians and improved diagnostic facilities.

Incidence rates for childhood cancers in Ibadan were published for 1960–69 (Junaid & Babalola, 1988) and for 1985–92 (Thomas & Aghadiuno, 1998) (Table 6). The most recent data from the registry, for 1993–99, are shown in Table 7.

Lymphomas, and specifically Burkitt lymphoma, have remained the commonest childhood cancer throughout the period. However, as suggested by the analysis of relative frequencies, there seems to have been a decline in incidence of Burkitt lymphoma between the 1960s and the 1990s. The recorded incidence decreased from 79.4 per million in 1960–69 to 18 per million in 1985–92 and 22.6 per million in 1993–99. The pattern of tumour presentation has also shown some changes, with fewer occurrences of the typical jaw tumour and more abdominal mass presentation. This declining trend has been associated with better hygiene and an improved standard of living. In support of this is the variation in frequency patterns between different parts of the country.

The most frequent solid tumour (excluding the lymphomas) throughout the period has been retinoblastoma (with an extremely high rate recorded in the most recent period). The great majority of cases are sporadic (non-familial) unilateral tumours, with a mean age of occurrence of 3.2 years ± 20 months and a median of 2 years. Wilms tumour and soft-tissue sarcomas were also relatively frequent, but registration rates for all other diagnostic groups were lower than in western populations. The frequency (and incidence rate) of neuroblastomas is low, especially in the two more recent periods, while there has been an increase in the frequency of recorded central nervous system cancers, probably related to improved diagnostic facilities. No cases of Kaposi sarcoma were

Table 2. Relative frequencies of the six most common tumours in Ibadan in two time periods: 1960–80 and 1981–95

1960–80		1981–95	
Site	Frequency (%)	Site	Frequency (%)
Non-Hodgkin lymphoma (incl. Burkitt)	15.1	Breast	14.8
Cervix	10.3	Cervix	12.7
Liver	6.5	Non-Hodgkin lymphoma (incl. Burkitt)	7.4
Breast	6.0	Liver	6.4
Connective tissue	4.5	Prostate	4.7
Choriocarcinoma	4.4	Colorectal	3.8

registered in 1993–99, despite the moderately high prevalence of childhood HIV infection in Nigeria (0.24% at the end of 1999) and the reports of increased rates elsewhere in Africa.

Reviews of frequency series of childhood tumours from Jos, Plateau State (Obafunwa *et al.*, 1992) and Enugu, Eastern Nigeria (Obioha *et al.*, 1989) noted the predominance of lymphomas, with frequencies of 34% and 39.7% respectively. These frequencies are lower that from Ibadan. Also significant are the comparatively higher frequencies of leukaemia (20% and 12.6%) observed in both centres, with overall lower frequencies of Burkitt lymphomas (11.4% and 26.5%). This difference in the Burkitt lymphoma/leukaemia ratio has been related to regional climatic differences and socioeconomic status. Jos, in the highland plateau region, has a lower ambient temperature and drier climate than Ibadan. Unpublished observations indicate that Burkitt lymphoma is less common in Lagos (a more urbanized area) than in Ibadan, although they are in the same geographical zone.

References

Abioye, A.O. (1981) Ibadan cancer registry, 1960-1980. In: Olatunbosun, D.A., ed., *Proceedings: Cancer in Africa. Workshop of West Africa College of Physicians*

Afolayan, E.A.O. (1992) Cancer registration in Nigeria. In: Solanke, T.F., ed., *Report of the Workshop on National Cancer Control Programme (NCCP) for Nigeria, Lagos*, Nigeria, December 13-17, 1992, p. 17

Akang, E.E.U. (1996) Childhood tumours in Ibadan (1973-1990). Pediatr. *Pathol. Lab. Med.*, **16**, 791–800

Awojobi, O. (1996) Malignant tumours in rural western Nigeria. In: Solanke, T.F. & Adebamowo, C.A., eds, *Report of the Workshop on State of the Art in Oncology in Ibadan and Ife*, pp. 13–16

Babarinsa, I.A., Akang, E.E.U. & Adewole, I.F. (1998) Pattern of gynaecological malignancies at the Ibadan Cancer Registry (1976-1995). *Niger. Q. J. Hosp. Med.*, **8**, 103–106

Cederquist, R. & Attah, E.B. (1986) Zaria Cancer Registry, 1976-1978. In: Parkin, D.M., ed., *Cancer Occurrence in Developing Countries* (IARC Scientific Publications No. 75), Lyon, IARC, pp. 68–73

Edington, G.M. & MacLean, C.M.V. (1965) A cancer rate survey in Ibadan, western Nigeria 1960-1963. *Br. J. Cancer*, **19**, 471–481

Enakem, I.-O. (1996) *Cancer Registry Report, 1979-1994*, Department of Pathology, College of Medical Sciences, University of Calabar

Iliyasu, Y., Ladipo, J.K., Akang, E.E.U., Adebamowo, C.A., Ajao, O.G. & Aghadiuno, P.U. (1996) A twenty year review of malignant coorectal neoplasms at the University College Hospital, Ibadan Nigeria. *Dis. Colon Rectum*, **39**, 536–540

Junaid, T.A. & Babalola, B.O. (1988) Nigeria: Ibadan Cancer Registry, 1960–1984. In: Parkin, D.M., Stiller, C.A., Draper, G.J., Bieber, C.A., Terracini, B. & Young, J.L., eds, *International Incidence of Childhood Cancer* (IARC Scientific Publications No. 87), Lyon, IARC, pp. 37–41

Obafunwa, J.O., Asagba, G.O. & Ezechukwu, C.C. (1992) Paediatric malignancies in Plateau State, Nigeria. *Cancer J.*, **5**, 211–215

Obianyo, N.E.N. (1992) Cancer registration in Nigeria. In: Solanke, T.F., ed., *Report of the Workshop on National Cancer Control Programme (NCCP) for Nigeria, Lagos*, Nigeria, December 13-17, 1992, p. 16.

Obioha, F.I., Kaine, W.N., Ikerionwu, S.E., Obi, G.O. & Ulasi, T.O. (1989) The pattern of childhood malignancy in eastern Nigeria. *Ann. Trop. Paediatr.*, **9** 261–265

Ojo, O.S. (1996) Cancer in Ife-Ijesha area of South Western Nigeria – Experience at the Ife-Ijesha Cancer Registry. In: Solanke, T.F. & Adebamowo, C.A., eds, *Report of the Workshop on State of the Art in Oncology in Ibadan and Ife*

Olisa, E.G., Chandra, R., Jackson, M.A. Kennedy, J. & Williams, A.O. (1975) Malignant tumours in American Black and Nigerian children: a comparative study. *J. Natl Cancer Inst.*, **55**, 281–284

Thomas, J.O. & Aghadiuno, P.U. (1998) Nigeria.: Ibadan Cancer Registry, 1985–1992. In: Parkin, D.M., Kramárová, E., Draper, G.J., Masuyer, E., Michaelis, J., Neglia, J, Qureshi, S. & Stiller, C.A., eds, *International Incidence of Childhood Cancer*, vol. II (IARC Scientific Publications No. 144), Lyon, IARC, pp. 43–45

UNAIDS (2000) Nigeria: Epidemiological Fact Sheets 2000 Update (revised). http:/www.unaids.org

Williams, A.O. (1975) Tumours of childhood in Ibadan, Nigeria. *Cancer*, **36**, 370–378

Table 3. Nigeria, Ibadan (1998-1999)

NUMBER OF CASES BY AGE GROUP AND SUMMARY RATES OF INCIDENCE - MALE

SITE	ALL AGES	AGE UNK	MV (%)	0-	15-	25-	35-	45-	55-	65+	CRUDE RATE	%	CR 64	ASR (W)	ICD (10th)
Mouth	9	0	78	-	2	1	1	3	-	3	0.6	1.9	0.05	1.1	C00-06
Salivary gland	5	0	80	-	-	-	-	3	2	-	0.3	1.0	0.06	0.6	C07-08
Nasopharynx	12	0	83	-	1	3	3	5	-	-	0.8	2.5	0.10	1.1	C11
Other pharynx	3	0	100	-	1	1	-	-	2	-	0.2	0.6	0.05	0.4	C09-10,C12-14
Oesophagus	7	0	29	-	-	1	1	1	1	4	0.5	1.4	0.03	1.1	C15
Stomach	9	0	56	-	-	-	3	2	2	2	0.6	1.9	0.09	1.2	C16
Colon, rectum and anus	29	0	72	1	1	-	7	7	10	3	2.0	6.0	0.35	3.8	C18-21
Liver	56	0	32	1	1	5	10	10	10	19	3.8	11.6	0.43	7.7	C22
Gallbladder etc.	1	0	0	-	-	-	-	-	-	1	0.1	0.2	0.00	0.2	C23-24
Pancreas	6	0	33	-	-	1	-	-	3	2	0.4	1.2	0.07	0.9	C25
Larynx	11	0	82	-	1	1	1	2	3	3	0.7	2.3	0.10	1.5	C32
Trachea, bronchus and lung	5	0	60	-	-	-	-	2	1	1	0.3	1.0	0.05	0.7	C33-34
Bone	19	0	74	2	6	4	2	1	4	-	1.3	3.9	0.15	1.6	C40-41
Melanoma of skin	5	0	80	-	-	1	-	3	-	2	0.3	1.0	0.03	0.7	C43
Other skin	12	0	92	-	1	1	5	3	-	1	0.8	2.4	0.10	1.3	C44
Mesothelioma	0	0	-	-	-	-	-	-	-	-	0.0	0.0	0.00	0.0	C45
Kaposi sarcoma	3	0	67	-	-	1	2	-	-	-	0.2	0.6	0.02	0.2	C46
Peripheral nerves	4	0	100	-	-	-	-	-	2	1	0.3	0.8	0.05	0.6	C47
Connective and soft tissue	18	0	72	3	2	5	5	2	-	1	1.2	3.7	0.10	1.4	C49
Breast	7	0	71	-	2	-	-	2	2	5	0.5	1.4	0.04	1.3	C50
Penis	0	0	-	-	-	-	-	-	-	-	0.0	0.0	0.00	0.0	C60
Prostate	115	0	70	-	-	-	1	11	33	70	7.7	23.8	0.84	19.8	C61
Testis	3	0	100	1	-	-	-	-	1	-	0.2	0.6	0.03	0.3	C62
Kidney	3	0	67	2	-	-	-	1	-	-	0.2	0.6	0.01	0.2	C64
Renal pelvis, ureter and other urinary	0	0	-	-	-	-	-	-	-	-	0.0	0.0	0.00	0.0	C65-66,C68
Bladder	16	0	75	1	-	2	-	2	6	4	1.1	3.3	0.17	2.3	C67
Eye	15	0	60	11	1	1	-	2	-	-	1.0	3.1	0.03	1.3	C69
Brain, nervous system	7	0	43	2	2	1	-	2	-	3	0.5	1.4	0.04	0.5	C70-72
Thyroid	6	0	100	-	-	1	-	3	-	2	0.4	1.2	0.04	0.8	C73
Hodgkin disease	7	0	57	1	4	-	-	-	2	-	0.5	1.4	0.06	0.6	C81
Non-Hodgkin lymphoma	50	0	46	15	4	5	6	6	8	6	3.4	10.3	0.35	4.9	C82-85,C96
Multiple myeloma	1	0	0	-	-	-	-	-	-	1	0.1	0.2	0.00	0.2	C90
Lymphoid leukaemia	2	0	0	-	2	-	1	-	-	-	0.1	0.4	0.01	0.1	C91
Myeloid leukaemia	9	0	22	2	2	2	1	1	-	1	0.6	1.9	0.04	0.7	C92-94
Leukaemia, unspecified	3	0	0	1	-	-	1	-	1	-	0.2	0.6	0.03	0.3	C95
Other and unspecified	38	0	58	4	3	3	5	7	10	6	2.6	7.9	0.36	4.6	O&U
All sites	496	0	61	48	34	41	55	73	104	141	33.4	100.0	3.87	63.9	ALL
All sites but C44	484	0	60	48	33	40	50	70	103	140	32.6	100.0	3.77	62.6	ALLbC44
Average annual population				312528	162347	108462	71599	45666	23425	19159					

Table 3. Nigeria, Ibadan (1998-1999)

NUMBER OF CASES BY AGE GROUP AND SUMMARY RATES OF INCIDENCE - FEMALE

SITE	ICD (10th)	ALL AGES	AGE UNK	MV (%)	0-	15-	25-	35-	45-	55-	65+	CRUDE RATE	%	CR 64	ASR (W)
Mouth	C00-06	2	0	50	-	-	-	-	-	1	1	0.1	0.3	0.02	**0.3**
Salivary gland	C07-08	4	0	75	-	-	-	-	1	1	-	0.3	0.6	0.04	**0.4**
Nasopharynx	C11	6	0	83	1	-	-	1	1	-	-	0.4	0.9	0.04	**0.6**
Other pharynx	C09-10,C12-14	1	0	0	1	-	-	1	-	-	1	0.1	0.2	0.00	**0.1**
Oesophagus	C15	2	0	0	-	-	1	-	1	1	-	0.1	0.3	0.03	**0.3**
Stomach	C16	11	0	55	-	-	3	1	2	6	2	0.7	1.7	0.13	**1.4**
Colon, rectum and anus	C18-21	24	0	75	-	2	3	4	4	6	5	1.6	3.7	0.22	**2.8**
Liver	C22	19	0	32	1	-	2	3	3	3	6	1.3	3.0	0.13	**2.1**
Gallbladder etc.	C23-24	1	0	100	-	-	-	-	-	1	-	0.1	0.2	0.02	**0.2**
Pancreas	C25	7	0	14	-	-	1	-	-	3	3	0.5	1.1	0.07	**1.0**
Larynx	C32	2	0	0	-	-	-	-	-	-	-	0.1	0.3	0.00	**0.3**
Trachea, bronchus and lung	C33-34	2	0	100	-	-	-	1	1	1	2	0.1	0.3	0.04	**0.3**
Bone	C40-41	7	0	57	-	3	-	1	2	-	1	0.5	1.1	0.04	**0.6**
Melanoma of skin	C43	4	0	75	1	-	1	-	2	1	-	0.3	0.6	0.04	**0.4**
Other skin	C44	9	0	100	-	-	1	-	3	2	3	0.6		0.07	**1.1**
Mesothelioma	C45	0	0	-	-	-	-	-	-	-	-	0.0	0.0	0.00	**0.0**
Kaposi sarcoma	C46	1	0	100	-	-	-	-	-	-	-	0.1	0.2	0.00	**0.1**
Peripheral nerves	C47	0	0	-	-	-	-	-	-	-	-	0.0	0.0	0.00	**0.0**
Connective and soft tissue	C49	7	0	100	3	-	1	1	1	1	-	0.5	1.1	0.05	**0.6**
Breast	C50	227	0	80	-	1	32	60	68	41	25	15.0	35.3	2.19	**25.3**
Vulva	C51	7	0	71	-	2	-	2	1	1	1	0.5	1.1	0.05	**0.7**
Vagina	C52	4	0	100	-	1	-	-	-	-	2	0.3	0.6	0.03	**0.5**
Cervix uteri	C53	157	0	75	-	1	7	27	42	42	38	10.4	24.4	1.53	**19.9**
Uterus	C54-55	17	0	76	-	-	1	3	5	5	3	1.1	2.6	0.17	**2.0**
Ovary	C56	30	0	73	1	1	2	8	8	5	5	2.0	4.7	0.24	**3.2**
Placenta	C58	4	0	50	-	-	1	3	-	-	-	0.3	0.6	0.02	**0.3**
Kidney	C64	9	0	67	2	2	1	-	-	2	1	0.6	1.4	0.07	**0.9**
Renal pelvis, ureter and other urinary	C65-66,C68	0	0	-	-	-	-	-	-	-	-	0.0	0.0	0.00	**0.0**
Bladder	C67	3	0	67	-	-	-	-	2	-	-	0.2	0.5	0.03	**0.3**
Eye	C69	7	0	71	6	1	-	-	-	-	-	0.5	1.1	0.03	**0.5**
Brain, nervous system	C70-72	10	0	40	2	-	1	-	3	1	1	0.7	1.6	0.08	**1.0**
Thyroid	C73	9	0	78	-	-	2	2	1	1	4	0.6	1.4	0.04	**1.0**
Hodgkin disease	C81	1	0	100	-	-	-	-	1	-	-	0.1	0.2	0.01	**0.1**
Non-Hodgkin lymphoma	C82-85,C96	26	0	69	3	2	4	2	4	7	4	1.7	4.0	0.22	**2.7**
Multiple myeloma	C90	5	0	20	-	-	-	1	1	2	1	0.3	0.8	0.05	**0.6**
Lymphoid leukaemia	C91	2	0	0	-	-	-	-	-	1	1	0.1	0.3	0.03	**0.2**
Myeloid leukaemia	C92-94	3	0	0	1	-	-	1	-	-	-	0.2	0.5	0.01	**0.3**
Leukaemia, unspecified	C95	2	0	0	-	1	-	1	-	-	-	0.1	0.3	0.01	**0.1**
Other and unspecified	O&U	20	0	85	1	1	1	6	4	5	2	1.3	3.1	0.20	**2.2**
All sites	ALL	652	0	73	22	20	64	129	162	142	113	43.2	100.0	5.95	**74.5**
All sites but C44	ALLbC44	643	0	72	21	20	64	129	159	140	110	42.6	100.0	5.88	**73.4**

| Average annual population | | | | | 301303 | 165688 | 118256 | 74698 | 43593 | 25271 | 25848 | | | | |

Table 4. Nigeria: cancer registry data

Site	Ife-Ijesha, 1993–95 (Ojo, 1996)					Eruwa, Oyo State, 1986–95 (Awojobi, 1996)					Calabar Cancer Registry, 1979–88 (Enakem, 1996)					Enugu Cancer Registry, 1988–92 (Obianyo, 1992)				
	Male		Female		%HV	Male		Female		%HV	Male		Female		%HV	Male		Female		%HV
	No.	%	No.	%		No.	%	No.	%		No.	%	No.	%		No.	%	No.	%	
Oral cavity	9	4.8%	3	1.4%		2	1.2	3	1.4	20										
Nasopharynx																				
Other pharynx																				
Oesophagus	2	1.1%	2	0.9%		5	3.0%	6	2.9%	0							8.9%			
Stomach	9	4.8%	7	3.3%		3	1.8%	3	1.4%	33.3	38	14.9%	31	5.4%						
Colon/rectum	8	4.3%	10	4.7%		12	7.3%	11	5.3%	26.1										
Liver	13	7.0%	13	6.1%		28	17.0%	22	10.5%	22	42	16.5%	28	4.9%			19.7%		6.2%	
Pancreas	1	0.5%				6	3.6%	1	0.5%	28.6										
Lung	3	1.6%	2	0.9%																
Melanoma	4	2.1%	3	1.4%							22	8.6%	15	2.6%						
Other skin	2	1.1%	4	1.9%		4	2.4%			100	33	12.9%	29	5.1%			9.2%		4.6%	
Kaposi sarcoma						4	2.4%	2	1.0%	33.3										
Breast			60	28.2%		1	0.6%	37	17.7%	52.6			170	29.8%					44.5%	
Cervix uteri			29	13.6%				52	24.9%	7.7			211	37.0%					23.0%	
Corpus uteri			1	0.5%																
Ovary etc.			4	1.9%				11	5.3%	63.6			43	7.5%						
Prostate	48	25.7%				32	19.4%			84.4	73	28.6%					29.0%			
Penis																				
Bladder	6	3.2%	3	1.4%		14	8.5%	1	0.5%	40										
Kidney etc.	2	1.1%	2	0.9%		4	2.4%	9	4.3%	38.5										
Eye	2	1.1%	4	1.9%																
Brain, nervous system	0	0.0%																		
Thyroid			8	3.8%		4	2.4%	12	5.7%	18.8										
Non-Hodgkin lymphoma	32	17.1%	15	7.0%		5	3.0%	7	3.3%	91.7	39	15.3%	16	2.8%						
Hodgkin disease	4	2.1%	4	1.9%		18	10.9%	12	5.7%	60										
Myeloma	1	0.5%	1	0.5%																
Leukaemia	8	4.3%	7	3.3%		3	1.8%	2	1.0%	0										
ALL SITES	187	100.0%	213	100.0%		165	100.0%	209	100.0%		255	100.0%	570	100.0%						

Table 5. Nigeria: Zaria Cancer Registry

Site	Zaria Cancer Registry, 1976–78 (Cederquist & Attah, 1986)					%HV	Zaria Cancer Registry, 1991–92 (Afolayan, 1992)					%HV
	Male		Female		%HV	Male		Female		%HV
	No.	%	No.	%		No.	%	No.	%	
Oral cavity[1]	57	6.9%	30	4.0%	100					
Nasopharynx	3	0.4%	0	0.0%	100					
Other pharynx		0.0%	8	1.1%	100					
Oesophagus	2	0.2%	0	0.0%	100					
Stomach	12	1.5%	8	1.1%	100					
Colon/rectum	18	2.2%	16	2.1%	100	8	3.5%	7	2.3%	
Liver	69	8.4%	16	2.1%	100	45	19.9%	19	6.3%	
Pancreas	2	0.2%	0	0.0%	100					
Lung	1	0.1%	1	0.1%	100					
Melanoma	22	2.7%	14	1.9%	100					
Other skin	72	8.7%	39	5.2%	100					
Kaposi sarcoma	16	1.9%	0	0.0%	100					
Breast	2	0.2%	80	10.7%	100			62	20.5%	
Cervix uteri			148	19.7%	100			75	24.8%	
Corpus uteri			13	1.7%	100			10	3.3%	
Ovary etc.			61	8.1%	100					
Prostate	22	2.7%			100	17	7.5%			
Penis	2	0.2%			100					
Bladder	47	5.7%	7	0.9%	100	21	9.3%			
Kidney etc.	11	1.3%	12	1.6%	100					
Eye	47	5.7%	25	3.3%	100					
Brain,nervous system	1	0.1%	0	0.0%	100					
Thyroid	14	1.7%	33	4.4%	100					
Non-Hodgkin lymphoma	189	22.9%	78	10.4%	100	36	15.9%	24	7.9%	
Hodgkin disease	51	6.2%	20	2.7%	100	12	5.3%			
Myeloma	3	0.4%	4	0.5%	100					
Leukaemia	71	8.6%	51	6.8%	100					
ALL SITES	825	100.0%	750	100.0%	100	226	100.0%	302	100.0%	

[1] Includes salivary gland tumours

Table 6. Nigeria, Ibadan Cancer Registry: childhood cancers, 1960–92

Cancer	1960–84 (Junaid & Babalola, 1988)			1985–92 (Thomas & Aghadiuno, 1998)		
	No.	%	ASR*	No.	%	ASR
Leukaemia	86	9.0%	11.8	46	12.0%	8.3
Acute lymphocytic leukaemia	33	3.4%	3.9	15	3.9%	2.6
Lymphoma	539	56.3%	96.8	152	39.7%	27.1
Burkitt lymphoma	446	46.6%	79.4	102	26.6%	18.0
Hodgkin disease	35	3.7%	6.7	18	4.7%	3.3
Brain and spinal neoplasms	47	4.9%	4.9	61	15.9%	11.1
Neuroblastoma	41	4.3%	6.0	1	0.3%	0.2
Retinoblastoma	67	7.0%	7.6	37	9.7%	7.4
Wilms tumour	67	7.0%	10.3	24	6.3%	4.7
Bone tumours	7	0.7%	2.8	11	2.9%	2.1
Soft-tissue sarcomas	46	4.8%	8.7	29	7.6%	5.4
Kaposi sarcoma	1	0.1%	0.6	0	0.0%	0
Other	57	6.0%	6.7	22	5.7%	4.2
Total	957	100.0%	155.6	383	100.0%	70.5

* ASR based on 282 cases registered in 1960–69

Table 7. Childhood cancer, Nigeria, Ibadan (1993-1999)

	NUMBER OF CASES					REL. FREQ.(%)	RATES PER MILLION					
	0-4	5-9	10-14	All	M/F	Overall	0-4	5-9	10-14	Crude	ASR	%MV
Leukaemia	1	2	2	5	1.5	2.8	2.0	3.6	3.6	3.1	3.0	20.0
Acute lymphoid leukaemia	0	0	0	0	-	-	-	-	-	-	-	-
Lymphoma	10	24	25	59	1.7	33.5	20.3	42.7	44.9	36.6	34.7	6.7
Hodgkin disease	0	1	4	5	-	2.8	-	1.8	7.2	3.1	2.7	-
Burkitt lymphoma	5	19	15	39	1.8	22.2	10.2	33.8	27.0	24.2	22.6	10.3
Brain and spinal neoplasms	7	7	4	18	2.6	10.2	14.2	12.4	7.2	11.2	11.6	11.1
Neuroblastoma	2	1	0	3	2.0	1.7	4.1	1.8	-	1.9	2.1	100.0
Retinoblastoma	22	3	0	25	1.5	14.2	44.7	5.3	-	15.5	19.0	40.0
Wilms tumour	3	1	1	5	0.7	2.8	6.1	1.8	1.8	3.1	3.5	40.0
Bone tumours	1	1	2	4	3.0	2.3	2.0	1.8	3.6	2.5	2.4	25.0
Soft tissue sarcomas	2	2	5	9	0.8	5.1	4.1	3.6	9.0	5.6	5.3	44.4
Kaposi sarcoma	0	0	0	0	-	-	-	-	-	-	-	-
Germ cell tumours	2	1	2	5	1.5	2.8	4.1	1.8	3.6	3.1	3.2	20.0
Other	21	7	15	43	1.9	24.4	42.6	12.4	27.0	26.7	28.3	20.9
All	71	49	56	176	1.7	100.0	144.1	87.1	100.7	109.2	113.1	21.6

3.2.14 Senegal

Background

Climate: Tropical; hot, humid; rainy season (May to November) with strong south-east winds; dry season (December to April) dominated by hot, dry, harmattan wind

Terrain: Generally low, rolling, plains rising to foothills in south-east

Ethnic groups: Wolof 36%, Fulani 17%, Serer 17%, Toucouleur 9%, Diola 9%, Mandingo 9%, European and Lebanese 1%, other 2%

Religions: Muslim 92%, indigenous beliefs 6%, Christian 2% (mostly Roman Catholic)

Economy—overview: Private activity accounts for 82% of GDP and in recent years information technology-based services have become important. However, Senegal faces deep-seated urban problems of chronic unemployment, juvenile delinquency and drug addiction.

Industries: Agricultural and fish processing, phosphate mining, fertilizer production, petroleum refining, construction materials

Agriculture—products: Peanuts, millet, corn, sorghum, rice, cotton, tomatoes, green vegetables; cattle, poultry, pigs; fish

Cancer registration

In 1968, a cancer registry was set up in the capital, Dakar, as a joint undertaking between IARC and the Pathology Department of the Hôpital Dantec in Dakar (Tuyns & Quenum, 1982). The registry was designed as population-based, covering the region of Cap Vert. The majority of the educational and medical services were concentrated in the Dakar area, serving the former French colony, but considerable expansion of specialized medical facilities subsequently took place in other regions of Senegal.

Four pathology departments in Dakar acted as the major diagnostic units at the time, for the entire country. It was stated that most of the cases of cancer diagnosed in Dakar were likely to be confirmed by histology. The pathology departments contributed most of the data recorded in the cancer registry. Data on clinically diagnosed malignancies obtained from the various departments of the hospitals serving the population were included as well. Registration of cancer was conducted for the period 1968–73 by one of the principal investigators, assisted by a secretary and a registry clerk, who checked the data for duplicate registrations based on patient identification parameters which included residence, mainly obtained from the patients themselves. To determine usual residence in the registration area, use was made of the national identity card. During the period of data collection by the registry (1968–73), there was no systematic registration of deaths in place in Cap Vert province.

The data items recorded included patient names, sex, age, usual residence, site and histology. These were transcribed onto a list and forwarded to IARC. After consistency checks conducted at the registry in Dakar, the data were subjected to a further systematic check for errors and duplicates at IARC. Such procedures resulted in the elimination of about 12% of the registrations. Furthermore, efforts to thoroughly check eligibility in terms residence in the Cap Vert Province left only 48% of the registrations for analysis.

Population: The figures obtained during the 1970–71 census were used in the calculation of population at risk. For the Cap Vert Province, the census was conducted based on sampling. Population estimates noted a total of 349 247 males and 349 700 females.

Review of data

Cancer registry

The available report on cancer incidence in Senegal is that from the registry of Dakar (Cap Vert) for the years 1969–74 (Tuyns & Quenum, 1982). The population at risk was estimated from the 1970–71 census. Table 1 shows that a total of 1893 malignant tumours were recorded.

The pattern of tumours in males was similar to those of neighbouring West African countries. Liver cancer (ASR 25.6 per 100 000) was the most common cancer in the male population, followed by skin cancers other than melanomas (ASR 10.3), prostate cancer (ASR 4.3), lymphomas and malignancies of the stomach.

In females, cervix cancer ranked first (ASR 17.2); followed by breast (ASR 11.8), liver (ASR 9.0), skin (excluding melanomas) (ASR 7.9) and ovarian cancers (ASR 4.3).

Since these data were essentially derived from four pathology laboratories, care is needed in interpretation. Although the quality of the data in terms of the proportion with histology is high, there is the possibility of over-representation of some easily accessible tumours and under-reporting of deep-sited ones.

Unlike recent series from neighbouring countries, the data from Senegal exhibit an unusually high incidence of non-melanoma skin cancers for the male population (ASR 10.3). Whether this is a reflection of a difference in registration practices for multiple skin tumours or a real difference due to an underlying carcinogenic exposure is unclear (Camain *et al.*, 1972).

References

Camain, R., Tuyns, A.J., Sarret, H., Quenum, C. & Faye, I. (1972) Cutaneous cancer in Dakar. *J. Natl Cancer Inst.*, **48**, 33–49

Tuyns, A.J. & Quenum, C. (1982) Senegal, Dakar. In: Waterhouse, J., Muir, C.S., Shanmugaratnam, K. & Powell, J. eds *Cancer Incidence in Five Continents*, Vol. IV (IARC Scientific Publications No. 42), Lyon, IARC, pp. 210–213

Table 1. Senegal, Dakar (1969–74)

Site	Male	(%)	ASR(w)	Female	(%)	ASR(w)
Lip	3	0.3	0.2	4	0.5	0.4
Tongue	10	1.0	0.9	4	0.5	0.3
Salivary gland	4	0.4	0.5	0	0.0	0
Mouth	12	1.2	1	11	1.3	1.3
Pharynx	8	0.8	0.6	0	0.0	0
Oesophagus	3	0.3	0.2	2	0.2	0.2
Stomach	44	4.3	3.7	19	2.2	2
Small intestine	0	0.0	0	3	0.3	0.3
Colon	8	0.8	0.6	10	1.2	0.7
Rectum	17	1.7	1.5	11	1.3	1
Liver and intrahepatic bile ducts, primary	378	36.8	25.6	116	13.4	9
Gallbladder and bile ducts	0	0.0	0	2	0.2	0.2
Pancreas	12	1.2	1	9	1.0	1
Nose, sinuses etc.	3	0.3	0.3	3	0.3	0.3
Larynx	12	1.2	1.3	2	0.2	0.1
Trachea, bronchus, lung	15	1.5	1.1	1	0.1	0.1
Bone	4	0.4	0.2	5	0.6	0.3
Connective tissue	39	3.8	2.7	19	2.2	1.5
Melanoma of skin	13	1.3	1.2	11	1.3	1.3
Other skin	127	12.4	10.3	88	10.2	7.9
Breast	7	0.7	0.7	127	14.7	11.8
Cervix uteri	0	0.0	0	182	21.0	17.2
Chorionepithelioma	0	0.0	0	16	1.8	0.9
Corpus uteri	0	0.0	0	13	1.5	1.5
Ovary etc.	0	0.0	0	52	6.0	4.3
Prostate	36	3.5	4.3	0	0.0	0
Testis	4	0.4	0.2	0	0.0	0
Penis	5	0.5	0.4	0	0.0	0
Bladder	36	3.5	3	17	2.0	1.7
Kidney, other urinary	13	1.3	0.5	10	1.2	0.6
Eye	22	2.1	1.5	11	1.3	0.9
Brain, central nervous system	34	3.3	2	18	2.1	1.3
Thyroid	6	0.6	0.6	13	1.5	1.1
Other endocrine	1	0.1	0.1	0	0.0	0
Hodgkin disease	23	2.2	1.4	13	1.5	0.7
Non-Hodgkin lymphoma	59	5.7	3.5	23	2.7	1.2
Multiple myeloma	3	0.3	0.2	2	0.2	0.2
Leukaemia	10	1.0	0.7	4	0.5	0.2
Other and unspecified sites	57	5.5	4.4	44	5.1	4.6
All sites	1028	100.0	76.3	865	100.0	75.8

3.2.15 Sierra Leone

Background

Climate: Tropical; hot, humid; summer rainy season (May to December); winter dry season (December to April)

Terrain: Coastal belt of mangrove swamps, wooded hill country, upland plateau, mountains in east

Ethnic groups: 20 native African tribes 90% (Temne 30%, Mende 30%, other 30%), Creole 10% (descendants of freed Jamaican slaves who were settled in the Freetown area in the late eighteenth century), refugees from Liberia's recent civil war, small numbers of Europeans, Lebanese, Pakistanis and Indians

Religions: Muslim 60%, indigenous beliefs 30%, Christian 10%

Economy—overview: Sierra Leone has substantial mineral, agricultural and fishery resources. However, the economic and social infrastructure is not well developed, and the continuing civil war has totally arrested economic development. About two thirds of the working-age population engages in subsistence agriculture. Manufacturing consists mainly of the processing of raw materials and of light manufacturing for the domestic market. Bauxite and rutile mines have been shut down by civil strife. The major source of hard currency is the mining of diamonds, the large majority of which are smuggled out of the country.

Industries: Mining (diamonds); small-scale manufacturing (beverages, textiles, cigarettes, footwear); petroleum refining

Agriculture—products: Rice, coffee, cocoa, palm kernels, palm oil, peanuts; poultry, cattle, sheep, pigs; fish

Cancer registration

There has been no cancer registration in the country.

Review of data

There are no published accounts of the cancer profile in the country.

3.2.16 Togo

Background

Climate: Tropical; hot, humid in south; semi-arid in north

Terrain: Gently rolling savanna in north; central hills; southern plateau; low coastal plain with extensive lagoons and marshes

Ethnic groups: Native African (37 tribes; largest and most important are Ewe, Mina and Kabre) 99%, European and Syrian-Lebanese less than 1%

Religions: Indigenous beliefs 70%, Christian 20%, Muslim 10%

Economy—overview: The economy is heavily dependent on both commercial and subsistence agriculture, which provides employment for more than 60% of the labour force. Cocoa, coffee and cotton together generate about 30% of export earnings. Togo is self-sufficient in basic foodstuffs when harvests are normal, with occasional regional supply difficulties. In the industrial sector, phosphate mining is by far the most important activity, but has suffered from the collapse of world phosphate prices and increased foreign competition. Togo serves as a regional commercial and trade centre.

Industries: Phosphate mining, agricultural processing, cement; handicrafts, textiles, beverages

Agriculture—products: Coffee, cocoa, cotton, yams, cassava (tapioca), corn, beans, rice, millet, sorghum; meat; annual fish catch of 10 000–14 000 tons

Cancer registration

There has been no cancer registration in Togo.

Review of data

We have identified no publication on the cancer profile in the country.

3.3 Central Africa

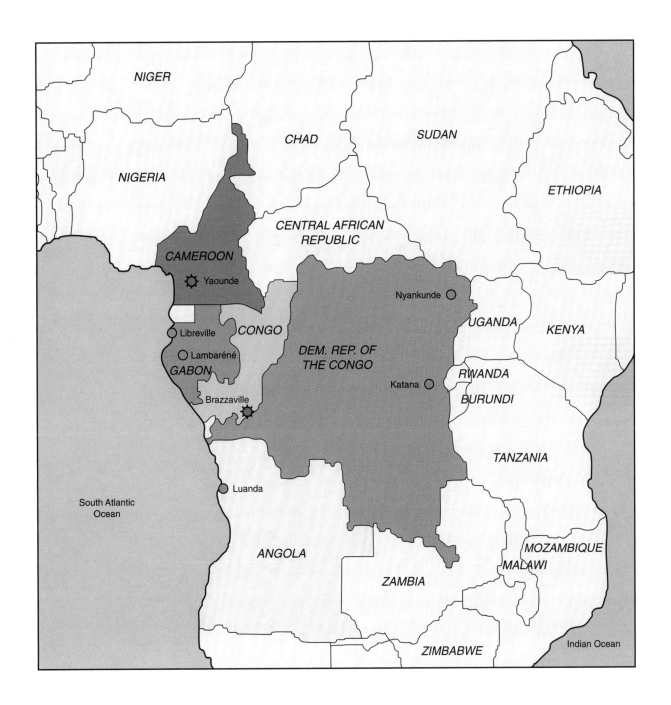

3.3.1 Angola

Background

Climate: Semiarid in south and along coast to Luanda; north has cool, dry season (May to October) and hot, rainy season (November to April)

Terrain: Narrow coastal plain rises abruptly to vast interior plateau

Ethnic groups: Ovimbundu 37%, Kimbundu 25%, Bakongo 13%, mestico (mixed European and native African) 2%, European 1%, other 22%

Religions: Indigenous beliefs 47%, Roman Catholic 38%, Protestant 15% (1998 est.)

Economy—overview: Angola has an economy in disarray because of more than 20 years of nearly continuous warfare. Despite its abundant natural resources, output per capita is among the world's lowest. Subsistence agriculture provides the main livelihood for 85% of the population. Oil production and the supporting activities are vital to the economy, contributing about 50% to GDP. Notwithstanding the signing of a peace accord in November 1994, sporadic violence continues, millions of land mines remain, and many farmers are reluctant to return to their fields. As a result, much of the country's food must still be imported. Despite the high inflation and political difficulties, total output grew an estimated 9% in 1996, largely due to increased oil production and higher oil prices.

Industries: Petroleum, diamonds, iron ore, phosphates, feldspar, bauxite, uranium, gold; cement; basic metal products; fish processing; food processing; brewing; tobacco products; sugar; textiles

Agriculture—products: Bananas, sugar cane, coffee, sisal, corn, cotton, manioc (tapioca), tobacco, vegetables, plantains; livestock; forest products; fish

Cancer registration

The National Cancer Registry was created in 1987, located in the Centro Nacional de Oncologia in Luanda. Previously, the only available statistics on cancer were derived from the Department of Pathology in the major university hospital (Americo Boavida). A report of the first four years of registration (1987–90) was published in 1990. The major source of notification to the registry remains the pathology departments of three hospitals in Luanda (including the Oncology Centre) (85% of recorded cases with histology), and the other cases registered are primarily from the same hospitals. Only 2% of registrations come from laboratories outside Luanda Province.

Review of data

Data from the Department of Pathology, University Hospitals, Luanda for the years 1977–1980 were published earlier (da Silva Lopes, 1986). The more recently published results from the National Cancer Registry are shown in Table 1, and it is these that have been used in preparing national estimates of incidence.

There is a small excess of cases in females, in whom cervix cancer is the major cancer (23.3%), followed by cancer of the breast (15.6%), skin (8.2%), stomach (5.1%) and non-Hodgkin lymphomas (4.5%). In men, the principal cancers are skin (10.2%), stomach (9.5%), non-Hodgkin lymphomas (6.9%), liver (5.6%) and Kaposi sarcoma (5.0%).

These results have to be interpreted cautiously, because of the high percentage of cases derived from pathology departments. Nevertheless, the high frequency of stomach cancer is noteworthy (85% with histology). Liver cancer (61% of cases with histology) is probably underestimated.

The age distribution of the Kaposi sarcoma cases was not available, so it is difficult to be certain whether they are AIDS-related or not. However, the high sex ratio (37:6) and the fact that Kaposi sarcoma was observed to be 'frequent' in the 1977–80 data (da Silva Lopes, 1986) suggests that many are of the 'endemic' type.

Reference

da Silva Lopes, C.A. (1986) Angola. Department of Pathology, University Hospitals, Luanda, 1977–1980. In: Parkin, D.M., ed., *Cancer Occurrence in Developing Countries* (IARC Scientific Publications No. 75), Lyon, IARC, pp. 33–35

Table 1. Angola 1987–90: frequency data

Site	Male		Female		%HV
	No.	%	No.	%	
Oral cavity	35	4.7%	20	2.5%	93
Nasopharynx	4	0.5%	6	0.7%	70
Other pharynx	15	2.0%	11	1.4%	77
Oesophagus	32	4.3%	3	0.4%	77
Stomach	71	9.5%	41	5.1%	85
Colon/rectum	22	3.0%	15	1.9%	86
Liver	42	5.6%	17	2.1%	61
Pancreas	9	1.2%	1	0.1%	90
Larynx	19	2.6%	4	0.5%	74
Lung	30	4.0%	9	1.1%	67
Melanoma	15	2.0%	17	2.1%	100
Other skin	76	10.2%	66	8.2%	97
Kaposi sarcoma	37	5.0%	6	0.7%	100
Breast	3	0.4%	126	15.6%	82
Cervix uteri			188	23.3%	87
Corpus uteri			25	3.1%	88
Ovary etc.			34	4.2%	76
Prostate	30	4.0%			93
Penis					
Testis	5	0.7%			80
Bladder	28	3.8%	9	1.1%	89
Kidney etc.	8	1.1%	12	1.5%	90
Eye					
Brain, nervous system	3	0.4%	4	0.5%	57
Thyroid	7	0.9%	16	2.0%	96
Non Hodgkin lymphoma	51	6.9%	36	4.5%	98
Hodgkin disease	12	1.6%	1	0.1%	100
Myeloma	2	0.3%	0	0.0%	100
Leukaemia	12	1.6%	9	1.1%	100
ALL SITES	744	100.0%	808	100.0%	86
ALL SITES excl. other skin	668		742		

Source: Relatorio Annual, Centro Nacional de Cancro, Registro Nacional de Cancro, 1990

3.3.2 Cameroon

Background

Climate: Varies with terrain, from tropical along coast to semiarid and hot in north

Terrain: Diverse, with coastal plain in southwest, dissected plateau in centre, mountains in west, plains in north

Ethnic groups: Cameroon Highlanders 31%, Equatorial Bantu 19%, Kirdi 11%, Fulani 10%, Northwestern Bantu 8%, Eastern Nigritic 7%, other African 13%, non-African less than 1%

Religions: Indigenous beliefs 51%, Christian 33%, Muslim 16%

Economy—overview: Because of its oil resources and favourable agricultural conditions, Cameroon has one of the best-endowed primary commodity economies in sub-Saharan Africa. Still, it faces many of the serious problems facing other under-developed countries, such as a top-heavy civil service and a generally unfavourable climate for business enterprise. The development of the oil sector led to rapid economic growth between 1970 and 1985. Growth came to an abrupt halt in 1986, precipitated by steep declines in the prices of major exports: petroleum, coffee and cocoa. Export earnings were cut by almost one third, and inefficiencies in fiscal management were exposed. Inflation, which rose to 48% after the devaluation of 1994, has been brought under control.

Industries: Petroleum production and refining, food processing, light consumer goods, textiles, lumber

Agriculture—products: Coffee, cocoa, cotton, rubber, bananas, oilseed, grains, root starches; livestock; timber

Cancer registration

A cancer registry was established in the Anti-Cancer Centre in the Central Hospital, Yaounde, in 1994. The objective was to collect data on cancer cases for the resident population of the city (estimated as 561 600 males and 517 300 females in mid-1995).

Review of data

The results of the first two years of operation in the Anti-Cancer Centre, Yaounde are shown in Table 1. The great majority of cases (80%) were identified in the two principal hospitals of the city (Central Hospital and University Teaching Hospital), and all had a histologically-based diagnosis. Calculation of incidence rates for this two-year period suggests a very low crude rate (24.1 per 100 000 in males and 33.7 per 100 000 in women). These figures imply considerable underascertainment, notably of cancer cases not diagnosed via the pathology laboratory, so that the calculated incidence rates are not presented.

The most common cancer in males is liver cancer (38.2%) followed by prostate (15.5%). In females, the most common cancers are cervix (30.7%), breast (27.1%), liver (10.3%) and ovary (6.7%). The category "skin" includes Kaposi sarcoma—it comprises 12.1% of cancers in men and 5.4% in women.

Previously, the most comprehensive picture of the cancer profile of Cameroon was the description of the series from the pathology laboratory of the Institut Pasteur, Yaounde, from the years 1969–73 (Table 2) (Jensen *et al.*, 1978). During these years, this was the only pathology laboratory in the country, and it recorded 3077 cancer cases (Table 2). As in all pathology series, superficial cancers are very evident (skin cancers and, in men, Kaposi sarcoma). Other than these, non-Hodgkin lymphoma (11.5%) and cancers of the liver (9.6%) are the most frequent in men, and cancers of the cervix (18.4%), breast (11.7%) and non-Hodgkin lymphoma (6.7%) in women.

Mbakop *et al.* (1992) provides some later information about histologically diagnosed cancers from 1986–91 (presumably from the authors' laboratory in Yaounde). This paper gives no breakdown by sex, but the most common sites are reported as liver (20%), skin (15%), cervix (11%), breast (11%) and lymph nodes (8%). The equality of the frequency of breast and cervix cancers is noteworthy.

References

Jensen, O.M., Tuyns, A.J. & Ravisse, P. (1978) Cancer in Cameroon: a relative frequency study. *Rev. Epid. Santé Publ.*, **26**, 147–159

Mbakop, A., Essame Oyono, J.L., Ngbangako, M.C. & Abondo, A. (1992) Epidémiologie actuelle des cancers au Cameroun (Afrique Centrale). *Bull. Cancer*, **79**, 1101–1104

Table 1. Cameroon, Yaounde (1995-1996)

NUMBER OF CASES BY AGE GROUP - MALE

SITE	ICD (10th)	ALL AGES	AGE UNK	MV (%)	0-	15-	25-	35-	45-	55-	65+	%
Mouth	C00-06	10	0	100	-	1	1	1	3	2	2	4.2
Salivary gland	C07-08	3	0	100	-	-	-	-	2	1	-	1.3
Nasopharynx	C11	7	0	100	1	2	1	2	1	-	-	2.9
Other pharynx	C09-10,C12-14	4	0	100	-	2	-	1	1	-	-	1.7
Oesophagus	C15	2	0	100	-	-	-	-	1	1	-	0.8
Stomach	C16	1	0	100	-	-	-	1	-	-	-	0.4
Colon, rectum and anus	C18-21	11	0	100	2	-	2	-	5	2	-	4.6
Liver	C22	91	2	100	6	5	9	15	15	18	21	38.2
Gallbladder etc.	C23-24	7	0	100	-	-	1	1	-	5	-	2.9
Pancreas	C25	1	0	100	-	-	-	-	-	1	-	0.4
Larynx	C32	8	0	100	-	-	-	1	-	3	4	3.4
Trachea, bronchus and lung	C33-34	6	0	100	-	-	1	-	-	5	-	2.5
Bone	C40-41	2	0	100	-	1	1	-	-	-	-	0.8
Melanoma of skin	C43	1	0	100	-	-	1	-	-	-	-	0.4
Other skin	C44	33	2	100	1	2	5	7	6	7	3	-
Mesothelioma	C45	0	0	-	-	-	-	-	-	-	-	0.0
Kaposi sarcoma	C46	0	0	-	-	-	-	-	-	-	-	0.0
Peripheral nerves	C47	0	0	-	-	-	-	-	-	-	-	0.0
Connective and soft tissue	C49	0	0	-	-	-	-	-	-	-	-	0.0
Breast	C50	0	0	-	-	-	-	-	-	-	-	0.0
Penis	C60	0	0	-	-	-	-	-	-	-	-	0.0
Prostate	C61	37	1	100	-	-	-	-	3	12	21	15.5
Testis	C62	0	0	-	-	-	-	-	-	-	-	0.0
Kidney	C64	1	0	100	1	-	-	-	-	-	-	0.4
Renal pelvis, ureter and other urinary	C65-66,C68	0	0	-	-	-	-	-	-	-	-	0.0
Bladder	C67	0	0	-	-	-	-	-	-	-	-	0.0
Eye	C69	2	0	100	2	-	-	-	-	-	-	0.8
Brain, nervous system	C70-72	0	0	-	-	-	-	-	-	-	-	0.0
Thyroid	C73	2	0	100	-	-	-	1	1	-	-	0.8
Hodgkin disease	C81	0	0	-	-	-	-	-	-	-	-	0.0
Non-Hodgkin lymphoma	C82-85,C96	1	0	100	-	-	-	-	-	-	1	0.4
Multiple myeloma	C90	0	0	-	-	-	-	-	-	-	-	0.0
Lymphoid leukaemia	C91	1	0	100	1	-	-	-	-	-	-	0.4
Myeloid leukaemia	C92-94	1	0	100	1	-	-	-	-	-	-	0.4
Leukaemia, unspecified	C95	0	0	-	-	-	-	-	-	-	-	0.0
Other and unspecified	O&U	39	0	100	8	2	5	3	6	4	11	16.4
All sites	ALL	271	5	100	23	15	27	33	44	61	63	
All sites but C44	ALLbC44	238	3	100	22	13	22	26	38	54	60	100.0

Table 1. Cameroon, Yaounde (1995-1996)

NUMBER OF CASES BY AGE GROUP - FEMALE

SITE	ICD (10th)	ALL AGES	AGE UNK	MV (%)	0-	15-	25-	35-	45-	55-	65+	%
Mouth	C00-06	6	0	100	1	1	-	3	1	-	-	1.8
Salivary gland	C07-08	1	0	100	-	-	-	-	-	1	-	0.3
Nasopharynx	C11	1	0	100	-	-	1	-	-	-	-	0.3
Other pharynx	C09-10,C12-14	3	1	100	-	1	1	-	-	-	-	0.9
Oesophagus	C15	0	0	-	-	-	-	-	-	-	-	0.0
Stomach	C16	8	0	100	-	-	2	1	2	2	1	2.4
Colon, rectum and anus	C18-21	12	0	100	-	-	1	-	7	4	-	3.6
Liver	C22	34	1	100	6	2	1	4	3	11	6	10.3
Gallbladder etc.	C23-24	1	0	-	-	-	-	-	-	1	-	0.3
Pancreas	C25	1	1	100	-	-	-	-	-	-	-	0.3
Larynx	C32	3	0	100	-	-	-	-	-	3	-	0.9
Trachea, bronchus and lung	C33-34	1	0	100	-	-	-	-	-	1	-	0.3
Bone	C40-41	5	0	100	1	-	-	2	-	1	1	1.5
Melanoma of skin	C43	0	0	-	-	-	-	-	-	-	-	0.0
Other skin	C44	19	0	100	-	2	-	3	4	5	5	0.0
Mesothelioma	C45	0	0	-	-	-	-	-	-	-	-	0.0
Kaposi sarcoma	C46	0	0	-	-	-	-	-	-	-	-	0.0
Peripheral nerves	C47	0	0	-	-	-	-	-	-	-	-	0.0
Connective and soft tissue	C49	0	0	-	-	-	-	-	-	-	-	0.0
Breast	C50	89	2	100	-	3	18	20	18	19	9	27.1
Vulva	C51	0	0	-	-	-	-	-	-	-	-	0.0
Vagina	C52	6	1	100	-	4	-	1	-	-	-	1.8
Cervix uteri	C53	101	3	100	-	4	9	14	36	27	8	30.7
Uterus	C54-55	5	0	100	-	-	2	-	2	1	-	1.5
Ovary	C56	22	1	100	-	4	3	5	7	2	-	6.7
Placenta	C58	0	0	-	-	-	-	-	-	-	-	0.0
Kidney	C64	1	0	100	-	-	-	-	-	1	-	0.3
Renal pelvis, ureter and other urinary	C65-66,C68	0	0	-	-	-	-	-	-	-	-	0.0
Bladder	C67	0	0	-	-	-	-	-	-	-	-	0.0
Eye	C69	0	0	-	-	-	-	-	-	-	-	0.0
Brain, nervous system	C70-72	0	0	-	-	-	-	-	-	-	-	0.0
Thyroid	C73	2	0	100	-	-	-	-	2	-	-	0.6
Hodgkin disease	C81	0	0	-	-	-	-	-	-	-	-	0.0
Non-Hodgkin lymphoma	C82-85,C96	0	0	-	-	-	-	-	-	-	-	0.0
Multiple myeloma	C90	0	0	-	-	-	-	-	-	-	-	0.0
Lymphoid leukaemia	C91	0	0	-	-	-	-	-	-	-	-	0.0
Myeloid leukaemia	C92-94	1	0	100	-	-	-	1	-	-	-	0.3
Leukaemia, unspecified	C95	0	0	-	-	-	-	-	-	-	-	0.0
Other and unspecified	O&U	27	2	100	3	5	1	1	3	7	5	8.2
All sites	ALL	348	12	100	11	22	39	54	85	90	35	100.0
All sites but C44	ALLbC44	329	12	100	11	20	39	51	81	85	30	

Table 2. Cameroon: case series

Site	Pasteur Institute, Yaounde,1968–73 (Jensen *et al.*, 1978)				%HV
	Male		Female		
	No.	%	No.	%	
Oral cavity	66	4.4%	31	2.0%	100
Nasopharynx	6	0.4%	4	0.3%	100
Other pharynx	23	1.5%	8	0.5%	100
Oesophagus	5	0.3%	0	0.0%	100
Stomach	41	2.7%	37	2.4%	100
Colon/rectum	49	3.2%	30	1.9%	100
Liver	146	9.6%	45	2.9%	100
Pancreas	6	0.4%	4	0.3%	100
Lung	34	2.2%	8	0.5%	100
Melanoma	55	3.6%	73	4.7%	100
Other skin	288	19.0%	240	15.4%	100
Kaposi sarcoma	157	10.4%	14	0.9%	100
Breast	28	1.8%	182	11.7%	100
Cervix uteri			287	18.4%	100
Corpus uteri			58	3.7%	100
Ovary etc.			83	5.3%	100
Prostate	44	2.9%			100
Penis	10	0.7%			100
Bladder	36	2.4%	14	0.9%	100
Kidney etc.	15	1.0%	15	1.0%	100
Eye	22	1.5%	13	0.8%	
Brain, nervous system	7	0.5%	4	0.3%	100
Thyroid	4	0.3%	22	1.4%	100
Non-Hodgkin lymphoma	174	11.5%	104	6.7%	100
Hodgkin disease	31	2.0%	13	0.8%	100
Myeloma	5	0.3%	3	0.2%	100
Leukaemia	10	0.7%	3	0.2%	100
ALL SITES	1515	100.0%	1562	100.0%	100

3.3.3 Central African Republic

Background

Climate: tropical; hot, dry winters; mild to hot, wet summers

Terrain: vast, flat to rolling, monotonous plateau; scattered hills in northeast and southwest

Ethnic groups: Baya 34%, Banda 27%, Sara 10%, Mandjia 21%, Mboum 4%, M'Baka 4%, Europeans 6500 (including 3600 French)

Religions: indigenous beliefs 24%, Protestant 25%, Roman Catholic 25%, Muslim 15%, other 11%. Note: animistic beliefs and practices strongly influence the Christian majority

Economy—overview: Subsistence agriculture, together with forestry, remains the backbone of the economy of the Central African Republic, with more than 70% of the population living in outlying areas. The agricultural sector generates half of the GDP. Timber has accounted for about 16% of export earnings and the diamond industry for nearly 54%.

Industries: diamond mining, sawmills, breweries, textiles, footwear, assembly of bicycles and motorcycles

Agriculture—products: cotton, coffee, tobacco, manioc (tapioca), yams, millet, corn, bananas, timber

Cancer registration

There has been no organized cancer registration in the country.

Review of data

We could trace no description of the cancer profile in the country.

3.3.4 Chad

Background

Climate: Tropical in south, desert in north

Terrain: Broad, arid plains in centre, desert in north, mountains in northwest, lowlands in south

Ethnic groups: Muslims (Arabs, Toubou, Hadjerai, Fulbe, Kotoko, Kanembou, Baguirmi, Boulala, Zaghawa, and Maba), non-Muslims (Sara, Ngambaye, Mbaye, Goulaye, Moundang, Moussei, Massa), non-indigenous 150 000 (of whom 1000 are French)

Religions: Muslim 50%, Christian 25%, indigenous beliefs (mostly animism) 25%

Economy—overview: Landlocked Chad's economic development suffers from its geographic remoteness, drought, lack of infrastructure, and political turmoil. About 85% of the population depends on agriculture, including the herding of livestock.

Industries: Cotton textiles, meat packing, beer brewing, natron (sodium carbonate), soap, cigarettes, construction materials

Agriculture—products: Cotton, sorghum, millet, peanuts, rice, potatoes, manioc (tapioca); cattle, sheep, goats, camels

Cancer registration

There has been no organized cancer registration in the country.

Review of data

We could trace no description of the cancer profile in the country.

3.3.5 Congo

Background

Climate: Tropical; rainy season (March to June); dry season (June to October); constantly high temperatures and humidity; particularly enervating climate astride the Equator

Terrain: Coastal plain, southern basin, central plateau, northern basin

Ethnic groups: Kongo 48%, Sangha 20%, M'Bochi 12%, Teke 17%

Religions: Christian 50%, animist 48%, Muslim 2%

Economy—overview: The economy is a mixture of village agriculture and handicrafts, and an industrial sector based largely on oil and related support services. Oil has supplanted forestry as the mainstay of the economy, providing about 90% of government revenues and exports. In the early 1980s, rapidly rising oil revenues enabled the government to finance large-scale development projects with GDP growth averaging 5% annually, one of the highest rates in Africa. Subsequently, falling oil prices cut GDP growth by half

Industries: Petroleum extraction, cement kilning, lumbering, brewing, sugar milling, palm oil, soap, cigarette making

Agriculture—products: Cassava (tapioca) accounts for 90% of food output, sugar, rice, corn, peanuts, vegetables, coffee, cocoa; forest products

Cancer registration

A population-based cancer registry was established in 1995, in the Department of Medical Oncology, situated in the largest hospital in the capital, Brazzaville. The registry aimed to register cases among the population of the city of Brazzaville. Before 1995, a register of cases attending the medical oncology service had been maintained. The registry functions by active case-finding through visits to all hospitals in the city, and collection of all pathology reports mentioning cancer. A few cases are notified by private practitioners.

The outbreak of civil war in 1997 caused a major disruption to medical and laboratory services, and a cessation of registry activity. However, this was able to restart towards the end of the year. The results presented in Table 1 are for three years, 1996 and 1998–99.

Review of data

1449 cases were registered in the three-year period, 51% of which had microscopically verified diagnosis. Table 1 presents incidence data based on the estimated population of Brazzaville. The calculated incidence rates are likely to be underestimates, given the social and political instability and consequent disruption to medical services.

In males, liver cancer is the most commonly registered tumour (26.4%) with 34% microscopic verification, followed by prostate (7.9%) non-Hodgkin lymphoma (6.9%) and Kaposi sarcoma (6.5%). In women, cervix cancer predominates (32.8% cancers). The age-standardized incidence, even though an underestimate, is rather high (31.7 per 100 000). Breast cancer is second in frequency (24.1%) with an estimated (minimum) ASR of 22.5 per 100 000. Liver is third in frequency (8.9%) and ovary (5.9%) fourth.

It is interesting to compare these results with the series compiled in 1965–66 from various hospitals and the Department of Pathology at the Institut Pasteur. There were 505 cases, most (70%) from Brazzaville, and 53% had a pathological diagnosis (Tuyns & Ravisse, 1970) (see Table 2).

At that time, the most frequently diagnosed cancers were, in males, liver (40.7%), prostate (9.5%), skin (9.1%), non-Hodgkin lymphoma (7%), and in women, cervix (21.8%), breast (14.1%), liver (13.4%) and skin (9.2%). The profile is similar to the more recent one, with the exception of the high apparent relative frequency of skin cancer. Burkitt's lymphoma was noted to be 'infrequent'.

Reference

Tuyns, A.J. & Ravisse, P. (1970) Cancer in Brazzaville, the Congo. *J. Natl Cancer Inst.*, **44**, 1121–1127

Table 1. Congo, Brazzaville (1996-1999)

NUMBER OF CASES BY AGE GROUP AND SUMMARY RATES OF INCIDENCE - MALE

SITE	ALL AGES	AGE UNK	MV (%)	0-	15-	25-	35-	45-	55-	65+	CRUDE RATE	%	CR 64	ASR (W)	ICD (10th)
Mouth	9	0	44	-	-	-	3	-	4	2	0.7	1.6	0.10	1.2	C00-06
Salivary gland	5	0	60	1	-	-	-	2	1	-	0.4	0.9	0.05	0.5	C07-08
Nasopharynx	3	0	100	-	-	-	-	2	1	-	0.2	0.5	0.04	0.4	C11
Other pharynx	13	0	62	-	1	1	1	5	3	3	1.1	2.3	0.13	1.7	C09-10,C12-14
Oesophagus	4	0	75	-	-	-	1	-	-	1	0.3	0.7	0.04	0.5	C15
Stomach	15	0	47	-	-	2	1	3	5	4	1.2	2.6	0.15	2.0	C16
Colon, rectum and anus	34	0	38	-	-	1	10	7	4	12	2.8	6.0	0.25	4.4	C18-21
Liver	150	0	34	1	17	33	35	21	20	23	12.4	26.4	1.23	17.2	C22
Gallbladder etc.	1	0	0	-	-	-	-	-	1	-	0.1	0.2	0.02	0.2	C23-24
Pancreas	16	0	6	-	-	2	2	3	6	3	1.3	2.8	0.17	2.1	C25
Larynx	15	0	67	-	-	-	-	2	2	6	1.2	2.6	0.15	2.2	C32
Trachea, bronchus and lung	28	0	36	-	-	-	3	6	11	8	2.3	4.9	0.29	3.9	C33-34
Bone	22	0	73	1	2	11	4	2	2	-	1.8	3.9	0.18	2.2	C40-41
Melanoma of skin	8	0	75	1	-	1	-	2	3	2	0.7	1.4	0.09	1.1	C43
Other skin	12	0	33	-	-	-	3	3	3	1	1.0	2.1	0.12	1.4	C44
Mesothelioma	0	0	-	-	-	-	-	-	-	-	0.0	0.0	0.00	0.0	C45
Kaposi sarcoma	37	0	76	1	1	4	15	10	3	3	3.1	6.5	0.34	4.3	C46
Peripheral nerves	0	0	-	-	-	-	-	-	-	-	0.0	0.0	0.00	0.0	C47
Connective and soft tissue	24	0	63	3	2	2	5	7	1	3	2.0	4.2	0.20	2.8	C49
Breast	4	0	25	-	2	-	2	-	1	1	0.3	0.7	0.03	0.5	C50
Penis	0	0	-	-	-	-	-	-	-	-	0.0	0.0	0.00	0.0	C60
Prostate	45	0	58	-	-	1	-	3	18	23	3.7	7.9	0.36	6.4	C61
Testis	4	0	50	1	-	-	2	2	1	-	0.3	0.7	0.04	0.4	C62
Kidney	8	0	0	4	-	2	1	-	-	-	0.7	1.4	0.05	0.7	C64
Renal pelvis, ureter and other urinary	0	0	-	-	-	-	-	-	-	-	0.0	0.0	0.00	0.0	C65-66,C68
Bladder	3	0	33	-	-	-	1	1	2	-	0.2	0.5	0.04	0.4	C67
Eye	6	0	50	3	-	-	-	-	-	2	0.5	1.1	0.02	0.6	C69
Brain, nervous system	2	0	0	-	1	1	1	1	-	-	0.2	0.4	0.01	0.2	C70-72
Thyroid	2	0	50	-	-	1	-	1	-	-	0.2	0.4	0.02	0.2	C73
Hodgkin disease	2	0	100	-	-	-	-	-	-	2	0.2	0.4	0.02	0.3	C81
Non-Hodgkin lymphoma	39	0	92	8	4	3	8	9	5	2	3.2	6.9	0.32	4.1	C82-85,C96
Multiple myeloma	9	0	56	-	-	-	-	4	5	3	0.7	1.6	0.08	1.2	C90
Lymphoid leukaemia	18	0	94	5	3	1	5	1	2	1	1.5	3.2	0.13	1.8	C91
Myeloid leukaemia	9	0	100	-	3	4	-	-	1	1	0.7	1.6	0.06	0.9	C92-94
Leukaemia, unspecified	9	0	100	1	2	2	1	-	2	1	0.7	1.6	0.06	0.9	C95
Other and unspecified	25	0	32	2	3	10	3	3	3	1	2.1	4.4	0.21	2.6	O&U
All sites	581	0	52	32	38	83	107	101	114	106	48.0	100.0	4.99	69.2	ALL
All sites but C44	569	0	52	31	38	82	104	98	111	105	47.1		4.87	67.7	ALLbC44
Average annual population				130895	59256	37934	26555	21572	14490	11606					

Table 1. Congo, Brazzaville (1996-1999)

NUMBER OF CASES BY AGE GROUP AND SUMMARY RATES OF INCIDENCE - FEMALE

SITE	ALL AGES	AGE UNK	MV (%)	0-	15-	25-	35-	45-	55-	65+	CRUDE RATE	%	CR 64	ASR (W)	ICD (10th)
Mouth	13	0	31	-	-	-	-	3	6	4	1.1	1.5	0.12	1.6	C00-06
Salivary gland	5	0	20	1	-	-	2	1	1	-	0.4	0.6	0.04	0.5	C07-08
Nasopharynx	2	0	100	1	-	-	1	-	-	-	0.2	0.2	0.01	0.2	C11
Other pharynx	5	0	60	1	-	-	-	1	2	1	0.4	0.6	0.04	0.5	C09-10,C12-14
Oesophagus	1	0	100	-	-	-	-	1	-	-	0.1	0.1	0.00	0.1	C15
Stomach	11	0	64	-	-	-	1	4	3	3	0.9	1.3	0.10	1.3	C16
Colon, rectum and anus	25	0	24	-	-	6	4	7	5	3	2.1	2.9	0.23	2.8	C18-21
Liver	76	0	37	1	4	9	17	19	11	15	6.3	8.9	0.61	8.4	C22
Gallbladder etc.	0	0	-	-	-	-	-	-	-	-	0.0	0.0	0.00	0.0	C23-24
Pancreas	9	0	0	-	-	1	2	1	2	3	0.7	1.1	0.07	1.1	C25
Larynx	0	0	-	-	-	-	-	-	-	-	0.0	0.0	0.00	0.0	C32
Trachea, bronchus and lung	4	0	0	-	-	-	1	1	1	1	0.3	0.5	0.03	0.5	C33-34
Bone	12	0	42	-	3	2	2	2	2	1	1.0	1.4	0.09	1.2	C40-41
Melanoma of skin	9	0	100	-	-	1	1	1	1	5	0.7	1.1	0.04	1.1	C43
Other skin	17	0	41	-	-	7	5	1	-	4	1.4		0.10	1.8	C44
Mesothelioma	0	0	-	-	-	-	-	-	-	-	0.0	0.0	0.00	0.0	C45
Kaposi sarcoma	14	0	86	-	1	6	4	1	1	1	1.2	1.6	0.11	1.4	C46
Peripheral nerves	0	0	-	-	-	-	-	-	-	-	0.0	0.0	0.00	0.0	C47
Connective and soft tissue	10	0	60	1	2	2	-	-	2	3	0.8	1.2	0.06	1.0	C49
Breast	205	0	48	-	10	35	64	54	34	8	17.0	24.1	1.95	22.5	C50
Vulva	4	0	75	-	1	-	-	1	-	2	0.3	0.5	0.02	0.4	C51
Vagina	1	0	100	-	1	-	-	-	-	-	0.1	0.1	0.01	0.1	C52
Cervix uteri	279	0	56	-	2	19	49	90	77	42	23.1	32.8	2.67	31.7	C53
Uterus	10	0	30	-	1	1	2	2	2	2	0.8	1.2	0.08	1.1	C54-55
Ovary	50	0	10	-	8	10	13	7	7	5	4.1	5.9	0.40	5.2	C56
Placenta	1	0	100	-	-	1	-	-	-	-	0.1	0.1	0.01	0.1	C58
Kidney	6	0	33	3	-	-	1	-	1	1	0.5	0.7	0.03	0.5	C64
Renal pelvis, ureter and other urinary	0	0	-	-	-	-	-	-	-	-	0.0	0.0	0.00	0.0	C65-66,C68
Bladder	3	0	0	-	1	-	1	1	-	-	0.2	0.4	0.03	0.3	C67
Eye	9	0	33	6	-	-	1	-	1	1	0.7	1.1	0.04	0.7	C69
Brain, nervous system	0	0	-	-	-	-	-	-	-	-	0.0	0.0	0.00	0.0	C70-72
Thyroid	5	0	80	-	-	4	1	-	-	-	0.4	0.6	0.04	0.5	C73
Hodgkin disease	2	0	100	-	-	-	1	1	-	-	0.2	0.2	0.02	0.2	C81
Non-Hodgkin lymphoma	26	0	88	10	3	6	3	2	2	-	2.2	3.1	0.17	2.2	C82-85,C96
Multiple myeloma	12	0	75	-	-	-	1	4	5	2	1.0	1.4	0.12	1.4	C90
Lymphoid leukaemia	19	0	100	-	1	1	4	3	6	4	1.6	2.2	0.17	2.2	C91
Myeloid leukaemia	6	0	100	-	-	-	1	4	1	-	0.5	0.7	0.07	0.7	C92-94
Leukaemia, unspecified	7	0	100	-	2	3	1	-	1	-	0.6	0.8	0.05	0.6	C95
Other and unspecified	10	0	10	-	1	4	4	1	-	-	0.8	1.2	0.08	1.0	O&U
All sites	868	0	50	24	40	120	186	212	173	113	72.0	100.0	7.60	94.9	ALL
All sites but C44	851	0	50	24	40	113	181	211	173	109	70.6	100.0	7.50	93.1	ALLbC44
Average annual population				123377	57910	38009	26009	24557	17120	14324					

Table 2. Congo, 1965–66: case series

Site	Brazzaville, 1965-66 (Tuyns & Ravisse, 1970)				%HV
	Male		Female		
	No.	%	No.	%	
Oral cavity					
Nasopharynx	5	2.1%	3	1.1%	64
Other pharynx					
Oesophagus					
Stomach					
Colon/rectum					
Liver	99	40.7%	35	13.4%	28
Pancreas					
Lung	5	2.1%	2	0.8%	14
Melanoma	6	2.5%	14	5.3%	91
Other skin	22	9.1%	24	9.2%	82
Kaposi sarcoma					
Breast			37	14.1%	51
Cervix uteri			57	21.8%	53
Corpus uteri			16	6.1%	56
Ovary etc			12	4.6%	67
Prostate	23	9.5%			61
Penis					
Bladder					
Kidney etc.					
Eye					
Brain, nervous system					
Thyroid					
Non Hodgkin lymphoma	17	7.0%	8	3.1%	72
Hodgkin disease					
Myeloma					
Leukaemia					
ALL SITES	243	100.0%	262	100.0%	53

3.3.6 Democratic Republic of the Congo (formerly Zaire)

Background

Climate: Tropical; hot and humid in equatorial river basin; cooler and drier in southern highlands; cooler and wetter in eastern highlands; north of equator – wet season April to October, dry season December to February; south of equator – wet season November to March, dry season April to October

Terrain: Vast central basin is a low-lying plateau; mountains in east

Ethnic groups: Over 200 African ethnic groups of which the majority are Bantu; the four largest tribes—Mongo, Luba, Kongo (all Bantu), and the Mangbetu-Azande (Hamitic) make up about 45% of the population

Religions: Roman Catholic 50%, Protestant 20%, Kimbanguist 10%, Muslim 10%, other syncretic sects and traditional beliefs 10%

Economy—overview: The economy of the Democratic Republic of the Congo—a nation endowed with vast potential wealth—has declined significantly since the mid-1980s. Most individuals and families survive through subsistence farming or petty trade. A barter economy flourishes in all but the largest cities.

Industries: Mining, mineral processing, consumer products (including textiles, footwear, cigarettes, processed foods and beverages), cement, diamonds

Agriculture—products: Coffee, sugar, palm oil, rubber, tea, quinine, cassava (tapioca), palm oil, bananas, root crops, corn, fruits; wood products

Cancer registration

There has been no organized cancer registration in the country.

Review of data

Several case series have been reported, giving an insight into the cancer profile of this vast country. Thijs (1957) published results from the pathology laboratory in Stanleyville (modern Kisangani) from the years 1939–1955. There were 2418 cancer cases, with specimens coming from hospitals all over the country, but mainly from Orientale province (44.6%) and Kivu (16.6%). Since sex was unknown for about one fifth of cases, the relative frequencies are a little difficult to interpret, but there were clearly high frequencies of liver cancer in males (15.9% of cancers), and cervix and breast cancers in females (17.9% and 12% respectively). Kaposi sarcoma was very frequent, 13.4% cancers in men, 2% in women.

Oates *et al.* (1984) and Oates (1986) described a histopathology series, based on biopsies performed in the surgical department of the Centre Médical Evangelique (C.M.E.) hospital, Nyankunde, Orientale Province, taken during 1971–83. The 794 malignant cancers detected (Table 1) showed, as might be expected, a considerable excess of superficial tumours, and deficit of poorly accessible cancers (the authors commented that the low frequency of liver cancer was surely an underestimate of true frequency). Of interest is the high relative frequency of Kaposi sarcoma (16.4% cancers in males); the authors noted that these occurred at younger ages than melanomas (the median age appears to be about 35 years), and that no increase in frequency was noted in the 13-year period. Breast cancer (17.9%) was more common than cervix cancer (10.8%) in women. Of interest too were the 25 eye cancers, 15 of which were squamous cell cancers, and 14 cases of Burkitt lymphoma (10 male, 4 female) among the 70 cases of non-Hodgkin lymphoma.

A more representative series was reported from a hospital at Katana, on the western shores of Lake Kivu (Kivu province), representing all cancer cases diagnosed in 1983-1986 (Bourdeaux *et al.*, 1988). In all, there were 494 cancer cases (six with sex not recorded) (Table 1); 73% were diagnosed with histology. Liver cancer is the most common cancer in both sexes, followed by Kaposi sarcoma in men (17.4%) and cervix cancer in women (12.1%). Stomach cancer was the third most common cancer in both sexes. The authors also provide tabulations for the 272 cases diagnosed among the residents of the four health districts served by the hospital (a total population of 204 000). For males, the profile is similar to that of the total series, while for females, stomach cancer appeared to be the most frequent (17.8%), followed by liver (16.8%) and cervix (13.1%). The crude incidence rate (all sites) for the resident cases was 40.7 per 100 000 for males and 26.4 per 100 000 for females. The authors note that the high frequency of stomach cancer had been noted previously in this region (Ceuterick, 1960), while Gigase *et al.* (1984) had drawn attention to the high frequency of Kaposi sarcoma. At the time this case series was collected (1983–1986), very few cases of Kaposi sarcoma were associated with HIV infection.

In a study of liver cancer, Kashala *et al.* (1992) observed the familiar association with chronic carriage of hepatitis B virus (HBV) (56.7% of 40 liver cancer cases HBsAg-positive, compared with 7.4% of 68 controls), and also noted higher levels of serum alpha-fetoprotein in the HBV-positive cases, compared with those HBV-negative.

Childhood cancer

A report from the C.M.E. hospital, Nyankunde, described 73 biopsied cancers among children from 1983–1988 (Fischer *et al.*, 1990). Lymphomas were the most common malignant tumour (38.4%), of which just over half were Burkitt lymphoma (Table 2).

References

Ceuterick, J., (1960) Cancer of the stomach in the Katana region. *Trop. Geogr. Med.*, **12**, 119–126

Gigase, P.L., de Muynck A. & de Feyter, M. (1984) Kaposi sarcoma in Zaire. In: Williams, A.O., O'Conor, G.T., De Thé, G.T. & Johnson, C.A., eds, *Virus-Associated Cancers in Africa* (IARC Scientific Publications No. 63), Lyon, IARC, pp. 549–557

Kashala, L.O., Kapanci, Y., Frei, P.C., Lambert, P.H., Kalengayi, M.R. & Essex, M. (1992) Hepatitis B virus, alpha-fetoprotein synthesis, and hepatocellular carcinoma in Zaire. *Liver*, **12**, 330–340

Thijs A (1957) Considérations sur les tumeurs malignes des indigènes du Congo belge et du Ruanda-Urundi. A propos de 2,536 cas. *Ann. Soc. Belge Med. Trop.*, **37**, 483–514

Table 1. Democratic Republic of the Congo: case series

Site	C.M.E. Nyankunde, 1971–83 (Oates *et al.*, 1984)					Katana, 1983–86 (Bourdeaux *et al.*, 1988)				
	Male		Female		%HV	Male		Female		%HV
	No.	%	No.	%		No.	%	No.	%	
Oral cavity*	22	6.1%	27	7.1%	100	5	1.8%	3	1.5%	88
Nasopharynx	18	5.0%	10	2.6%	100	2	0.7%	0	0.0%	100
Other pharynx	0	0.0%	0	0.0%	100	1	0.4%	0	0.0%	100
Oesophagus	1	0.3%	0	0.0%	100	1	0.4%	0	0.0%	100
Stomach*	19	5.3%	9	2.4%	100	32	11.3%	24	11.7%	64
Colon/rectum*	11	3.1%	8	2.1%	100	2	0.7%	5	2.4%	100
Liver	9	2.5%	11	2.9%	100	76	27.0%	35	17.0%	54
Pancreas*	2	0.6%	1	0.3%	100	3	1.1%	7	3.4%	60
Lung	0	0.0%	0	0.0%	100	0	0.0%	0	0.0%	
Melanoma	28	7.8%	22	5.8%	100	5	1.8%	3	1.5%	100
Other skin	51	14.2%	26	6.8%	100	16	5.7%	18	8.7%	91
Kaposi sarcoma	59	16.4%	6	1.6%	100	49	17.4%	9	4.4%	84
Breast	3	0.8%	68	17.9%	100	2	0.7%	16	7.8%	89
Cervix uteri			41	10.8%	100		0.0%	25	12.1%	76
Corpus uteri			1	0.3%	100		0.0%	4	1.9%	100
Ovary etc.			31	8.2%	100		0.0%	5	2.4%	80
Prostate	17	4.7%		0.0%	100	20	7.1%		0.0%	75
Penis	6	1.7%		0.0%	100	4	1.4%		0.0%	75
Bladder	9	2.5%	1	0.3%	100	2	0.7%	0	0.0%	100
Kidney etc.	6	1.7%	5	1.3%	100	6	2.1%	5	2.4%	54
Eye*	11	3.1%	14	3.7%	100	2	0.7%	3	1.5%	80
Brain, nervous system	0	0.0%	0	0.0%	100	1	0.4%	0	0.0%	0
Thyroid	6	1.7%	11	2.9%	100	3	1.1%	3	1.5%	83
Non-Hodgkin lymphoma	42	11.7%	28	7.4%	100	17	6.0%	16	7.8%	88
Hodgkin disease	6	1.7%	2	0.5%	100					
Myeloma*	1	0.3%	2	0.5%	100					
Leukaemia	3	0.8%	2	0.5%	100	3	1.1%	2	1.0%	40
ALL SITES	359	100.0%	380	100.0%	100	282	100.0%	206	100.0%	73

* Distribution between males and females estimated from subtotals

Table 2. Democratic Republic of the Congo: childhood case series

Cancer	Nyankunde, 1983–88 (Fischer *et al.*, 1990)	
	No.	%
Leukaemia	0	0.0%
Acute lymphocytic leukaemia		0.0%
Lymphoma	28	38.4%
Burkitt lymphoma	15	20.5%
Hodgkin disease	3	4.1%
Brain and spinal neoplasms	0	0.0%
Neuroblastoma	2	2.7%
Retinoblastoma	5	6.8%
Wilms tumour	6	8.2%
Bone tumours		0.0%
Soft-tissue sarcomas		0.0%
Kaposi sarcoma	5	6.8%
Other	27	37.0%
Total	73	100.0%

3.3.7 Equatorial Guinea

Background

Climate: Tropical; always hot, humid

Terrain: Coastal plains rise to interior hills; islands are volcanic

Ethnic groups: Bioko (primarily Bubi, some Fernandinos), Rio Muni (primarily Fang), Europeans less than 1000, mostly Spanish

Religions: Nominally Christian and predominantly Roman Catholic, pagan practices

Economy—overview: The discovery and exploitation of large oil reserves have contributed to dramatic economic growth in recent years. Farming, forestry, and fishing are also major components of GDP. Subsistence farming predominates.

Undeveloped natural resources include titanium, iron ore, manganese, uranium and alluvial gold.

Industries: Fishing, sawmilling

Agriculture—products: Coffee, cocoa, rice, yams, cassava (tapioca), bananas, palm oil nuts, manioc; livestock; timber

Cancer registration

There has been no organized cancer registration in the country.

Review of data

We could trace no description of the cancer profile in the country.

3.3.8 Gabon

Background

Climate: Tropical; always hot, humid

Terrain: Narrow coastal plain; hilly interior; savanna in east and south

Ethnic groups: Bantu tribes including four major tribal groupings (Fang, Eshira, Bapounou, Bateke), other Africans and Europeans 154 000, including 6000 French and 11 000 persons of dual nationality

Religions: Christian 55–75%, Muslim less than 1%, animist

Economy—overview: Gabon enjoys a per capita income four times that of most nations of sub-Saharan Africa. This has supported a sharp decline in extreme poverty, but because of high income inequality a large proportion of the population remains poor. Gabon depended on timber and manganese until oil was discovered offshore in the early 1970s. The oil sector now accounts for 50% of GDP. Gabon continues to face fluctuating prices for its oil, timber, manganese and uranium exports.

Industries: Food and beverages; textile; lumber and plywood; cement; petroleum extraction and refining; manganese, uranium and gold mining; chemicals; ship repair

Agriculture—products: Cocoa, coffee, sugar, palm oil; rubber; okoume (a tropical softwood); cattle; small fishing operations (which provide a catch of about 30 000 metric tons)

Cancer registration

There has been no population-based cancer registration in the country, although there is a pathology-based register in the capital, Libreville, which has published its results (see below).

Review of data

Denues and Munz (1967) published the results of an analysis of the 196 histologically-proved malignancies seen in the Dr Schweitzer Hospital, Lambaréné, between 1950 and 1965 (Table 1). Other than the usual finding in histology series of large numbers of skin cancers, the commonest cancers in men were liver (14.6%), prostate (8.3%) and non-Hodgkin lymphoma (8.3%), and in women, cervix (18%), ovary (11%) and non-Hodgkin lymphoma

(6%). The authors noted that only one case of Burkitt lymphoma was observed among the non-Hodgkin lymphoma cases, a male aged 24 years.

Walter *et al.* (1986) published the results from the Department of Pathology, Centre for Health Sciences, Libreville, for the years 1978–84. The series comprises surgical biopsy results (excluding, therefore, haematological malignancies) (Table 1). Ignoring cutaneous malignancies, the most common cancers in men were prostate (13.2%), non-Hodgkin lymphoma (12.1%), oral cavity (10.8%) and liver (4.8%), and in women, cervix (27.1%), breast (13.8%) and ovary (5.8%). The authors commented that the low frequency of liver cancer reflected reluctance to perform biopsies, rather than a low incidence of this cancer. Burkitt lymphoma comprised 80% of the childhood non-Hodgkin lymphoma (10/13 cases in boys, 2/2 in girls), and accounted for one third of childhood cancers. Kaposi sarcoma was more common in men, affecting mainly the lower limb (25/27 cases), but surprisingly was most frequent in the 25–34-year age group in men (7/30 cancers), and unusual in older men (only 5/167 cancers aged 55 years or more).

Nze-Nguema *et al.* (1996) published a sequential series (1984–93) from the same source (Table 1). The basic profile was unchanged, other than the emergence of oral cavity cancers (tongue and mouth) as the most common cancers in males (9.6% cases) and a rather higher frequency of liver cancers (8.9% in males, 3.9% in females). While the relative frequency of Kaposi sarcoma is much the same in the two series, cancers of the eye are much more frequent in the later period – 34 cases (26 in adults) in men (2.5% of cancers). In a separate analysis of childhood cancers (Table 2), the authors drew attention to the frequency of Burkitt lymphoma.

References

Denues, A.R.T. & Munz, W. (1967) Malignancies at the hospital of Doctor Albert Schweitzer, Lambaréné, Gabon, 1950-1965. *Int. J. Cancer*, **2**, 406–411

Walter, P.R., Philippe, E., Chamlian, A., Khalil, T. & Minko-mi-Etoua, D. (1986) Gabon. In: Parkin, D.M., ed., *Cancer Occurrence in Developing Countries* (IARC Scienific Publications No. 75), Lyon, IARC, pp. 43–46

Nze-Nguema, F., Sankaranarayanan, R., Barthelemy, M., Nguizi-Ogoula, S., Whelan, S., Minko-Mi-Etoua, D. (1996) Cancer in Gabon, 1984-1993: a pathology registry based relative frequency study. *Bull. Cancer*, **83**, 693–696

Table 1. Gabon: case series

Site	A. Schweitzer Hospital, Lambarene, 1950–65 (Denues & Munz, 1967)					Dept. of Pathology, Centre for Health Sciences, Libreville, 1978-84 (Walter et al., 1986)					Dept. of Pathology, Centre for Health Sciences, Libreville, 1984-93 (Nze-Nguema et al., 1996)				
	Male		Female		%HV	Male		Female		%HV	Male		Female		%HV
	No.	%	No.	%		No.	%	No.	%		No.	%	No.	%	
Oral cavity	3	3.1%	0	0.0%	100	58	10.8%	21	3.8%	100	131	9.6%	44	3.6%	100
Nasopharynx	0	0.0%	0	0.0%	100	7	1.3%	5	0.9%	100	3	0.2%	3	0.2%	100
Other pharynx	0	0.0%	0	0.0%	100	9	1.7%	0	0.0%	100	68	5.0%	6	0.5%	100
Oesophagus	0	0.0%	0	0.0%	100	6	1.1%	2	0.4%	100	42	3.1%	19	1.5%	100
Stomach	0	0.0%	0	0.0%	100	6	1.1%	10	1.8%	100	29	2.1%	16	1.3%	100
Colon/rectum	6	6.3%	5	5.0%	100	11	2.0%	16	2.9%	100	57	4.2%	57	4.6%	100
Liver	14	14.6%	2	2.0%	100	26	4.8%	6	1.1%	100	121	8.9%	48	3.9%	100
Pancreas	4	4.2%	0	0.0%	100	4	0.7%	0	0.0%	100	10	0.7%	3	0.2%	100
Larynx	1	1.0%	0	0.0%	100	21	3.9%	3	0.5%	100	57	4.2%	4	0.3%	100
Lung	2	2.1%	1	1.0%	100	33	6.1%	11	2.0%	100	94	6.9%	18	1.5%	100
Melanoma	5	5.2%	6	6.0%	100	23	4.3%	21	3.8%	100	16	1.2%	32	2.6%	100
Other skin	7	7.3%	17	17.0%	100	36	6.7%	32	5.8%	100	90	6.6%	54	4.4%	100
Kaposi sarcoma						24	4.5%	3	0.5%	100	61	4.5%	9	0.7%	100
Breast	0	0.0%	7	7.0%	100	5	0.9%	76	13.8%	100	21	1.5%	172	13.9%	100
Cervix uteri			18	18.0%	100			149	27.1%	100			325	26.3%	100
Corpus uteri			1	1.0%	100			24	4.4%	100					100
Ovary etc.			11	11.0%	100			32	5.8%	100			41	3.3%	100
Prostate	8	8.3%			100	71	13.2%			100	106	7.8%			100
Penis	2	2.1%			100	11	2.0%			100					100
Bladder	4	4.2%	0	0.0%	100	13	2.4%	4	0.7%	100	22	1.6%	8	0.6%	100
Kidney etc.	6	6.3%	1	1.0%	100	6	1.1%	6	1.1%	100	18	1.3%	16	1.3%	100
Brain, nervous system	2	2.1%	0	0.0%	100	0	0.0%	0	0.0%	100					100
Eye	2	2.1%	0	0.0%	100	0	0.0%	2	0.4%	100	34	2.5%	5	0.4%	100
Thyroid	0	0.0%	2	2.0%	100	3	0.6%	14	2.5%	100	7	0.5%	13	1.1%	100
Non-Hodgkin lymphoma	8	8.3%	6	6.0%	100	65	12.1%	20	3.6%	100	119	8.7%	88	7.1%	100
Hodgkin disease	4	4.2%	1	1.0%	100	3	0.6%	2	0.4%	100					100
Myeloma	0	0.0%	0	0.0%	100	4	0.7%	0	0.0%	100					100
Leukaemia	1	1.0%	0	0.0%	100	0	0.0%	2	0.4%	100	13	1.0%	13	1.1%	100
ALL SITES	96	100.0%	100	100.0%	100	539	100.0%	550	100.0%	100	1367	100.0%	1235	100.0%	100

* Distribution between males and females estimated from subtotals

Table 2. Gabon: childhood case series

Cancer	Dept of Pathology, Libreville, 1984–93 (Nze-nguema *et al.* 1996)	
	No.	%
Leukaemia	11	7.7%
Acute lymphocytic leukaemia		
Lymphoma	61	43.0%
Burkitt lymphoma	47	33.1%
Hodgkin disease	5	3.5%
Brain and spinal neoplasms	0	0.0%
Neuroblastoma	2	1.4%
Retinoblastoma	10	7.0%
Wilms tumour	27	19.0%
Bone tumours		
Soft-tissue sarcomas		
Kaposi sarcoma	3	2.1%
Other	28	19.7%
Total	142	100.0%

3.4 East Africa

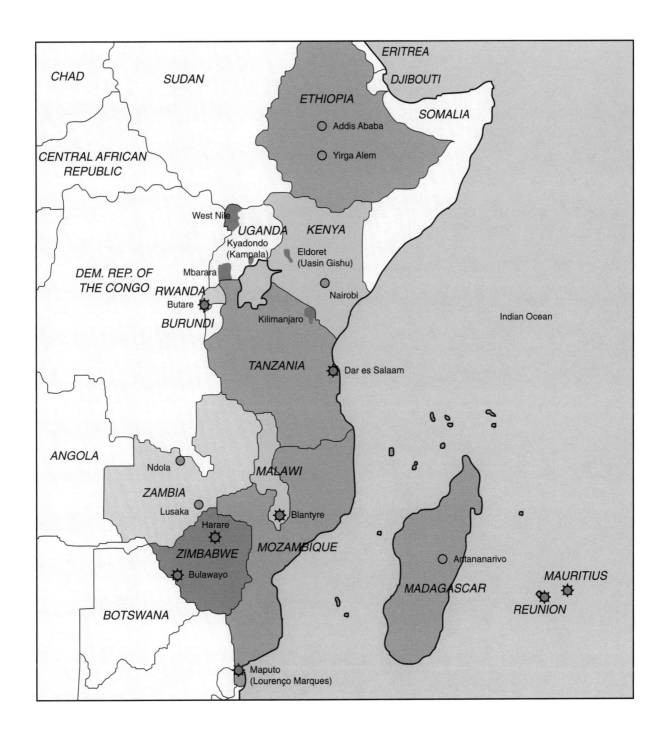

3.4.1 Burundi

Background

Climate: Equatorial; high plateau with considerable altitude variation (772 m to 2760 m); average annual temperature varies with altitude from 23 to 17 degrees centigrade, but is generally moderate as the average altitude is about 1700 m; average annual rainfall is about 150 cm; wet seasons from February to May and September to November, and dry seasons from June to August and December to January

Terrain: Hilly and mountainous, dropping to a plateau in east, some plains

Ethnic groups: Hutu (Bantu) 85%, Tutsi (Hamitic) 14%, Twa (Pygmy) 1%, Europeans 3000, South Asians 2000

Religions: Christian 67% (Roman Catholic 62%, Protestant 5%), indigenous beliefs 32%, Muslim 1%

Economy—overview: Burundi is a landlocked, resource-poor country in an early stage of economic development. The economy is predominantly agricultural, with roughly 90% of the population dependent on subsistence agriculture. Its economic health depends on the coffee crop, which accounts for 80% of foreign exchange earnings. The ability to pay for imports therefore rests largely on the vagaries of the climate and the international coffee market. Since October 1993, the nation has suffered from massive ethnic-based violence that has resulted in the death of perhaps 100 000 persons and the displacement of a million others. Foods, medicines and electricity remain in short supply.

Industries: Light consumer goods such as blankets, shoes, soap; assembly of imported components; public works construction; food processing

Agriculture—products: Coffee, cotton, tea, corn, sorghum, sweet potatoes, bananas, cassava (tapioca); meat, milk, hides

Cancer registration

There has been no systematic cancer registration in Burundi.

Review of data

Early reports of cancer include an analysis of 900 cases seen in seven hospitals in the region during 1956–60 (Clemmesen *et al.*, 1962) and a summary of 120 cases from four hospitals in Rwanda-Burundi in 1968–69 (Cook & Burkitt, 1971).

Kocheleff *et al.* (1984) conducted a systematic search for liver cancer cases during a one-year period in 19 hospitals located in three of the four natural regions of the country. Using alpha-fetoprotein (AFP) testing by counter-immunoelectrophoresis, with a cut-off of 200 ng/ml, they identified 87 AFP-positive cases, equivalent to a crude incidence rate of 5.2 per 100 000 (or 8.8 per 100 000 allowing for 60% sensitivity of the test). They postulated considerable geographical variation, although, since this was based on location of hospital, rather than place of residence of the subjects, the results may be questioned.

References

Clemmesen, J., Maisin, J. & Gigase P. (1962) *Cancer in Kivu and Rwanda-Urundi. A preliminary report.* Louvain, Institut du cancer, Université de Louvain

Cook, P.J. & Burkitt, D.P. (1971) Cancer in Africa. *Br. Med. Bull.*, **27**, 14–20

Kocheleff, P., Carteron, B., Constant, J.L., Bedere, C., Perrin, J., Kabondo, P. & Chiron, J.P. (1984) Incidence rate and geographic distribution of hepatoma in Burundi. *Ann. Soc. Belge Med. Trop.*, **64**, 299–307

3.4.2 Comoros

Background

Climate: Tropical marine; rainy season (November to May)

Terrain: Volcanic islands, interiors vary from steep mountains to low hills

Ethnic groups: Antalote, Cafre, Makoa, Amalsala, Sakalawa

Religions: Sunni Muslims 86%, Roman Catholic 14%

Economy—overview: Comoros is made up of three islands that have inadequate transportation links, a young and rapidly increasing population, and few natural resources. The low educational level of the labour force contributes to a subsistence level of economic activity, high unemployment and heavy dependence on foreign grants and technical assistance. Agriculture, including fishing, hunting and forestry, is the leading sector of the economy. It contributes 40% to GDP, employs 80% of the labour force, and provides most of the exports. The country is not self-sufficient in food production; rice, the main staple, accounts for the bulk of imports. The government is struggling to upgrade education and technical training, to privatize commercial and industrial enterprises, to improve health services, to diversify exports, to promote tourism, and to reduce the high population growth rate.

Industries: Tourism, perfume distillation, textiles, furniture, jewellery, construction materials, soft drinks

Agriculture—products: Vanilla, cloves, perfume essences, copra, coconuts, bananas, cassava (tapioca)

Cancer registration

There is no reported cancer registration in the whole of Comoros.

3.4.3 Djibouti

Background

Climate: Desert, torrid dry.

Terrain: Coastal plain and plateau separated by central mountains.

Ethnic groups: Somali 60%, Afar 35%, French, Arab, Ethiopian and Italian 5%.

Religion: Muslim 94%, Christian 6%.

Economy—Overview: The economy is based on service activities connected with the country's strategic location and status as a free trade zone in north-east Africa. Two thirds of the inhabitants live in the capital city, the remainder being mostly nomadic herders. Scanty rainfall limits crop production to fruits and vegetables, and most food must be imported. Djibouti provides services as both a transit port for the region and an international transshipment and refuelling centre. It has few natural resources and little industry. The nation is, therefore, heavily dependent on foreign assistance to support its balance of payments and to finance development projects. The unemployment rate is 40–50% and per capita consumption dropped an estimated 35% over the last seven years because of recession, civil war and a high population growth rate (including immigrants and refugees).

Industries: Limited to a few small-scale enterprises, such as dairy products and mineral-water bottling

Agriculture—products: Fruits, vegetables; goats, sheep, camels

Cancer registration

There has been no documented cancer registration in Djibouti.

3.4.4 Eritrea

Background

Climate: Hot, dry desert strip along Red Sea coast; cooler and wetter in the central highlands (up to 61 cm of rainfall annually); semi-arid in western hills and lowlands; rainfall heaviest during June–September except on coastal desert

Terrain: Dominated by extension of Ethiopian north–south trending highlands, descending on the east to a coastal desert plain, on the northwest to hilly terrain and on the southwest to flat-to-rolling plains

Ethnic groups: Ethnic Tigrinya 50%, Tigre and Kunama 40%, Afar 4%, Saho (Red Sea coast dwellers) 3%

Religions: Muslim, Coptic Christian, Roman Catholic, Protestant

Economy—overview: With independence from Ethiopia in 1993, Eritrea faced the economic problems of a small, desperately poor African country. The economy is largely based on subsistence agriculture, with over 70% of the population involved in farming and herding. The small industrial sector consists mainly of light industries with outmoded technology. Domestic output (GDP) is substantially augmented by worker remittances from abroad. Government revenues come from custom duties and taxes on income and sales. Road construction is a top domestic priority. Eritrea has inherited the entire coastline of Ethiopia and has long-term prospects for revenues from the development of offshore oil-fields, offshore fishing and tourism.

Industries: Food processing, beverages, clothing and textiles

Agriculture—products: Sorghum, lentils, vegetables, maize, cotton, tobacco, coffee, sisal (for making rope); livestock (including goats); fish

Cancer registration

There is no information on any form of cancer registration in Eriteria.

128

3.4.5 Ethiopia

Background

Climate: Tropical monsoon with wide topographic-induced variation

Terrain: High plateau with central mountain range divided by Great Rift Valley

Ethnic groups: Oromo 40%, Amhara and Tigrean 32%, Sidamo 9%, Shankella 6%, Somali 6%, Afar 4%, Gurage 2%, other 1%

Religions: Muslim 45–50%, Ethiopian Orthodox 35–40%, animist 12%, other 3–8%

Economy—overview: The economy is based on agriculture, which accounts for more than half of GDP, 90% of exports, and 80% of total employment; coffee generates 60% of export earnings. The agricultural sector suffers from frequent periods of drought and poor cultivation practices, as well as poor internal security conditions. The manufacturing sector is heavily dependent on inputs from the agricultural sector.

Industries: Food processing, beverages, textiles, chemicals, metal processing, cement

Agriculture—products: Cereals, pulses, coffee, oilseed, sugar-cane, potatoes, other vegetables; hides, cattle, sheep, goats

Cancer registration

There has been no population-based cancer registration in Ethiopia.

Review of data

There is no information on cancer incidence in Ethiopia. The only data on the cancer profile derive from published series, principally from pathology departments (Table 1).

Lindtjorn (1987) reported on 1154 patients with histologically diagnosed cancer at three hospitals in the Sidamo and Gamu Gofa regions of southern Ethiopia, for periods between the mid-1960s and mid-1980s. Among men, the commonest malignancies were hepatocellular carcinoma (especially notable in a histology-based series), lymphomas and superficial malignancies (skin cancers including melanomas and superficial soft-tissue sarcomas), while among women cervical, breast and ovarian cancers predominated. There were 12 Kaposi sarcoma cases diagnosed (1% of the total); the sex distribution was not given. In childhood, Hodgkin disease and Burkitt lymphoma were the most common cancers.

Loutfi and Pickering (1992) analysed the cases diagnosed in two laboratories in Addis Ababa in 1979–88 and 1986–88. There were 4067 cases, an annual average of 219 in men and 396 in women. In men, the commonest cancers were lymphoma (19%), soft-tissue sarcoma (13%) and head and neck cancer (11%); the other sites are shown in Table 1. In women, cervix cancer and breast cancer accounted for over half of the cases.

Ashine and Lemma (1999) reported on 841 cases of cancer (8.1% in children) diagnosed histologically (at the Norwegian Radium Hospital, Oslo) at Yirga Alem Hospital, Sidama Zone, southern Ethiopia, in 1986–95. The most common sites recorded were, in men, non-Hodgkin lymphoma (13.9%), soft-tissue sarcoma (12.7%) and non-melanoma skin cancer (12.2%), and in women cervix cancer (25.8%) and breast cancer (12.5%) (Table 1). The authors commented on the low frequency of liver cancer in their biopsy series (diagnosis was mainly by ultrasound).

Patterns of malignant tumours in Ethiopian Jews migrating to Israel in 1984 were analysed by the Israel Cancer Registry (Iscovich *et al.*, 1993). This cohort of 8272 Ethiopian immigrants (4253 males and 4019 females, with 27 966 and 26 848 person-years observed for males and females respectively) had significantly lower overall cancer incidence than Jews born in Israel. The standardized incidence ratios (SIR) for cancers at all sites were 39% (95% CI 22–64) and 63% (95% CI 41–92) for males and females respectively. Male primary liver cancer and female thyroid cancer had high SIRs. All other sites had either average or low SIRs. There were no reported cases of respiratory system neoplasms. Digestive system neoplasms (other than primary liver cancer) were more common in females than males.

From these data, it seems fairly sure that liver cancer is relatively common in Ethiopia. Some clinical series have commented upon this (Pavlica & Samuel, 1970; Tsega, 1977), and prevalence of hepatitis B surface antigen (HBsAg) in the general adult population has been variously estimated as between 6 (Tsega *et al.*, 1986) and 11% (Tsega *et al.*, 1987; Kefene *et al.*, 1988). The relatively high frequency of oesophageal cancer in Sidamo Regional Hospital (Table 1) was further investigated by Madebo *et al.* (1994). They found that, among patients attending this hospital for gastrointestinal symptoms, a significantly higher proportion of those from the Bale highlands had oesophageal or gastric cancer, compared with patients from elsewhere.

Two series of childhood cancer cases have been described. Ahmed (1984) reported on 122 cases of childhood cancer, diagnosed by pathology or haematology, in the main teaching hospital of Addis Ababa, between 1974 and 1981, and Teka (1992) a series of 71 cases, similarly diagnosed, in the Gonder College of Medical Sciences (north-west Ethiopia) between 1981 and 1990 (Table 2). Both show that lymphomas are the most commonly diagnosed childhood cancer, with one third of cases Burkitt lymphoma. Neuroblastomas do not appear to be rare.

Daniel (1990) described 39 cases of Burkitt lymphoma admitted to an Addis Ababa hospital and noted that the majority came from areas of high altitude (> 1500 m) without endemic malaria.

References

Ahmed, B. (1984) Incidence of malignancies in infancy and childhood in an Addis Ababa hospital. *Ethiop. Med. J.*, **23**, 35–38

Ashine, S. & Lemma, B. (1999) Malignant tumours at Yirga-Alem Hospital. *Ethiop. Med. J.*, **37**, 163–172

Daniel, E. (1990) Burkitt's lymphoma in Ethiopian children. *Trop. Geogr. Med.*, **42**, 255–260

Iscovich, J, Steinitz, R. & Andrew, V. (1993) Descriptive epidemiology of malignant tumours in Ethiopian Jews immigrant to Israel; 1984-89. *Isr. J. Med. Sci.*, **29**, 364–367

Kefene, H., Rapicetta, M., Rossi, G.B., Bisanti, L., Bekura, D., Morace, G. *et al.* (1988) Ethiopian National Hepatitis B study. *J. Med. Virol.*, **24**, 75–83

Lindtjorn, B. (1987) Cancer in southern Ethiopia. *J. Trop. Med. Hyg.*, **90**, 181–187

Loutfi, A. & Pickering, J.L. (1992) The distribution of cancer specimens from two pathology centers in Ethiopia. *Ethiop. Med. J.*, **30**, 13–17

Madebo, T., Lindtjorn, B. & Henriksen, T.-H. (1994) High incidence of oesophagus and stomach cancers in the Bale highlands of south Ethiopia. *Trans. R. Soc. Trop. Med. Hyg.*, **88**, 415

Pavlica, D. & Samuel, I. (1970) Primary carcinoma of the liver in Ethiopia. A study of 38 cases proved at post-mortem examination. *Br. J. Cancer*, **25**, 22–29

Table 1. Ethiopia: case series

Site	Three hospitals in S. Ethiopia (Lindtjorn, 1987)						Two laboratories in Addis Ababa (Loutfi & Pickering, 1992)					Yirga Alem Hospital, Sidama, Ethiopia, 1986–95 (Ashine & Lemma, 1999)				
	Male		Female		%HV		Male		Female		%HV	Male		Female		%HV
	No.	%	No.	%			No.²	%	No.²	%		No.	%	No.	%	
Oral cavity	24	3.9%	22	4.1%	100							21	5.1%	17	3.9%	100
Other pharynx¹	7	1.1%	2	0.4%	100							1	0.2%	0	0.0%	100
Oesophagus							6	2.7%		0.0%		42	10.2%	13	3.0%	100
Stomach	23	3.7%	13	2.4%	100		16	7.3%	13	3.3%	100	24	5.9%	14	3.2%	100
Colon/rectum	24	3.9%	10	1.9%	100		21	9.6%	14	3.5%	100	20	4.9%	13	3.0%	100
Liver	60	9.8%	7	1.3%	100		20	9.1%	11	2.8%	100	10	2.4%	1	0.2%	100
Pancreas	3	0.5%	2	0.4%	100							2	0.5%	1	0.2%	100
Lung	11	1.8%	6	1.1%	100							2	0.5%	2	0.5%	100
Melanoma	40	6.5%	29	5.4%	100		9	4.1%	5	1.3%	100	26	6.3%	21	4.9%	100
Other skin	85	13.8%	33	6.1%	100		26	11.9%	19	4.8%	100	50	12.2%	38	8.8%	100
Kaposi sarcoma					100							15	3.7%	2	0.5%	100
Breast	11	1.8%	77	14.3%	100				91	23.0%	100	9	2.2%	54	12.5%	100
Cervix uteri			118	21.9%	100				126	31.8%	100			111	25.8%	100
Corpus uteri			8	1.5%	100				15	3.8%	100			12	2.8%	100
Ovary etc.			54	10.0%	100				28	7.1%	100			38	8.8%	100
Prostate	7	1.1%			100		9	4.1%				3	0.7%			100
Penis	26	4.2%			100							5	1.2%			100
Bladder	6	1.0%	2	0.4%	100		9	4.1%			100	1	0.2%	0	0.0%	100
Kidney etc.	9	1.5%	6	1.1%	100							5	1.2%	5	1.2%	100
Eye	33	5.4%	20	3.7%	100							18	4.4%	12	2.8%	
Brain,nervous system																
Thyroid	12	2.0%	7	1.3%	100							6	1.5%	6	1.4%	100
Non-Hodgkin lymphoma	58	9.4%	20	3.7%	100		30	13.7%	14	3.5%	100	57	13.9%	15	3.5%	100
Hodgkin disease	26	4.2%	5	0.9%	100		12	5.5%	3	0.8%	100	6	1.5%	0	0.0%	100
Myeloma					100											
Leukaemia	7	1.1%	2	0.4%	100											
ALL SITES	614	100.0%	540	100.0%	100		219	100.0%	396	100.0%	100	410	100.0%	431	100.0%	100

¹ Includes nasopharynx
² Average annual number

Table 2. Ethiopia: childhood case series

Cancer	Ahmed, 1984		Teka, 1992	
	No.	%	No.	%
Leukaemia	29	23.8%	8	11.3%
Acute lymphocytic leukaemia			7	9.9%
Lymphoma	34	27.9%	18	25.4%
Burkitt lymphoma	11	9.0%	6	8.5%
Hodgkin disease	6	4.9%		
Brain and spinal neoplasms	0	0.0%		
Neuroblastoma	9	7.4%	6	8.5%
Retinoblastoma	3	2.5%	11	15.5%
Wilms tumour	15	12.3%	5	7.0%
Bone tumours	4	3.3%	14	19.7%
Soft-tissue sarcomas	13	10.7%		
Kaposi sarcoma	0	0.0%		
Other	15	12.3%	9	12.7%
Total	122	100.0%	71	100.0%

Teka, T. (1992) Childood malignancies in an Ethiopian teaching hospital. *Ethiop. Med. J.*, **30**, 159–162

Tsega, E. (1977) Hepatocellular carcinoma in Ethiopia. A prospective clinical study of 100 patients. *E. Afr. Med. J.*, **54**, 281–292

Tsega, E., Mengesha, B., Hansson, B.G., Lindberg, J. & Nordenfeld, E. (1986) Hepatitis A, B, and delta infection in Ethiopia: a serologic survey with demographic data. *Am. J. Epidemiol.*, **123**, 344–351

Tsega, E., Mengesha, B., Nordenfeld, E., Hansson, B.G., Lindberg, J. (1987) Prevalence of hepatitis B virus markers among Ethiopian blood donors; is HbsAg screening necessary? *Trop. Geogr. Med.*, **39**, 336–340

3.4.6 Kenya

Background

Climate: Varies from tropical along coast to arid in interior

Terrain: Low plains rise to central highlands bisected by Great Rift Valley; fertile plateau in west

Ethnic groups: Kikuyu 22%, Luhya 14%, Luo 13%, Kalenjin 12%, Kamba 11%, Kisii 6%, Meru 6%, other African 15%, non-African (Asian, European, and Arab) 1%

Religions: Protestant (including Anglican) 38%, Roman Catholic 28%, indigenous beliefs 26%, Muslim 6%, other 2%

Economy—overview: Economic liberalization and reform were introduced in 1993 and this included removal of import licensing and price controls, and removal of foreign exchange controls.

Industries: Small-scale consumer goods (plastic, furniture, batteries, textiles, soap, cigarettes, flour), processing agricultural products; oil refining, cement; tourism

Agriculture—products: Coffee, tea, corn, wheat, sugar-cane, fruit, vegetables; dairy products, beef, pork, poultry, eggs

Cancer registration

Until very recently, there was no population-based cancer registration in Kenya, but a pathology-based registry existed since 1962, based in the pathology department of the main government teaching hospital (Kenyatta National Hospital) in Nairobi.

The Eldoret Cancer Registry, established in 1999, is located in the Faculty of Medical Sciences of Moi University. The registry records details of all cancer patients diagnosed and treated in hospitals of Eldoret town and aims to be population-based for the district of Uasin Gishu, in the Rift Valley Region of Kenya (population in 1999: 623 000). As well as the Director, the registry has two full-time staff: a registrar and secretary, plus three part-time staff for data collection and data entry. Case-finding is active, using hospital records departments, pathology and death certificates. There are five hospital sources. The most important is Moi Teaching Hospital, which also acts as the District General Hospital. Cases are identified from the disease index (completed by records staff in ICD-10) and details of cases abstracted from case records. This method is supplemented by ward visits by medical students, which serve to identify cases not found through the medical records department. The registrar visits four private hospitals and the Eldoret Hospice regularly to identify cancer cases. There is only one pathology laboratory serving the District (in Moi University Faculty of Medical Sciences). Haematological malignancies are all diagnosed by the registry director (Department of Haematology).

Death registration is virtually universal, although deaths at home are certified by the village chief, and are of questionable accuracy.

Cases are coded in the registry, and data entry and management is by CANREG-3.

Review of data

The results from Eldoret for the three-year period 1998–2000 (Table 1) show that, in this highland area, cancer of the oesophagus is the most common cancer of men, with the moderately high ASR of 24.5 per 100 000, while it is fourth in frequency in women, with an incidence rate around half that in men. This implies that the area of high incidence of this cancer in Kenya is rather more extensive than

was proposed based on earlier studies. For example, Ahmed and Cook (1969), on the basis of an analysis of records from Kisumu hospital, suggested that the area of high incidence was localized in Central Nyanza district, close to Lake Victoria. Gatei *et al.* (1978), using data from the histopathology register at Kenyatta National Hospital, noted that a relatively high proportion of cases occurred among individuals from the Luo and Luhya tribes, who originate from western Kenya (around Lake Victoria), while < 1% of oesophageal cancers in their register were from the Kalenjin, the majority people around Eldoret. Linsell (1967a, b), examining data from the same source, earlier noted rather low frequencies of both oesophageal and gastric cancers among the Kalenjin tribe. Stomach cancer incidence is, in fact, moderate in Eldoret (ASR 10.4 per 100 000 in men and 7.8 per 100 000 in women). Incidence of liver cancer in this registry is moderately high; the rates (ASR 10.0 in men and 7.3 in women) are based on cases diagnosed by all methods, not just histology, so that the relative importance of liver cancer is greater than in earlier data from Kenya, which were based on pathology reports (see below). Currently, the incidence of Kaposi sarcoma is moderately high; these are presumably related to AIDS, since Kaposi sarcoma was not particularly common in Kenya before the epidemic. Nasopharyngeal cancer also appears to be relatively common (ASR 3.9 in males and 2.9 in females). A relatively high incidence has been reported previously from the highland area of central Kenya (Clifford, 1965).

Linsell (1967a) reported histologically diagnosed cancers among Africans, from the Medical Research laboratory in Nairobi, for the years 1957–63 (Table 2).

Cook and Burkitt (1971) reported on the records of three hospitals in western Kenya (Central Nyanza, 1965–66; Maseno, 1950–65; Kaimosi, 1966–69) with respect to the frequency of 12 common cancers in Africa: oesophagus, stomach, colon, liver, lung, penis, cervix, breast, bladder, skin, Kaposi sarcoma and Burkitt lymphoma. A total of 371 cases in men and 206 in women were included. The commonest cancer in men was cancer of the oesophagus, and in women cancer of the cervix in all the three hospitals. Kaposi sarcoma was relatively uncommon at that time (4% of cancers in men).

The results from the National Cancer Registry (based on the records of the pathology department in Kenyatta National Hospital, Nairobi) for the years 1968–78 were published by Kungu (1986) (Table 2). Excluding non-melanoma skin cancer, the most commonly recorded cancer was cervix cancer (22.4% of cases in women), followed by the lymphomas. Cancers of liver, oesophagus and nasopharynx were relatively common.

Chopra *et al.* (1975) compared the frequencies and types of cancer among Asians (from the Indian subcontinent) resident in Kenya with those in indigenous Africans. Higher risks of lung, breast and colon cancer were found in the Asians (Table 2).

Cameron and Warwick (1977) earlier investigated primary cancer of the liver in Kenyan children. In a nine-year period they reported 34 examples of primary liver cancer diagnosed in the first two decades of life and 29 of these were hepatocellular carcinoma; those diagnosed in the second decade were associated with liver cirrhosis. Peers and Linsell (1973) had reported a statistically significant association between estimated levels of aflatoxin ingestion and liver cancer in some parts of Kenya. Pettigrew *et al.* (1977) reported that 77% of a series of Kenyan patients with chronic persistent hepatitis or chronic active hepatitis or liver cirrhosis had hepatitis B surface antigen compared with 15% of a control group, and deduced that HBV was probably responsible for the high prevalence of hepatocellular carcinoma.

Table 1. Kenya, Eldoret (1998-2000)

NUMBER OF CASES BY AGE GROUP AND SUMMARY RATES OF INCIDENCE - MALE

SITE	ALL AGES	AGE UNK	MV (%)	0-	15-	25-	35-	45-	55-	65+	CRUDE RATE	%	CR 64	ASR (W)	ICD (10th)
Mouth	16	0	100	1	-	2	2	6	3	2	1.7	2.3	0.31	**3.7**	C00-06
Salivary gland	3	0	67	1	-	-	1	1	-	-	0.3	0.4	0.03	**0.4**	C07-08
Nasopharynx	20	0	90	1	1	4	4	6	2	2	2.1	2.9	0.32	**3.9**	C11
Other pharynx	5	0	100	-	1	2	1	1	-	1	0.5	0.7	0.05	**0.9**	C09-10,C12-14
Oesophagus	89	0	40	-	1	1	11	20	25	31	9.5	12.8	1.66	**24.5**	C15
Stomach	36	0	33	-	-	-	2	9	8	17	3.8	5.2	0.58	**10.4**	C16
Colon, rectum and anus	24	0	54	-	-	1	6	5	5	7	2.6	3.4	0.45	**6.3**	C18-21
Liver	44	0	45	-	-	6	8	14	7	8	4.7	6.3	0.75	**10.0**	C22
Gallbladder etc.	1	0	0	-	-	-	-	-	1	-	0.1	0.1	0.04	**0.3**	C23-24
Pancreas	16	0	25	-	-	-	1	-	8	7	1.7	2.3	0.40	**5.4**	C25
Larynx	14	0	71	-	-	1	2	3	5	4	1.5	2.0	0.33	**4.1**	C32
Trachea, bronchus and lung	15	0	53	-	-	1	2	2	5	5	1.6	2.2	0.28	**4.0**	C33-34
Bone	22	0	41	2	11	1	2	2	-	4	2.3	3.2	0.15	**3.2**	C40-41
Melanoma of skin	2	0	100	-	1	-	-	-	-	1	0.2	0.3	0.00	**0.4**	C43
Other skin	19	0	79	-	-	2	2	2	6	7	2.0		0.36	**5.3**	C44
Mesothelioma	0	0	-	-	-	-	-	-	-	-	0.0	0.0	0.00	**0.0**	C45
Kaposi sarcoma	35	0	83	3	-	9	13	5	4	1	3.7	5.0	0.51	**5.8**	C46
Peripheral nerves	1	0	100	-	-	1	-	-	-	-	0.1	0.1	0.04	**0.3**	C47
Connective and soft tissue	11	0	91	2	-	-	2	3	1	2	1.2	1.6	0.15	**2.2**	C49
Breast	3	0	67	-	-	-	1	-	-	2	0.3	0.4	0.01	**0.8**	C50
Penis	2	0	50	-	-	-	-	-	1	1	0.2	0.3	0.05	**0.7**	C60
Prostate	54	0	30	-	-	-	-	7	13	34	5.8	7.7	0.77	**16.8**	C61
Testis	3	0	0	-	-	-	1	1	-	-	0.3	0.4	0.08	**0.7**	C62
Kidney	14	0	71	9	1	-	-	-	2	2	1.5	2.0	0.14	**2.2**	C64
Renal pelvis, ureter and other urinary	1	0	100	-	-	-	-	-	-	-	0.1	0.1	0.05	**0.4**	C65-66,C68
Bladder	10	0	30	-	-	-	2	1	3	4	1.1	1.4	0.19	**2.9**	C67
Eye	9	0	100	2	2	1	4	-	-	-	1.0	1.3	0.07	**0.9**	C69
Brain, nervous system	34	0	6	6	2	4	5	9	7	1	3.6	4.9	0.65	**6.7**	C70-72
Thyroid	2	0	100	-	-	-	-	1	1	-	0.2	0.3	0.07	**0.6**	C73
Hodgkin disease	15	0	100	3	4	-	3	4	-	1	1.6	2.2	0.17	**2.4**	C81
Non-Hodgkin lymphoma	55	0	84	16	7	9	7	6	2	8	5.9	7.9	0.46	**8.2**	C82-85,C96
Multiple myeloma	8	0	75	-	-	-	-	3	2	2	0.9	1.1	0.17	**2.2**	C90
Lymphoid leukaemia	21	0	90	6	2	2	-	3	3	5	2.2	3.0	0.24	**4.1**	C91
Myeloid leukaemia	16	0	94	3	3	6	1	1	2	-	1.7	2.3	0.19	**2.2**	C92-94
Leukaemia, unspecified	4	0	75	2	-	-	-	1	-	-	0.4	0.6	0.03	**0.5**	C95
Other and unspecified	92	0	16	2	3	11	10	18	16	32	9.8	13.2	1.30	**22.3**	O&U
All sites	716	0	52	58	39	67	92	134	135	191	76.2	100.0	11.07	**165.6**	ALL
All sites but C44	697	0	52	58	39	65	90	132	129	184	74.2	100.0	10.70	**160.3**	ALLbC44
Average annual population				136931	68617	48245	28045	15529	7889	7764					

Table 1. Kenya, Eldoret (1998-2000)

NUMBER OF CASES BY AGE GROUP AND SUMMARY RATES OF INCIDENCE - FEMALE

SITE	ALL AGES	AGE UNK	MV (%)	0-	15-	25-	35-	45-	55-	65+	CRUDE RATE	%	CR 64	ASR (W)	ICD (10th)
Mouth	5	0	80	-	-	-	1	2	1	1	0.5	0.8	0.11	1.4	C00-06
Salivary gland	3	0	67	-	-	-	-	1	1	1	0.3	0.5	0.04	0.7	C07-08
Nasopharynx	13	0	85	1	3	1	1	1	4	2	1.4	2.0	0.24	2.9	C11
Other pharynx	0	0	-	-	-	-	-	-	-	-	0.0	0.0	0.00	0.0	C09-10,C12-14
Oesophagus	51	0	35	-	-	1	10	12	17	11	5.6	7.8	1.36	15.5	C15
Stomach	26	0	35	-	-	-	3	8	7	8	2.8	4.0	0.59	7.8	C16
Colon, rectum and anus	10	0	80	-	-	-	4	2	-	4	1.1	1.5	0.09	2.2	C18-21
Liver	29	0	24	-	-	4	7	7	6	5	3.2	4.4	0.60	7.3	C22
Gallbladder etc.	5	0	60	-	1	-	3	-	-	1	0.5	0.8	0.07	1.1	C23-24
Pancreas	12	0	25	-	-	1	2	5	1	3	1.3	1.8	0.20	3.0	C25
Larynx	2	0	100	-	1	1	-	-	-	-	0.2	0.3	0.04	0.4	C32
Trachea, bronchus and lung	10	0	60	-	-	1	-	4	2	3	1.1	1.5	0.24	3.0	C33-34
Bone	9	0	33	1	3	1	2	2	-	-	1.0	1.4	0.11	1.3	C40-41
Melanoma of skin	14	0	93	1	1	-	1	6	1	4	1.5	2.1	0.18	3.2	C43
Other skin	8	0	75	-	1	3	1	1	1	1	0.9		0.13	1.6	C44
Mesothelioma	1	0	100	-	-	-	-	1	-	-	0.1	0.2	0.02	0.2	C45
Kaposi sarcoma	15	0	87	-	3	5	5	1	-	1	1.6	2.3	0.21	2.4	C46
Peripheral nerves	0	0	-	-	-	-	-	-	-	-	0.0	0.0	0.00	0.0	C47
Connective and soft tissue	20	0	95	2	3	5	6	2	-	2	2.2	3.1	0.22	3.2	C49
Breast	59	0	93	-	3	10	14	14	13	5	6.5	9.0	1.30	14.3	C50
Vulva	1	0	100	-	-	-	-	-	1	-	0.1	0.2	0.04	0.3	C51
Vagina	0	0	-	-	-	-	-	-	-	-	0.0	0.0	0.00	0.0	C52
Cervix uteri	93	0	71	-	-	9	17	21	28	18	10.2	14.2	2.22	25.9	C53
Uterus	29	0	72	-	1	3	7	7	4	7	3.2	4.4	0.50	7.1	C54-55
Ovary	39	0	74	-	5	7	7	3	7	10	4.3	6.0	0.59	8.7	C56
Placenta	8	0	63	-	4	1	3	-	-	-	0.9	1.2	0.08	1.1	C58
Kidney	10	0	40	6	1	2	1	-	-	-	1.1	1.5	0.06	1.0	C64
Renal pelvis, ureter and other urinary	0	0	-	-	-	-	-	-	-	-	0.0	0.0	0.00	0.0	C65-66,C68
Bladder	5	0	80	-	-	-	-	-	1	4	0.5	0.8	0.04	1.4	C67
Eye	5	0	100	2	1	-	2	-	-	-	0.5	0.8	0.04	0.6	C69
Brain, nervous system	26	0	4	5	3	7	5	1	3	2	2.8	4.0	0.32	4.2	C70-72
Thyroid	7	0	43	1	-	-	3	1	-	3	0.8	1.1	0.05	1.5	C73
Hodgkin disease	8	0	88	1	1	2	2	2	-	-	0.9	1.2	0.12	1.4	C81
Non-Hodgkin lymphoma	34	0	76	14	3	5	4	3	3	2	3.7	5.2	0.41	5.3	C82-85,C96
Multiple myeloma	3	0	100	-	1	-	-	-	-	2	0.3	0.5	0.00	0.6	C90
Lymphoid leukaemia	5	0	100	1	1	-	2	2	-	-	0.5	0.8	0.12	1.2	C91
Myeloid leukaemia	19	0	84	4	1	4	2	3	4	1	2.1	2.9	0.35	3.9	C92-94
Leukaemia, unspecified	2	0	0	1	1	-	-	-	-	-	0.2	0.3	0.01	0.2	C95
Other and unspecified	76	0	8	2	3	11	10	10	15	25	8.3	11.6	1.21	18.7	O&U
All sites	662	0	58	42	43	85	125	120	122	125	72.5	100.0	11.89	154.4	ALL
All sites but C44	654	0	58	42	43	82	123	119	121	124	71.6		11.76	152.7	ALLbC44
Average annual population				135433	72081	44362	24030	13064	7333	8214					

Table 2. Kenya: case series

Site	Medical Research Laboratory Nairobi, 1957–63 (Linsell, 1967)						National Cancer Registry, 1968–78 (Kungu, 1986)						3 Nairobi hospitals: Asians, 1967–71 (Chopra, 1975)				
	Male		%HV	Female		%HV	Male		%HV	Female		%HV	Male		Female		%HV
	No.	%		No.	%		No.	%		No.	%		No.	%	No.	%	
Oral cavity[1]	85	3.7%	100	112	5.9%	100	383	4.3%	100	390	4.4%	100	13	7.6%	4	2.4%	100
Nasopharynx	97	4.2%	100	26	1.4%	100	487	5.5%	100	225	2.5%	100	2	1.2%	2	1.2%	100
Other pharynx	3	0.1%	100	1	0.1%	100	11	0.1%	100	5	0.1%	100	3	1.8%	2	1.2%	100
Oesophagus	175	7.6%	100	10	0.5%	100	803	9.1%	100	112	1.3%	100	3	1.8%	4	2.4%	100
Stomach	57	2.5%	100	43	2.3%	100	381	4.3%	100	212	2.4%	100	4	2.3%	6	3.6%	100
Colon/rectum	69	3.0%	100	37	1.9%	100	217	2.5%	100	126	1.4%	100	26	15.2%	10	6.0%	100
Liver	160	6.9%	100	58	3.1%	100	806	9.2%	100	335	3.8%	100	7	4.1%	5	3.0%	100
Pancreas	12	0.5%	100	6	0.3%	100	78	0.9%	100	40	0.5%	100	2	1.2%	1	0.6%	100
Lung	24	1.0%	100	7	0.4%	100	69	0.8%	100	33	0.4%	100	21	12.3%	1	0.6%	100
Melanoma	94	4.1%	100	100	5.3%	100	337	3.8%	100	378	4.3%	100	1	0.6%	0	0.0%	100
Other skin	279	12.1%	100	319	16.8%	100	855	9.7%	100	1010	11.4%	100	2	1.2%	1	0.6%	100
Kaposi sarcoma	92	4.0%	100	15	0.8%	100	390	4.4%	100	55	0.6%	100					100
Breast	23	1.0%	100	174	9.2%	100	110	1.2%	100	829	9.4%	100	1	0.6%	58	34.9%	100
Cervix uteri				270	14.2%	100				1985	22.4%	100			16	9.6%	100
Corpus uteri				23	1.2%	100				161	1.8%	100			10	6.0%	100
Ovary etc.				51	2.7%	100				341	3.9%	100			7	4.2%	100
Prostate	44	1.9%	100				387	4.4%	100				8	4.7%			100
Penis	42	1.8%	100				0	0.0%	100				3	1.8%			100
Bladder	30	1.3%	100	14	0.7%	100	118	1.3%	100	55	0.6%	100	4	2.3%			100
Kidney etc.	20	0.9%	100	26	1.4%	100	126	1.4%	100	124	1.4%	100	4	2.3%	0	0.0%	100
Eye	54	2.3%	100	36	1.9%	100	162	1.8%	100	123	1.4%	100	0	0.0%	0	0.0%	100
Brain, nervous system	15	0.7%	100	9	0.5%	100	187	2.1%	100	113	1.3%	100	7	4.1%	4	2.4%	100
Thyroid	22	1.0%	100	22	1.2%	100	61	0.7%	100	200	2.3%	100	0	0.0%	3	1.8%	100
Non-Hodgkin lymphoma	349	15.1%	100	152	8.0%	100	957	10.9%	100	552	6.2%	100	5	2.9%	3	1.8%	100
Hodgkin disease	85	3.7%	100	23	1.2%	100	337	3.8%	100	94	1.1%	100	4	2.3%	3	1.8%	100
Myeloma	15	0.7%	100	3	0.2%	100	34	0.4%	100	21	0.2%	100	3	1.8%	0	0.0%	100
Leukaemia	10	0.4%	100	5	0.3%	100	154	1.7%	100	129	1.5%	100	14	8.2%	8	4.8%	100
ALL SITES	2305	100.0%	100	1901	100.0%	100	8808	100.0%	100	8846	100.0%	100	171	100.0%	166	100.0%	100

[1] Includes salivary gland tumours

Table 3. Kenya: childhood case series

Cancer	Kungu, 1984		Makata et al., 1996	
	No.	%	No.	%
Leukaemia		0.0%		0.0%
Acute lymphocytic leukaemia		0.0%		0.0%
Lymphoma	751	49.3%	356	59.3%
Burkitt lymphoma	367	24.1%	201	33.5%
Hodgkin disease	136	8.9%	25	4.2%
Brain and spinal neoplasms	56	3.7%	0	0.0%
Neuroblastoma	2	0.1%	3	0.5%
Retinoblastoma	119	7.8%	69	11.5%
Wilms tumour	134	8.8%	27	4.5%
Bone tumours	81	5.3%	18	3.0%
Soft-tissue sarcomas	154	10.1%	84	14.0%
Kaposi sarcoma	28	1.8%	37	6.2%
Other	225	14.8%	43	7.2%
Total	1522	100.0%	600	100.0%

In a recent retrospective survey of the records of eight hospitals serving the population of the four districts of Greater Meru in Eastern province, McFarlane *et al.* (2001) identified 200 cases of gastric carcinoma diagnosed in 1991–93. Most had been diagnosed by laparotomy (52%) or endoscopy (24%), but histology was available for only 18 cases (9%). The estimated age-standardized incidence rates were 14.3 per 100 000 in men and 7.1 per 100 000 in women.

Childhood cancer

Kungu (1984) provided data on 1522 histologically confirmed cases of childhood cancer in Kenya between 1968 and 1980 (Table 3). No haematological malignancies are included in the series. Childhood cancers accounted for 10% of the total number of all cancers registered in that registry and lymphoma accounted for 49.3% of all childhood cancers. Burkitt lymphoma was the most frequent type of lymphoma (48.9%), occurring mainly in the age range 3–8 years, with a male:female ratio of 1.7:1. 45% of cases involved the face, maxilla or mandible. The Luo tribe, from a lowland area near Lake Victoria, seemed to be the most affected, accounting for 30% of cases of Burkitt lymphoma. Hodgkin disease was much more frequent in boys (ratio 4.6:1).

Makata *et al.* (1996) identified 676 surgical histological specimens in three hospitals of western Kenya (in Nakuru, Kisumu and Eldoret), diagnosed in the sixteen-year period 1979–94. The distribution of the 600 cases for which information was considered adequate is shown in Table 3. Burkitt lymphoma was the most commonly identified solid tumour. The frequency was rather different in the three hospitals, however, being 51.6% of biopsies in Kisumu, in the humid tropical zone around Lake Victoria, but only 23.4% in the cooler, highland Rift Valley province (Eldoret).

Neither of these two series included leukaemia cases. In two small case series of childhood cancer, leukaemias were found to comprise 21% of cases in Kenyatta Hospital (Macharia, 1996) and 12.8% in data from eight hospitals (including Kenyatta) in 1997 (Mwanda, 1999).

References

Ahmed, N. & Cook, P. (1969) The incidence of cancer of the oesophagus in west Kenya. *Br. J. Cancer*, **23**, 302–312

Cameron, H.M. & Warwick, G.P. (1977) Primary cancer of the liver in Kenyan children. *Br. J. Cancer*, **36**, 793–803

Chopra, S.A., Linsell, C.A., Peers, F.G. & Chopra, F.S. (1975) Cancer of Asians in Kenya. *Int. J. Cancer*, **15**, 684–693

Clifford, P. (1965) Carcinoma of the nasopharynx in Kenya. *E. Afr. Med. J.*, **42**, 373–396

Cook, P.J. & Burkitt, D.P. (1971) Cancer in Africa. *Br. Med. Bull.*, **27**, 14–20

Gatei, D.G., Odhiambo, P.A., Orinda, D.A., Muruka, F.J. & Wasunna, A. (1978) Retrospective study of carcinoma of the oesophagus in Kenya. *Cancer Res.*, **38**, 303–307

Kungu, A. (1984) Childhood cancers in Kenya: a histopathological and epidemiological study. *E. Afr. Med. J.*, **61**, 11–24

Kungu, A. (1986) National Cancer Registry, 1968-1978. In: Parkin, D.M., ed., *Cancer Occurrence in Developing Countries* (IARC Scientific Publications No. 75), Lyon, IARC, pp. 47–53

Linsell, C.A. (1967a) Cancer incidence in Kenya 1957-63. *Br. J. Cancer*, **21**, 465–473

Linsell, C.A. (1967b) Tumours of the alimentary tract in Kenyans. *Natl Cancer Inst. Monogr.*, **25**, 49–55

Macharia, W.M. (1996) Childhood cancers in a referral hospital in Kenya; a review. *E. Afr. Med. J.*, **73**, 647–650

Makata, A.M., Toriyama, K., Kamidigo, N.O., Eto, H. & Itakura, H. (1996) The pattern of pediatric solid malignant tumours in Western Kenya, East Africa, 1979-1994; an analysis based on histopathologic study (sic). *Am. J. Trop. Med. Hyg.*, **54**, 343–347

McFarlane, G., Forman, D., Sitas, F. & Lachlan, G. (2001) A minimum estimate for the incidence of gastric cancer in Eastern Kenya. *Br. J. Cancer*, **85**, 1322–1325

Mwanda, O.W. (1999) Cancers in children younger than age 16 in Kenya. *E. Afr. Med. J.*, **76**, 3–9

Peers, F.G. & Linsell, C.A. (1973) Dietary aflatoxins and liver cancer – a population based study in Kenya. *Br. J. Cancer*, **27**, 473–484

Pettigrew, N.M., Bagshawe, A.F., Cameron, H.M., Cameron, C.H., Dorman, J.M. & MacSween, R.N. (1977) Hepatitis b surface antigenaemia in Kenyans with chronic liver disease. *Trans. R. Soc. Trop. Med. Hyg.*, **70**, 462–465

3.4.7 Madagascar

Background

Climate: Tropical along coast, temperate inland, arid in south

Terrain: Narrow coastal plain, high plateau and mountains in centre

Ethnic groups: Malayo-Indonesian (Merina and related Betsileo), Cotiers (mixed African, Malayo-Indonesian, and Arab ancestry—Betsimisaraka, Tsimihety, Antaisaka, Sakalava), French, Indian, Creole, Comoran

Religions: Indigenous beliefs 52%, Christian 41%, Muslim 7%

Economy—overview: Madagascar suffers from chronic malnutrition, under-funded health and education facilities, a roughly 3% annual population growth rate, and severe loss of forest cover, accompanied by erosion. Agriculture, including fishing and forestry, is the mainstay of the economy, accounting for 33% of GDP and contributing more than 70% to export earnings.

Industries: Meat processing, soap, breweries, tanneries, sugar, textiles, glassware, cement, automobile assembly plant, paper, petroleum, tourism

Agriculture—products: Coffee, vanilla, sugarcane, cloves, cocoa, rice, cassava (tapioca), beans, bananas, peanuts; livestock products

Cancer registration

There has been no cancer registration in Madagascar.

Review of data

A description of 11 151 malignant tumours diagnosed in the anatomo-pathology service of the Institut Pasteur of Madagascar in 1954–78 was reported by Coulanges *et al.* (1979); this showed a high frequency of skin cancer (17%), lymphoma (9.8%) and melanoma of skin (8.2%) among males, while in females cevical cancer (31.5%) and breast cancer (12.3%) were the most frequent. A further report, for the years 1979–81 was published in 1986 (Table 1). Raharisolo Vololonantenaina *et al.* (1998) described a further case series, from the same pathology laboratory, for the period 1992–96. Cancer of the cervix remained the most common cancer of women (38%), followed by breast cancer (17%). In men, the most common cancers appear to have been colon-rectum (11.3%) and stomach cancer (10.3%) – a situation very different from that reported ten years earlier (Table 1).

References

Coulanges, P., Rakotonirina-Randriambeloma, P.J., Gueguen, A. & Randriamalala, J.C. (1979) Le cancer à Madagascar. *Arch. Inst. Pasteur Madagascar*, **48**, 171–212

Coulanges, P. (1986) Anatamo-pathology Laboratory, Institut Pasteur, 1979-1981. In Parkin, D.M., ed., *Cancer Incidence in Developing Countries* (IARC Scientific Publications No 75), Lyon, IARC, pp. 59–62

Raharisolo Vololonantenaina, C., Pecarrere, J.L. & Roux, J.F. (1998) Le cancer à Madagascar. Expérience de l'Institut Pasteur de Madagascar de début septembre 1992 à fin juin 1996. *Bull. Soc. Pathol. Exot.*, **91**, 17–21

Table 1. Madagascar: case series

Site	Institut Pasteur, pathology data, 1979–81 (Coulanges, 1986)				
	Male		Female		%HV
	No.	%	No.	%	
Oral cavity[1]	28	7.4%	15	2.5%	100
Nasopharynx	0	0.0%	2	0.3%	100
Other pharynx	1	0.3%	0	0.0%	100
Oesophagus	0	0.0%	0	0.0%	
Stomach	5	1.3%	3	0.5%	100
Colon/rectum	25	6.6%	17	2.8%	100
Liver	5	1.3%	2	0.3%	100
Pancreas	0	0.0%	1	0.2%	100
Lung	8	2.1%	2	0.3%	100
Melanoma	31	8.2%	13	2.2%	100
Other skin	64	17.0%	29	4.8%	100
Kaposi sarcoma	20	5.3%	1	0.2%	100
Breast	2	0.5%	74	12.3%	100
Cervix uteri			190	31.5%	100
Corpus uteri			7	1.2%	100
Ovary etc.			50	8.3%	100
Prostate	16	4.2%			100
Penis etc.	14	3.7%			
Bladder	6	1.6%	4	0.7%	100
Kidney etc.	3	0.8%	9	1.5%	100
Eye	16	4.2%	12	2.0%	100
Brain, nervous system	1	0.3%	1	0.2%	100
Thyroid	5	1.3%	20	3.3%	100
Non-Hodgkin lymphoma	37	9.8%	39	6.5%	100
Hodgkin disease	8	2.1%	7	1.2%	100
Myeloma	0	0.0%	0	0.0%	
Leukaemia	1	0.3%	0	0.0%	100
ALL SITES	377	100.0%	604	100.0%	100

[1] Includes salivary gland

3.4.8 Malawi

Background

Climate: Tropical; rainy season (November to May); dry season (May to November)

Terrain: Narrow elongated plateau with rolling plains, rounded hills, some mountains

Ethnic groups: Chewa, Nyanja, Tumbuko, Yao, Lomwe, Sena, Tonga, Ngoni, Ngonde, Asian, European

Religions: Protestant 55%, Roman Catholic 20%, Muslim 20%, traditional indigenous beliefs

Economy—overview: The economy is predominantly agricultural, with about 90% of the population living in rural areas. Agriculture accounts for 45% of GDP and 90% of export revenues. The economy depends on substantial inflows of economic assistance from the International Monetary Fund, the World Bank, and individual donor nations. The government faces strong challenges to spur exports, to improve educational and health facilities and to deal with environmental problems of deforestation and erosion.

Industries: Tea, tobacco, sugar, sawmill products, cement, consumer goods

Agriculture—products: Tobacco, sugarcane, cotton, tea, corn, potatoes, cassava (tapioca), sorghum, pulses; cattle, goats

Cancer registration

The Malawi National Cancer registry was established in 1989. Initially it was a histopathology-based registry, recording data on cancer cases diagnosed in the pathology laboratory in Queen Elizabeth's Hospital (QEH), Blantyre, which received specimens from hospitals throughout the country. In 1993, the registry began to record cases from all hospitals and clinics serving the population of Blantyre District (Urban and Rural), however diagnosed. This was achieved by a programme of regular visits by a cancer registrar and registry clerk to hospital records departments and clinical services where cases might have been diagnosed or treated. The majority of cases (76%) were from QEH – the main government hospital – with smaller numbers from other hospitals run by religious orders or privately. There is no comprehensive death registration in Malawi, so that death certificates cannot be used as a source of information on cancer cases. The number of cases recorded among residents of the Districts remained more or less constant in the five-year period 1994–98 at 400–500 per year.

In 1999, a new registry director was appointed and extra staff were employed. This allowed more frequent visits to hospitals for case-finding and visits to hospitals in neighbouring districts were scheduled. In addition, medical record staff in local hospitals were asked to record details of any cancer cases seen in out-patient departments. This resulted in a marked increase in cases from Blantyre district recorded by the registry, to an average of 735 per year in 1999–2001.

Review of data

Results are presented for a recent two-year period (2000–2001), corresponding to the years in which the enhanced case-finding described above were employed (Table 1). The incidence rates are rather higher than in the data from the first five years of registration (1994–98) published by Banda *et al.* (2001). In this earlier data-set, the age-standardized incidence for all sites was 92.0 per 100 000 in

men and 88.8 per 100 000 in women. The authors commented that there was probably underascertainment of cases during these years; the results are therefore summarized as relative frequencies of different cancers in Table 2.

The overall incidence rates for the period 2000–2001 were 128.2 per 100 000 in men and 151.3 per 100 000 in women (Table 1). Only a minority of cases were registered on the basis of microscopic evidence; this largely reflects the very high incidence of Kaposi sarcoma: 53.5% of all cancers in men (ASR, 49.9) and 32.3% in women (ASR, 31.7) and relatively few of these cases were diagnosed on the basis of histology. Following Kaposi sarcoma, the most common cancers of men are oesophageal cancer (10%, ASR 17.4), prostate cancer (4.2%, ASR 10.7), non-Hodgkin lymphomas (5.8%, ASR 6.0) and bladder cancer (2.2%, ASR 3.4). In women, the most common cancers (after Kaposi sarcoma) are cervix cancer, (30.7%, ASR 53.1), breast cancer (6.6%, ASR 12.0) and oesophageal cancer (5.2%, ASR 10.7).

The pattern is very similar to that in the earlier data (Table 2), although, as noted, the incidence rates are higher.

The only comprehensive analysis of the cancer profile in Malawi previously published was a histopathology series from 1976–80; in this period, there was no local histopathology service in Malawi, and biopsies from all over the country were sent to St Thomas's Hospital, London, UK (Hutt, 1986). The most frequent cancers (other than skin) in males were oesophagus (12.8%), bladder (7.4%) non-Hodgkin lymphomas (7.1%) and Kaposi sarcoma (6.6%) (Table 2). In women, the most common cancers were cervix (36.6%), bladder (6.8%) and breast (6.7%). Burkitt lymphomas comprised 22.2% of childhood cancers.

The frequency of bladder cancer in Malawi, and the fact that it is predominantly squamous cell in type, which is related to schistosomiasis (endemic in Malawi) was noted by Lucas (1982). Bladder cancer appears to be proportionally less common in the 1994–98 data (3.1% in males and females). This may be partly due to increases in numbers of other cancers (especially Kaposi sarcoma) or to restriction to subjects resident in Blantyre; however, it is possible that the prevalence of schistosomiasis has also declined over time. In the older series, the high sex ratio (8.5:1) and age distribution of the Kaposi sarcoma cases suggest that few were HIV-related at this time, and the overall frequency was much as it had been (4.2%) in the early 1970s (O'Connell *et al.*, 1977). The large increase in frequency of Kaposi sarcoma in the most recent registry data almost certainly reflects the effects of the epidemic of AIDS; Malawi is one of the most affected countries on the continent, with an estimated adult prevalence of HIV infection at the end of 1997 of 14.9%.

Childhood cancer

The numbers of cases of childhood cancer registered have varied little from year to year, probably because the majority of cancers in this age group have been diagnosed histologically. Table 3 shows the cases recorded among residents of Blantyre district in the period 1991–2001. Burkitt lymphoma is by far the most common cancer of boys and girls (ASR 25.9 per million), followed by Kaposi sarcoma (11.8), retinoblastoma (6.8) and Wilms tumour (5.7). Only nine leukaemias and one brain cancer were recorded, and there was just one case of neuroblastoma.

Three reports have detailed the profile of childhood cancer cases diagnosed in the national pathology series, from 1967–76 (Molyneux, 1979), from 1985–93 (Mukiibi *et al.*, 1995), and from 1991–95 (Banda & Liomba 1999), as shown in Table 4. All demonstrate the overwhelming importance of Burkitt lymphoma in

Table 1. Malawi, Blantyre (2000-2001)

NUMBER OF CASES BY AGE GROUP AND SUMMARY RATES OF INCIDENCE - MALE

SITE	ALL AGES	AGE UNK	MV (%)	0-	15-	25-	35-	45-	55-	65+	CRUDE RATE	%	CR 64	ASR (W)	ICD (10th)
Mouth	4	2	75	-	-	-	-	1	1	-	0.4	0.6	0.08	0.8	C00-06
Salivary gland	2	1	100	-	-	-	-	-	1	-	0.2	0.3	0.11	0.9	C07-08
Nasopharynx	1	0	100	-	-	-	1	-	-	-	0.1	0.1	0.01	0.1	C11
Other pharynx	0	0	-	-	-	-	-	-	-	-	0.0	0.0	0.00	0.0	C09-10,C12-14
Oesophagus	72	7	26	-	-	6	19	13	14	13	8.0	10.0	1.28	17.4	C15
Stomach	9	0	67	-	-	2	2	1	1	3	1.0	1.3	0.12	2.3	C16
Colon, rectum and anus	11	0	82	-	-	2	2	2	1	4	1.2	1.5	0.12	2.7	C18-21
Liver	28	3	64	4	4	2	5	5	2	3	3.1	3.9	0.35	5.1	C22
Gallbladder etc.	0	0	-	-	-	-	-	-	-	-	0.0	0.0	0.00	0.0	C23-24
Pancreas	2	0	0	-	-	-	-	1	-	1	0.2	0.3	0.02	0.6	C25
Larynx	3	0	100	-	-	-	-	1	1	1	0.3	0.4	0.04	0.8	C32
Trachea, bronchus and lung	9	1	44	-	-	-	1	3	1	3	1.0	1.3	0.13	2.5	C33-34
Bone	9	1	89	-	2	2	-	2	2	-	1.0	1.3	0.18	1.7	C40-41
Melanoma of skin	3	1	100	-	-	-	-	2	-	-	0.3	0.4	0.05	0.6	C43
Other skin	16	2	94	-	1	1	-	5	3	4	1.8	2.2	0.29	4.4	C44
Mesothelioma	0	0	-	-	-	-	-	-	-	-	0.0	0.0	0.00	0.0	C45
Kaposi sarcoma	385	38	11	9	28	142	110	45	11	2	42.8	53.5	4.15	49.9	C46
Peripheral nerves	0	0	-	-	-	-	-	-	-	-	0.0	0.0	0.00	0.0	C47
Connective and soft tissue	7	0	100	-	1	2	1	1	1	1	0.8	1.0	0.12	1.5	C49
Breast	5	0	100	-	-	1	-	-	-	4	0.6	0.7	0.04	1.7	C50
Penis	4	1	25	-	2	1	-	-	-	-	0.4	0.6	0.02	0.3	C60
Prostate	30	8	47	-	-	-	-	3	7	12	3.3	4.2	0.57	10.7	C61
Testis	1	0	100	-	-	-	1	-	-	-	0.1	0.1	0.02	0.2	C62
Kidney	9	2	-	3	-	-	1	1	2	-	1.0	1.3	0.15	1.6	C64
Renal pelvis, ureter and other urinary	0	0	100	-	-	-	-	-	-	-	0.0	0.0	0.00	0.0	C65-66,C68
Bladder	16	3	31	-	-	5	4	2	3	2	1.8	2.2	0.26	3.4	C67
Eye	18	4	83	3	-	5	3	1	2	-	2.0	2.5	0.10	2.5	C69
Brain, nervous system	1	0	0	1	-	-	-	-	-	-	0.1	0.1	0.00	0.1	C70-72
Thyroid	1	0	0	-	-	1	-	-	-	-	0.1	0.1	0.02	0.2	C73
Hodgkin disease	5	0	60	3	-	1	-	1	-	-	0.6	0.7	0.06	0.6	C81
Non-Hodgkin lymphoma	42	3	81	12	2	9	5	9	1	1	4.7	5.8	0.45	6.0	C82-85,C96
Multiple myeloma	2	0	100	-	-	-	1	1	-	-	0.2	0.3	0.05	0.4	C90
Lymphoid leukaemia	0	0	-	-	-	-	-	-	-	-	0.0	0.0	0.00	0.0	C91
Myeloid leukaemia	2	0	50	-	-	-	-	1	1	-	0.2	0.3	0.01	0.2	C92-94
Leukaemia, unspecified	3	0	33	1	2	-	-	-	-	-	0.3	0.4	0.08	0.8	C95
Other and unspecified	35	1	43	1	1	6	4	8	9	5	3.9	4.9	0.76	8.9	O&U
All sites	735	78	34	37	44	183	160	108	64	61	81.8	100.0	9.60	128.2	ALL
All sites but C44	719	76	32	37	43	182	160	103	61	57	80.0		9.31	123.9	ALLbC44
Average annual population				172918	103703	83683	42468	25486	11401	9655					

Table 1. Malawi, Blantyre (2000-2001)

NUMBER OF CASES BY AGE GROUP AND SUMMARY RATES OF INCIDENCE - FEMALE

SITE	ALL AGES	AGE UNK	MV (%)	0-	15-	25-	35-	45-	55-	65+	CRUDE RATE	%	CR 64	ASR (W)	ICD (10th)
Mouth	7	0	86	-	2	1	2	1	-	-	0.8	1.0	0.13	1.3	C00-06
Salivary gland	0	0	-	-	-	-	-	-	-	-	0.0	0.0	0.00	0.0	C07-08
Nasopharynx	1	0	100	-	-	-	-	-	1	-	0.1	0.1	0.05	0.4	C11
Other pharynx	0	0	-	-	-	-	-	-	-	-	0.0	0.0	0.00	0.0	C09-10,C12-14
Oesophagus	38	7	13	-	1	2	6	11	4	7	4.4	5.2	0.79	10.7	C15
Stomach	3	0	100	-	-	1	-	1	1	-	0.3	0.4	0.10	0.9	C16
Colon, rectum and anus	13	0	69	-	2	2	4	1	-	4	1.5	1.8	0.12	2.7	C18-21
Liver	2	1	50	-	-	-	-	-	-	1	0.2	0.3	0.00	0.6	C22
Gallbladder etc.	1	1	100	-	-	-	-	-	-	-	0.1	0.1	0.00	0.0	C23-24
Pancreas	4	0	50	-	2	2	2	-	-	1	0.5	0.6	0.05	0.9	C25
Larynx	0	0	-	-	-	-	-	-	-	-	0.0	0.0	0.00	0.0	C32
Trachea, bronchus and lung	1	0	0	-	1	-	-	-	1	-	0.1	0.1	0.06	0.5	C33-34
Bone	6	1	50	1	1	1	2	-	-	-	0.7	0.8	0.05	0.7	C40-41
Melanoma of skin	4	0	100	-	-	1	-	-	2	1	0.5	0.6	0.13	1.4	C43
Other skin	17	2	100	-	3	-	7	7	3	1	2.0		0.46	4.9	C44
Mesothelioma	0	0	-	-	-	-	-	-	-	-	0.0	0.0	0.00	0.0	C45
Kaposi sarcoma	234	23	11	7	53	78	50	19	4	-	27.0	32.3	2.58	31.7	C46
Peripheral nerves	0	0	-	-	-	-	-	-	-	-	0.0	0.0	0.00	0.0	C47
Connective and soft tissue	8	0	75	-	2	1	2	2	-	-	0.9	1.1	0.16	1.6	C49
Breast	48	2	77	-	3	8	12	12	7	4	5.5	6.6	1.07	12.0	C50
Vulva	2	0	100	-	-	2	-	-	-	-	0.2	0.3	0.02	0.2	C51
Vagina	3	0	100	-	-	-	1	-	-	-	0.3	0.4	0.03	0.7	C52
Cervix uteri	222	19	48	-	2	41	68	47	26	19	25.6	30.7	4.47	53.1	C53
Uterus	7	1	71	-	1	1	1	1	3	-	0.8	1.0	0.24	2.4	C54-55
Ovary	10	0	80	1	2	1	3	3	-	1	1.2	1.4	0.12	1.8	C56
Placenta	0	0	-	-	-	-	-	-	-	-	0.0	0.0	0.00	0.0	C58
Kidney	2	0	50	2	-	-	-	-	-	-	0.2	0.3	0.01	0.2	C64
Renal pelvis, ureter and other urinary	0	0	-	-	-	-	-	-	-	-	0.0	0.0	0.00	0.0	C65-66,C68
Bladder	16	0	56	-	1	1	6	3	3	2	1.8	2.2	0.35	4.1	C67
Eye	25	2	84	2	1	8	8	1	2	1	2.9	3.5	0.34	4.2	C69
Brain, nervous system	0	0	-	-	-	-	-	-	-	-	0.0	0.0	0.00	0.0	C70-72
Thyroid	6	0	67	-	-	2	-	2	1	1	0.7	0.8	0.12	1.5	C73
Hodgkin disease	3	0	67	1	1	-	-	1	-	-	0.3	0.4	0.01	0.2	C81
Non-Hodgkin lymphoma	25	0	80	2	4	5	6	5	2	1	2.9	3.5	0.41	4.9	C82-85,C96
Multiple myeloma	1	0	100	-	-	-	-	-	-	-	0.1	0.1	0.06	0.5	C90
Lymphoid leukaemia	2	0	50	1	-	-	1	-	-	-	0.2	0.3	0.04	0.4	C91
Myeloid leukaemia	0	0	-	-	-	-	-	-	-	-	0.0	0.0	0.00	0.0	C92-94
Leukaemia, unspecified	3	0	33	2	1	-	-	-	-	-	0.3	0.4	0.01	0.2	C95
Other and unspecified	27	6	74	3	1	2	5	5	3	2	3.1	3.7	0.54	6.3	O&U
All sites	741	66	44	22	81	159	175	124	66	48	85.6	100.0	12.56	151.3	ALL
All sites but C44	724	64	43	22	78	158	175	117	63	47	83.6	100.0	12.11	146.4	ALLbC44
Average annual population				180541	112151	66987	33833	19556	9018	10790					

Table 2. Malawi: case series

Site	Pathology series: Malawi 1976–80 (Hutt, 1986)					Malawi Cancer Registry: Blantyre District, 1994–98 (Banda *et al.*, 2001)				
	Male		Female		%HV	Male		Female		%HV
	No.	%	No.	%		No.	%	No.	%	
Oral cavity[1]	90	5.0%	71	3.6%	100	14	1.1%	8	0.8%	86
Nasopharynx	9	0.5%	2	0.1%	100	2	0.2%	0	0.0%	50
Other pharynx	1	0.1%	1	0.1%	100	1	0.1%	0	0.0%	100
Oesophagus	232	12.8%	36	1.8%	100	154	12.4%	77	7.7%	20
Stomach	38	2.1%	7	0.4%	100	11	0.9%	3	0.3%	72
Colon/rectum	41	2.3%	26	1.3%	100	16	1.3%	10	1.0%	65
Liver	101	5.6%	32	1.6%	100	52	4.2%	20	2.0%	29
Pancreas	1	0.1%	2	0.1%	100	3	0.2%	3	0.3%	17
Lung	6	0.3%	3	0.2%	100	8	0.6%	0	0.0%	100
Melanoma	55	3.0%	63	3.2%	100	7	0.6%	14	1.4%	86
Other skin	226	12.5%	130	6.7%	100	24	1.9%	23	2.3%	79
Kaposi sarcoma	119	6.6%	14	0.7%	100	674	54.1%	274	27.3%	17
Breast	14	0.8%	108	5.5%	100	3	0.2%	74	7.4%	70
Cervix uteri			712	36.6%	100			251	25.0%	48
Corpus uteri			71	3.6%	100			14	1.4%	86
Ovary etc.			61	3.1%	100			11	1.1%	82
Prostate	64	3.5%			100	45	3.6%			33
Penis	46	2.5%			100	8	0.6%			38
Bladder	133	7.4%	132	6.8%	100	39	3.1%	31	3.1%	33
Kidney etc.	20	1.1%	21	1.1%	100	5	0.4%	7	0.7%	75
Eye	1	0.1%	0	0.0%	100	29	2.3%	31	3.1%	100
Brain, nervous system	41	2.3%	38	2.0%	100	3	0.2%	1	0.1%	19
Thyroid	17	0.9%	39	2.0%	100	7	0.6%	19	1.9%	92
Non-Hodgkin lymphoma	128	7.1%	87	4.5%	100	69	5.5%	58	5.8%	69
Hodgkin disease	17	0.9%	1	0.1%	100	7	0.6%	4	0.4%	91
Myeloma	10	0.6%	4	0.2%	100	0	0.0%	2	0.2%	100
Leukaemia	6	0.3%	3	0.2%	100	9	0.7%	11	1.1%	70
ALL SITES	1808	100.0%	1946	100.0%	100	1245	100.0%	1003	100.0%	39

[1] Includes salivary gland tumours

Table 3. Childhood cancer, Malawi, Blantyre (1991-2001)

	NUMBER OF CASES					REL. FREQ.(%)	RATES PER MILLION					
	0-4	5-9	10-14	All	M/F	Overall	0-4	5-9	10-14	Crude	ASR	%MV
Leukaemia	0	4	5	9	0.5	3.4	-	3.3	4.8	2.5	2.5	28.6
Acute lymphoid leukaemia	0	1	1	2	1.0	0.8	-	0.8	1.0	0.6	0.5	50.0
Lymphoma	20	75	34	129	2.0	49.0	15.4	61.1	32.8	36.2	35.2	79.2
Hodgkin disease	0	5	5	10	9.0	3.8	-	4.1	4.8	2.8	2.7	70.0
Burkitt lymphoma	16	61	18	95	2.2	36.1	12.4	49.7	17.4	26.7	25.9	67.4
Brain and spinal neoplasms	0	1	0	1	-	0.4	-	0.8	-	0.3	0.3	100.0
Neuroblastoma	0	1	0	1	-	0.4	-	0.8	-	0.3	0.3	-
Retinoblastoma	20	3	0	23	0.8	8.7	15.4	2.4	-	6.5	6.8	82.6
Wilms tumour	12	7	1	20	1.5	7.6	9.3	5.7	1.0	5.6	5.7	85.0
Bone tumours	2	0	4	6	1.0	2.3	1.5	-	3.9	1.7	1.7	16.7
Soft tissue sarcomas	16	12	18	46	1.6	17.5	12.4	9.8	17.4	12.9	13.0	100.0
Kaposi sarcoma	14	11	17	42	1.6	16.0	10.8	9.0	16.4	11.8	11.8	45.2
Germ cell tumours	1	0	2	3	-	1.1	0.8	-	1.9	0.8	0.9	100.0
Other	5	8	12	25	0.9	9.5	3.9	6.5	11.6	7.0	7.0	84.0
All	76	111	76	263	1.4	100.0	58.7	90.4	73.3	73.9	73.2	67.7

Table 4. Malawi: childhood case series

Cancer	Malawi 1967–76 (Molyneux, 1979)		Malawi 1985–93 (Mukiibi et al., 1995)		Malawi 1991–95 (Banda & Liomba, 1999)	
	No.	%	No.	%	No.	%
Leukaemia	0	0.0%	18	2.3%	6	1.1%
Acute lymphocytic leukaemia		0.0%	10	1.3%	1	0.2%
Lymphoma	187	45.9%	472	59.7%	283	51.7%
Burkitt lymphoma	121	29.7%	368	46.5%	199	36.4%
Hodgkin disease	11	2.7%	38	4.8%	22	4.0%
Brain and spinal neoplasms	0	0.0%	6	0.8%	1	0.2%
Neuroblastoma	13	3.2%	0	0.0%	0	0.0%
Retinoblastoma	56	13.8%	89	11.3%	46	8.4%
Wilms tumour	27	6.6%	50	6.3%	27	4.9%
Bone tumours	14	3.4%	16	2.0%	16	2.9%
Soft-tissue sarcomas	48	11.8%	66	8.3%	120	21.9%
Kaposi sarcoma	18	4.4%	32	4.0%	88	16.1%
Other	62	15.2%	74	9.4%	48	8.8%
Total	407	100.0%	791	100.0%	547	100.0%

this age group, and the most recent data show the rise in importance of Kaposi sarcoma, in line with the evolution of the epidemic of AIDS.

References

Banda, L.T. & Liomba, N.G. (1999) Malawi National Cancer Registry 1991–1995. In: Parkin, D.M., Kramárová, E., Draper, G.J., Masuyer, E., Michaelis, J., Neglia, J, Qureshi, S. & Stiller, C.A., eds, *International Incidence of Childhood Cancer,* vol. II (IARC Scientific Publications No. 144), Lyon, IARC, pp. 31–34

Banda, L.T., Parkin, D.M., Dzamalala, C.P. & Liomba, N.G. (2001) Cancer incidence in Blantyre, Malawi 1994–1998. *Trop. Med. Int. Health,* 6, 296–304

Hutt, M.S.R. (1986) Malawi: Register of Tumour Pathology, 1976–1980. In: Parkin, D.M., ed., *Cancer Occurrence in Developing Countries* (IARC Scientific Publications No 75), Lyon, IARC, pp. 63–66

Lucas, S.B. (1982) Bladder tumours in Malawi. *Br. J. Urol.,* 54, 275–279

O'Connell, K.M., Borgstein, J. & Hutt, M.S.R. (1977) Kaposi's sarcoma in Malawi: clinico-epidemiological features. *E. Afr. J. Med. Res.,* 4, 59–63

Molyneux, E.M. (1979) Childhood malignancies in Malawi 1967-1976. *E. Afr. Med. J.,* 56, 15–21

Mukiibi, J.M., Banda, L., Liomba, N.G., Sungani, F.C.M. & Parkin, D.M. (1995) Spectrum of childhood cancers in Malawi 1985-1993. *E. Afr. Med. J.,* 72, 25–29

3.4.9 Mauritius

Background

Climate: Tropical, modified by southeast trade winds; warm, dry winter (May to November); hot, wet, humid summer (November to May)

Terrain: Small coastal plain rising to discontinuous mountains encircling central plateau

Ethnic groups: Indo-Mauritian 68%, Creole 27%, Sino-Mauritian 3%, Franco-Mauritian 2%

Religions: Hindu 52%, Christian 28.3% (Roman Catholic 26%, Protestant 2.3%), Muslim 16.6%, other 3.1%

Economy—overview: Since independence in 1968, Mauritius has developed from a low-income, agriculturally based economy to a middle-income diversified economy with growing industrial, financial services and tourist sectors. For most of the period, annual growth has been of the order of 5–6%. This remarkable achievement has been reflected in increased life expectancy, lowered infant mortality and a much improved infrastructure. Sugar-cane is grown on about 90% of the cultivated land area and accounts for 25% of export earnings. The government's development strategy centres on industrialization (with a view to modernization and to exports), agricultural diversification, and tourism.

Industries: Food processing (largely sugar milling), textiles, clothing; chemicals, metal products, transport equipment, non-electrical machinery; tourism

Agriculture—products: Sugar-cane, tea, corn, potatoes, bananas, pulses; cattle, goats; fish

Cancer registration

A cancer registry was established in Mauritius in 1986. Since 1989, information has been collected from the radiotherapy patient register, the Central Pathology Laboratory, hospital inpatient records, the Overseas Treatment unit and the civil status office. Notification from the private sector is voluntary. Responsibility for the registry was transferred to the Mauritius Institute of Health in 1996. Duplicate registrations are eliminated by manual search of the patient register.

The first results, for 1989–93 were published in 1998 (Manraj *et al.*, 1998). A more detailed report for the period 1989–96 was published in May 1999 as a locally prepared monograph: *Cancer Study in Mauritius* (1989–1996), by Manraj, S.S., Poorun, S. & Burhoo.

Review of data

Table 1 and Table 2 have been extracted from the 1999 report, which presents registrations for the years 1989–96. There was a progressive increase in the number of cases registered each year from 1989 (736 cases) to 1993 (1010 cases), but the number was more stable in the later four years. The mortality to incidence (M:I) ratios also suggest some underregistration (85% for males, 59% for females). 82% of cases were histologically verified.

Table 1 shows that in men lung cancer is the most common tumour, although the actual recorded incidence (ASR 11.8 per 100 000) and mortality:incidence (M:I) ratio (1.3) is modest. There are moderately elevated rates for cancers of the oral cavity, and stomach.

In women, cancer of the breast is the most commonly diagnosed cancer (ASR 26.4; M:I ratio 0.37), followed by cervix (ASR 22.4; M:I 0.58).

Childhood cancer

In children (Table 2), lymphomas appear to be relatively uncommon, compared with leukaemias, and there is a relatively high percentage of brain and nervous system neoplasms (18%).

Reference

Manraj, S.S., Mustun, H., Ghurburrun, P., Laniece, C. & Salamon, R. (1998) Incidence des cancers Maurice en 1989-1993. *Bull. Soc. Pathol. Exotique*, **91**, 9–12

Table 1. Mauritius:1989-1996: annual incidence per 100 000 by age group (years)

Site		Age group					All	%	Crude rate	ASR (world)
		0–14	15–44	45–54	55–64	65+				
Male										
Oral cavity and pharynx	C00–C14	0	32	50	93	114	298	9.6%	7	9.3
Oesophagus	C15	0	2	23	43	44	114	3.7%	2.7	3.7
Stomach	C16	0	21	28	82	134	266	8.6%	6.3	8.7
Colon/rectum	C18–21	0	45	35	76	100	258	8.3%	6.1	7.9
Liver	C22	1	11				51	1.6%	1.2	1.5
Pancreas	C25	0	8				45	1.5%	1.1	1.4
Larynx	C32						116	3.7%	2.7	3.8
Lung	C33–34	0	32	52	120	159	373	12.1%	8.8	11.8
Melanoma of skin	C43	2	21	13	25	62	14	0.5%	0.3	0.5
Other skin	C44						111	3.6%	2.6	3.5
Kaposi sarcoma	C46							0.0%		
Penis	C60						47	1.5%	1.1	1.3
Prostate	C61	0	2	7	33	153	200	6.5%	4.7	6.7
Testis	C62						36	1.2%	0.8	0.8
Bladder	C67	0	8	34	61	108	184	5.9%	4.3	6.1
Kidney etc.	C64–66	5	5				40	1.3%	0.9	1.3
Brain	C71–72	21					121	3.9%	2.9	2.7
Thyroid	C73						8	0.3%	0.2	0.2
Non-Hodgkin lymphoma	C82–85, C96	8	44	19	19	23	79	2.6%	2.2	3.1
Hodgkin disease	C81						37	1.2%	0.8	
Myeloma	C90	0	48	10	21	27	27	0.9%	0.6	4.6
Leukaemia	C91–95	62					156	5.0%	3.7	
Other sites	Other						514	16.6%	12.1	14.6
All sites	ALL	151	500	388	770	1199	3095	100.0%	73	93.5
Female										
Oral cavity and pharynx	C00–C14	0	28	16	27	48	125	2.9%	2.9	3.1
Oesophagus	C15	0	5	7	21	38	76	1.7%	1.7	1.9
Stomach	C16	0	22	19	39	70	151	3.5%	3.6	4
Colon/rectum	C18–21	0	48	52	63	95	261	6.0%	6.2	7
Liver	C22	0	9				42	1.0%	1	1.1
Pancreas	C25	0	4				40	0.9%	1	1.1
Larynx	C32						22	0.5%	0.5	0.6
Lung	C33–34	0	11	12	17	23	65	1.5%	1.5	1.7
Melanoma of skin	C43	1	19	19	23	56	14	0.3%	0.3	0.4
Other skin	C44						106	2.4%	2.5	2.7
Kaposi sarcoma	C46							0.0%		
Breast	C50	1	382	259	191	220	1085	25.0%	25.5	26.4
Cervix	C53	0	159	216	216	247	855	19.7%	20.1	22.4
Corpus	C54	0	14				113	2.6%	2.7	3
Ovary	C56	0	75	58	53	49	245	5.6%	5.8	6.2
Bladder	C67	1	3	13	25	44	69	1.6%	1.6	1.8
Kidney etc.	C64–66	4	5				26	0.6%	0.6	0.7
Brain	C71–72	26					124	2.9%	3	3.2
Thyroid	C73						48	1.1%	1.1	1.2
Non-Hodgkin lymphoma	C82–85, C96	10	33	12	13	22	68	1.6%	1.6	2.3
Hodgkin disease	C81						25	0.6%	0.8	
Myeloma	C90	0	38	16	21	24	33	0.8%	0.8	3.4
Leukaemia	C91–95	35					110	2.5%	2.6	
Other sites	Other						641	14.8%	15.1	16.2
All sites	ALL	117	1048	853	952	1272	4344	100.0%	102	110.4

Source: Cancer Study in Mauritius (1989–1996). Report of the National Cancer Registry, Ministry of Health and Quality of Life, Mauritius Institute of Health (May 1999)

Table 2. Mauritius, 1989–96: childhood case series

Cancer	No.	%
Leukaemia	97	36%
Acute lymphocytic leukaemia		
Lymphoma	18	7%
Burkitt lymphoma		
Hodgkin disease		
Brain and spinal neoplasms	47	18%
Neuroblastoma	22	8%
Retinoblastoma	15	6%
Wilms tumour	5	2%
Bone tumours	29	11%
Soft-tissue sarcomas		
Kaposi sarcoma		
Other	35	13%
Total	268	100%

3.4.10 Mozambique

Background

Climate: Tropical to subtropical

Terrain: Mostly coastal lowlands, uplands in centre, high plateaux in northwest, mountains in west

Ethnic groups: Indigenous tribal groups 99.66% (Shangaan, Chokwe, Manyika, Sena, Makua, and others), Europeans 0.06%, Euro-Africans 0.2%, Indians 0.08%

Religions: Indigenous beliefs 50%, Christian 30%, Muslim 20%

Economy—overview: Before the peace accord of October 1992, Mozambique was devastated by civil war and was one of the poorest countries in the world. Prospects subsequently improved, and Mozambique has begun to exploit its sizeable agricultural, hydropower and transportation resources. Foreign assistance programmes help supply the foreign exchange required to support the budget and pay for import of goods and services.

Industries: Food, beverages, chemicals (fertilizer, soap, paints), petroleum products, textiles, cement, glass, asbestos, tobacco

Agriculture—products: Cotton, cashew nuts, sugar-cane, tea, cassava (tapioca), corn, rice, tropical fruits; beef, poultry

Cancer registration

A 'cancer survey' for the population of Lourenço Marques (now Maputo) was organized from the Department of Pathology, Hospital Central Miguel Bombarda, between May 1956 and April 1961, supported financially by the Portuguese Government and the National Cancer Association of South Africa (Prates & Torres,1965). Cases were registered by medical staff from hospital inpatients and outpatients, radiotherapy departments, pathology departments, death certificates and doctors attending cases at home. Cases were also identified from autopsy records, the Department of Statistics, two mission hospitals, three private nursing homes, twelve state or municipal or company outpatient clinics, the Medical Officer of Health for Lourenço Marques and from the Port Health Authority. Registration was stated to be more than 90% complete.

The registry covered the area of the city of Lourenço Marques and a peri-urban area of 60 square kilometres. The population at risk was estimated from a sample survey as 99 030, and comprised 60% Thonga (Ronga) Shangana group, 30% Bitonga and Chope people, 10% other tribes including Chuabos and Macuas. 51% were Catholic, 23% Protestant, 4% Muslim and 22% had other religions (African) or no religion. The majority of the population (76%) were engaged in agriculture

Review of data

The results from the registry of Lourenço Marques (Maputo) for the period 1956–60 are shown in Table 1. Of the 600 cases registered, 87.3% were morphologically verified (90.7% in men, 81.7% in women). Liver cancer was by far the most common cancer of men (65.5% of cases, ASR 101.7 per 100 000), followed by cancers of the bladder (6% of cases, ASR 17.1) and non-Hodgkin lymphomas (4.5% of cases, ASR 5.2). In women, liver cancer was first in importance (31% of cases, ASR 31.4) followed by cancers of the cervix (21.3% of cases, ASR 29.1) and bladder (10.7% of cases, ASR 14.0). The almost equal incidence of bladder cancer in males and females and the observation (Prates & Torres, 1965) that the

majority (56%) were squamous-cell cancers indicates that the majority were related to schistosomiasis. 18 of the 24 cases of non-Hodgkin lymphomas were Burkitt lymphoma, but only four cases (2 boys, 2 girls) were in the childhood age group. In contrast to neighbouring parts of South Africa and Malawi, cancer of the oesophagus was rare, as were respiratory and gastrointestinal cancers in general.

In a later report from the pathology department of the same hospital, based on cases diagnosed by histology, cytology or autopsy, Bijlsma (1981) noted that the relative frequency of liver cancer in men had declined from 51.8% of cases in 1956–61 to 35.3% in 1977; there was no change in the relative frequency in women.

Another source of information on cancer patterns and trends in Mozambique derives from the studies of cancer patterns among gold miners in South Africa. The first report, for the period 1964–71 (Harington *et al.*, 1975) confirmed the very high incidence of liver cancer in these men (crude incidence, considered equivalent to an age-specific rate for age group 25–34 years, was 80.4 per 100 000), and the low rates for cancers of the oesophagus and lung. Later reports (Bradshaw *et al.*, 1982; Harington *et al.*, 1983) showed quite marked declines in incidence of liver cancer, to 40.8 per 100 000 in 1972–79 and 29.9 per 100 000 in 1981. There was also a suggestion of a decline in the incidence of bladder cancer (Bradshaw *et al.*, 1982). Considerable variation was present in the incidence of liver cancer in miners from different regions of Mozambique, with the highest incidence in those from coastal districts, and low rates in men from inland areas to the west (Bradshaw *et al.*, 1982). A later study (van Rensburg *et al.*, 1985) included systematic registration of all liver cancers (histologically verified) from hospitals in the coastal province of Inhambane between 1968 and 1974. Incidence rates were calculated, based on the census of 1970. The overall (crude) incidence for the province was 25.5 per 100 000 in men and 13.0 per 100 000 in women (the corresponding ASRs are 23.2 and 7.9 per 100 000). The maximum recorded incidence was in age group 30–39 years, with a decline thereafter. There was considerable variation in the rates between different districts of the province (e.g., in men, from 9.3 per 100 000 in Massinga to 60.7 per 100 000 in Panda), which was correlated with aflatoxin intake (as estimated from food samples obtained from villages in the different districts).

References

Bijlsma, F. (1981) Malignant tumours in Mozambiquan Africans with special reference to primary liver carcinoma. *Trans. R. Soc. Trop. Med. Hyg.*, **75**, 451–454

Bradshaw, E., McGlashan, N.D., Fitzgerald, D. & Harington, J.S. (1982) Analyses of cancer incidence in black gold miners from Southern Africa (1964-79). *Br. J. Cancer;* **46**, 737–748

Harington, J.S., McGlashan, N.D., Bradshaw, E., Geddes, E.W. & Purves, L.R. (1975) A spatial and temporal analysis of four cancers in African gold miners from Southern Africa. *Br. J. Cancer,* **31**, 665–678

Harington, J.S., Bradshaw, E.M. & McGlashan, N.D. (1983) Changes in primary liver and oesophageal cancer rates among black goldmines, 1964-1981. *S. Afr. Med. J.*, **64**, 650

Prates, M.D. & Torres, F.O. (1965) A cancer survey in Laurenco Marques. *J. Natl Cancer Inst.*, **35**, 729–757

van Rensburg, S.J., Cook-Mozaffari, P., van Schalkwyk, D.J., van der Watt, J.J., Vincent, T.J. & Purchase, I.F. (1985) Hepatocellular carcinoma and dietary aflatoxin in Mozambique and Transkei. *Br. J. Cancer,* **51**, 713–726

Table 1. Mozambique, Lourenco Marques (1956-1960)

NUMBER OF CASES BY AGE GROUP AND SUMMARY RATES OF INCIDENCE - MALE

SITE	ALL AGES	AGE UNK	0-	10-	20-	30-	40-	50-	60+	CRUDE RATE	%	ASR (W)	ICD (10th)
Mouth	6	0	-	1	-	-	-	3	1	2.2	1.5	3.6	C00-C08
Nasopharynx	3	0	-	-	-	1	-	1	1	1.1	0.7	2.2	C11
Other pharynx	0	0	-	-	-	-	-	-	-	0.0	0.0	0.0	C09-C10,C12-C14
Oesophagus	7	0	-	-	-	2	1	3	1	2.6	1.7	4.4	C15
Stomach	3	0	-	-	-	-	-	1	2	1.1	0.7	3.0	C16
Colon, rectum and anus	4	0	-	-	1	-	-	-	-	1.5	1.0	1.8	C18-C21
Liver	264	2	1	51	90	53	47	12	8	98.2	65.5	101.7	C22
Pancreas	2	0	-	-	1	-	-	-	1	0.7	0.5	1.5	C25
Larynx	2	0	-	1	-	-	1	1	-	0.7	0.5	1.1	C32
Trachea, bronchus and lung	6	0	-	-	-	-	2	1	2	2.2	1.5	4.3	C33-C34
Melanoma of skin	0	0	-	-	-	-	-	-	-	0.0	0.0	0.0	C43
Other skin	13	0	-	-	1	5	2	3	2	4.8		7.6	C44
Kaposi sarcoma	0	0	-	-	-	-	-	-	-	0.0	0.0	0.0	C46
Breast	0	0	-	-	-	-	-	-	-	0.0	0.0	0.0	C50
Penis	5	0	-	-	-	1	2	2	-	1.9	1.2	2.6	C60
Prostate	10	0	-	-	-	1	-	4	5	3.7	2.5	9.0	C61
Kidney etc.	2	0	-	-	2	-	-	-	2	0.7	0.5	2.4	C64-C66,C68
Bladder	24	0	-	-	2	3	5	7	7	8.9	6.0	17.1	C67
Eye	4	0	2	-	-	2	-	-	-	1.5	1.0	1.5	C69
Brain, nervous system	6	0	-	3	3	-	-	-	-	2.2	1.5	1.6	C70-C72
Thyroid	2	0	-	-	-	1	-	-	1	0.7	0.5	1.8	C73
Hodgkin disease	0	0	-	-	-	-	-	-	-	0.0	0.0	0.0	C81
Non-Hodgkin lymphoma	18	0	1	8	7	2	-	-	-	6.7	4.5	5.2	C82-C85,C96
Multiple myeloma	0	0	-	-	-	-	-	-	-	0.0	0.0	0.0	C90
Leukaemia	7	0	1	2	1	1	-	-	2	2.6	1.7	3.9	C91-C95
Other and unspecified	15	0	1	4	2	2	2	2	2	5.6	3.7	7.4	O&U
All sites	403	2	6	70	109	74	63	42	37	149.9	100.0	184.0	ALL
All sites but C44	390	2	6	70	108	69	61	39	35	145.1	96.8	176.4	ALLbC44
Average annual population			12600	14800	10800	6000	4900	2850	1820				

Source: Cancer Incidence in Five Continents volume 1

Table 1. Mozambique, Lourenco Marques (1956-1960)

NUMBER OF CASES BY AGE GROUP AND SUMMARY RATES OF INCIDENCE - FEMALE

SITE	ALL AGES	AGE UNK	0-	10-	20-	30-	40-	50-	60+	CRUDE RATE	%	ASR (W)	ICD (10th)
Mouth	10	0	-	2	2	-	1	3	2	4.4	5.1	7.0	C00-C08
Nasopharynx	0	0	-	-	-	-	-	-	-	0.0	0.0	0.0	C11
Other pharynx	0	0	-	-	-	-	-	-	-	0.0	0.0	0.0	C09-C10,C12-C14
Oesophagus	0	0	-	-	-	-	-	-	-	0.0	0.0	0.0	C15
Stomach	2	0	-	-	-	-	-	-	2	0.9	1.0	2.4	C16
Colon, rectum and anus	2	0	-	-	-	-	-	1	1	0.9	1.0	2.0	C18-C21
Liver	61	0	-	5	21	10	15	5	5	27.0	31.0	31.4	C22
Pancreas	2	0	-	-	-	-	-	1	1	0.9	1.0	2.0	C25
Larynx	2	0	-	-	-	2	-	-	-	0.9	1.0	1.1	C32
Trachea, bronchus and lung	2	0	-	-	-	-	2	-	-	0.9	1.0	1.6	C33-C34
Melanoma of skin	0	0	-	-	-	-	-	-	-	0.0	0.0	0.0	C43
Other skin	9	0	1	-	-	1	1	2	4	4.0		7.6	C44
Kaposi sarcoma		0	-	-	-	-	-	-	-				C46
Breast	5	0	-	-	-	-	2	3	-	2.2	2.5	3.5	C50
Cervix uteri	42	1	-	-	4	8	11	9	9	18.6	21.3	29.1	C53
Uterus	4	0	-	-	-	3	-	-	1	1.8	2.0	2.3	C54-C55
Ovary etc.	0	0	-	-	-	-	-	-	-	0.0	0.0	0.0	C56-C57
Kidney etc.	2	0	-	-	1	-	-	1	-	0.9	1.0	0.6	C64-C66,C68
Bladder	21	0	-	-	4	2	5	7	3	9.3	10.7	14.0	C67
Eye	6	0	2	1	1	1	1	-	-	2.7	3.0	2.7	C69
Brain, nervous system	4	0	1	-	2	-	-	1	-	1.8	2.0	1.5	C70-C72
Thyroid	3	0	-	-	1	-	-	1	1	1.3	1.5	2.3	C73
Hodgkin disease	0	0	-	-	-	-	-	-	-	0.0	0.0	0.0	C81
Non-Hodgkin lymphoma	6	0	1	1	-	2	-	1	1	2.7	3.0	2.7	C82-C85,C96
Multiple myeloma	0	0	-	-	-	-	-	-	-	0.0	0.0	0.0	C90
Leukaemia	4	0	-	-	1	2	-	-	1	1.8	2.0	2.3	C91-C95
Other and unspecified	10	0	2	2	2	1	1	-	2	4.4	5.1	6.1	O&U
All sites	197	1	7	11	39	32	39	35	33	87.1	100.0	122.2	ALL
All sites but C44	188	1	6	11	39	31	38	33	29	83.1	95.4	114.6	ALLbC44
Average annual population			13310	7090	10180	6340	4240	2250	1850				

Source: Cancer Incidence in Five Continents volume 1

3.4.11 Réunion

Background

Climate: Tropical, but temperature moderates with elevation; cool and dry from May to November, hot and rainy from November to April

Terrain: Mostly rugged and mountainous; fertile lowlands along coast

Ethnic groups: French, African, Malagasy, Chinese, Pakistani, Indian

Religions: Roman Catholic 94%, Hindu, Islam, Buddhist

Economy—overview: The economy has traditionally been based on agriculture. Sugarcane has been the primary crop for more than a century, and in some years it accounts for 85% of exports. The government has been pushing the development of a tourist industry to relieve high unemployment. The gap in Réunion between the well-off and the poor is large; the white and Indian communities are substantially better off than other segments of the population, often approaching European standards, whereas indigenous groups suffer the poverty and unemployment typical of the poorer nations of the African continent. The economic well-being of Réunion depends heavily on continued financial assistance from France.

Industries: Sugar, rum, cigarettes, handicraft items, flower oil extraction

Agriculture—products: Sugar-cane, vanilla, tobacco, tropical fruits, vegetables, corn

Cancer registration

Collection of data on cancer morbidity was initiated on the island of La Réunion in 1983. The population-based registry was established in 1988, with the aim of establishing the burden and patterns of cancer among residents of the island, whether diagnosed locally or elsewhere.

Registration is active. The first step involves collecting information from the principal sources, the public and private pathology and haematology laboratories. These data are then linked and supplemented with data from the treating physician. This step permits the removal of cases diagnosed in previous years, recurrences or metastases from a cancer already registered, as well as cases among non-residents. The data are coded using ICD-O-1 for topography and morphology; IARC/IACR rules are used for multiple tumours. Basal-cell carcinomas of the skin are registered but excluded from analysis of the data.

Review of data

A preliminary retrospective survey was performed in 1981, before the establishment of the population-based registry (Julvez & Vaillant, 1985). The results from the first five years of cancer regsistration (1988–92) were published in *Cancer Incidence in Five Continents*, volume VII (Parkin *et al.*, 1997) and by Grizeau *et al.* (1998).

The data published in this volume update this material with registrations from an additional two years (1993, 1994). The incidence rates, especially the age standardized rates, are rather higher for the period 1988–94 than in the previously published 1988–92 data. This results from both an increased number of registrations (an average of 843 per year in 1993–94, compared with 905 in 1988–92), a change in the estimate of the population (the more recent data take account of the census performed in 2000) and calculation of the ASR using 65+ as upper age category. The percentage of cases with morphological verification of diagnosis is relatively high (97% in both sexes); it was 98% in 1988–92 (Parkin *et al.*, 1997). The ratio between cases registered and deaths from cancer (M:I ratio) was 0.72 in males and 0.53 in females in 1988–92 (Grizeau *et al.*, 1998).

In males, the most common cancer registered is lung cancer, with an ASR of 34.4 per 100 000. This is one of the highest rates recorded in contemporary Africa, but lower than those observed in metropolitan France (Chapter 4.9, Table 1). The incidence in females is low (3.3 per 100 000), and equivalent to that recorded in populations of non-smokers. The incidence of cancer of prostate is moderately high, as are the rates of stomach cancer and oesophageal cancer. The sex ratio for cancers of the oesophagus is 10:1, suggesting that the high rates relate to tobacco and alcohol consumption; Grizeau *et al.* (1998) allude to the high consumption of locally produced rum. These habits may well account for the moderately high rates of cancers of the mouth and pharynx among men but not women.

In females, the main cancers are breast and cervix uteri, with the rates for the former being somewhat higher. Both are possibly underestimates, given the high percentage of cases with histological proof of diagnosis (99%).

Childhood cancer

122 childhood cancers were registered in the seven-year period. Leukaemias were the most common childhood cancers (ASR 30.1 per million), of which the majority (74%) were acute lymphocytic. Lymphomas comprised 16.4% of childhood cancers, with an ASR of 16.7 per million. CNS tumours were third in frequency (11.5%).

References

Grizeau, P., Vaillant, J.Y. & Begue. A. (1998) Le registre des cancers à la Réunion: données des cinq premières années d'enregistrement. *Bull. Soc. Pathol. Exotique*, **91**, 13–16

Julvez, J. & Vaillant, J.Y. (1985) Le cancer à la Réunion: résultats d'une enquête préalable à la création d'un registre des tumeurs. *Rev. Epidemiol. Santé Publ.*, **33**, 39–42

Parkin, D.M., Whelan, S.L., Ferlay, J., Raymond, L. & Young, J., eds (1997) *Cancer Incidence in Five Continents*, Vol. VII (IARC Scientific Publications No. 143), Lyon, IARC

Table 1. France, La Reunion (1988-1994)

NUMBER OF CASES BY AGE GROUP AND SUMMARY RATES OF INCIDENCE - MALE

SITE	ALL AGES	AGE UNK	MV (%)	0-	15-	25-	35-	45-	55-	65+	CRUDE RATE	%	CR 64	ASR (W)	ICD (10th)
Mouth	205	0	100	-	-	5	29	68	62	41	9.8	6.2	1.00	12.5	C00-06
Salivary gland	8	0	100	-	-	2	2	3	-	1	0.4	0.2	0.03	0.4	C07-08
Nasopharynx	11	0	100	1	1	-	3	2	3	1	0.5	0.3	0.05	0.6	C11
Other pharynx	228	0	99	-	-	3	27	82	75	41	10.9	6.9	1.16	13.9	C09-10,C12-14
Oesophagus	362	0	98	-	-	4	30	97	135	96	17.3	11.0	1.76	22.8	C15
Stomach	340	0	99	1	-	6	22	58	97	156	16.2	10.3	1.21	21.8	C16
Colon, rectum and anus	199	0	98	-	2	7	20	36	42	92	9.5	6.0	0.65	12.6	C18-21
Liver	47	0	79	-	-	2	6	11	12	16	2.2	1.4	0.19	2.9	C22
Gallbladder etc.	21	0	81	-	-	-	2	-	6	13	1.0	0.6	0.05	1.4	C23-24
Pancreas	49	0	71	-	-	-	3	8	20	18	2.3	1.5	0.22	3.2	C25
Larynx	115	0	100	-	-	3	7	33	33	39	5.5	3.5	0.49	7.2	C32
Trachea, bronchus and lung	522	0	96	-	-	5	17	87	151	262	24.9	15.8	1.80	34.4	C33-34
Bone	22	0	95	4	9	1	1	3	1	3	1.0	0.7	0.06	1.1	C40-41
Melanoma of skin	28	0	100	-	-	4	5	6	8	5	1.3	0.8	0.13	1.6	C43
Other skin	136	0	99	1	-	5	7	20	40	63	6.5		0.48	8.8	C44
Mesothelioma	8	0	100	-	-	-	1	2	1	4	0.4	0.2	0.02	0.5	C45
Kaposi sarcoma	9	0	44	-	-	6	1	1	1	-	0.4	0.3	0.03	0.4	C46
Peripheral nerves	1	0	100	1	-	-	-	-	-	-	0.0	0.0	0.00	0.0	C47
Connective and soft tissue	20	0	100	2	3	2	3	2	3	5	1.0	0.6	0.06	1.1	C49
Breast	10	0	90	-	-	-	-	-	6	4	0.5	0.3	0.05	0.6	C50
Penis	14	0	100	-	-	1	2	2	3	6	0.7	0.4	0.05	0.9	C60
Prostate	353	0	98	-	-	-	-	6	55	292	16.8	10.7	0.50	24.5	C61
Testis	23	0	100	1	3	14	4	1	-	-	1.1	0.7	0.07	0.9	C62
Kidney	35	0	97	3	-	1	4	8	9	10	1.7	1.1	0.14	2.1	C64
Renal pelvis, ureter and other urinary	7	0	100	-	-	1	1	2	1	2	0.3	0.2	0.03	0.4	C65-66,C68
Bladder	154	0	99	-	-	-	7	24	39	84	7.3	4.7	0.48	10.2	C67
Eye	7	0	100	3	-	1	-	-	-	3	0.3	0.2	0.01	0.4	C69
Brain, nervous system	40	0	93	8	-	6	6	8	8	4	1.9	1.2	0.17	2.3	C70-72
Thyroid	12	0	100	-	-	3	-	4	2	3	0.6	0.4	0.05	0.7	C73
Hodgkin disease	21	0	100	-	6	5	3	2	1	4	1.0	0.6	0.07	1.0	C81
Non-Hodgkin lymphoma	94	0	99	11	8	5	10	14	21	25	4.5	2.8	0.35	5.5	C82-85,C96
Multiple myeloma	52	0	94	-	-	-	2	7	17	26	2.5	1.6	0.18	3.4	C90
Lymphoid leukaemia	32	0	97	12	7	2	1	-	6	4	1.5	1.0	0.11	1.8	C91
Myeloid leukaemia	59	0	100	4	7	5	6	6	10	21	2.8	1.8	0.18	3.4	C92-94
Leukaemia, unspecified	7	0	100	2	1	-	-	-	-	4	0.3	0.2	0.01	0.4	C95
Other and unspecified	185	0	93	5	5	8	10	39	47	71	8.8	5.6	0.68	11.6	O&U
All sites	3436	0	97	59	54	106	242	641	917	1417	164.0		12.51	217.3	ALL
All sites but C44	3300	0	97	58	54	101	235	621	877	1354	157.5	100.0	12.03	208.5	ALLbC44
Average annual population				90022	60012	52262	38796	26334	17635	14325					

Table 1. France, La Reunion (1988-1994)

NUMBER OF CASES BY AGE GROUP AND SUMMARY RATES OF INCIDENCE - FEMALE

SITE	ALL AGES	AGE UNK	MV (%)	0-	15-	25-	35-	45-	55-	65+	CRUDE RATE	%	CR 64	ASR (W)	ICD (10th)
Mouth	17	0	100	-	-	1	1	5	4	6	0.8	0.7	0.06	0.9	C00-06
Salivary gland	5	0	100	-	-	1	2	1	2	-	0.2	0.2	0.03	0.2	C07-08
Nasopharynx	4	0	100	-	2	-	1	1	-	1	0.2	0.2	0.01	0.2	C11
Other pharynx	16	0	100	-	-	3	-	6	5	1	0.7	0.6	0.08	0.8	C09-10,C12-14
Oesophagus	36	0	100	1	-	-	1	6	10	19	1.7	1.5	0.11	1.9	C15
Stomach	158	0	98	1	-	5	11	15	30	96	7.3	6.4	0.36	7.8	C16
Colon, rectum and anus	199	0	97	1	5	9	19	37	35	93	9.2	8.1	0.58	10.0	C18-21
Liver	32	0	78	-	-	-	3	5	9	15	1.5	1.3	0.11	1.6	C22
Gallbladder etc.	53	0	92	-	-	-	3	6	9	35	2.4	2.2	0.11	2.6	C23-24
Pancreas	35	0	69	-	-	1	4	2	11	17	1.6	1.4	0.11	1.8	C25
Larynx	6	0	100	-	-	-	-	1	1	3	0.3	0.2	0.02	0.3	C32
Trachea, bronchus and lung	64	0	89	-	-	-	3	5	18	38	3.0	2.6	0.17	3.3	C33-34
Bone	15	0	100	2	2	2	4	-	2	3	0.7	0.6	0.04	0.7	C40-41
Melanoma of skin	40	0	100	2	2	11	8	2	6	9	1.8	1.6	0.12	1.8	C43
Other skin	127	0	100	-	-	1	10	17	21	78	5.9		0.29	6.3	C44
Mesothelioma	5	0	100	-	-	-	1	-	1	3	0.2	0.2	0.01	0.2	C45
Kaposi sarcoma	0	0	-	-	-	-	-	-	-	-	0.0	0.0	0.00	0.0	C46
Peripheral nerves	2	0	100	1	-	-	1	-	-	-	0.1	0.1	0.01	0.1	C47
Connective and soft tissue	16	0	100	2	2	3	2	3	2	3	0.7	0.6	0.05	0.8	C49
Breast	566	0	99	-	2	33	109	156	110	156	26.2	23.0	2.18	29.2	C50
Vulva	18	0	100	-	-	1	1	2	4	11	0.8	0.7	0.04	0.9	C51
Vagina	6	0	100	-	-	-	1	1	1	2	0.3	0.2	0.02	0.3	C52
Cervix uteri	447	0	99	-	3	55	101	108	85	95	20.7	18.2	1.74	22.3	C53
Uterus	104	0	99	-	-	5	9	17	18	55	4.8	4.2	0.27	5.1	C54-55
Ovary	101	0	99	1	5	9	10	20	22	34	4.7	4.1	0.35	5.1	C56
Placenta	3	0	100	-	1	-	2	-	-	-	0.1	0.1	0.01	0.1	C58
Kidney	25	0	92	9	1	3	3	2	4	3	1.2	1.0	0.09	1.3	C64
Renal pelvis, ureter and other urinary	5	0	100	-	-	-	1	2	2	-	0.2	0.2	0.02	0.3	C65-66,C68
Bladder	35	0	97	-	-	-	1	2	5	27	1.6	1.4	0.05	1.7	C67
Eye	7	0	86	5	-	-	-	-	-	2	0.3	0.3	0.03	0.4	C69
Brain, nervous system	41	0	93	7	7	7	2	4	6	8	1.9	1.7	0.13	1.9	C70-72
Thyroid	33	0	100	-	3	9	5	6	5	5	1.5	1.3	0.12	1.6	C73
Hodgkin disease	12	0	100	-	4	-	3	3	-	3	0.6	0.5	0.03	0.5	C81
Non-Hodgkin lymphoma	75	0	95	6	2	8	6	5	6	42	3.5	3.0	0.14	3.5	C82-85,C96
Multiple myeloma	64	0	97	-	-	-	4	1	13	46	3.0	2.6	0.12	3.1	C90
Lymphoid leukaemia	29	0	97	13	1	1	-	2	4	8	1.3	1.2	0.08	1.5	C91
Myeloid leukaemia	51	0	100	4	6	1	2	6	9	20	2.4	2.1	0.14	2.5	C92-94
Leukaemia, unspecified	3	0	67	-	-	1	-	-	-	2	0.1	0.1	0.00	0.1	C95
Other and unspecified	134	0	96	9	5	5	7	21	28	59	6.2	5.4	0.40	6.9	O&U
All sites	2589	0	97	63	51	184	338	465	490	998	119.6		8.21	129.7	ALL
All sites but C44	2462	0	97	63	51	183	328	448	469	920	113.8	100.0	7.92	123.4	ALLbC44
Average annual population				88123	60455	53653	39114	26687	19231	21855					

Table 2. Childhood cancer, France, La Réunion (1988-1994)

	NUMBER OF CASES				REL. FREQ.(%)	RATES PER MILLION					
	0-4	5-9	10-14	**All**	*M/F*	Overall	0-4	5-9	10-14	Crude	**ASR**	%MV
Leukaemia	18	11	5	**34**	*1.0*	27.9	48.3	24.9	11.6	27.3	**30.1**	100.0
Acute lymphoid leukaemia	13	8	4	**25**	*0.9*	20.5	34.9	18.1	9.3	20.0	**22.0**	96.0
Lymphoma	8	6	6	**20**	*2.3*	16.4	21.5	13.6	13.9	16.0	**16.7**	90.9
Hodgkin disease	2	0	1	**3**	-	2.5	5.4	-	2.3	2.4	**2.7**	100.0
Burkitt lymphoma	2	2	2	**6**	-	4.9	5.4	4.5	4.6	4.8	**4.9**	83.3
Brain and spinal neoplasms	7	2	5	**14**	*1.3*	11.5	18.8	4.5	11.6	11.2	**12.1**	100.0
Neuroblastoma	6	1	0	**7**	*0.4*	5.7	16.1	2.3	-	5.6	**7.0**	100.0
Retinoblastoma	5	0	0	**5**	*0.3*	4.1	13.4	-	-	4.0	**5.2**	80.0
Wilms tumour	9	3	0	**12**	*0.3*	9.8	24.1	6.8	-	9.6	**11.5**	100.0
Bone tumours	1	1	4	**6**	*2.0*	4.9	2.7	2.3	9.3	4.8	**4.5**	83.3
Soft tissue sarcomas	1	0	2	**3**	*0.5*	2.5	2.7	-	4.6	2.4	**2.4**	100.0
Kaposi sarcoma	0	0	0	**0**	-	-	-	-	-	-	**-**	-
Germ cell tumours	4	1	0	**5**	*1.5*	4.1	10.7	2.3	-	4.0	**4.9**	100.0
Other	6	5	5	**16**	*0.6*	13.1	16.1	11.3	11.6	12.8	**13.2**	93.8
All	65	30	27	**122**	*0.9*	100.0	174.4	67.8	62.5	97.8	**107.5**	95.1

3.4.12 Rwanda

Background

Climate: Temperate; two rainy seasons (February to April, November to January); mild in mountains with frost and snow possible

Terrain: Mostly grassy uplands and hills; relief is mountainous with altitude declining from west to east

Ethnic groups: Hutu 80%, Tutsi 19%, Twa (Pygmoid) 1%

Religions: Roman Catholic 65%, Protestant 9%, Muslim 1%, indigenous beliefs and other 25%

Economy—overview: Rwanda has suffered bitterly from ethnic-based civil war. The agricultural sector dominates the economy; coffee and tea normally make up 80–90% of exports. The amount of fertile land is limited, however, and deforestation and soil erosion continue to reduce the production potential. Manufacturing focuses mainly on the processing of agricultural products. A structural adjustment programme with the World Bank began in October 1990. Civil war in 1990 devastated wide areas, especially in the north, and displaced hundreds of thousands of people. A peace accord in mid-1993 temporarily ended most of the fighting, but resumption of large-scale violence and genocide in April 1994 in the capital city Kigali and elsewhere took 500 000 lives in that year alone and severely damaged already poor economic prospects. In 1994–96, peace was restored throughout much of the country. In 1996–97, most of the refugees who fled the war returned to Rwanda. Sketchy data suggest that GDP dropped 50% in 1994 and recovered partially, by 25%, in 1995. Plentiful rains helped agriculture in 1996, and outside aid continued to support this desperately poor economy.

Industries: Mining of cassiterite (tin ore) and wolframite (tungsten ore), tin, cement, processing of agricultural products, small-scale beverage production, soap, furniture, shoes, plastic goods, textiles, cigarettes

Agriculture—products: Coffee, tea, pyrethrum (insecticide made from chrysanthemums), bananas, beans, sorghum, potatoes; livestock

Cancer registration

A cancer registry was established in the Department of Pathology at the University Hospital, Butare, in 1991. This registry began active data collection, through regular visits by registry staff, to collect data on cancer cases diagnosed in all four hospitals in the prefecture of Butare (population 765 000) in May 1991. The Department of Pathology itself served as an important source of information. The registry continued to function until the Rwandan genocide of April 1994. Here we present the results for the first 32 months of operation, May 1991–December 1993. These have been published as part of a paper examining the distribution, and some determinants, of cancer in Rwanda (Newton *et al.*, 1996). The calculated incidence rates are very low (age standardized rates for all cancers combined of 27.4 per 100 000 in men and 28.1 in women). These are clearly underestimates, presumably the result of underascertainment of cases, and the percentage of cases with morphological verification of diagnosis seems rather high (83.4%). However, the relative frequencies of different cancers may be a more or less true reflection of reality (Table 1). They suggest that the main cancers of men are liver (20.5%), Kaposi sarcoma (9.4%) and stomach (8.8%), and in women cervix (22.1%), stomach (9.6%), liver (8.7%) and breast (7.7%).

Review of data

Early reports of cancer in Rwanda included an analysis of 900 cases seen in seven hospitals in the period 1956–60 (Clemmesen *et al.*, 1962) and a summary of 120 cases from four hospitals in Rwanda-Burundi in 1968–69 (Cook & Burkitt, 1971). More recently, Ngendahayo (1986) and Ngendahayo & Parkin (1986) reported on cancer cases diagnosed in the Department of Pathology at the University Hospital, Butare, in 1982–84 (Table 2).

A more detailed analysis of 119 Kaposi sarcoma cases diagnosed histologically in 1979–86 (Ngendahayo *et al.*, 1989) showed that, at that time, the sex ratio remained high (6.4:1) and that incidence appeared to show a progressive increase with age. Nevertheless, 28 cases were "generalized", either cutaneous or affecting lymph nodes, or gastrointestinal tract. All eight of the generalized cases tested for anti-HIV antibody were positive, while none of the 10 localized cutaneous cases were. By 1991–93, 61% of the 18 cases of Kaposi sarcoma tested for HIV antibody were positive (Newton *et al.*, 1995).

Ngendahayo & Schmauz (1992) provided more detail of the 115 lymphoma cases diagnosed in 1979–87. There were 19 cases of Hodgkin disease, five under age 20 years, and the majority (11 cases) of mixed cellularity type. 91/96 non-Hodgkin lymphoma cases were B-cell lymphomas, with about equal numbers of high and low grade, nodal and extra-nodal cases. There were 12 cases of Burkitt lymphoma (9 abdominal), all aged <20 years (46.2% of non-Hodgkin lymphoma cases in this age group).

References

Clemmesen, J., Maisin, J. & Gigase P. (1962) Cancer in Kivu and Rwanda-Urundi. A preliminary report. Louvain, Institut du Cancer, Université de Louvain

Cook, P.J. & Burkitt, D.P. (1971) Cancer in Africa. *Br. Med. Bull.*, **27**, 14–20

Ngendahayo P. & Parkin D.M. (1986) Le cancer au Rwanda. Etude de fréquence relative. *Bull. Cancer*, **73**, 155–164

Ngendahayo P. (1986) Rwanda. In: Parkin D.M., ed., *Cancer Occurrence in Developing Countries* (IARC Scientific Publications, No. 75), Lyon, IARC, pp. 77–80

Ngendahayo, P. & Schmauz, R. (1992) Pattern of malignant lymphomas in Rwanda. *Bull. Cancer*, **79**, 1087–1096

Ngendahayo, P., Mets, T., Bugingo, G. & Parkin, D.M. (1989) Le sarcome de Kaposi au Rwanda. Aspects clinico-pathologiques et épidémiologiques. *Bull. Cancer*, **76**, 383–394

Newton, R., Grulich, A., Beral, V., Sindikubwabo, B., Ngilimana, P.J., Nganyira, A. & Parkin, D.M. (1995) Cancer and HIV infection in Rwanda. *Lancet*, **345**, 1378–1379

Newton, R., Ngilimana, P.J., Grulich, A., Beral, V., Sindikubwabo, B., Nganyira, A. & Parkin, D.M. (1996) Cancer in Rwanda. *Int. J. Cancer*, **66**, 75–81

Table 1. Rwanda, Butare (1991-1993)
NUMBER OF CASES BY AGE GROUP - MALE

SITE	ICD (10th)	%	65+	55-	45-	35-	25-	15-	0-	MV (%)	AGE UNK	ALL AGES
Mouth	C00-06	1.8	2	1	-	-	-	-	-	100	0	3
Salivary gland	C07-08	1.2	-	-	-	1	1	-	-	100	0	2
Nasopharynx	C11	0.0	-	-	-	-	-	-	-	-	0	0
Other pharynx	C09-10,C12-14	1.8	-	1	-	1	-	1	-	100	0	3
Oesophagus	C15	0.0	-	-	-	-	-	-	-	-	0	0
Stomach	C16	8.8	1	-	7	4	3	-	-	60	0	15
Colon, rectum and anus	C18-21	2.3	2	-	-	1	1	-	-	100	0	4
Liver	C22	20.5	5	13	5	4	2	6	-	51	0	35
Gallbladder etc.	C23-24	0.0	-	-	-	-	-	-	-	-	0	0
Pancreas	C25	1.8	1	1	-	1	-	-	-	67	0	3
Larynx	C32	0.6	1	-	-	-	-	-	-	100	0	1
Trachea, bronchus and lung	C33-34	1.2	-	-	-	2	-	-	-	0	0	2
Bone	C40-41	3.5	2	1	-	1	1	1	-	33	0	6
Melanoma of skin	C43	1.2	-	-	2	-	-	-	-	100	0	2
Other skin	C44	0.0	2	-	4	3	4	1	-	100	0	14
Mesothelioma	C45	0.0	-	-	-	-	-	-	-	-	0	0
Kaposi sarcoma	C46	9.4	3	-	-	6	6	1	-	100	0	16
Peripheral nerves	C47	0.0	-	-	-	-	-	-	-	-	0	0
Connective and soft tissue	C49	2.9	2	-	1	1	-	-	1	100	0	5
Breast	C50	0.6	-	-	-	-	-	1	-	100	0	1
Penis	C60	2.9	3	1	1	-	-	-	-	100	0	5
Prostate	C61	2.9	4	1	-	-	-	-	-	100	0	5
Testis	C62	0.0	-	-	-	-	-	-	-	-	0	0
Kidney	C64	1.8	-	-	-	2	-	-	1	67	0	3
Renal pelvis, ureter and other urinary	C65-66,C68	0.0	-	-	-	-	-	-	-	-	0	0
Bladder	C67	2.3	3	-	-	1	-	-	-	50	0	4
Eye	C69	2.3	-	-	-	-	1	1	2	100	0	4
Brain, nervous system	C70-72	0.6	-	-	-	-	-	1	-	100	0	1
Thyroid	C73	0.0	-	-	-	-	-	-	-	-	0	0
Hodgkin disease	C81	1.8	-	-	1	-	1	-	1	100	0	3
Non-Hodgkin lymphoma	C82-85,C96	5.8	-	-	-	1	3	1	4	100	1	10
Multiple myeloma	C90	0.6	1	-	-	-	-	-	-	100	0	1
Lymphoid leukaemia	C91	0.0	-	-	-	-	-	-	-	-	0	0
Myeloid leukaemia	C92-94	0.6	-	-	-	1	-	-	-	100	0	1
Leukaemia, unspecified	C95	0.6	-	-	-	-	-	-	1	100	0	1
Other and unspecified	O&U	20.5	2	5	7	6	6	3	5	80	1	35
All sites	ALL		34	24	28	36	29	17	15	78	2	185
All sites but C44	ALLbC44	100.0	32	24	24	33	25	16	15	77	2	171

Table 1. Rwanda, Butare (1991-1993)

NUMBER OF CASES BY AGE GROUP - FEMALE

SITE	ICD (10th)	ALL AGES	AGE UNK	MV (%)	0-	15-	25-	35-	45-	55-	65+	%
Mouth	C00-06	1	0	100	-	-	-	-	-	1	-	0.5
Salivary gland	C07-08	0	0	-	-	-	-	-	-	-	-	0.0
Nasopharynx	C11	0	0	-	-	-	-	-	-	-	-	0.0
Other pharynx	C09-10,C12-14	2	0	100	-	-	1	-	-	1	-	1.0
Oesophagus	C15	1	0	0	-	-	1	-	-	-	-	0.5
Stomach	C16	20	1	75	-	-	-	4	6	1	8	9.6
Colon, rectum and anus	C18-21	6	0	83	-	-	-	2	1	1	2	2.9
Liver	C22	18	0	78	-	1	2	4	4	6	1	8.7
Gallbladder etc.	C23-24	0	0	-	-	-	-	-	-	-	-	0.0
Pancreas	C25	3	0	0	-	-	2	-	1	-	-	1.4
Larynx	C32	1	0	0	-	-	1	-	-	-	-	0.5
Trachea, bronchus and lung	C33-34	0	0	-	-	-	-	-	-	-	-	0.0
Bone	C40-41	5	0	80	1	2	1	1	-	-	-	2.4
Melanoma of skin	C43	4	0	100	-	1	-	-	-	-	3	1.9
Other skin	C44	12	0	100	1	3	-	3	3	1	1	
Mesothelioma	C45	0	0	-	-	-	-	-	-	-	-	0.0
Kaposi sarcoma	C46	3	0	100	-	-	1	2	-	-	-	1.4
Peripheral nerves	C47	0	0	-	-	-	-	-	-	-	-	0.0
Connective and soft tissue	C49	7	0	100	2	1	1	-	1	-	2	3.4
Breast	C50	16	0	94	-	1	4	6	3	-	2	7.7
Vulva	C51	1	0	100	-	-	-	-	1	-	-	0.5
Vagina	C52	1	0	100	-	-	-	-	-	1	-	0.5
Cervix uteri	C53	46	0	100	-	-	4	9	18	11	4	22.1
Uterus	C54-55	11	1	100	-	-	3	1	1	2	3	5.3
Ovary	C56	5	0	80	-	-	-	-	3	2	-	2.4
Placenta	C58	0	0	-	-	-	-	-	-	-	-	0.0
Kidney	C64	1	0	100	-	-	-	-	1	-	-	0.5
Renal pelvis, ureter and other urinary	C65-66,C68	0	0	-	-	-	-	-	-	-	-	0.0
Bladder	C67	3	0	100	-	-	-	-	-	1	2	1.4
Eye	C69	10	0	80	5	1	1	-	3	-	-	4.8
Brain, nervous system	C70-72	1	0	100	-	-	1	-	-	-	-	0.5
Thyroid	C73	3	0	67	-	-	-	1	1	1	-	1.4
Hodgkin disease	C81	2	0	100	1	1	-	-	-	-	-	1.0
Non-Hodgkin lymphoma	C82-85,C96	5	0	80	2	-	2	-	-	1	-	2.4
Multiple myeloma	C90	0	0	-	-	-	-	-	-	-	-	0.0
Lymphoid leukaemia	C91	1	0	100	-	-	-	1	-	-	-	0.5
Myeloid leukaemia	C92-94	3	0	100	-	-	-	1	-	1	1	1.4
Leukaemia, unspecified	C95	0	0	-	-	-	-	-	-	-	-	0.0
Other and unspecified	O&U	28	0	82	2	3	4	3	9	4	3	13.5
All sites	ALL	220	2	88	14	16	26	40	57	33	32	100.0
All sites but C44	ALLbC44	208	2	87	13	13	26	37	54	32	31	

Table 2. Rwanda: case series

Site	Department of Pathology, University Hospital, Butare (1982–84) (Ngendahayo & Parkin, 1986)				%HV
	Male		Female		
	No.	%	No.	%	
Oral cavity	38	9.7%	16	3.8%	100
Nasopharynx	3	0.8%	1	0.2%	100
Other pharynx	0	0.0%	0	0.0%	100
Oesophagus	2	0.5%	0	0.0%	100
Stomach	39	9.9%	27	6.5%	100
Colon/rectum	10	2.5%	11	2.6%	100
Liver	26	6.6%	3	0.7%	100
Pancreas	1	0.3%	0	0.0%	100
Larynx	1	0.3%	0	0.0%	100
Lung	0	0.0%	0	0.0%	100
Melanoma	18	4.6%	12	2.9%	100
Other skin	52	13.2%	43	10.3%	100
Kaposi sarcoma	45	11.5%	8	1.9%	100
Breast	2	0.5%	70	16.8%	100
Cervix uteri			89	21.4%	100
Corpus uteri			6	1.4%	100
Ovary etc.			18	4.3%	100
Prostate	9	2.3%			100
Penis	18	4.6%			100
Bladder	1	0.3%	1	0.2%	100
Kidney etc.	5	1.3%	5	1.2%	100
Brain, nervous system	0	0.0%	0	0.0%	100
Eye	6	1.5%	7	1.7%	100
Thyroid	3	0.8%	10	2.4%	100
Non-Hodgkin lymphoma	32	8.1%	17	4.1%	100
Hodgkin disease	10	2.5%	3	0.7%	100
Myeloma	5	1.3%	0	0.0%	100
Leukaemia	2	0.5%	0	0.0%	100
ALL SITES	393	100.0%	416	100.0%	100

[1]Lip and tongue

3.4.13 Somalia

Background

Climate: Principally desert; December to February—northeast monsoon, moderate temperatures in north and very hot in south; May to October—southwest monsoon, torrid in the north and hot in the south, irregular rainfall, hot and humid periods (tangambili) between monsoons

Terrain: Mostly flat to undulating plateau rising to hills in north

Ethnic groups: Somali 85%, Bantu and other non-somali (including Arabs 30 000)

Religions: Sunni Muslim

Economy—overview: Somalia has few resources. Much of the economy has been devastated by civil war. Agriculture is the most important sector, with livestock accounting for about 40% of GDP and about 65% of export earnings. Nomads and semi-nomads, who are dependent upon livestock for their livelihood, make up a large portion of the population. Crop production generates only 10% of GDP and employs about 20% of the work force. After livestock, bananas are the principal export; sugar, sorghum, corn and fish are produced for the domestic market. The small industrial sector, based on the processing of agricultural products, accounts for less than 10% of GDP; most facilities have been shut down because of the civil strife. Moreover, continuing civil disturbances in Mogadishu and outlying areas interfere with any substantial economic advance.

Industries: A few small industries, including sugar refining, textiles, petroleum refining (mostly shut down)

Agriculture—products: Bananas, sorghum, corn, sugar-cane, mangoes, sesame seeds, beans; cattle, sheep, goats; fishing potential largely unexploited

Cancer registration

No cancer registration is being conducted in Somalia.

3.4.14 Tanzania, United Republic of

Background

Climate: Varies from tropical along coast to temperate in highlands

Terrain: Plains along coast; central plateau; highlands in north and south

Ethnic groups: Mainland—native African 99% (of which 95% are Bantu consisting of more than 130 tribes), other 1% (consisting of Asian, European and Arab). Zanzibar—Arab, native African, mixed Arab and native African

Religions: Mainland—Christian 45%, Muslim 35%, indigenous beliefs 20%. Zanzibar—more than 99% Muslim

Economy—overview: Tanzania is one of the poorest countries in the world. The economy is heavily dependent on agriculture, which accounts for 57% of GDP, provides 85% of exports and employs 90% of the work force. Topography and climatic conditions, however, limit cultivated crops to only 4% of the land area. Industry accounts for 17% of GDP and is mainly limited to processing agricultural products and light consumer goods. In the last 10 years there has been a substantial increase in output of minerals, led by gold. Natural gas exploration in the Rufiji Delta looks promising and production could start by 2002.

Industries: Primarily agricultural processing (sugar, beer, cigarettes, sisal twine), diamond and gold mining, oil refining, shoes, cement, textiles, wood products, fertilizer, salt

Agriculture—products: Coffee, sisal, tea, cotton, pyrethrum (insecticide made from chrysanthemums), cashews, tobacco, cloves (Zanzibar), corn, wheat, cassava (tapioca), bananas, fruits, vegetables; cattle, sheep, goats

Cancer registration

The Tanzania Cancer Registry was established in 1966 and is located in the Pathology Department of Muhumbili Medical Centre. It is a pathology-based cancer registry for cases diagnosed at all the hospitals in the central and southern parts of the Republic of Tanzania. However, the registry is also occasionally notified of histopathologically diagnosed cases from Mwanza Hospital, which acts a reference hospital to the northern and eastern parts of the country.

Kilimanjaro Cancer Registry is located in the Department of Pathology of the Kilimanjaro Christian Medical Centre (KCMC), in Moshi, north-western Tanzania. KCMC is a 420-bed hospital where all the major specialties are present and which provides specialist services for the north-western regions of the country. The registry was started in 1974 and recorded pathology-based data between 1975 and 1981 (Lauren & Kitinya, 1986). Approximately half of the cases at that time were from KCMC, the remainder coming from many other hospitals in the northern part of the country.

In 1998, the registry was restarted as a population-based registry, covering four districts (Moshi, urban and rural, Rombo, Hai) in Kilimanjaro region, with a population of about 840 386. Data collection is not only from the pathology department, but also by scheduled visits to all of the hospitals within these four districts by the cancer registrar.

A hospital cancer registry is present in the Ocean Road Cancer Centre in Dar es Salaam, the only specialized treatment centre for cancer in the whole country.

Review of data

Two sets of data are presented in this volume: from the Tanzania (Dar es Salaam) Cancer Registry, for the years 1990–91 (Table 1) and from the Kilimanjaro Cancer Registry (Table 2). The data from the Tanzania Cancer Registry represent 1881 cases diagnosed histologically only. In men, the most common cancers were Kaposi sarcoma (17.5% of cases, excluding non-melanoma skin cancers), oesophagus (9.5%) and non-Hodgkin lymphoma (9.1%), and in women, cervix cancer (46.9%) and breast cancer (12.7%).

These results can be compared with previous reports from this registry, from 1969–73 (Hiza, 1976) and from 1980–81 (Shaba & Owor, 1986) (Table 3). The latter report includes separate tables for cases notified to the National Registry from the pathology departments in Muhimbili Medical Centre, Dar es Salaam (2384 cases) and from Mwanza Hospital in the north-east of the country, south of Lake Victoria (422 cases). In males the frequency of cancer of the oesophagus is notable, and relatively constant between the series. The frequency of liver cancer, based only on histologically confirmed cases, is underestimated. Kaposi sarcoma comprised 3.6% cases in males in the 1980–81 data from Muhimbili Medical Centre and over two thirds of the cases with age recorded were over 45 years. The frequency in Mwanza was noted to be higher (18/191 cases in men, 9.4%). However, it is clear that there was a considerable increase in frequency by 1990–91, and two thirds of cases in men are now aged less than 45 years.

The Kilimanjaro Cancer Registry recorded 1204 cases in 1998–2000, 72% with a diagnosis based upon histology or cytology (Table 2). There are no recent census data, to permit calculation of incidence rates, so the results are presented simply as frequencies of the different cancers. The most frequently diagnosed cancer in men is cancer of the prostate (20.2% of cases), followed by stomach (12.4%), liver (8.8%), oesophagus (7.8%) and Kaposi sarcoma (6.5%). In women, the principal cancers are cervix (29.8%) and breast (12.2%). Cancers of the eye were also common in both sexes; the cases in adults were predominantly squamous cell carcinomas of the conjunctiva (Chapter 4.5, Table 3).

These results are rather different from the earlier series from the registry, for the years 1975-1979 (Table 3), in paricular, in the increased frequency of prostate and oesophageal cancers. The frequency of KS was not reported. Cervix cancer was still the most common cancer of women; Kitinya and Lauren (1988) also estimated age adjusted incidence rates of cervical cancer among the two main tribal groups, and found a higher rate in the Pare ethnic group compared to Chagga. They ascribed this to differences in sexual lifestyles. The relatively high frequency of stomach cancer in the data from Kilimanjaro has also been commented on (Kitinya et al, 1988), with respect to the larger proportion of tumours of intestinal-type histology than in lower-risk areas, and the possible role of volcanic soils in the aetiology.

Childhood cancer

The cases of childhood cancer recorded in the Tanzania Cancer Registry (histology-based) in 1990–91 are shown in Table 4. Earlier series (Table 5) are essentially from the same source. Shaba (1988) reported a series of 258 cases of childhood cancer diagnosed histologically in three government referral hospitals (Mwanza, Kilimanjaro Christian Medical Centre (Moshi) and Muhimbili Medical Centre in Dar es Salaam) during 1980–81. The series reported by Carneiro et al. represents the childhood cancer cases collected by the Department of Pathology at Muhimbili Medical Centre in Dar es Salaam over a period of 22 years (1973–95), a total of 1874 cases.

Table 1. Tanzania, Dar Es Salaam (1990-1991)

NUMBER OF CASES BY AGE GROUP - MALE

SITE	ALL AGES	AGE UNK	MV (%)	0-	15-	25-	35-	45-	55-	65+	%	ICD (10th)
Mouth	26	2	100	-	1	3	1	4	12	3	4.0	C00-06
Salivary gland	7	1	100	-	-	1	-	2	1	1	1.1	C07-08
Nasopharynx	19	0	100	-	4	2	3	6	2	2	2.9	C11
Other pharynx	12	1	100	-	-	-	1	4	2	4	1.8	C09-10,C12-14
Oesophagus	62	2	100	-	-	4	5	18	18	15	9.5	C15
Stomach	8	1	100	-	-	-	-	1	5	1	1.2	C16
Colon, rectum and anus	21	1	100	-	1	2	5	5	3	4	3.2	C18-21
Liver	12	3	100	-	1	-	5	1	2	-	1.8	C22
Gallbladder etc.	0	0	-	-	-	-	-	-	-	-	0.0	C23-24
Pancreas	0	0	-	-	-	-	-	-	-	-	0.0	C25
Larynx	22	1	100	1	1	1	1	6	9	3	3.4	C32
Trachea, bronchus and lung	6	0	100	1	-	-	-	2	3	-	0.9	C33-34
Bone	17	2	100	1	5	4	1	-	3	1	2.6	C40-41
Melanoma of skin	5	1	100	-	-	-	1	-	1	-	0.8	C43
Other skin	54	9	100	2	7	16	2	8	5	5		C44
Mesothelioma	0	0	-	-	-	-	-	-	-	-	0.0	C45
Kaposi sarcoma	114	15	99	-	7	32	27	14	5	14	17.5	C46
Peripheral nerves	6	1	100	2	-	-	-	2	1	-	0.9	C47
Connective and soft tissue	24	4	100	4	4	4	5	2	-	1	3.7	C49
Breast	0	0	-	-	-	-	-	-	-	-	0.0	C50
Penis	8	0	100	1	-	1	-	1	-	1	1.2	C60
Prostate	42	10	100	-	-	-	-	2	10	20	6.5	C61
Testis	4	2	100	-	-	1	-	1	-	-	0.6	C62
Kidney	3	0	100	2	-	1	1	-	-	-	0.5	C64
Renal pelvis, ureter and other urinary	1	0	100	-	-	-	-	-	-	1	0.2	C65-66,C68
Bladder	29	5	100	-	1	2	2	5	6	9	4.5	C67
Eye	39	8	100	9	5	5	6	4	1	1	6.0	C69
Brain, nervous system	2	0	100	1	1	-	1	-	-	-	0.3	C70-72
Thyroid	6	0	100	-	1	1	-	-	2	1	0.9	C73
Hodgkin disease	8	0	100	4	2	2	-	-	-	-	1.2	C81
Non-Hodgkin lymphoma	59	5	100	31	10	3	3	5	2	-	9.1	C82-85,C96
Multiple myeloma	3	0	100	-	-	-	1	1	1	-	0.5	C90
Lymphoid leukaemia	25	0	100	8	4	-	4	4	2	3	3.8	C91
Myeloid leukaemia	22	0	100	4	5	2	6	2	2	1	3.4	C92-94
Leukaemia, unspecified	2	0	100	2	-	-	-	-	-	-	0.3	C95
Other and unspecified	36	7	100	2	1	3	4	5	5	9	5.5	O&U
All sites	704	81	100	74	60	89	89	105	107	99		ALL
All sites but C44	650	72	100	72	53	73	87	97	102	94	100.0	ALLbC44

Table 1. Tanzania, Dar Es Salaam (1990-1991)

NUMBER OF CASES BY AGE GROUP - FEMALE

SITE	ICD (10th)	%	65+	55-	45-	35-	25-	15-	0-	MV (%)	AGE UNK	ALL AGES
Mouth	C00-06	3.0	1	8	14	4	2	2	1	100	2	34
Salivary gland	C07-08	0.6	-	-	-	1	2	1	2	100	1	7
Nasopharynx	C11	0.8	-	2	3	2	-	1	1	100	0	9
Other pharynx	C09-10,C12-14	0.8	2	1	-	1	2	1	-	100	2	9
Oesophagus	C15	2.2	5	7	4	4	1	2	-	100	2	25
Stomach	C16	0.8	4	2	-	1	1	-	-	100	2	9
Colon, rectum and anus	C18-21	1.7	-	10	2	3	1	-	-	100	3	19
Liver	C22	0.4	-	-	1	1	-	2	-	100	1	4
Gallbladder etc.	C23-24	0.1	-	-	1	-	-	-	-	100	0	1
Pancreas	C25	0.0	-	-	-	-	-	-	-	-	0	0
Larynx	C32	0.5	-	-	3	-	1	-	1	100	0	6
Trachea, bronchus and lung	C33-34	0.3	-	-	-	3	-	-	-	100	0	3
Bone	C40-41	1.2	1	2	1	1	1	6	2	100	1	14
Melanoma of skin	C43	0.6	1	1	3	1	-	-	-	86	0	7
Other skin	C44		8	9	5	8	6	4	-	100	7	47
Mesothelioma	C45	0.0	-	-	-	-	-	-	-	-	0	0
Kaposi sarcoma	C46	3.7	2	3	1	8	13	8	1	100	6	42
Peripheral nerves	C47	0.4	-	-	-	-	-	-	2	100	0	4
Connective and soft tissue	C49	1.6	-	4	-	7	7	4	1	100	1	18
Breast	C50	12.7	20	24	36	30	17	3	1	100	12	143
Vulva	C51	0.8	1	2	6	-	-	-	-	100	0	9
Vagina	C52	0.5	-	-	3	2	2	-	-	100	1	6
Cervix uteri	C53	46.9	41	87	144	115	56	3	1	100	83	530
Uterus	C54-55	3.5	2	7	8	10	4	2	-	100	7	40
Ovary	C56	1.0	1	2	1	3	2	2	-	100	0	11
Placenta	C58	0.0	-	-	-	-	-	-	-	-	0	0
Kidney	C64	0.2	-	-	-	1	1	1	1	100	0	2
Renal pelvis, ureter and other urinary	C65-66,C68	0.4	-	1	-	2	2	-	2	100	0	5
Bladder	C67	2.1	-	10	2	3	3	1	2	100	3	24
Eye	C69	2.6	3	1	4	1	5	3	9	100	3	29
Brain, nervous system	C70-72	0.1	-	-	-	-	-	1	-	100	0	1
Thyroid	C73	0.1	-	1	-	-	-	-	-	100	0	1
Hodgkin disease	C81	0.4	-	-	-	3	2	-	-	100	0	5
Non-Hodgkin lymphoma	C82-85,C96	3.5	2	4	2	2	3	3	23	100	1	40
Multiple myeloma	C90	0.2	1	1	-	-	-	-	-	100	0	2
Lymphoid leukaemia	C91	0.7	1	3	3	3	-	-	-	100	0	8
Myeloid leukaemia	C92-94	1.2	-	-	2	2	4	2	5	100	0	14
Leukaemia, unspecified	C95	0.2	-	-	-	1	-	-	-	100	0	2
Other and unspecified	O&U	4.2	3	6	11	10	6	4	2	100	5	47
All sites	ALL	100.0	98	198	260	222	144	56	55	100	144	1177
All sites but C44	ALLbC44		90	189	255	214	138	52	55	100	137	1130

162

Table 2. Tanzania, Kilimanjaro (1998-2000)

NUMBER OF CASES BY AGE GROUP - MALE

SITE	ICD (10th)	ALL AGES	AGE UNK	MV (%)	0-	15-	25-	35-	45-	55-	65+	%
Mouth	C00-06	13	0	92	1	-	-	1	2	3	6	2.1
Salivary gland	C07-08	2	0	100	-	-	-	-	-	2	-	0.3
Nasopharynx	C11	7	0	100	-	3	1	1	1	1	1	1.1
Other pharynx	C09-10,C12-14	5	0	100	-	-	-	-	1	3	1	0.8
Oesophagus	C15	76	0	25	-	-	4	4	12	19	37	12.4
Stomach	C16	48	2	44	-	-	1	1	11	10	24	7.8
Colon, rectum and anus	C18-21	11	0	64	-	1	1	-	1	2	5	1.8
Liver	C22	54	1	37	-	2	8	6	14	8	15	8.8
Gallbladder etc.	C23-24	1	0	100	-	-	-	1	-	-	-	0.2
Pancreas	C25	10	0	10	-	-	3	-	1	-	5	1.6
Larynx	C32	17	0	82	-	-	-	-	2	5	10	2.8
Trachea, bronchus and lung	C33-34	5	0	20	-	-	-	-	1	-	4	0.8
Bone	C40-41	7	0	71	-	4	-	1	-	1	1	1.1
Melanoma of skin	C43	4	0	100	-	-	1	-	-	2	1	0.7
Other skin	C44	18	0	100	-	5	2	4	2	3	2	
Mesothelioma	C45	0	0	-	-	-	-	-	-	-	-	0.0
Kaposi sarcoma	C46	40	0	73	2	4	7	13	4	2	8	6.5
Peripheral nerves	C47	2	0	100	-	-	1	-	-	-	2	0.3
Connective and soft tissue	C49	5	0	100	-	1	-	2	-	-	1	0.8
Breast	C50	6	0	67	-	-	-	1	-	2	2	1.0
Penis	C60	2	0	100	-	-	-	-	1	1	-	0.3
Prostate	C61	124	3	96	-	-	-	-	4	16	101	20.2
Testis	C62	1	0	0	-	1	-	-	-	-	-	0.2
Kidney	C64	6	0	83	4	-	-	-	1	1	-	1.0
Renal pelvis, ureter and other urinary	C65-66,C68	1	0	100	1	-	-	-	-	-	-	0.2
Bladder	C67	22	1	82	-	-	-	-	2	5	13	3.6
Eye	C69	37	0	95	8	-	8	8	5	3	4	6.0
Brain, nervous system	C70-72	3	0	0	2	-	1	-	-	-	-	0.5
Thyroid	C73	5	0	100	2	-	-	-	1	1	1	0.8
Hodgkin disease	C81	4	0	100	1	-	1	1	-	-	-	0.7
Non-Hodgkin lymphoma	C82-85,C96	19	0	95	6	2	2	1	2	4	4	3.1
Multiple myeloma	C90	1	1	100	-	-	-	-	1	-	-	0.2
Lymphoid leukaemia	C91	7	0	100	1	1	-	-	-	1	4	1.1
Myeloid leukaemia	C92-94	8	0	100	2	-	2	3	-	1	-	1.3
Leukaemia, unspecified	C95	5	0	60	2	1	2	-	-	-	-	0.8
Other and unspecified	O&U	56	0	75	1	5	4	5	12	14	15	9.1
All sites	ALL	632	8	70	33	30	48	53	83	110	267	100.0
All sites but C44	ALLbC44	614	8	70	33	25	46	49	81	107	265	

Table 2. Tanzania, Kilimanjaro (1998-2000)
NUMBER OF CASES BY AGE GROUP - FEMALE

SITE	ICD (10th)	ALL AGES	AGE UNK	MV (%)	0-	15-	25-	35-	45-	55-	65+	%
Mouth	C00-06	7	0	86	-	-	-	1	1	3	2	1.2
Salivary gland	C07-08	1	0	100	-	-	1	-	-	-	-	0.2
Nasopharynx	C11	3	0	100	1	1	-	-	-	-	1	0.5
Other pharynx	C09-10,C12-14	2	0	100	-	-	-	2	-	-	-	0.4
Oesophagus	C15	24	2	17	-	-	-	2	8	5	7	4.3
Stomach	C16	34	0	41	-	-	2	6	5	8	13	6.0
Colon, rectum and anus	C18-21	13	1	54	-	-	-	1	5	2	4	2.3
Liver	C22	23	2	43	-	-	3	5	3	3	7	4.1
Gallbladder etc.	C23-24	1	0	0	-	-	-	-	1	-	-	0.2
Pancreas	C25	4	0	0	-	-	-	1	1	-	2	0.7
Larynx	C32	3	0	100	-	-	-	-	1	1	1	0.5
Trachea, bronchus and lung	C33-34	1	0	100	-	-	-	-	-	1	-	0.2
Bone	C40-41	3	0	67	-	1	2	-	-	-	-	0.5
Melanoma of skin	C43	5	0	100	-	-	1	1	-	1	2	0.9
Other skin	C44	8	0	100	-	-	-	2	3	1	2	-
Mesothelioma	C45	-	0	-	-	-	-	-	-	-	-	0.0
Kaposi sarcoma	C46	23	0	57	3	4	7	6	1	1	1	4.1
Peripheral nerves	C47	0	0	-	-	-	-	-	-	-	-	0.0
Connective and soft tissue	C49	10	0	100	1	2	2	1	1	1	2	1.8
Breast	C50	69	1	68	-	1	8	19	18	12	10	12.2
Vulva	C51	4	0	100	-	-	-	2	2	-	-	0.7
Vagina	C52	0	0	-	-	-	-	-	-	-	-	0.0
Cervix uteri	C53	168	1	89	-	-	13	48	54	30	22	29.8
Uterus	C54-55	14	0	86	-	2	4	1	3	2	2	2.5
Ovary	C56	29	0	79	1	1	6	7	8	2	4	5.1
Placenta	C58	0	0	-	-	-	-	-	-	-	-	0.0
Kidney	C64	8	0	100	7	-	-	1	-	-	-	1.4
Renal pelvis, ureter and other urinary	C65-66,C68	0	0	-	-	-	-	-	-	-	-	0.0
Bladder	C67	4	0	50	-	-	-	-	-	1	3	0.7
Eye	C69	29	0	100	5	-	11	8	2	-	3	5.1
Brain, nervous system	C70-72	0	0	-	-	-	-	-	-	-	-	0.0
Thyroid	C73	10	0	80	-	-	-	5	2	1	2	1.8
Hodgkin disease	C81	3	0	100	1	2	-	-	-	-	-	0.5
Non-Hodgkin lymphoma	C82-85,C96	11	0	64	3	1	2	-	1	2	2	2.0
Multiple myeloma	C90	1	0	100	-	-	-	-	-	-	1	0.2
Lymphoid leukaemia	C91	5	0	100	1	-	1	-	-	-	3	0.9
Myeloid leukaemia	C92-94	6	0	100	1	2	-	-	1	2	-	1.1
Leukaemia, unspecified	C95	7	0	71	3	2	-	-	1	-	1	1.2
Other and unspecified	O&U	39	3	82	-	1	4	4	4	6	17	6.9
All sites	ALL	572	10	75	27	20	67	123	125	86	114	100.0
All sites but C44	ALLbC44	564	10	75	27	20	67	121	122	85	112	

Table 3. Tanzania: case series

Site	Tanzania Cancer Registry, 1969–73 (Hiza,1976)					Tanzania Cancer Registry, 1980–81: Muhimbili M.C.(Shaba & Owor, 1986)					Kilimanjaro Cancer Registry, 1975–79 (Lauren & Kitinya, 1986)				
	Male		Female		%HV	Male		Female		%HV	Male		Female		%HV
	No.	%	No.	%		No.	%	No.	%		No.	%	No.	%	
Oral cavity[1]	139		116		100	73	7.2%	51	4.0%	100	44	8.6%	29	7.2%	100
Nasopharynx	13					13	1.3%	5	0.4%	100	20	3.9%	6	1.5%	100
Other pharynx			8		100	14	1.4%	3	0.2%	100	5	1.0%	0	0.0%	100
Oesophagus	106		8		100	97	9.5%	18	1.4%	100	19	3.7%	5	1.2%	100
Stomach	135		65		100	17	1.7%	19	1.5%	100	44	8.6%	40	9.9%	100
Colon/rectum	93		60		100	26	2.6%	31	2.4%	100	9	1.8%	6	1.5%	100
Liver	236		66		100	68	6.7%	35	2.7%	100	78	15.3%	15	3.7%	100
Pancreas	11		10		100	1	0.1%	1	0.1%	100	5	1.0%	1	0.2%	100
Lung						4	0.4%	4	0.3%	100	5	1.0%	0	0.0%	100
Melanoma						32	3.1%	23	1.8%	100	9	1.8%	11	2.7%	100
Other skin						115	11.3%	90	7.1%	100	26	5.1%	20	4.9%	100
Kaposi sarcoma						37	3.6%	10	0.8%	100					
Breast	33		328		100	20	2.0%	119	9.3%	100	3	0.6%	49	12.1%	100
Cervix uteri								482	37.8%	100			85	21.0%	100
Corpus uteri								18	1.4%	100			8	2.0%	100
Ovary etc.								33	2.6%	100			20	4.9%	100
Prostate	149				100	59	5.8%			100	57	11.2%			100
Penis	116				100	25	2.5%			100	4	0.8%			100
Bladder	154		70		100	50	4.9%	23	1.8%	100	15	2.9%	4	1.0%	100
Kidney etc.						5	0.5%	12	0.9%	100	6	1.2%	9	2.2%	100
Eye						32	3.1%	18	1.4%	100	9	1.8%	7	1.7%	100
Brain, nervous system						0	0.0%	0	0.0%	100	6	1.2%	3	0.7%	100
Thyroid						7	0.7%	15	1.2%	100	3	0.6%	3	0.7%	100
Non-Hodgkin lymphoma						64	6.3%	44	3.5%	100	39	7.7%	17	4.2%	100
Hodgkin disease						33	3.2%	7	0.5%	100	15	2.9%	10	2.5%	100
Myeloma						10	1.0%	1	0.1%	100	2	0.4%	0	0.0%	100
Leukaemia						30	2.9%	30	2.4%	100	4	0.8%	1	0.2%	100
ALL SITES						1019	100.0%	1275	100.0%	100	509	100.0%	405	100.0%	100

[1] Includes salivary gland tumours

Table 4. Childhood cancer, Tanzania, Dar Es salaam (1990-1991)

	NUMBER OF CASES				M/F	REL. FREQ.(%)	RATES PER MILLION					
	0-4	5-9	10-14	All	M/F	Overall	0-4	5-9	10-14	Crude	ASR	%MV
Leukaemia	2	6	11	19	2.8	14.7	-	-	-	-	-	100.0
Acute lymphoid leukaemia	1	1	5	7	-	5.4	-	-	-	-	-	100.0
Lymphoma	10	38	10	58	1.5	45.0	-	-	-	-	-	100.0
Hodgkin disease	1	3	0	4	-	3.1	-	-	-	-	-	100.0
Burkitt lymphoma	6	23	2	31	0.9	24.0	-	-	-	-	-	100.0
Brain and spinal neoplasms	0	0	1	1	-	0.8	-	-	-	-	-	100.0
Neuroblastoma	2	1	1	4	3.0	3.1	-	-	-	-	-	100.0
Retinoblastoma	9	5	0	14	0.8	10.9	-	-	-	-	-	100.0
Wilms tumour	2	0	0	2	-	1.6	-	-	-	-	-	100.0
Bone tumours	0	0	3	3	0.5	2.3	-	-	-	-	-	100.0
Soft tissue sarcomas	2	2	2	6	2.0	4.7	-	-	-	-	-	100.0
Kaposi sarcoma	0	1	0	1	-	0.8	-	-	-	-	-	100.0
Germ cell tumours	0	0	0	0	-	-	-	-	-	-	-	-
Other	5	8	9	22	0.6	17.1	-	-	-	-	-	100.0
All	32	60	37	129	1.3	100.0	-	-	-	-	-	100.0

Table 5. Tanzania: childhood case series

Cancer	Shaba, 1988		Carneiro et al., 1998	
	No.	%	No.	%
Leukaemia	12	4.7%	85	4.5%
Acute lymphocytic leukaemia	4	1.6%		
Lymphoma	115	44.6%	728	38.8%
Burkitt lymphoma	53	20.5%	388	20.7%
Hodgkin disease	33	12.8%	126	6.7%
Brain and spinal neoplasms	1	0.4%	6	0.3%
Neuroblastoma	1	0.4%	31	1.7%
Retinoblastoma	26	10.1%	207	11.0%
Wilms tumour	15	5.8%	109	5.8%
Bone tumours	7	2.7%	32	1.7%
Soft-tissue sarcomas	51	19.8%	245	13.1%
Kaposi sarcoma	26	10.1%	90	4.8%
Other	30	11.6%	431	23.0%
Total	258	100.0%	1874	100.0%

The results are shown in Table 5. Lymphomas predominate in all these series, with about half the cases being Burkitt lymphomas.

References

Carneiro, P.M.R., Kalokola, F.M. & Kaaya, E.E. (1998) Paediatric malignancies in Tanzania. *E. Afr. Med. J.*, **75**, 533–535

Hiza, P.R. (1976) Malignant disease in Tanzania. *E. Afr. Med. J.*, **53**, 82–95

Kitinya, J.N., Lauren, P.A. & Kajembe, A.H. (1988a) Differential rates of carcinoma of cervix uteri among the chagga and pares of Kilimanjaro region, Tanzania. *Int. J. Gynaecol. Obstet.*, **27**, 395–399

Kitinya, J.N., Lauren, P.A., Jones, M.E. & Paljarvi, L. (1988b) Epidemiology of intestinal and diffuse types of gastric carcinoma in the Mount Kilimanjaro area, Tanzania. *Afr. J. Med. Sci.*, **17**, 89–95

Lauren, P. & Kitinya, J. (1986) Kilimanjaro Cancer Registry, 1975–1979. In: Parkin, D.M., ed., *Cancer Occurrence in Developing Countries* (IARC Scientific Publications No. 75), Lyon, IARC, pp. 108–110

Shaba, J. & Owor, R. (1986) Tanzania Cancer registry, 1980-1981. In: Parkin, D.M., ed., *Cancer Occurrence in Developing Countries* (IARC Scientific Publications No. 75), Lyon, IARC, pp. 107–108

Shaba J. (1988) Tanzania Cancer Registry, 1980–1981. In: Parkin, D.M., Stiller, C.A., Draper, G.J., Bieber, C.A., Terracini, B. & Young, J.L., eds, *International Incidence of Childhood Cancer* (IARC Scientific Publications No. 87), Lyon, IARC, pp. 49–51

3.4.15 Uganda

Background

Climate: Tropical; generally rainy with two dry seasons (December to February, June to August); semi-arid in north-east

Terrain: Mostly plateau with rim of mountains

Ethnic groups: Baganda 17%, Karamojong 12%, Basogo 8%, Iteso 8%, Langi 6%, Rwanda 6%, Bagisu 5%, Acholi 4%, Lugbara 4%, Bunyoro 3%, Batobo 3%, non-African (European, Asian, Arab) 1%, other 23%

Religions: Roman Catholic 33%, Protestant 33%, Muslim 16%, indigenous beliefs 18%

Economy—overview: Uganda has substantial natural resources, including fertile soils, regular rainfall and sizable mineral deposits of copper and cobalt. Agriculture is the most important sector of the economy, employing over 80% of the work force. Coffee is the major export crop and accounts for the bulk of export revenues.

Industries: The limited manufacturing industry is concentrated in a few towns and involved mainly in repacking of merchandise, sugar, brewing, tobacco, cotton textiles, cement

Agriculture—products: Coffee, tea, cotton, tobacco, cassava (tapioca), potatoes, corn, millet, pulses; beef, goat meat, milk, poultry

Cancer registration

Uganda has had well established cancer registration since the early 1950s. An account of the development of statistical data on cancer, since the early observations of Sir Albert Cook in 1901 to the early 1970s, is provided by Templeton and Hutt (1972).

Kampala Cancer Registry was established in 1954, in the Department of Pathology of Makerere University Medical School. The aim was to obtain information on cancer occurrence in the population of Kyadondo County, in which the capital city of Kampala is situated. The registry functioned continuously both before and after independence (1962), until the coup d'état of General Idi Amin Dada in 1971. Thereafter, full population coverage was not possible, although a register was maintained within the Department of Pathology until 1980, when all registration ceased. With the return of political stability, the registry restarted in 1989 and has functioned continuously since.

Initially, the registry used request/result forms of the Department of Pathology, redesigned specifically to permit registration of cancers. Thus, they contained demographic information on the patient, as well as the source of the specimen and the results of the examination. In addition to data collected in this way, tumour registrars have been employed to search for cancer cases admitted to, or treated in, the four main hospitals in Kampala (and, in recent years, the Uganda Hospice) and, for individuals resident in Kyadondo County, to extract somewhat more extensive information onto special notification forms.

Between 1954 and 1980, registration was manual, apart from the period 1964–68, when the data were transferred to punched cards (Templeton, 1973), which are no longer available in Uganda. The details of all patients were entered into a large register. Since 1989 the registration process has been computerized, using the CanReg system of IARC.

West Nile Cancer Registry was essentially a hospital cancer registry, based in Kuluva Hospital, in the West Nile District, in the far northwest of the country. The registry functioned between 1961 and 1978, and provided a basis for a variety of research studies on the epidemiology of Burkitt lymphoma.

Mbarara: Cancer registration for Mbarara district in the south-west of Uganda was initiated in 2000, based on the department of pathology in Mbarara University Teaching Hospital (MUTH). The registry depended upon case-finding by the pathologist, and was based upon cancers diagnosed in the department of pathology, but also those traced via the medical records department in MUTH and in several smaller hospitals in Mbarara and neighbouring districts, as well as Mbarara hospice. Data collection was retrospective, beginning in 1997.

Review of data

Reports of cancer in Uganda date back to end of 19th century, when the first missionary doctor established western medicine in Uganda. Davies *et al.* (1964) reviewed the hospital records of Mengo Hospital (in Kyadondo County) from 1897 to 1956. Although the frequency of different cancers was not available by sex, they noted that the general pattern of malignant diseases admitted to the hospital changed little during the period.

Kampala Cancer Registry

The most complete set of data comes from the Kampala Cancer Registry.

Registry data for the whole country were analysed by Templeton (1973) and published as a monograph. The focus was on the 6956 cases of cancer histologically diagnosed in the Department of Pathology during the years 1964–68, although 391 cases clinically diagnosed in the Kampala hospitals were also included. Because the observed incidence rates are markedly affected by differing referral/biopsy rates (Templeton & Bianchi, 1972), much of the analysis of regional and ethnic variation is based on proportions. These serve to suggest variations in the cancer patterns in different regions or ethnic groups, with, for example, relatively high frequencies of stomach cancer among Rwandans, penile cancer among the Bunyoro, bladder cancer among Baganda, and Burkitt lymphoma among the Lugbara.

Incidence rates for the population of Kyadondo County have been published for the periods 1954–60 (Davies *et al.*, 1962, 1965), 1968–70 (Templeton *et al.*, 1972), 1989–91 (Wabinga *et al.*, 1993) and 1991–93 (in Parkin *et al.*, 1997). In addition, frequency data, from the period when population coverage was incomplete (1971–80), were published by Owor (1986). The results presented in this monograph represent a recent five-year period, 1993–97 (Table 1). Table 2 shows the results for the period 1954–1960, as published in *Cancer Incidence in Five Continents*, Vol. I (Doll *et al.*, 1966). A complete review of the data set, for four time periods (1960–66, 1967–71, 1991–94, 1995–97) has been published by Wabinga *et al.* (2000). Table 3 shows the summary age-standardized incidence rates for the major sites, for the four different periods.

The most striking feature is the very high incidence of Kaposi sarcoma (KS), the most common cancer of men (41.3% cases), with an age-standardized incidence (ASR 37.7 per 100 000), about double that in women (20.5 per 100 000). These high rates reflect the effects of the epidemic of AIDS, Uganda being one of the first countries in Africa to have been affected, and incidence rates have been more or less stable throughout the 1990s (Parkin *et al.*, 1999). As seen in the earlier data reported here, KS has always been observed in the Ugandan population, although before the AIDS epidemic it was of the typical 'endemic' pattern, involving the skin,

Table 1. Uganda, Kyadondo County (1993-1997)

NUMBER OF CASES BY AGE GROUP AND SUMMARY RATES OF INCIDENCE - MALE

SITE	ALL AGES	AGE UNK	MV (%)	0-	15-	25-	35-	45-	55-	65+	CRUDE RATE	%	CR 64	ASR (W)	ICD (10th)
Mouth	23	2	91	-	1	2	7	6	2	3	0.8	1.1	0.14	2.1	C00-06
Salivary gland	4	0	75	-	-	-	2	2	-	1	0.1	0.2	0.01	0.3	C07-08
Nasopharynx	33	0	82	4	2	14	6	3	4	-	1.2	1.6	0.18	1.8	C11
Other pharynx	17	2	65	-	2	3	2	5	4	1	0.6	0.8	0.16	1.8	C09-10,C12-14
Oesophagus	106	2	40	-	2	7	14	34	19	28	3.8	5.2	0.82	13.3	C15
Stomach	57	1	51	2	2	6	7	10	11	18	2.0	2.8	0.39	7.2	C16
Colon, rectum and anus	68	2	59	-	3	9	13	10	9	22	2.4	3.3	0.39	8.0	C18-21
Liver	74	5	36	2	6	15	16	9	12	9	2.6	3.6	0.48	6.5	C22
Gallbladder etc.	0	0		-	-	-	-	-	-	-	0.0	0.0	0.00	0.0	C23-24
Pancreas	8	0	25	-	-	1	1	1	1	4	0.3	0.4	0.04	1.1	C25
Larynx	10	0	90	-	-	-	2	4	1	1	0.4	0.5	0.12	1.3	C32
Trachea, bronchus and lung	33	3	61	-	-	4	9	5	7	5	1.2	1.6	0.28	3.6	C33-34
Bone	24	0	67	5	8	4	1	3	1	2	0.9	1.2	0.08	1.4	C40-41
Melanoma of skin	11	0	91	-	1	-	1	6	-	3	0.4	0.5	0.06	1.3	C43
Other skin	32	0	81	3	1	3	2	9	4	10	1.1		0.19	3.8	C44
Mesothelioma	0	0		-	-	-	-	-	-	-	0.0	0.0	0.00	0.0	C45
Kaposi sarcoma	843	31	83	81	63	343	225	62	24	14	30.0	41.3	2.94	37.7	C46
Peripheral nerves	0	0		-	-	-	-	-	-	-	0.0	0.0	0.00	0.0	C47
Connective and soft tissue	35	3	91	7	4	3	10	4	2	2	1.2	1.7	0.16	2.2	C49
Breast	10	0	70	-	1	1	-	4	-	3	0.4	0.5	0.04	1.1	C50
Penis	34	2	76	-	1	4	6	6	1	14	1.2	1.7	0.12	4.1	C60
Prostate	215	20	77	-	-	-	1	17	40	135	7.6	10.5	1.19	38.6	C61
Testis	6	0	50	2	3	-	-	1	2	-	0.2	0.3	0.06	0.5	C62
Kidney	21	0	71	13	-	3	1	1	1	1	0.7	1.0	0.06	0.9	C64
Renal pelvis, ureter and other urinary	1	0	100	-	-	-	-	-	-	-	0.0	0.0	0.02	0.2	C65-66,C68
Bladder	17	0	53	-	-	-	3	2	3	11	0.6	0.8	0.09	2.9	C67
Eye	76	3	74	14	10	30	10	8	2	-	2.7	3.7	0.22	2.9	C69
Brain, nervous system	11	0	64	3	2	-	3	1	2	-	0.4	0.5	0.08	0.8	C70-72
Thyroid	6	1	100	1	-	2	-	-	2	-	0.2	0.3	0.06	0.6	C73
Hodgkin disease	18	0	94	5	3	4	1	2	1	2	0.6	0.9	0.06	1.1	C81
Non-Hodgkin lymphoma	141	0	79	84	16	13	14	9	1	4	5.0	6.9	0.33	5.7	C82-85,C96
Multiple myeloma	2	0	100	-	-	-	-	-	-	-	0.1	0.1	0.01	0.1	C90
Lymphoid leukaemia	6	0	33	3	2	1	-	-	-	-	0.2	0.3	0.01	0.2	C91
Myeloid leukaemia	8	0	50	4	-	3	1	-	-	-	0.3	0.4	0.02	0.2	C92-94
Leukaemia, unspecified	9	0	44	2	1	2	-	-	-	-	0.3	0.4	0.04	0.4	C95
Other and unspecified	115	10	69	11	9	14	15	19	15	22	4.1	5.6	0.67	11.2	O&U
All sites	2074	87	74	246	141	495	374	242	174	315	73.7		9.47	163.3	ALL
All sites but C44	2042	87	74	243	140	492	372	233	170	305	72.6	100.0	9.28	159.5	ALLbC44
Average annual population				228305	135021	112285	47364	22622	9270	7312					

Table 1. Uganda, Kyadondo County (1993-1997)

NUMBER OF CASES BY AGE GROUP AND SUMMARY RATES OF INCIDENCE - FEMALE

SITE	ALL AGES	AGE UNK	MV (%)	0-	15-	25-	35-	45-	55-	65+	CRUDE RATE	%	CR 64	ASR (W)	ICD (10th)
Mouth	16	0	81	-	-	2	2	5	2	5	0.6	0.7	0.11	1.8	C00-06
Salivary gland	9	0	56	-	-	1	3	1	2	1	0.3	0.4	0.07	0.8	C07-08
Nasopharynx	30	0	73	4	6	10	6	2	2	-	1.0	1.3	0.12	1.4	C11
Other pharynx	6	0	67	-	-	1	1	1	3	-	0.2	0.3	0.08	0.7	C09-10,C12-14
Oesophagus	91	0	42	-	-	2	11	18	20	40	3.1	4.1	0.68	12.1	C15
Stomach	47	2	45	-	1	3	6	14	15	6	1.6	2.1	0.51	5.6	C16
Colon, rectum and anus	61	1	67	-	4	5	8	14	12	17	2.1	2.7	0.47	7.0	C18-21
Liver	59	4	39	2	4	9	12	13	9	6	2.0	2.6	0.46	5.5	C22
Gallbladder etc.	1	0	0	-	-	-	-	1	-	-	0.0	0.0	0.01	0.1	C23-24
Pancreas	9	0	22	-	-	-	3	-	5	1	0.3	0.4	0.12	1.1	C25
Larynx	8	1	88	-	-	1	-	1	-	5	0.3	0.4	0.02	1.0	C32
Trachea, bronchus and lung	23	1	65	-	2	6	2	4	5	3	0.8	1.0	0.20	2.3	C33-34
Bone	16	0	63	5	6	1	2	-	-	2	0.6	0.7	0.03	0.7	C40-41
Melanoma of skin	13	0	62	-	-	-	-	1	5	7	0.4	0.6	0.12	2.0	C43
Other skin	12	1	75	-	-	6	-	2	1	2	0.4	0.5	0.07	1.0	C44
Mesothelioma	0	0	-	-	-	-	-	-	-	-	0.0	0.0	0.00	0.0	C45
Kaposi sarcoma	533	11	85	46	129	243	72	22	4	6	18.4	23.9	1.49	20.5	C46
Peripheral nerves	1	0	100	-	-	-	1	-	-	-	0.0	0.0	0.00	0.0	C47
Connective and soft tissue	46	2	85	7	4	13	5	9	3	3	1.6	2.1	0.24	3.1	C49
Breast	224	6	63	-	13	34	68	44	30	29	7.7	10.0	1.62	21.0	C50
Vulva	5	2	80	-	-	1	-	-	1	1	0.2	0.2	0.04	0.6	C51
Vagina	8	0	63	2	-	-	1	3	-	2	0.3	0.4	0.04	0.5	C52
Cervix uteri	465	13	64	-	15	102	146	99	47	43	16.1	20.9	3.26	40.7	C53
Uterus	48	2	83	-	5	4	7	17	9	4	1.7	2.2	0.46	5.1	C54-55
Ovary	75	1	55	3	7	15	19	11	10	9	2.6	3.4	0.50	6.4	C56
Placenta	16	1	75	-	7	4	1	3	-	-	0.6	0.7	0.07	0.8	C58
Kidney	17	0	76	7	2	2	2	3	-	1	0.6	0.8	0.10	1.1	C64
Renal pelvis, ureter and other urinary	5	0	60	-	-	1	2	1	-	1	0.2	0.2	0.03	0.4	C65-66,C68
Bladder	8	0	25	-	-	-	2	1	2	3	0.3	0.4	0.05	1.1	C67
Eye	64	1	58	9	12	25	11	4	2	-	2.2	2.9	0.23	2.8	C69
Brain, nervous system	6	0	100	1	1	-	2	2	-	-	0.2	0.3	0.03	0.4	C70-72
Thyroid	47	2	81	1	3	6	11	14	8	2	1.6	2.1	0.41	4.5	C73
Hodgkin disease	20	1	90	4	3	9	3	1	3	4	0.7	0.9	0.05	0.7	C81
Non-Hodgkin lymphoma	110	2	83	61	16	17	6	1	3	4	3.8	4.9	0.25	4.1	C82-85,C96
Multiple myeloma	9	0	22	-	-	-	1	3	2	3	0.3	0.4	0.08	1.2	C90
Lymphoid leukaemia	7	0	14	4	1	-	1	1	-	-	0.2	0.3	0.05	0.5	C91
Myeloid leukaemia	7	0	71	1	1	-	1	1	2	1	0.2	0.3	0.06	0.6	C92-94
Leukaemia, unspecified	10	0	10	4	3	-	1	1	-	2	0.3	0.4	0.02	0.5	C95
Other and unspecified	109	7	66	8	11	20	18	17	14	14	3.8	4.9	0.69	9.2	O&U
All sites	2241	60	69	169	258	543	436	331	224	220	77.4	100.0	12.83	169.0	ALL
All sites but C44	2229	59	69	169	258	537	436	329	223	218	77.0	100.0	12.76	168.0	ALLbC44
Average annual population				251703	158288	95571	35540	18232	9673	9771					

Table 2. Uganda, Kyadondo (1954-1960)

NUMBER OF CASES BY AGE GROUP AND SUMMARY RATES OF INCIDENCE - MALE

SITE	ALL AGES	AGE UNK	0-	15-	25-	35-	45-	55-	65+	CRUDE RATE	%	ASR (W)	ICD (10th)
Mouth	2	0	–	–	–	1	1	–	–	0.2	0.6	0.2	C00-C08
Nasopharynx	0	0	–	–	–	–	–	–	–	0.0	0.0	0.0	C11
Other pharynx	2	0	–	–	–	1	–	1	–	0.2	0.6	0.4	C09-C10,C12-C14
Oesophagus	8	0	–	–	1	–	4	3	–	1.0	2.5	1.8	C15
Stomach	13	0	–	–	3	3	4	3	–	1.6	4.0	2.3	C16
Colon, rectum and anus	5	0	–	–	–	2	1	1	1	0.6	1.5	1.4	C18-C21
Liver	46	0	–	3	17	12	10	1	3	5.6	14.2	6.3	C22
Pancreas	7	0	–	–	2	1	1	3	–	0.8	2.2	1.4	C25
Larynx	3	0	–	–	1	–	–	1	1	0.4	0.9	0.9	C32
Trachea, bronchus and lung	7	0	1	1	1	3	1	–	–	0.8	2.2	0.9	C33-C34
Melanoma of skin	6	0	–	1	–	–	1	2	2	0.7	1.8	1.5	C43
Other skin	40	0	–	4	9	10	8	5	4	4.9	12.3	6.7	C44
Kaposi sarcoma	–	–	–	–	–	–	–	–	–				C46
Breast	1	0	–	–	–	–	–	1	–	0.1	0.3	0.3	C50
Penis	31	0	–	1	2	7	10	6	5	3.8	9.5	6.6	C60
Prostate	16	0	–	–	–	–	6	5	5	1.9	4.9	4.5	C61
Kidney etc.	1	0	1	–	–	–	–	–	–	0.1	0.3	0.1	C64-C66,C68
Bladder	26	0	–	–	–	4	4	10	7	3.2	8.0	6.8	C67
Eye	8	0	2	2	1	1	2	–	–	1.0	2.5	1.0	C69
Brain, nervous system	2	0	1	–	1	–	–	–	–	0.2	0.6	0.2	C70-C72
Thyroid	1	0	–	–	1	–	–	–	–	0.1	0.3	0.1	C73
Hodgkin disease	13	0	2	2	6	1	–	1	1	1.6	4.0	1.5	C81
Non-Hodgkin lymphoma	24	1	6	6	3	3	4	1	–	2.9	7.4	3.2	C82-C85,C96
Multiple myeloma	2	0	–	–	–	–	–	1	1	0.2	0.6	0.5	C90
Leukaemia	19	0	4	7	2	2	3	1	–	2.3	5.8	2.5	C91-C95
Other and unspecified	42	0	8	4	8	5	8	5	4	5.1	12.9	7.1	O&U
All sites	325	1	25	31	59	56	68	51	34	39.4	100.0	58.1	ALL
All sites but C44	285	1	25	27	50	46	60	46	30	34.6	87.7	51.4	ALLbC44
Average annual population			33640	27120	28250	14490	7580	3830	2900				

Source: Cancer Incidence in Five Continents volume 1

Table 2. Uganda, Kyadondo (1954-1960)

NUMBER OF CASES BY AGE GROUP AND SUMMARY RATES OF INCIDENCE - FEMALE

SITE	ALL AGES	AGE UNK	0-	15-	25-	35-	45-	55-	65+	CRUDE RATE	%	ASR (W)	ICD (10th)
Mouth	8	0	-	1	1	4	1	1	-	1.3	2.7	1.8	C00-C08
Nasopharynx	0	0	-	-	-	-	-	-	-	0.0	0.0	0.0	C11
Other pharynx	1	0	-	-	-	-	-	-	1	0.2	0.3	0.5	C09-C10,C12-C14
Oesophagus	3	0	-	-	-	-	2	1	-	0.5	1.0	1.1	C15
Stomach	3	0	-	-	-	1	2	-	-	0.5	1.0	0.9	C16
Colon, rectum and anus	12	0	1	-	6	3	2	-	-	2.0	4.1	3.0	C18-C21
Liver	10	0	-	-	3	3	2	1	1	1.7	3.4	2.2	C22
Pancreas	4	0	-	-	1	1	1	1	-	0.7	1.4	1.0	C25
Larynx	0	0	-	-	-	-	-	-	-	0.0	0.0	0.0	C32
Trachea, bronchus and lung	0	0	-	-	-	-	-	-	-	0.0	0.0	0.0	C33-C34
Melanoma of skin	0	0	-	-	-	-	-	-	-	0.0	0.0	0.0	C43
Other skin	12	0	-	-	4	2	4	1	1	2.0	4.1	3.1	C44
Kaposi sarcoma			-	-	-	-	-	-	-				C46
Breast	32	1	-	-	8	7	7	7	2	5.3	10.9	8.8	C50
Cervix uteri	76	1	-	3	11	21	22	14	4	12.6	25.9	21.4	C53
Uterus	10	0	-	1	2	1	2	1	3	1.7	3.4	3.1	C54-C55
Ovary etc.	26	0	-	-	1	12	6	6	1	4.3	8.8	7.6	C56-C57
Kidney etc.	1	0	1	-	-	-	-	-	-	0.2	0.3	0.1	C64-C66,C68
Bladder	5	0	-	-	-	2	2	1	-	0.8	1.7	1.5	C67
Eye	6	0	-	-	1	3	1	-	1	1.0	2.0	1.6	C69
Brain, nervous system	1	0	-	-	-	-	1	-	-	0.2	0.3	0.2	C70-C72
Thyroid	10	0	-	2	1	2	3	2	-	1.7	3.4	2.6	C73
Hodgkin disease	4	0	-	1	2	1	-	-	-	0.7	1.4	0.7	C81
Non-Hodgkin lymphoma	12	0	7	-	-	1	1	1	2	2.0	4.1	2.9	C82-C85,C96
Multiple myeloma	0	0	-	-	-	-	-	-	-	0.0	0.0	0.0	C90
Leukaemia	12	0	3	1	1	2	2	-	3	2.0	4.1	3.2	C91-C95
Other and unspecified	46	0	3	9	7	10	9	6	2	7.6	15.6	10.9	O&U
All sites	294	2	15	18	49	73	72	44	21	48.7	100.0	78.1	ALL
All sites but C44	282	2	15	18	45	71	68	43	20	46.8	95.9	75.0	ALLbC44
Average annual population			31010	20360	17050	8210	4560	2880	2090				

Source: Cancer Incidence in Five Continents volume 1

Table 3. Incidence of the major cancers in Kyadondo County, Uganda, in four time periods

Site	1960–66			1967–71			1991–94			1995–97		
	No.	ASR	(standard error)	No.	ASR	(standard error)	No.	ASR	(standard error)	No.	ASR	(standard error)
Males												
Nasopharynx	3	0.3	(0.2)	9	1.8	(0.7)	11	0.7	(0.2)	26	2.3	(0.6)++
Oesophagus	8	1.7	(0.6)	25	5.1	(1.1)+++	83	15.8	(1.9)+++	68	13.0	(1.8)
Stomach	14	2.7	(0.8)	20	4.7	(1.1)	31	4.7	(1.0)	37	7.6	(1.4)
Colon/rectum	14	3.0	(0.8)	23	4.8	(1.1)	52	8.3	(1.3)+	38	6.8	(1.4)
Liver	44	6.0	(1.1)	75	11.7	(1.6)+++	73	9.8	(1.4)-	41	5.9	(1.2)-
Lung	5	0.8	(0.4)	10	2.1	(0.8)	25	4.1	(1.0)	19	3.2	(1.0)
Melanoma	1	0.1	(0.1)	8	1.3	(0.6)+	7	1.5	(0.7)	7	1.1	(0.5)
Skin	26	3.7	(0.8)	27	4.3	(0.9)	18	2.5	(0.7)--	20	4.1	(1.0)
Kaposi sarcoma	28	3.2	(0.7)	29	3.7	(0.8)	670	39.3	(2.1)+++	513	39.3	(2.3)
Prostate	13	3.1	(0.9)	27	6.8	(1.4)+	113	26.3	(2.6)+++	139	39.2	(3.7)+
Penis	29	5.5	(1.1)	30	6.3	(1.2)	18	2.9	(0.8)--	23	4.4	(1.1)
Bladder	24	5.2	(1.1)	27	5.9	(1.2)	13	2.5	(0.8)---	10	2.9	(0.9)
Eye	5	0.4	(0.2)	12	1.1	(0.4)	43	2.3	(0.4)+	47	3.0	(0.6)
Hodgkin disease	16	1.9	(0.6)	17	1.7	(0.5)	8	0.8	(0.4)---	11	1.3	(0.6)
Non-Hodgkin lymphoma	32	3.9	(0.8)	32	3.6	(0.7)	76	3.6	(0.5)	95	7.4	(1.1)++
Leukaemia	22	2.2	(0.6)	24	3.2	(0.9)	13	0.7	(0.2)---	16	1.1	(0.3)
ALL	352	54.2	(3.3)	478	81.2	(4.3)	1456	149.1	(5.2)	1290	166.6	(6.2)
ALL (except KS)	324	51.0		449	77.5		780	109.8		777	127.3	
Females												
Nasopharynx	3	0.7	(0.4)	2	0.3	(0.2)	13	0.9	(0.3)	21	1.6	(0.4)+
Oesophagus	9	2.6	(0.9)	31	7.9	(1.5)+++	55	9.4	(1.3)	63	14.2	(1.9)+
Stomach	4	0.8	(0.5)	14	3.4	(1.0)+	22	3.2	(0.7)	28	5.6	(1.1)
Colon/rectum	11	2.7	(0.9)	22	6.3	(1.5)+	36	5.7	(1.1)	34	6.6	(1.2)
Liver	9	1.8	(0.6)	21	5.0	(1.3)	42	5.1	(1.0)	35	6.3	(1.3)
Lung	3	0.6	(0.4)	6	1.4	(0.6)	7	0.7	(0.3)	18	3.2	(0.9)++
Melanoma	7	1.8	(0.7)	9	2.5	(0.8)	8	1.3	(0.5)	8	2.2	(0.8)
Skin	16	4.0	(1.1)	15	3.1	(0.9)	12	1.4	(0.5)-	8	1.0	(0.4)
Kaposi sarcoma	1	0.1	(0.1)	2	0.2	(0.1)	360	17.9	(1.2)+++	335	21.8	(1.5)
Breast	52	11.7	(1.8)	45	9.8	(1.6)	161	19.1	(1.8)+++	146	22.0	(2.1)
Cervix uteri	84	17.7	(2.2)	109	22.5	(2.5)	341	39.7	(2.5)+++	296	44.1	(3.0)
Corpus uteri	14	3.1	(0.9)	18	4.6	(1.3)	30	4.1	(0.9)	21	4.0	(0.9)
Ovary	26	5.7	(1.3)	19	3.2	(0.8)	62	6.9	(1.1)	41	5.3	(1.0)
Vulva/vagina	8	1.8	(0.7)	10	2.1	(0.8)	7	0.6	(0.3)	11	1.6	(0.6)
Eye	4	0.3	(0.2)	3	0.2	(0.1)	37	1.7	(0.4)+++	45	3.4	(0.7)+
Thyroid	5	1.3	(0.6)	12	3.0	(1.0)	22	2.6	(0.7)	34	5.6	(1.1)
Hodgkin disease	2	0.6	(0.5)	7	0.7	(0.3)	7	0.2	(0.1)	13	0.9	(0.3)
Non-Hodgkin lymphoma	14	2.2	(0.7)	15	2.2	(0.7)	48	2.1	(0.4)	82	5.7	(0.9)+++
Leukaemia	13	2.3	(0.7)	20	2.8	(0.7)	17	1.2	(0.4)---	17	1.9	(0.6)
ALL	338	73.0	(4.4)	469	98.9	(5.3)	1508	146.8	(4.8)	1421	179.7	(6.0)
ALL (except KS)	337	72.9		467	98.7		1148	128.9		1086	157.9	

Significant increase since preceding period: + p < 0.05; ++ p < 0.01; +++ p < 0.001

Significant decrease since preceding period: - p < 0.05; -- p < 0.05; --- p < 0.001

Source: Wabinga *et al.* (2000)

particularly the legs, and affecting principally males, with the risk rising progressively with age (Taylor *et al.*, 1971; Templeton, 1981). The results from the 1990s indicate an enormous increase in incidence of KS, together with the narrowing of the sex ratio (from 18:1 in 1960–71 to 1.7:1 in the 1990s). Ziegler and Katangole-Mbidde (1996) have drawn attention to the dramatic increase in the incidence of KS in children. The age-specific incidence of KS now corresponds closely to the age-specific reporting rates for AIDS, which are highest at ages 30–44 years for men and 25–34 years for women (Table 1). Current evidence suggests that human herpes virus 8 (HHV8) is the etiological agent responsible for KS (IARC, 1998). HHV8 has been identified in over 85% of KS tissue specimens in Uganda (Chang *et al.*, 1996). Seroprevalence studies suggest a relatively high prevalence of infection by HHV8 in the general population of Uganda – considerably higher than in the United States and Europe, which would be consistent with the elevated frequency of 'endemic' KS which preceded the AIDS epidemic (Gao *et al.*, 1996; Simpson *et al.*, 1996).

The incidence of oesophageal cancer is relatively high, and the rates in women are similar to those in men. This would seem to exclude tobacco and alcohol as major risk factors in this population. It is possible that the risk relates to some type of dietary deficiency. The other major cancers of the gastrointestinal tract – stomach and large bowel – have long been remarked to be relatively infrequent in Uganda (Hutt *et al.*, 1967; Burkitt, 1971). Templeton (1973) noted the very different relative frequency of stomach cancer in the different tribes, with the highest frequency among Rwandans, from the southwest of the country. The variation appears to be due to pyloric tumours, of intestinal-type histology. The rather higher incidence rates of gastric cancer in the more recent periods possibly reflect better diagnosis because of the availability of gastroscopy, although incidence remains low. This is not the result of a low prevalence of *Helicobacter pylori* since infection appears to be common, at least in the western part of Uganda (Wabinga, 1996).

The reported rates of liver cancer in Uganda are low in comparison with other parts of sub-Saharan Africa. The reasons for this are not clear. The prevalence of chronic carriage of hepatitis B in Uganda is similar to that in other countries, and aflatoxin contamination of foodstuffs appears to be common (Sebunya & Yourtee, 1990), though less perhaps in Kampala than in other parts of the country (Alpert *et al.*, 1971).

The incidence rate of cervix cancer in women is high, and the rates have increased markedly between the 1950s and 60s, and the 1990s. This increase is unlikely to be related to the epidemic of AIDS. It is possible that the social disruption of the Amin dictatorship and the subsequent civil wars (1972–86) favoured the spread of human papillomavirus (HPV), like other sexually transmitted diseases; HPV is present in the great majority of cervix cancers in Uganda, with HPV type 16 in 53% (Bosch *et al.*, 1995).

Non-Hodgkin lymphomas are relatively frequent. Burkitt lymphomas of childhood are responsible for about one third of the cases (see below). The incidence remained relatively stable in Kyadondo County until the early 1990s, but by 1995–97 there appeared to have been a significant increase in incidence in both males and females (Wabinga *et al.*, 2000). This may relate to improved survival of patients with HIV infection as other opportunistic infections are controlled, permitting a more prolonged duration of immunosuppression and the development of more clinically-evident lymphomas.

The absolute incidence of breast cancer is relatively low, but the incidence appears to have increased twofold since the 1960s. It is possible that some of the increase is related to declines in fertility.

The incidence of cancer of the prostate is one of the highest recorded in Africa. The rate has increased remarkably, from an ASR of 3–6 per 100 000 in the 1950s and 60s, to 40 per 100 000 in the late 1990s. Most of this increase is in elderly men, aged 65 years or over, although the actual rates are not exceptionally high compared with those reported in Europe and North America. The increase in Uganda is certainly not due to screening, although it is quite likely that increased awareness, a greater readiness to perform prostatectomy for urinary symptoms in elderly men, and histological examination of operative biopsies have played a role; the level of histological confirmation of diagnosis has certainly increased over time (Wabinga *et al.*, 2000).

The incidence of cancer of the penis is relatively high: the age-standardized rate is 4.1 per 100 000 in Kampala compared with 0.8 in the black population in the United States SEER registries (Parkin *et al.*, 1997). However, the rate is lower than in the 1960s. Penile cancer was clearly very frequent in the early case series from Kampala (Davies *et al.*, 1964) and Dodge *et al.* (1973) found it 'the commonest tumour registered in males' in 1964–68. In the 1964–68 registry data, there appears to have been considerable variation in the frequency of penile cancer between different tribes, with the highest percentages in the Bunyoro (41.4% cancers) and Toro (31.2%) from the west of the country (Dodge *et al.*, 1973). The decline in incidence since that time is probably real, since penile cancer is easily diagnosed and probably always brought for medical attention. Penile cancer has been related to genital hygiene (Kyalwazi, 1966) and the decline in incidence may be related to improved hygiene as a consequence of urbanization and greater availability of piped water supplies.

Bladder cancer incidence is also significantly lower in the 1990s than in the 1960s. In Uganda, bladder cancer has been linked to the presence of urethral stricture. Dodge (1964) found that 30% of bladder cancer cases had such strictures and Owor (1975) found 4% of patients with strictures developed bladder cancer. Since strictures are a sequel to gonococcal infection, it is possible that better treatment for sexually transmitted diseases may have reduced their prevalence. Kyadondo County is not an endemic area for *Schistosoma haematobium* (Bradley *et al.*, 1967).

Eye cancers are relatively frequent (3.7% in men, 2.9% in women). Although some are retinoblastomas, the majority are now squamous-cell carcinomas of the conjunctiva. The large increase in incidence of eye cancers is the consequence of increasing incidence of these conjunctival tumours, from 4/17 eye cancers (23.5%) in men in 1960–71 (none of the 7 eye cancers in women), to 32/45 (71% in men) and 34/40 (85%) in women in 1995–97 (Wabinga *et al.*, 2000). These cancers have been recognized for many years as more common in Africans than in Europeans, but there is also a considerable (tenfold or more) increase in risk in the presence of HIV infection, and Ateenyi-Agaba (1995) reported a large increase in the numbers of cases presenting clinically in Kampala since the onset of the AIDS epidemic.

Registration rates are particularly low for melanoma, tumours of the brain and nervous system, and leukaemias.

West Nile Cancer Registry
The results have been presented by Williams (1988). The full series, from 1961 to 1978 (Table 4) is dominated by the high frequency of non-Hodgkin lymphomas. The great majority of these are Burkitt lymphomas (78% of non-Hodgkin lymphomas in males, 74% in females), most of which (95%) are in children. The West Nile district is well known for the high incidence of Burkitt lymphomas (Wright, 1973) and was the location for several studies on space–time clustering of Burkitt lymphomas (see chapter on Lymphomas).

The frequency of liver cancer (21% in men, 8% in women) appears to be rather higher than in Kampala; Williams (1986) noted that a rather high percentage of cases had morphological diagnosis – 60% by histology and 21% cytology of needle aspirate.

There were 50 cases of endemic KS (12% cancers) in men, but only two in women. Templeton (1973) confirmed the relatively high

Table 4. Uganda: West Nile Cancer Registry 1961–78

Site	Kuluva Hospital, West Nile, 1961–78 (Williams, 1988)				%HV
	Male		Female		
	No.	%	No.	%	
Oral cavity[1]	1	0.2%	4	1.3%	
Nasopharynx	13	3.1%	7	2.3%	
Other pharynx					
Oesophagus	4	0.9%	2	0.7%	
Stomach	2	0.5%	0	0.0%	
Colon/rectum	1	0.2%	2	0.7%	
Liver	91	21.4%	23	7.7%	
Pancreas	0	0.0%	0	0.0%	
Lung	8	1.9%	1	0.3%	
Melanoma	0	0.0%	0	0.0%	
Other skin	31	7.3%	24	8.1%	
Kaposi sarcoma	50	11.8%	2	0.7%	
Breast	4	0.9%	31	10.4%	
Cervix uteri			40	13.4%	
Corpus uteri			3	1.0%	
Ovary etc.			13	4.4%	
Prostate	4	0.9%			
Penis	13	3.1%			
Bladder	2	0.5%	0	0.0%	
Kidney etc.	4	0.9%	5	1.7%	
Eye	12	2.8%	11	3.7%	
Brain, nervous system	1	0.2%	2	0.7%	
Thyroid	1	0.2%	0	0.0%	
Non-Hodgkin lymphoma	111	26.1%	82	27.5%	
Hodgkin disease	5	1.2%	2	0.7%	
Myeloma	0	0.0%	1	0.3%	
Leukaemia	23	5.4%	18	6.0%	
ALL SITES	425	100.0%	298	100.0%	

[1] Includes salivary gland

frequency of KS in biopsies from northwest Uganda. McHardy *et al.* (1984) reported on geographical and tribal distribution of the tumour in the West Nile.

Mbarara Cancer Registry

Table 5 shows details of the 811 cases recorded in the Mbarara Cancer Registry (for district residents) in the years 1997–2000. Rather less than half of the cases (41%) had histological confirmation of diagnosis. Oesophageal cancer and Kaposi sarcoma are the most common cancers of males (13.2%), although Kaposi sarcoma appears to be relatively less frequent than in the data from Kampala (Table 1). The frequency of stomach cancer (10.1% of cases) is rather higher than in Kampala. In females, cervix cancer (30.0%) and breast cancer (12.0%) both outnumber Kaposi sarcoma (6.1%). The virtual absence of haematological malignancies (only one case of leukaemia recorded) must reflect the deficient diagnostic facilities in this region.

Childhood cancer

Table 6 shows the incidence of childhood cancer in Kyadondo County population for the period 1993–97. Results from the registry have been published as frequencies of all registered cases for the periods 1952–58 (O'Conor & Davies, 1960), 1964–68 (Davies, 1973), and 1968–82 (Owor, 1988), and as incidence rates for the Kyadondo population for 1968–82 (Owor, 1988 IICC1) and for 1992–95 (Wabinga *et al.*,1998). Frequency data from Kuluva Hospital, in West Nile district, have also been published (Williams, 1988) (Table 7).

The incidence of Burkitt lymphoma of childhood has remained relatively high. Data from Kampala Cancer Registry for 1959–68 were used to estimate the incidence of Burkitt lymphoma in Mengo district and its constituent counties (Morrow *et al.*, 1976). The age-standardized incidence was 19.1 per million in boys (0 to 14 years) and 12.1 per million in girls; however, rates in Kyadondo County were lower than for Mengo district as a whole (crude rate ratio 0.57). Table 8 shows a comparison of incidence rates of childhood cancers in 1960–71 and in 1991–97 (from Wabinga *et al.*, 2000). For Burkitt lymphoma, it does seem that that the incidence has increased since the 1960s. Three explanations appear possible. The first is that, with the economic and social disruption in Uganda in the 1970s and early 1980s, the make-up of the population of Kyadondo County changed markedly, with a higher representation of individuals from areas with high risk of Burkitt lymphoma. Although the frequency of Burkitt lymphoma varies markedly throughout the country, with very high frequencies in the north and northwest (Schmauz *et al.*, 1990), this seems unlikely to have been a cause for the change in incidence in young children; since other (non-Burkitt) lymphomas are also much more common in these areas, the incidence of other non-Hodgkin lymphomas would also have increased (which, as stated, it did not). A second possibility relates to a change in the endemicity of malaria; Morrow *et al.* (1976) observed a fall in incidence in Mengo district during the late 1960s which they ascribed to the increasing use of chloroquine. There are no data on malaria endemicity in Uganda over the last 20 to 30 years, but it seems quite likely that there has been an increase in prevalence and severity of infection. Finally, the AIDS epidemic may be responsible. In the United States and Europe, non-Hodgkin lymphomas are the most common malignancies in paediatric AIDS patients and about one third are Burkitt lymphomas. However, in a study in Uganda, Parkin *et al.* (2000) found that there was no increase in the risk of endemic, EBV-positive Burkitt lymphoma in HIV-infected children. A probable explanation is the poor survival of children infected perinatally with HIV – only 34% of HIV-infected children in Kampala survive to the age of three years (Marum *et al.*, 1997).

The case series from Kuluva Hospital, in West Nile district (Table 7), demonstrates the exceptionally high frequency of Burkitt

lymphoma in this area at the time (1961–78). West Nile district was the focus of a considerable amount of research into patterns of space-time clustering and the relationship of incidence of Burkitt lymphoma to infection with the Epstein–Barr virus and malaria (see Chapter 4.10, Burkitt lymphoma)

References

Alpert, M.E., Hutt, M.S.R., Wogan, G.N. & Davidson, C.S. (1971) Association between aflatoxin content of food and hepatoma frequency in Uganda. *Cancer*, **28**, 253–260

Ateenyi-Agaba, C. (1995) Conjunctival squamous-cell carcinoma associated with HIV infection in Kampala, Uganda. *Lancet*, **345**, 695–696

Bosch, F.X., Manos, M.M., Munoz, N., Sherman, M., Jansen, A.M., Peto, J., Schiffman, M.H., Moreno, V., Kurman, R. & Shah, K.V. (1995) Prevalence of human papillomavirus in cervical cancer: a worldwide perspective. International biological study on cervical cancer (IBSCC) Study Group. *J. Natl Cancer Inst.*, **87**, 796–802

Bradley, D.J., Sturrock, R.F. & Williams, P.N. (1967) The circumstantial epidemiology of Schistosoma haematobium in Lango district, Uganda. *E. Afr. Med. J.*, **44**, 193–204

Burkitt, D.P. (1971) Epidemiology of cancer of the colon and rectum. *Cancer*, **28**, 3–13

Chang, Y., Ziegler, J., Wabinga, H., Katangole-Mbidde, E., Bashoff, C., Schultz, T., Whitby, D., Maddelena, D., Jaffe, H.W., Weiss, R.A., the Uganda Kaposi's Sarcoma Study Group, Moore, P.S. (1996) Kaposi's sarcoma-associated herpesvirus and Kaposi's sarcoma in Africa. *Arch. Int. Med.*, **156**, 202–204

Davies, J.N., Wilson, B.A. & Knowelden, J. (1962) Cancer incidence of the African population of Kyadondo (Uganda). *Lancet*, **2**, 328–330

Davies, J.N.P., Elmes, S., Hutt, M.S.R., Mtimavalye, L.A.R., Owor, R. & Shaper, L. (1964) Cancer in an African community, 1897-1956. *Br. Med. J.*, **1**, 259–264

Davies, J.N.P., Knowelden, J. & Wilson, B.A. (1965) Incidence rates of cancer in Kyondondo county, Uganda 1954-1960. *J. Natl Cancer Inst.*, **35**, 789–821

Dodge, O.G. (1964) Tumours of the bladder and urethra associated with urinary retention in Ugandan Africans. *Cancer*, **17**, 1433–1436

Dodge, O.G., Owor, R. & Templeton, A.C. (1973) Tumours of the male genitalia. In: Templeton, A.C., ed., *Tumours in a Tropical Country. Recent Results in Cancer Control*, No. 41, Berlin, Springer Verlag

Gao, S.J., Kingsley, L., Li, M., *et al.* (1996) KSHV antibodies among Americans, Italians and Ugandans with and without Kaposi's sarcoma. *Nature Med.*, **2**, 925–928

Hutt, M.S.R., Burkitt, D.P., Shepherd, J.J., Wright, B., Mati, J.K.G. & Auma, S. (1967) Malignant tumours of the gastrointestinal tract in Africans. *Natl Cancer Inst. Monogr.*, **25**, 41–48

IARC (1998) IARC *Monographs on the Evaluation of Carcinogenic Risks to Humans. Volume 70, Epstein-Barr Virus and Kaposi's Sarcoma Herpesvirus/Human Herpesvirus 8*, Lyon, IARC

Kyalwazi, S.K. (1966) Carcinoma of the penis. A review of 153 patients admitted to Mulago Hospital, Kampala, Uganda. *E. Afr. Med. J.*, **43**, 415–425

Marum, L.H., Tindyebwa, D. & Gibb, B. (1997) Care of children with HIV infection and AIDS in Africa. *AIDS*, **11** (Suppl. B), S125–S134

McHardy, J., Williams, E.H., Geser, A., de-The, G., Beth, E. & Giraldo, G. 1984 Endemic Kaposi's sarcoma: incidence and risk factors in the West Nile District of Uganda. *Int. J. Cancer*, **33**, 203–212

Morrow, P.H., Kisube, A., Pike, M.C. & Smith, P.G. (1976) Burkitt's lymphoma in Mengo districts in Uganda: epidemiologic features and their relationship to malaria. *J. Natl Cancer Inst.*, **56**, 479–483

Owor, R. (1975) Carcinoma of bladder and urethra in patients with urethral strictures. *E. Afr. Med. J.*, **52**, 12–18

Table 5. Uganda, Mbarara (1997-2000)

NUMBER OF CASES BY AGE GROUP - MALE

SITE	ICD (10th)	ALL AGES	AGE UNK	MV (%)	0-	15-	25-	35-	45-	55-	65+	%
Mouth	C00-06	14	0	79	-	-	-	1	2	4	7	4.4
Salivary gland	C07-08	4	0	50	-	-	1	2	1	-	-	1.3
Nasopharynx	C11	1	0	0	1	-	-	-	-	-	-	0.3
Other pharynx	C09-10,C12-14	3	0	33	-	-	1	-	-	-	2	0.9
Oesophagus	C15	42	0	24	-	1	4	4	10	14	13	13.2
Stomach	C16	32	0	28	2	1	4	4	4	8	9	10.1
Colon, rectum and anus	C18-21	9	0	33	1	-	1	-	2	2	3	2.8
Liver	C22	21	0	0	-	-	4	3	8	2	4	6.6
Gallbladder etc.	C23-24	1	0	0	-	-	-	-	-	-	1	0.3
Pancreas	C25	4	0	0	-	-	-	-	1	-	3	1.3
Larynx	C32	2	0	0	-	-	-	-	-	2	-	0.6
Trachea, bronchus and lung	C33-34	1	0	0	-	1	-	-	-	-	-	0.3
Bone	C40-41	12	0	42	2	7	-	3	-	-	-	3.8
Melanoma of skin	C43	1	0	100	-	-	-	-	1	-	-	0.3
Other skin	C44	7	0	71	-	1	2	2	-	2	-	2.2
Mesothelioma	C45	0	0	-	-	-	-	-	-	-	-	0.0
Kaposi sarcoma	C46	42	0	67	3	4	9	12	1	8	5	13.2
Peripheral nerves	C47	1	0	100	-	-	-	1	-	-	-	0.3
Connective and soft tissue	C49	7	0	71	3	-	-	1	2	-	1	2.2
Breast	C50	4	0	0	-	-	-	1	2	-	1	1.3
Penis	C60	7	0	57	1	1	-	1	-	1	3	2.2
Prostate	C61	28	0	46	1	-	1	1	1	7	17	8.8
Testis	C62	0	0	-	-	-	-	-	-	-	-	0.0
Kidney	C64	4	0	0	2	-	-	-	-	-	2	1.3
Renal pelvis, ureter and other urinary	C65-66,C68	0	0	0	-	-	-	-	-	-	-	0.0
Bladder	C67	2	0	0	-	1	-	-	-	-	1	0.6
Eye	C69	10	0	100	4	1	-	3	2	-	-	3.2
Brain, nervous system	C70-72	1	0	0	-	-	-	1	-	-	-	0.3
Thyroid	C73	1	0	100	-	-	-	-	-	1	-	0.3
Hodgkin disease	C81	2	0	100	-	-	1	1	-	-	-	0.6
Non-Hodgkin lymphoma	C82-85,C96	33	0	58	22	4	3	2	1	-	1	10.4
Multiple myeloma	C90	1	0	0	-	1	-	-	-	-	-	0.3
Lymphoid leukaemia	C91	0	0	-	-	-	-	-	-	-	-	0.0
Myeloid leukaemia	C92-94	0	0	-	-	-	-	-	-	-	-	0.0
Leukaemia, unspecified	C95	0	0	-	-	-	-	-	-	-	-	0.0
Other and unspecified	O&U	27	0	44	5	-	-	5	5	6	6	8.5
All sites	ALL	324	0	44	47	21	29	46	43	59	79	100.0
All sites but C44	ALLbC44	317	0	43	47	20	27	44	43	57	79	

Table 5. Uganda, Mbarara (1997-2000)

NUMBER OF CASES BY AGE GROUP - FEMALE

SITE	ICD (10th)	ALL AGES	AGE UNK	MV (%)	0-	15-	25-	35-	45-	55-	65+	%
Mouth	C00-06	3	0	33	-	-	-	1	1	-	1	0.6
Salivary gland	C07-08	2	0	100	-	-	1	-	1	-	-	0.4
Nasopharynx	C11	0	0	0	-	-	-	-	-	-	-	0.0
Other pharynx	C09-10,C12-14	1	0	0	-	-	-	-	-	-	1	0.2
Oesophagus	C15	10	0	20	1	-	1	1	3	2	2	2.1
Stomach	C16	25	0	24	1	-	1	4	5	6	8	5.3
Colon, rectum and anus	C18-21	20	0	35	-	1	1	2	3	8	5	4.2
Liver	C22	20	0	10	1	1	2	2	3	9	2	4.2
Gallbladder etc.	C23-24	1	0	100	-	-	-	-	-	1	-	0.2
Pancreas	C25	0	0	-	-	-	-	-	-	-	-	0.0
Larynx	C32	0	0	-	-	-	-	-	-	-	-	0.0
Trachea, bronchus and lung	C33-34	0	0	-	-	-	-	-	-	-	-	0.0
Bone	C40-41	2	0	50	1	1	-	-	-	-	-	0.4
Melanoma of skin	C43	3	0	67	1	-	-	1	-	-	1	0.6
Other skin	C44	11	0	91	1	1	2	1	3	-	3	2.3
Mesothelioma	C45	0	0	-	-	-	-	-	-	-	-	0.0
Kaposi sarcoma	C46	29	0	59	2	6	16	4	-	1	-	6.1
Peripheral nerves	C47	0	0	-	-	-	-	-	-	-	-	0.0
Connective and soft tissue	C49	10	0	60	2	3	1	1	-	1	2	2.1
Breast	C50	57	0	40	3	4	8	13	15	7	7	12.0
Vulva	C51	3	0	0	-	1	-	-	2	-	-	0.6
Vagina	C52	3	0	0	-	-	-	1	-	1	1	0.6
Cervix uteri	C53	143	1	41	3	5	8	41	41	34	10	30.0
Uterus	C54-55	12	0	67	-	-	2	4	1	4	-	2.5
Ovary	C56	41	0	10	4	8	10	10	5	2	2	8.6
Placenta	C58	3	0	100	-	1	1	-	1	-	-	0.6
Kidney	C64	6	0	83	5	-	-	1	-	-	-	1.3
Renal pelvis, ureter and other urinary	C65-66,C68	0	0	-	-	-	-	-	-	-	-	0.0
Bladder	C67	0	0	-	-	-	-	-	-	-	-	0.0
Eye	C69	12	0	83	5	3	4	-	-	-	-	2.5
Brain, nervous system	C70-72	1	0	0	-	-	-	-	1	-	-	0.2
Thyroid	C73	2	0	50	-	1	-	-	1	-	-	0.4
Hodgkin disease	C81	0	0	-	-	-	-	-	-	-	-	0.0
Non-Hodgkin lymphoma	C82-85,C96	25	0	64	13	5	3	2	-	-	2	5.3
Multiple myeloma	C90	0	0	-	-	-	-	-	-	-	-	0.0
Lymphoid leukaemia	C91	1	0	0	-	1	-	-	-	-	-	0.2
Myeloid leukaemia	C92-94	0	0	-	-	-	-	-	-	-	-	0.0
Leukaemia, unspecified	C95	0	0	-	-	-	-	-	-	-	-	0.0
Other and unspecified	O&U	41	0	24	7	4	4	7	7	5	7	8.6
All sites	ALL	487	1	40	50	48	64	95	92	81	56	100.0
All sites but C44	ALLbC44	476	1	39	49	47	62	94	89	81	53	

Table 6. Childhood cancer, Uganda, Kyadondo County (1993-1997)

	NUMBER OF CASES					REL. FREQ.(%)	RATES PER MILLION					
	0-4	5-9	10-14	All	M/F	Overall	0-4	5-9	10-14	Crude	ASR	%MV
Leukaemia	2	8	8	18	1.0	4.3	2.0	11.4	11.9	7.5	7.9	33.3
Acute lymphoid leukaemia	1	2	3	6	0.5	1.4	1.0	2.8	4.5	2.5	2.6	-
Lymphoma	53	63	38	154	1.4	37.1	51.8	89.7	56.4	64.2	65.3	85.5
Hodgkin disease	4	4	1	9	1.3	2.2	3.9	5.7	1.5	3.7	3.8	88.9
Burkitt lymphoma	30	38	22	90	1.4	21.7	29.3	54.1	32.7	37.5	38.3	78.9
Brain and spinal neoplasms	0	3	1	4	3.0	1.0	-	4.3	1.5	1.7	1.8	50.0
Neuroblastoma	0	0	0	0	-	-	-	-	-	-	-	-
Retinoblastoma	18	1	1	20	1.5	4.8	17.6	1.4	1.5	8.3	7.7	65.0
Wilms tumour	13	3	2	18	2.0	4.3	12.7	4.3	3.0	7.5	7.2	94.4
Bone tumours	2	2	6	10	1.0	2.4	2.0	2.8	8.9	4.2	4.3	60.0
Soft tissue sarcomas	66	48	27	141	1.7	34.0	64.4	68.3	40.1	58.7	58.6	100.0
Kaposi sarcoma	62	45	20	127	1.8	30.6	60.5	64.0	29.7	52.9	52.7	92.1
Germ cell tumours	1	2	0	3	0.5	0.7	1.0	2.8	-	1.2	1.3	100.0
Other	15	13	19	47	1.4	11.3	14.6	18.5	28.2	19.6	19.8	61.7
All	170	143	102	415	1.5	100.0	166.0	203.5	151.5	172.9	173.9	79.8

Table 7. Uganda, West Nile: childhood cancers, 1961–78

Cancer	West Nile 1961–78 (Williams, 1988)	
	No.	%
Leukaemia	8	3.9%
Acute lymphocytic leukaemia	0	0.0%
Lymphoma	155	75.6%
Burkitt lymphoma	140	68.3%
Hodgkin disease	1	0.5%
Brain and spinal neoplasms	0	0.0%
Neuroblastoma	0	0.0%
Retinoblastoma	12	5.9%
Wilms tumour	9	4.4%
Bone tumours	2	1.0%
Soft-tissue sarcomas	6	2.9%
Kaposi sarcoma	1	0.5%
Other	13	6.3%
Total	205	100.0%

Table 8. Uganda, Kyadondo county: childhood cancer (age 0–14 years), 1960–71 and 1991–97

Cancer	1960–71				1991–97			
	No.	(%)	M:F	Age-stand. rate (per 10^6)	No.	(%)	M:F	Age-stand. rate (per 10^6)
Leukaemia	25	(18.4)	1.1	18.7	27	(4.9)	0.7	8.6
Hodgkin disease	11	(8.1)	2.7	8.7	9	(1.6)	1.3	2.8
Burkitt lymphoma	13	(9.6)	1.6	9.5	109	(19.7)	1.5	34.3
Other non-hodgkin lymphoma*	18	(13.4)	2.6	13.1	61	(11.1)	1.3	19.1
Brain & central nervous system	4	(2.9)	0.3	3.0	7	(1.3)	2.5	2.3
Neuroblastoma	5	(3.7)	1.5	2.9	1	(0.2)	-	0.3
Retinoblastoma	16	(11.8)	1.7	9.4	33	(6.0)	1.4	9.3
Wilms tumour	10	(7.4)	0.7	6.1	29	(5.3)	1.6	8.6
Osteosarcoma	5	(3.7)	1.5	4.2	6	(1.1)	4.0	1.9
Kaposi sarcoma	3	(2.2)	2.0	2.5	183	(33.2)	1.5	55.8
Other soft-tissue sarcoma	10	(7.4)	4.0	7.6	20	(3.6)	0.8	6.0
Carcinomas	9	(6.7)	2.0	7.4	18	(3.3)	1.3	5.7
Total	136	(100.0)	1.6	97.8	552	(100.0)	1.4	169.7

Owor, R. (1986) Kampala Cancer Registry, 1971-1980. In: Parkin, D.M., ed., *Cancer Occurrence in Developing Countries* (IARC Scientific Publications No. 75), Lyon, IARC, pp. 97–99

Owor, R. (1988) Kampala Cancer Registry, 1980–1981. In: Parkin, D.M., Stiller, C.A., Draper, G.J., Bieber, C.A., Terracini, B. & Young, J.L., eds, *International Incidence of Childhood Cancer* (IARC Scientific Publications No. 87), Lyon, IARC, pp. 57–61

Parkin, D.M., Whelan, S.L., Ferlay, J., Raymond, L. & Young, J., eds (1997) *Cancer Incidence in Five Continents,* Vol. VII (IARC Scientific Publications No. 143), Lyon, IARC

Parkin, D.M., Wabinga, H.R., Nambooze, S. & Wabwire-Mangen, F. (1999) AIDS-related cancers in Africa: maturation of the epidemic in Uganda. *AIDS*, **13**, 2563–2570

Parkin, D.M., Garcia-Giannoli, H., Raphaël, M., Martin, A., Katangole-Mbidde, E., Wabinga, H. & Ziegler, J. (2000) Non-Hodgkin lymphoma in Uganda: a case-control study. *AIDS*, **14**, 2929–2936

Schmauz, R., Mugerwa, J.W. & Wright, D.H. (1990) The distribution of non-Burkitt, non Hodgkin's lymphomas in Uganda in relation to malarial endemicity. *Int. J. Cancer*, **47**, 650–653

Sebunya, T.K. & Yourtee, D.M. (1990) Aflatoxigenic Aspergilli in foods and feeds in Uganda. *J. Food Quality*, **13**, 97–197

Simpson, G.R., Schulz, T.F., Whitby, D., Cook, P.M., Boshoff, C., Rainbow, L., Howard, M.R., Gao, S.J., Bohenzky, R.A., Simmonds, P., Lee, C., de Ruiter, A., Hatzakis, A., Tedder, R.S., Weller, I.V., Weiss, R.A. & Moore, P.S. (1996) Prevalence of Kaposi's sarcoma associated herpesvirus infection measured by antibodies to recombinant capsid protein and latent immunofluorescence antigen. *Lancet*, **348**, 1133–1138

Taylor, J.F., Templeton, A.C., Vogel, C.L., Ziegler, J.L. & Kyalwazi, S.K. (1971) Kaposi's sarcoma in Uganda: a clinico-pathological study. *Int. J. Cancer*, **8**, 122–135

Templeton, A.C., ed. (1973) *Tumours in a Tropical Country. Recent Results in Cancer Research* No. 41. Berlin, Springer Verlag

Templeton, A.C. (1981) Kaposi's sarcoma. *Pathol. Ann.*, **16**, 315–336

Templeton, A.C. & Bianchi A (1972) Bias in an African cancer registry. *Int. J. Cancer*, **10**, 186–193

Templeton, A.C. & Hutt, M.S.R. (1973) Introduction: Distribution of tumours in Uganda. In: Templeton, A.C., ed., *Tumours in a Tropical Country. Recent Results in Cancer Research* No. 41. Berlin, Springer Verlag

Templeton, A.C., Buxton, E. & Bianchi, A. (1972) Cancer in Kyadondo County, Uganda, 1968-1970. *J. Natl Cancer Inst.*, **48**, 865–874

Wabinga, H.R. (1996) Frequency of Helicobacter pylori in gastroscopic biopsy of Ugandan Africans. *E. Afr. Med. J.*, **73**, 691–693

Wabinga, H.R., Parkin, D.M., Wabwire-Mangen, F. & Mugerwa, J.W. (1993) Cancer in Kampala, Uganda, in 1989-91: changes in incidence in the era of AIDS. *Int. J. Cancer*, **54**, 26–36

Wabinga, H.R., Owor, R. & Nambooze, S. (1998) Kampala Cancer Registry 1992–1995. In: Parkin, D.M., Kramárová, E., Draper, G.J., Masuyer, E., Michaelis, J., Neglia, J, Qureshi, S. & Stiller, C.A., eds, *International Incidence of Childhood Cancer, vol. II* (IARC Scientific Publications No. 144), Lyon, IARC, pp. 31–34

Wabinga, H.R., Parkin, D.M., Wabwire-Mangen, F. & Nambooze, S. (2000) Trends in cancer incidence in Kyadondo County, Uganda, 1960-1997. *Br. J. Cancer*, **82**, 1585–1592

Williams, E.H. (1968) Variations in tumour distribution in the West Nile district of Uganda. In: Clifford, P., Linsell, C.A. & Timms, G.L., eds, *Cancer in Africa*, Nairobi, East African Publishing House, pp. 37–42

Williams, E.H. (1986) Kuluva Hospital, West Nile District, 1961-1978. In: Parkin, D.M., ed., Cancer Occurrence in Developing Countries (IARC Scientific Publications No. 75), Lyon, IARC, p. 100

Williams, E.H. (1988) Kuluva Hospital, West Nile District, 1961-1978. In: Parkin, D.M., Stiller, C.A., Draper, G.J., Bieber, C.A., Terracini, B. & Young, J.L., eds, *International Incidence of Childhood Cancer* (IARC Scientific Publications No. 87), Lyon, IARC, pp. 63–69

Wright, D.H. (1973) Lympho-reticular neoplasms. In: Templeton, A.C., ed., *Tumours in a Tropical Country. Recent Results in Cancer Research* No. 41. Berlin, Springer Verlag, pp. 270–291

Ziegler, J.L. & Katangole-Mbidde, E. (1996) Kaposi's sarcoma in childhood: an analysis of 100 cases from Uganda and relationship to HIV infection. *Int. J. Cancer*, **65**, 200–203

3.4.16 Zambia

Background

Climate: Tropical; modified by altitude; rainy season (October to April)

Terrain: Mostly high plateau with some hills and mountains, the lowest point being the Zambezi river at 329 m and the highest 2301 m.

Ethnic groups: African 98.7%, European 1.1%, other 0.2%

Religions: Christian 50–75%, Muslim and Hindu 24–49%, indigenous beliefs 1%

Economy—overview: Zambia is rich in copper, cobalt, zinc, lead, coal, emeralds, gold, silver and uranium. Agriculture contributes 23%, industry 40% and services 37% of the GDP. However, in 1993, 86% of the population was estimated to live below the poverty line. Zambia's copper mining sector accounts for over 80% of the nation's foreign currency. The main exports are copper, cobalt, zinc, lead and tobacco.

Industries: Copper mining and processing, construction, foodstuffs, beverages, chemicals, textiles, fertilizers

Agriculture—products: Corn, sorghum, rice, peanuts, sunflower seed, tobacco, cotton, sugarcane, cassava (tapioca); cattle, goats, pigs, poultry, beef, pork, poultry meat, milk, eggs, hides

Cancer registration

The Zambian National Cancer Registry, based in the Department of Community Health of the School of Medicine in Lusaka, operated for several years after its inception in November 1981. The registry relied upon voluntary notification of cases of cancer treated in all of the hospitals in Zambia, using a special notification form. The extent to which cancer patients were notified by different hospitals varied enormously, and registration was certainly very incomplete. Additional information on cancer cases was collected from records of cases of cancer diagnosed at the pathology laboratory of Lusaka, which handles specimens from all over the country, apart from hospitals in or near the Copperbelt region.

Review of data

Watts (1986) presented a report for 1981–83 from the National Cancer Registry for both sexes (see Table 1). 1250 malignant tumours (excluding carcinoma *in situ*) were registered; 64% of cases in males and 61% in females had histological verification of diagnosis.

Carcinoma of the cervix was by far the most commonly encountered cancer – 38% of all cancers in females – while breast cancer was second in importance in females, followed by cancers of the bladder, stomach and liver.

In males, primary cancer of the liver (16.4% of cases) was the most frequent cancer. Bladder cancer (8.2%) was also common; the majority were squamous-cell carcinomas, presumably related to schistosomiasis, which is endemic in Zambia, particularly in the east. Prostate cancer was third in frequency in males, followed by connective-tissue tumours, the majority of which were Kaposi

sarcoma, predominantly in young males (90% of cases were in males, of whom 70% were under 45 years of age) and mainly lesions of the lower limbs. Cancer of the penis accounted for 5.2% of cancers in men (in a pathology series from University Department of Pathology in 1970–74 (Naik, 1977), it accounted for 3%).

Non-Hodgkin lymphomas were about twice as frequent in males as in females, accounting for 6.2% of tumours in males; about one third were Burkitt lymphomas, which occur almost exclusively in children. Similar findings were reported from the pathology series (Naik & Bhagwandeen, 1977).

Patil *et al.* (1995) reviewed the pattern of cancers seen at the University Teaching Hospital histopathology laboratory between 1980 and 1989 (see Table 1). Kaposi sarcoma appears to have increased in relative frequency from about 2% of all cancers in the National Cancer Registry reports (Watts, 1986) to about 7% of all cancers in the histopathology data. Given that these data-sets overlap considerably, it is likely that the proportion of cases of Kaposi sarcoma was much higher in the later period.

Table 1 also shows the relative frequency of different cancers diagnosed in the pathology department of the hospital in Ndola, in north-central Zambia, during 1976–1979 (O'Riordan, 1986).

Childhood cancer

Two reports of the frequency of paediatric malignancies treated in the University Teaching Hospital have been published (Table 2). Patil *et al.* (1992) presented data on 525 cases diagnosed by histology, autopsy and haematology in 1980–89 (the estimated incidence rates are incorrect by a factor of 10). Chintu *et al.* (1995) compared the histopathologically diagnosed cases from 1980–82 (114 cases) and 1990–92 (200 cases), with a view to estimating the influence of the AIDS epidemic on the profile of childhood cancer. The frequency of Kaposi sarcoma increased from 2.6% of childhood cancers in 1980–82 to 19.5% in 1990–92, while the frequency of Burkitt lymphoma declined (15.8% to 5.5%).

References

Chintu, C., Athale, U.H. & Patil, P.S. (1995) Childhood cancers in Zambia before and after the HIV epidemic. *Arch. Dis. Child.*, **73**, 100–105

Naik, K.G (1977) Pattern of tumors of the male genitalia in Zambia. *Int. Surg.*, **62**, 356–357

Naik, K.G. & Bhagwandeen, S.B. (1977) Pattern of lymphomas in Zambia. *E. Afr. med. J.*, **54**, 491–496

O'Riordan, E.C. (1986) Department of Pathology, Ndola Central Hospital 1976-1979. In: Parkin, D.M., ed., Cancer Occurrence in Developing Countries (IARC Scientific Publications No. 75), Lyon, IARC, pp. 118–123

Patil, P., Elem, B., Gwavava, N.J.T. & Urban, M.I. (1992) Pattern of paediatric malignancy in Zambia (1980-1989): a hospital-based histopathological study. *J. Trop. Med. Hyg.*, **95**, 124–127

Patil, P., Elem, B. & Zumla, A. (1995) Pattern of adult malignancies in Zambia (1980-1989) in light of the human immunodeficiency virus type 1 epidemic. *J. Trop. Med. Hyg.*, **98**, 281–284

Watts, T. (1986b) Zambia: The cancer registry of Zambia, Lusaka, November 1981-May 1983. In: Parkin, D.M., ed., *Cancer Occurrence in Developing Countries* (IARC Scientific Publications No. 75), Lyon, IARC, pp. 117–121

Table 1. Zambia: case series

Site	Cancer Registry of Zambia 1981–83 (Watts, 1986)					Ndola, Dept, Pathology, 1976–79 (O'Riordan, 1986)					University Teaching Hospital, pathology data, 1980–89 (Patil et al., 1995)		
	Male		Female		%HV	Male		Female		%HV	Both sexes		%HV
	No.	%	No.	%		No.	%	No.	%		No.	%	
Oral cavity[1]	18	3.0%	2	0.3%		5	1.6%	1	0.3%	100	73	0.9%	100
Nasopharynx	2	0.3%	1	0.2%		0	0.0%	0	0.0%				
Other pharynx	2	0.3%	0	0.0%		1	0.3%	2	0.6%				
Oesophagus	30	5.0%	9	1.4%		13	4.1%	3	0.8%	100	205	2.6%	100
Stomach	30	5.0%	32	4.9%		9	2.8%	5	1.4%	100	202	2.6%	100
Colon/rectum	23	3.8%	14	2.1%		21	6.6%	4	1.1%	100	204	2.6%	100
Liver	98	16.4%	30	4.6%		32	10.0%	11	3.1%	100	452	5.8%	100
Pancreas	8	1.3%	6	0.9%		1	0.3%	0	0.0%	100		0.0%	100
Lung	31	5.2%	6	0.9%		1	0.3%	0	0.0%	100	91	1.2%	100
Melanoma	9	1.5%	11	1.7%		11	3.4%	10	2.8%	100	206	2.6%	100
Other skin	30	5.0%	32	4.9%		46	14.4%	10	2.8%	100	521	6.6%	100
Kaposi sarcoma	26	4.3%	3	0.5%		10	3.1%	0	0.0%	100	548	7.0%	100
Breast	2	0.3%	58	8.9%		4	1.3%	33	9.3%	100	347	4.4%	100
Cervix uteri			248	38.0%				141	39.8%	100	1533	19.6%	100
Corpus uteri			16	2.5%				11	3.1%	100	115	1.5%	100
Ovary etc.			18	2.8%				10	2.8%	100	86	1.1%	100
Prostate	48	8.0%		0.0%		0	0.0%			100	264	3.4%	100
Penis	31	5.2%		0.0%		0	0.0%			100	169	2.2%	100
Bladder	49	8.2%	42	6.4%		34	10.6%	17	4.8%	100	491	6.3%	100
Kidney etc.	9	1.5%	3	0.5%		5	1.6%	5	1.4%	100			100
Eye	12	2.0%	5	0.8%		8	2.5%	2	0.6%	100	165	2.1%	100
Brain, nervous system	1	0.2%	1	0.2%			0.0%	1	0.3%	100		0.0%	100
Thyroid	2	0.3%	7	1.1%		1	0.3%	7	2.0%	100		0.0%	100
Non-Hodgkin lymphoma	37	6.2%	19	2.9%		34	10.6%	11	3.1%	100	290	3.7%	100
Hodgkin disease	11	1.8%	3	0.5%		12	3.8%	2	0.6%	100	69	0.9%	100
Myeloma	3	0.5%	3	0.5%		1	0.3%	2	0.6%	100			100
Leukaemia	5	0.8%	13	2.0%		3	0.9%	0	0.0%	100			100
ALL SITES	598	100.0%	652	100.0%	63%	320	100.0%	354	100.0%	100	7836	100.0%	100

[1] Includes salivary gland

Table 2. Zambia: childhood case series

Cancer	1980–89 (Patil *et al.*, 1992)		1980–82 (Chintu *et al.*, 1995)		1990–92 (Chintu *et al.*, 1995)	
	No.	%	No.	%	No.	%
Leukaemia	42	8.0%	0	0.0%	0	0.0%
Acute lymphocytic leukaemia	21	4.0%				
Lymphoma	196	37.3%	48	42.1%	65	32.5%
Burkitt lymphoma	73	13.9%	18	15.8%	11	5.5%
Hodgkin disease	31	5.9%	6	5.3%	10	5.0%
Brain and spinal neoplasms	3	0.6%	0	0.0%	0	0.0%
Neuroblastoma	7	1.3%	0	0.0%	1	0.5%
Retinoblastoma	60	11.4%	7	6.1%	37	18.5%
Wilms tumour	31	5.9%	8	7.0%	24	12.0%
Bone tumours	16	3.0%				
Soft-tissue sarcomas	76	14.5%	17	14.9%	58	29.0%
Kaposi sarcoma	31	5.9%	3	2.6%	39	19.5%
Other	94	17.9%	34	29.8%	15	7.5%
Total	525	100.0%	114	100.0%	200	100.0%

3.4.17 Zimbabwe

Background

Climate: Tropical; moderated by altitude; rainy season (November to March)

Terrain: Mostly high plateau with higher central plateau (high veld); mountains in east

Ethnic groups: African 98% (Shona 71%, Ndebele 16%, other 11%), white 1%, mixed and Asian 1%

Religions: Syncretic (part Christian, part indigenous beliefs) 50%, Christian 25%, indigenous beliefs 24%, Muslim and other 1%

Economy—overview: Agriculture employs 27% of the labour force of this landlocked nation and supplies almost 25% of exports. Mining accounts for only 5% of both GDP and employment, but minerals and metals account for about 20% of exports. The country faces many economic problems. The annual inflation rate rose from 32% in 1998 to 59% in 1999. About 60% of the population lives below the poverty line.

In 1994, Zimbabwe ranked as the world's sixth largest producer of tobacco and the third largest exporter.

Industries: Mining (coal, clay, numerous metallic ores (chromium, gold, nickel, copper, iron, vanadium, lithium, tin and platinum) and chrysotile asbestos), copper, steel, nickel, tin, wood products, cement, chemicals, fertilizer, clothing and footwear, foodstuffs, beverages

Agriculture—products: corn, cotton, tobacco, wheat, coffee, sugarcane, peanuts; cattle, sheep, goats, pigs

Cancer registration

Following several reports of hospital and laboratory series, a population-based registry was established in Bulawayo in 1963, which functioned for 15 years. The Zimbabwe National Cancer Registry, established in 1985, covers the population of the city of Harare, and has continued until the present.

Bulawayo Cancer Registry

The cancer registry of Bulawayo was founded in 1963 and functioned for 15 years. It was located in the Mpilo Central Hospital which, in addition to providing the only hospital service to the black African population of the city of Bulawayo, also acted as the referral centre for cancer cases from the south-western part of Zimbabwe (until 1980, Rhodesia), including the provinces of Matabeleland (North and South), Masvingo (formerly Victoria) and Midlands. New cases of cancer were notified from all hospital wards and departments; case notes with a diagnosis of cancer or suspected cancer were sent to the registry on discharge or death. Copies of all histology and autopsy reports mentioning cancer were scrutinized monthly by the registrar. Since death certification before burial was mandatory in the city of Bulawayo, persons who died outside hospital were brought for autopsy before certification. This, together with the very high autopsy rate within the hospital, meant that, for the great majority of cases registered, histological information of diagnosis was available. An attempt was made to interview all cases notified; if the individuals themselves could not be questioned, the relatives were interviewed.

Zimbabwe National Cancer Registry

The Zimbabwe National Cancer Registry, established in 1985 as a result of a collaborative agreement between the Zimbabwean Ministry of Health and the International Agency for Research on Cancer, began operations in Harare in 1986. Acceptably complete coverage of the population of the city of Harare was achieved in 1990.

The Registry is situated in the Parirenyatwa Central Hospital complex, which provides most of the specialized cancer-management services for the northern part of the country and is the teaching hospital of the University of Zimbabwe School of Medicine. Registry staff make weekly visits to the inpatient wards and oncology outpatient clinics of the two government-referral hospitals (Harare and Parirenyatwa). In addition, they periodically collect information from: (i) medical records of discharged and deceased cancer patients, (ii) copies of histology reports of cancer patients from public and private histology laboratories, (iii) death certificates of cancer patients who die in the greater Harare area and (iv) records of specific cancer research studies including case series assembled by clinicians. Death certificate notifications are followed up to obtain additional information on the diagnosis and management of the cancer, and if this proves fruitless, cases are registered on the basis of the death certificate only.

The registry records all cases identified, but the population base for calculation of incidence rates includes only residents of the target population (Harare City), defined as people who have lived in the city for at least six months.

Review of data

Cancer patterns derived from a series of cases diagnosed histologically and by autopsy in 1939–46 from Salisbury (Harare) were described by Gelfand (1949), a series of 2000 histologically diagnosed cases from Bulawayo in 1948–61 by Tulloch (1963), a series of cases diagnosed histologically in Salisbury (Harare) in 1955–65 by Ross (1967a, b) and cases from Harare hospital and histopathology records from Parirenyatwa hospital in 1980–82 by Stein (1984a, b) (Table 1).

Bulawayo Cancer Registry

The results from the registry were published as incidence rates for the period 1963–72. The unilateral declaration of independence by the colony of Rhodesia in 1965 and the ensuing civil war meant that it was impossible to derive accurate population denominators, so that the data from the final quinquennium of registration (1973–77) were simply presented as relative frequencies (Skinner *et al.*, 1970, 1976, 1993; Skinner, 1986; Parkin *et al.*, 1994).

During the 10-year period (1963–72) for which reasonably valid estimates of the population at risk were available, 1281 cancers were registered among the residents of Bulawayo, 991 cases in men (corresponding to a crude annual incidence of 93.8 per 100 000) and 290 cases in women (39.5 per 100 000). Table 2 shows the age-specific, crude and age-standardized incidence rates by cancer site. Three cancers dominate the picture in men: liver, oesophagus, and lung, the precise ranking depending upon the index chosen. Thus, with the age-standardized (world) rate, oesophagus cancer is first in importance, although the high rate (ASR 55.6) is strongly influenced by 33 cases in the oldest age-group (65+), so that with the cumulative rate (0–64 years), liver cancer is first. Moderately high rates are also observed for cancers of the prostate (ASR 20.8) and bladder (ASR 15.8). In women, cervix cancer is the dominant malignant tumour (ASR 29.5), followed by cancers of the liver (ASR 20.1), breast (ASR 13.7), bladder (ASR 11.2) and oesophagus (ASR 6.9). A very high proportion of cancer cases had histological verification of diagnosis (94% overall).

The risk factors for various cancers were evaluated in case–control analyses in which other cancer cases (excluding tobacco-related cancers in men and hormone-related cancers in women) were considered as controls (Parkin et al., 1994; Vizcaino et al., 1994; Vizcaino et al., 1995).

The high rates of oesophageal cancer in men in Bulawayo are similar to those observed in the former Transkei region of South Africa, an area of known high oesophageal cancer risk. The incidence is some three times higher than in the more recent data from Harare (see below). In men, tobacco smoking was associated with increased risk (odds ratio (OR) = 5.7) in the highest consumption category (15 g of tobacco per day) compared with non-smokers. There was no independent effect of alcohol consumption (Vizcaino et al., 1995).

Lung cancer rates in men in Bulawayo in the 1960s are among the highest recorded in Africa (see Chapter 4.9, Table 1). Tulloch (1963) had earlier noted the higher frequency of lung cancer in Bulawayo than in Salisbury (Harare). The OR associated with the highest category of tobacco consumption (15 g of tobacco per day) was 5.2, compared with non-smokers. Although 41% of men at this period were smokers, consumption was not high: 86% of smokers were smoking less than 15 cigarettes daily. Osburn (1957) noted the frequency of lung cancer in the Gwanda area of Matabeleland and related this to the arsenic content of the local mines. Parkin et al. (1994) found that copper (OR 1.5), gold (OR 1.5) and nickel (OR 2.6) miners had increased risks of lung cancer and noted that the copper/nickel ore mined at Filabusi in Matabeleland contains varying amounts of arsenic. No increase in risk was found, however, among asbestos miners (OR 0.7). Previous studies had also failed to identify an excess of lung cancer in asbestos miners (Osburn, 1957; Mossop, 1983). The asbestos mined in Zimbabwe is chrysotile.

Squamous cell carcinomas were 71% of bladder cancers; the presence of schistosomiasis was associated with a significantly increased risk (OR 3.9 in men, 5.7 in women) (Vizcaino et al., 1994).

The risk of invasive cervical cancer increased with number of children—the estimated odds ratio was 1.8 in women with six or more births—but no consistent association was found for age at first intercourse. In postmenopausal women, the risk of breast cancer increased with age at first pregnancy (but not in the highly fertile) and decreased with high parity, if age at first pregnancy was 19 or more (Parkin et al., 1994).

Zimbabwe Cancer Registry
The first (non-population-based) series of data for 1986–89 was published by Bassett et al. (1992). The first population-based results for the two main ethnic groups (Africans and Europeans) for the period 1990–92 were reported separately in 1995 (Bassett et al., 1995a, b), and these data were reproduced in volume VII of *Cancer Incidence in Five Continents* (Parkin et al., 1997). An updated analysis for 1993–95 (Chokunonga et al., 2000) has also been published.

In this volume, three sets of tables are shown. For the African population, the rates for 1990–93 (Table 3) and 1994–97 (Table 4), and for the European population, the incidence over the full eight-year period 1990–97 (Table 5).

In the most recent period (1994–97), among the African population, the leading cancers in males were Kaposi sarcoma (41.8% of the total, ASR 50.9 per 100 000), cancer of the liver (9.2%, ASR 26.0), prostate (6.8%, ASR 28.5), oesophagus (5.5%, ASR 17.2) and lung (3.9%, ASR 12.1). In females, the principal cancers are cancer of the cervix (comprising 22.6% of all cancers, ASR 53.1), Kaposi's sarcoma (21.4% ASR 21.6), breast (8.2% ASR 19.8) and liver (3.7%, ASR 10.6) and stomach (3.1%, ASR 10.3).

Many of the features of the cancer profile are a consequence of the epidemic of AIDS, which is particularly severe in Zimbabwe

(Chokunonga et al., 1999). Kaposi sarcoma has always been observed in Zimbabwe, as the old series summarized in Table 1 testify. It was typically an indolent tumour affecting elderly men (Gordon, 1973). The data from Bulawayo (Table 2) show an incidence of 2.6 in men and 0.3 in women in 1963–72. The incidence in Harare is now much higher, and it has almost doubled between 1990–93 and 1994–97. The median ages at diagnosis, 35 and 32 years in men and women, respectively, reflect the difference in age-specific prevalence of HIV infection between the sexes. The relatively high rates for cancer of the eye in both sexes are a consequence of a high proportion of squamous-cell carcinoma of the conjunctiva (see Chapter 4.5). This tumour is recognized as an AIDS-related cancer in sub-Saharan Africa. There has also been an increase in the incidence of non-Hodgkin lymphoma between 1990–93 and 1994–97. Chokunonga et al. (1999) noted that most of this increase had been in adults (aged 15–54 years), with no significant change in the incidence in children.

The high incidence of liver cancer reflects a relatively high rate of infection with hepatitis B virus (Tswana, 1985). Blood-donor and community data do not suggest any major geographical variation in the prevalence of this infection in Zimbabwe. Aflatoxin exposure has been suggested to be important in determining geographical variations in incidence of liver cancer in southern Africa, but the prevalence of exposure appears to be low in Zimbabwe, based on analysis of urine samples (Nyathi et al., 1987).

The incidence of bladder cancer in the African population is moderately high, and squamous-cell tumours predominate (Chapter 4.1, Table 3), as in Bulawayo and in earlier Zimbabwean studies (Houston, 1964; Thomas et al., 1990). Several studies have linked infection with *Schistosoma haematobium* with bladder cancer. *S. haematobium* infection is endemic in Zimbabwe, its prevalence varying with the presence of standing water (Taylor & Makura, 1985) and regional variations in bladder cancer incidence within the country vary directly with the prevalence of infection (Thomas et al., 1990; Vizcaino et al., 1994). The lower incidence of bladder cancer recorded in Harare, compared with Bulawayo, is somewhat puzzling, because *S. haematobium* infection is more common in Mashonaland than in the semi-arid Matabeleland.

As noted in an earlier clinical series (Levy, 1984, 1988), myeloid leukaemia is more frequent than lymphoid in the African population of Zimbabwe. However, the age-specific incidence rates confirm the predominance of acute lymphocytic leukaemia in young children, and of chronic lymphocytic leukaemia in the elderly.

In the European-origin population (Table 5), most registered cases are non-melanoma skin cancers (61.4% of cases in men and 50.4% in women). Excluding these, the ASR per 100 000 was 372.6 in males and 340.3 in females. The incidence of malignant melanoma is very high (ASR 40.5 in men and 30.2 in women), somewhat higher than the rates among whites in Australia (ASR 36.7 in males and 28.4 in women (Parkin et al., 2002)). In men, other leading cancers are prostate (ASR 70.1), colon/rectum (ASR 49.8), and lung (ASR 38.4). In females, the leading cancers were breast (ASR 121.2), colon/rectum (ASR 35.5) and lung (ASR 24.5). The incidence of cancer of the liver is higher than that observed in western countries (in males 8.4 vs. 2.5 in England and 3.9 in US whites (Chapter 4.8, Table 1)). Similarly bladder cancer incidence rates are elevated (ASR 25.6) compared with western rates (e.g., ASR 19.8 in England (Chapter 4.1, Table 1)). Breast cancer appears to be more common in Harare whites than in Los Angeles (ASR 103.9 (Parkin et al., 2002)) and six times more common than in Harare black females (ASR 19.8).

Childhood cancer
Data on cancer in childhood from Bulawayo Cancer Registry were published by Skinner (1988). Tables of relative frequency for all 543 childhood cancers registered in 1963–97, as well as incidence rates for residents of Bulawayo (78 cases) were presented (Table 6).

Chokunonga *et al.* (1998) published data for residents of Harare (347 cases) diagnosed in 1990–94. The data shown in this volume (Table 7) update this material to the period 1990–97. In this series, the leading cancers among African children are leukaemia (19.4%, ASR 21.6 per million), Wilms tumour (12.7%, ASR 14.0 per million), and lymphoma (12.4%, ASR 13.8 per million). Among the lymphomas, Burkitt lymphoma is not especially frequent (only 6/48 cases), while Kaposi sarcoma now comprises 9.3% of childhood cancers. In a clinical series from the paediatric wards of Parirenyatwa Hospital, Chitsike and Siziya (1998) found that non-Hodgkin lymphomas comprised 22.4% of 64 cases and Kaposi sarcoma 15.8%. All of the 12 children with Kaposi sarcoma were HIV-positive, as were 9 out of 17 (53%) non-Hodgkin lymphoma cases, compared with only 6 of 34 (17.6%) children with other tumours.

References

Bassett, M.T., Levy, L.M., Chetsanga, C., Chokunonga, E. (1992) Zimbabwe National Cancer Registry: summary data 1986-1989. National Cancer Registry Advisory Committee. *Cent. Afr. J. Med.*, **38**, 91–94.

Bassett, M.T., Chokunonga, E., Mauchaza, B., Levy, L., Ferlay, J. & Parkin, D.M. (1995) Cancer in the African population of Harare, Zimbabwe, 1990-1992. *Int. J. Cancer*, **63**, 29–36

Bassett, M.T., Levy, L., Chokunonga, E., Mauchaza, B., Ferlay, J. & Parkin, D.M. (1995b) Cancer in the European population of Harare, Zimbabwe, 1990-1992. *Int. J. Cancer*, **63**, 24–28.

Chitsike, I. & Siziya, S. (1998) Seroprevalence of human immunodeficiency virus type 1 infection in childhood malignancy in Zimbabwe. *Cent. Afr. J. Med.*, **44**, 242–245

Chokunonga, E., Mauchaza, B.G., Levy, L.M., Chetsanga, N.J.T., Bassett, M.T., Abayomi, A., Nyakabau, A. & Chitsike, I. (1998) Zimbabwe: Zimbabwe National Cancer Registry, 1990-1994 In: Parkin, D.M., Kramárová, E., Draper, G.J., Masuyer, E., Michaelis, J., Neglia, J, Qureshi, S. & Stiller, C.A., eds, *International Incidence of Childhood Cancer,* vol. II (IARC Scientific Publications No. 144), Lyon, IARC, pp. 57–59

Chokunonga, E., Levy, L.M., Bassett, M.T., Borok, M.Z., Mauchaza, B.G., Chirenje, M.Z. & Parkin, D.M. (1999) AIDS and cancer in Africa: the evolving epidemic in Zimbabwe. *AIDS*, **13**, 2583–2588

Chokunonga, E., Levy, L.M., Bassett, M.T., Mauchaza, B.G., Thomas, D.B. & Parkin, D.M. (2000) Cancer incidence in the African population of Harare, Zimbabwe: second results from the cancer registry 1993-1995. *Int. J. Cancer*, **85**, 54–59.

Gelfand, M. (1949) Malignancy in the African. *S. Afr. Med. J.*, **23**, 1010–1016

Gordon, J.A. (1973) Clinical features of Kaposi's sarcoma amongst Rhodesian Africans. *Cent. Afr. J. Med.*, **19**, 1–6

Houston, W. (1964) Carcinoma of the bladder in Southern Rhodesia. *Br. J. Urol.*, **36**, 71–76

Levy, L.M. (1984) The pattern of leukaemia in adult Zimbabweans. *Cent. Afr. J. Med.*, **30**, 57–63

Levy, L.M. (1988) The pattern of haematological and lymphoreticular malignancy in Zimbabwe. *Trop. Geogr. Med.*, **40**, 109–114

Mossop, R.T. (1983) Asbestos hazards in Zimbabwe. *Cent. Afr. J. Med.*, **29**, 117–118

Nyathi, C.B., Mutiro, C.F., Hasler, J.A. & Chetsanga, C.J. (1987) A survey of urinary aflatoxin in Zimbabwe. *Int. J. Epidemiol.*, **16**, 516–519

Osburn, H.S. (1957) Cancer of the lung in Gwanda. *Cent. Afr. J. Med.*, **3**, 215–223

Parkin, D.M., Vizcaino, A.P., Skinner, M.E. & Ndhlovu, A. (1994) Cancer patterns and risk factors in the African population of southwestern Zimbabwe, 1963-1977. *Cancer Epidemiol. Biomarkers Prev.*, **3**, 537–547

Parkin, D.M., Whelan, S.L., Ferlay, J., Raymond, L. & Young, J., eds (1997) *Cancer Incidence in Five Continents,* Vol. VII (IARC Scientific Publications No. 143), Lyon, IARC

Parkin, D.M., Whelan, S.L., Ferlay, J., Teppo, L. & Thomas, D.B., eds (2002) *Cancer Incidence in Five Continents,* Vol. VIII (IARC Scientific Publications No. 155), Lyon, IARC

Ross, M.D. (1967a) Tumours in Mashonaland Africans. *Cent. Afr. J. Med.*, **13**, 107–116

Ross, M.D. (1967b) Tumours in Mashonaland Africans. II. *Cent. Afr. J. Med.*, **13**, 139–145

Skinner, M.E.G. (1986) Zimbabwe: Bulawayo Cancer Registry, 1963-1977. In: Parkin, D.M., ed., *Cancer Occurrence in Developing Countries* (IARC Scientific Publications No. 75), Lyon, IARC, pp. 125–129

Skinner, M.E.G. (1988) Zimbabwe: Bulawayo Cancer Registry, 1963-1977. In: Parkin, D.M., Stiller, C.A., Draper, G.J., Bieber, C.A., Terracini, B. & Young, J.L., eds, *International Incidence of Childhood Cancer* (IARC Scientific Publications No. 87), Lyon, IARC, pp. 67–71

Skinner, M.E.G., Parker, D.A., Flegg, M.H. & Fraser, R.W. (1970) Cancer incidence in Bulawayo, 1963-1967. In: Doll, R., Muir, C. & Waterhouse, J., eds, *Cancer Incidence in Five Continents, Vol II*, Berlin, Springer Verlag (for UICC), pp. 94-97

Skinner, M.E.G., Parker, D.A. & Chamisa, C. (1976) Cancer Incidence in Rhodesia: Bulawayo, 1969-1972. In: Waterhouse, J., Muir, C., Correa, P. & Powell, J., eds, *Cancer Incidence in Five Continents, Vol III* (IARC Scientific Publications No. 15), Lyon, IARC, pp. 120–123

Skinner, M.E.G., Parkin, D.M., Vizcaino, A.P. & Ndhlovu, A. (1993) *Cancer in the African Population of Bulawayo, Zimbabwe, 1963-1977* (IARC Technical Report No. 15), Lyon, IARC

Stein, C.M. (1984a) The pattern of malignancy in Mashonaland. *Cent Afr J Med.*, **30**, 64–68

Stein, C.M. (1984b) The pattern of malignancy in Mashonaland. Part II. *Cent. Afr. J. Med.*, **30**, 84–86

Taylor, P. & Makura, O. (1985) Prevalence and distribution of schistosomiasis in Zimbabwe. *Ann. Trop. Med. Parasitol.*, **79**, 287–299

Thomas, J.E., Bassett, M.T., Sigola, L.B. & Taylor, P. (1990) Relationship between bladder cancer incidence, Schistosoma haematobium infection, and geographical region in Zimbabwe. *Trans. R. Soc. Trop. Med. Hyg.*, **84**, 551–553

Tswana, S.A. (1985) Serologic survey of hepatitis B surface antigen among the healthy population in Zimbabwe. *Cent. Afr. J. Med.*, **31**, 45–49

Tulloch, B.S. (1963) MD Thesis, University of St Andrews (reported in Ross, 1967)

Vizcaino, A.P., Parkin, D.M., Boffeta, P. & Skinner, M.E.G. (1994) Bladder cancer: epidemiology and risk factors in Bulawayo, Zimbabwe. *Cancer Causes Control*, **5**, 517–522

Vizcaino, A.P., Parkin, D.M. & Skinner, M.E.G. (1995) Risk factors associated with oesophageal cancer in Bulawayo, Zimbabwe. *Br. J. Cancer*, **72**, 769–773

WHO (2001) Tobacco or Health. A Global Status Report. Country profile: Zimbabwe. (www.cdc.gov/nccdphp/osh/who/zimbabwe.htm)

Table 1. Zimbabwe: case series

Site	Pathology cases (histology and autopsy) (Gelfand, 1949) Both sexes			Histologically diagnosed cases, Salisbury (Harare), 1955-65 (Ross, 1967a, b) Male		Female		%HV	Harare hospital and pathology cases (Parirenyatwa Hospital) (Stein,1984 a, b) Both sexes		%HV
	No.	%	%HV	No.	%	No.	%		No.	%	
Oral cavity[a]	9	2.7%		70	2.7%	28	1.9%	100	52	0.9%	65.4
Nasopharynx									270	4.6%	54.4
Other pharynx										0.0%	
Oesophagus	2	0.6%		226	8.7%	8	0.6%	100	624	10.6%	43.3
Stomach	5	1.5%		99	3.8%	33	2.3%	100	233	4.0%	42.9
Colon/rectum	11	3.3%		81	3.1%	19	1.3%	100	140	2.4%	50.0
Liver	25	7.5%		175	6.8%	25	1.7%	100	369	6.3%	42.0
Pancreas	3	0.9%		15	0.6%	4	0.3%	100	30	0.5%	6.7
Lung	7	2.1%		134[b]	5.2%	12	0.8%	100	395	6.7%	42.0
Melanoma	29	8.7%		55	2.1%	65	4.5%	100	82	1.4%	76.8
Other skin	89	26.6%		289	11.2%	146	10.1%	100	239	4.1%	86.2
Kaposi sarcoma	2	0.6%		128	4.9%	4	0.3%	100	55	0.9%	100
Breast	10	3.0%		6	0.2%	100	6.9%	100	214	3.6%	55.6
Cervix uteri	4	1.2%			0.0%	323	22.4%	100	1034	17.5%	52.0
Corpus uteri	2	0.6%			0.0%	16	1.1%	100	83	1.4%	59.0
Ovary etc.					0.0%	54	3.7%	100	57	1.0%	59.7
Prostate	1	0.3%		96	3.7%		0.0%	100	168	2.8%	51.2
Penis				105	4.1%		0.0%	100	83	1.4%	68.7
Bladder				245	9.5%	109	7.5%	100	317	5.4%	49.2
Kidney etc.	9	2.7%		31	1.2%	28	1.9%	100	74	1.3%	28.4
Eye	1	0.3%		113	4.4%	53	3.7%	100	63	1.1%	31.8
Brain, nervous system				27	1.0%	19	1.3%	100	52	0.9%	59.6
Thyroid	1	0.3%		38	1.5%	44	3.0%	100	82	1.4%	45.1
Non-Hodgkin lymphoma				180	7.0%	55	3.8%	100	99	1.7%	54.6
Hodgkin disease				48	1.9%	8	0.6%	100	51	0.9%	21.6
Myeloma				8	0.3%	2	0.1%	100	71	1.2%	28.2
Leukaemia				5	0.2%	3	0.2%	100	88	1.5%	100
ALL SITES	334	100.0%		2587	100.0%	1444	100.0%	100	5895	100.0%	50.2

[a] Includes salivary gland

Table 2. Zimbabwe, Bulawayo: African (1963-1972)

NUMBER OF CASES BY AGE GROUP AND SUMMARY RATES OF INCIDENCE - MALE

SITE	ALL AGES	AGE UNK	0-	15-	25-	35-	45-	55-	65+	CRUDE RATE	%	ASR (W)	ICD (10th)
Mouth	16	0	-	1	4	5	4	-	2	1.5	1.6	3.2	C00-C08
Nasopharynx	2	0	-	-	1	1	-	-	-	0.2	0.2	0.1	C11
Other pharynx	8	0	-	-	-	2	2	4	-	0.8	0.8	1.7	C09-C10,C12-C14
Oesophagus	164	0	-	-	3	27	60	41	33	15.5	16.5	55.6	C15
Stomach	36	0	-	-	1	6	16	9	4	3.4	3.6	9.4	C16
Colon, rectum and anus	28	0	-	2	5	6	8	3	4	2.7	2.8	6.8	C18-C21
Liver	261	0	-	11	41	56	87	45	21	24.7	26.3	53.7	C22
Pancreas	23	0	-	-	1	3	9	6	4	2.2	2.3	7.3	C25
Larynx	16	0	-	-	1	4	4	4	3	1.5	1.6	5.1	C32
Trachea, bronchus and lung	121	0	-	-	6	10	38	42	25	11.5	12.2	44.1	C33-C34
Melanoma of skin	6	0	-	3	1	3	1	-	1	0.6	0.6	1.4	C43
Other skin	18	0	-	3	4	2	3	3	3	1.7		4.9	C44
Kaposi sarcoma	17	0	-	2	5	4	4	1	1	1.6	1.7	2.6	C46
Breast	2	0	-	-	-	1	1	-	-	0.2	0.2	0.4	C50
Penis	12	0	-	-	1	1	3	6	3	1.1	1.2	5.1	C60
Prostate	37	0	-	-	-	-	9	12	16	3.5	3.7	20.8	C61
Kidney etc.	14	0	3	-	-	4	4	1	1	1.3	1.4	2.7	C64-C66,C68
Bladder	63	0	-	1	7	20	14	13	8	6.0	6.4	15.8	C67
Eye	7	1	2	2	1	-	-	1	-	0.7	0.7	0.9	C69
Brain, nervous system	7	0	4	1	-	-	1	1	-	0.7	0.7	0.9	C70-C72
Thyroid	5	0	-	-	1	1	-	2	1	0.5	0.5	1.7	C73
Hodgkin disease	23	0	1	4	7	4	6	1	-	2.2	2.3	2.2	C81
Non-Hodgkin lymphoma	19	0	4	2	3	6	3	1	-	1.8	1.9	1.9	C82-C85,C96
Multiple myeloma	8	0	-	-	1	1	1	4	1	0.8	0.8	2.5	C90
Leukaemia	30	0	6	6	6	5	3	3	1	2.8	3.0	4.1	C91-C95
Other and unspecified	48	0	5	7	8	8	7	12	1	4.5	4.8	7.8	O&U
All sites	991	1	25	42	108	180	285	217	133	93.8	100.0	263.0	ALL
All sites but C44	973	1	25	39	104	178	282	214	130	92.1	98.2	258.0	ALLbC44
Average annual population			30963	20040	25829	17285	8295	2507	709				

Source: Cancer Incidence in Five Continents volume 2 and 3

Table 2. Zimbabwe, Bulawayo: African (1963-1972)

NUMBER OF CASES BY AGE GROUP AND SUMMARY RATES OF INCIDENCE - FEMALE

SITE	ALL AGES	AGE UNK	0-	15-	25-	35-	45-	55-	65+	CRUDE RATE	%	ASR (W)	ICD (10th)
Mouth	2	0	2	-	-	-	-	-	-	0.3	0.7	0.2	C00-C08
Nasopharynx	1	0	-	-	-	-	-	1	-	0.1	0.3	1.1	C11
Other pharynx	0	0	-	-	-	-	-	-	-	0.0	0.0	0.0	C09-C10,C12-C14
Oesophagus	10	0	-	1	1	3	2	3	1	1.4	3.4	6.9	C15
Stomach	9	0	-	-	1	2	3	2	1	1.2	3.1	6.1	C16
Colon, rectum and anus	6	0	-	-	1	1	1	3	-	0.8	2.1	3.8	C18-C21
Liver	33	0	-	-	8	8	8	5	4	4.5	11.4	20.1	C22
Pancreas	4	0	-	-	1	1	1	-	1	0.5	1.4	3.1	C25
Larynx	3	0	-	-	1	1	-	1	-	0.4	1.0	1.5	C32
Trachea, bronchus and lung	6	0	-	-	-	1	4	1	-	0.8	2.1	2.8	C33-C34
Melanoma of skin	5	0	-	1	2	-	1	1	-	0.7	1.7	1.7	C43
Other skin	6	0	-	1	2	3	1	-	-	0.8		1.1	C44
Kaposi sarcoma	3	0	1	1	1	-	-	-	-	0.4	1.0	0.3	C46
Breast	30	0	-	-	7	9	9	3	2	4.1	10.3	13.7	C50
Cervix uteri	60	0	-	-	10	22	15	9	4	8.2	20.7	29.5	C53
Uterus	11	0	-	-	2	2	4	2	1	1.5	3.8	6.6	C54-C55
Ovary etc.	11	0	-	-	1	3	3	2	2	1.5	3.8	8.6	C56-C57
Kidney etc.	3	0	1	-	-	1	1	-	-	0.4	1.0	0.7	C64-C66,C68
Bladder	14	0	-	2	2	5	1	-	4	1.9	4.8	11.2	C67
Eye	4	0	3	-	-	1	-	-	-	0.5	1.4	0.5	C69
Brain, nervous system	9	1	5	1	1	1	1	-	-	1.2	3.1	1.2	C70-C72
Thyroid	6	0	-	1	-	2	3	-	-	0.8	2.1	1.6	C73
Hodgkin disease	1	0	-	1	-	-	-	-	-	0.1	0.3	0.1	C81
Non-Hodgkin lymphoma	6	0	3	-	2	1	-	-	-	0.8	2.1	0.6	C82-C85,C96
Multiple myeloma	3	0	-	-	-	-	2	-	1	0.4	1.0	3.2	C90
Leukaemia	15	0	4	1	4	1	1	2	2	2.0	5.2	8.4	C91-C95
Other and unspecified	29	0	4	4	11	5	2	-	3	4.0	10.0	10.7	O&U
All sites	290	1	24	12	58	70	64	35	26	39.5	100.0	145.8	ALL
All sites but C44	284	1	24	12	56	67	63	35	26	38.7	97.9	144.8	ALLbC44
Average annual population	30700		16058	15172	7630	2725	760	291					

Source: Cancer Incidence in Five Continents volume 2 and 3

Table 3. Zimbabwe, Harare: African (1990-1993)

NUMBER OF CASES BY AGE GROUP AND SUMMARY RATES OF INCIDENCE - MALE

SITE	ALL AGES	AGE UNK	MV (%)	0-	15-	25-	35-	45-	55-	65+	CRUDE RATE	%	CR 64	ASR (W)	ICD (10th)
Mouth	17	1	82	-	2	-	2	5	4	3	0.7	0.7	0.10	1.7	C00-06
Salivary gland	7	0	86	-	-	-	2	2	1	2	0.3	0.3	0.02	0.7	C07-08
Nasopharynx	14	0	86	-	1	5	1	2	1	4	0.6	0.6	0.04	1.4	C11
Other pharynx	6	0	67	-	1	-	-	1	2	2	0.3	0.3	0.03	0.8	C09-10,C12-14
Oesophagus	212	0	52	-	-	1	24	43	78	66	8.9	9.1	1.38	27.9	C15
Stomach	90	0	49	-	-	3	10	21	20	36	3.8	3.9	0.44	12.6	C16
Colon, rectum and anus	84	0	62	1	6	7	13	20	20	17	3.5	3.6	0.47	8.5	C18-21
Liver	289	0	22	2	10	38	46	59	66	68	12.2	12.4	1.51	30.7	C22
Gallbladder etc.	4	0	50	-	-	-	1	1	1	1	0.2	0.2	0.02	0.5	C23-24
Pancreas	44	0	27	-	-	4	2	8	14	16	1.9	1.9	0.25	6.1	C25
Larynx	37	1	73	-	-	-	1	7	18	10	1.6	1.6	0.28	4.8	C32
Trachea, bronchus and lung	156	0	37	-	-	6	7	33	60	50	6.6	6.7	1.03	20.9	C33-34
Bone	21	0	90	4	10	-	2	1	3	1	0.9	0.9	0.09	1.3	C40-41
Melanoma of skin	18	0	94	-	2	2	3	3	5	3	0.8	0.8	0.10	1.7	C43
Other skin	28	2	93	-	2	2	6	3	4	9	1.2		0.11	3.4	C44
Mesothelioma	0	0	-	-	-	-	-	-	-	-	0.0	0.0	0.00	0.0	C45
Kaposi sarcoma	679	4	73	11	44	299	183	76	48	14	28.6	29.1	2.45	31.3	C46
Peripheral nerves	0	0	-	-	-	-	-	-	-	-	0.0	0.0	0.00	0.0	C47
Connective and soft tissue	26	0	96	3	6	4	6	2	3	2	1.1	1.1	0.10	1.6	C49
Breast	5	0	80	-	-	-	1	3	1	-	0.2	0.2	0.04	0.4	C50
Penis	17	0	71	-	-	-	2	4	5	6	0.7	0.7	0.10	2.3	C60
Prostate	161	4	65	-	-	-	3	18	56	80	6.8	6.9	0.88	26.9	C61
Testis	6	0	50	-	1	1	1	1	1	1	0.3	0.3	0.03	0.5	C62
Kidney	19	0	95	11	1	-	1	3	1	2	0.8	0.8	0.06	1.3	C64
Renal pelvis, ureter and other urinary	0	0	-	-	-	-	-	-	-	-	0.0	0.0	0.00	0.0	C65-66,C68
Bladder	95	0	61	1	1	3	8	27	23	32	4.0	4.1	0.53	12.5	C67
Eye	17	0	94	10	1	2	1	2	-	1	0.7	0.7	0.05	1.0	C69
Brain, nervous system	32	0	28	9	6	5	5	2	4	1	1.3	1.4	0.12	1.7	C70-72
Thyroid	11	0	64	1	1	1	5	-	1	2	0.5	0.5	0.08	1.2	C73
Hodgkin disease	18	0	100	4	2	3	4	3	1	1	0.8	0.8	0.08	0.9	C81
Non-Hodgkin lymphoma	73	0	86	15	5	16	13	12	9	3	3.1	3.1	0.30	4.2	C82-85,C96
Multiple myeloma	27	0	93	-	-	2	5	7	9	4	1.1	1.2	0.18	2.6	C90
Lymphoid leukaemia	26	0	92	12	3	1	1	1	3	5	1.1	1.1	0.08	2.2	C91
Myeloid leukaemia	38	0	92	9	6	9	5	6	2	1	1.6	1.6	0.13	1.9	C92-94
Leukaemia, unspecified	2	0	50	-	-	-	1	-	1	1	0.1	0.1	0.01	0.4	C95
Other and unspecified	86	4	57	4	7	5	12	11	27	16	3.6	3.7	0.52	8.8	O&U
All sites	2365	16	61	97	117	420	371	388	497	459	99.6	100.0	11.61	224.7	ALL
All sites but C44	2337	14	60	97	115	418	365	385	493	450	98.4		11.50	221.3	ALLbC44
Average annual population				192913	140631	122669	70844	39116	20277	7334					

Table 3. Zimbabwe, Harare: African (1990-1993)

NUMBER OF CASES BY AGE GROUP AND SUMMARY RATES OF INCIDENCE - FEMALE

SITE	ALL AGES	AGE UNK	MV (%)	0-	15-	25-	35-	45-	55-	65+	CRUDE RATE	%	CR 64	ASR (W)	ICD (10th)
Mouth	5	0	100	-	-	-	1	2	-	2	0.2	0.3	0.03	1.0	C00-06
Salivary gland	6	0	100	-	1	3	1	-	-	1	0.3	0.4	0.01	0.5	C07-08
Nasopharynx	7	0	86	-	4	-	1	-	1	1	0.3	0.4	0.04	0.7	C11
Other pharynx	4	0	75	-	-	-	-	2	1	1	0.2	0.3	0.06	0.9	C09-10,C12-14
Oesophagus	36	0	36	-	-	2	2	4	14	14	1.7	2.3	0.48	8.6	C15
Stomach	67	0	57	-	-	3	6	18	10	30	3.1	4.3	0.58	15.1	C16
Colon, rectum and anus	47	1	66	-	4	4	10	12	10	6	2.2	3.0	0.53	7.1	C18-21
Liver	93	0	24	2	2	10	12	17	35	15	4.4	5.9	1.39	17.1	C22
Gallbladder etc.	3	0	67	-	-	-	1	1	-	1	0.1	0.2	0.04	0.7	C23-24
Pancreas	27	0	19	-	-	2	2	2	8	13	1.3	1.7	0.28	6.7	C25
Larynx	3	0	67	-	1	-	-	-	-	2	0.1	0.2	0.03	0.9	C32
Trachea, bronchus and lung	32	0	41	-	1	2	4	4	7	14	1.5	2.0	0.29	7.2	C33-34
Bone	14	0	86	2	6	-	5	-	-	-	0.7	0.9	0.07	0.8	C40-41
Melanoma of skin	17	0	88	1	-	2	2	1	6	5	0.8	1.1	0.22	3.5	C43
Other skin	21	0	90	-	3	1	3	1	4	9	1.0		0.16	4.4	C44
Mesothelioma	0	0	-	-	-	-	-	-	-	-	0.0	0.0	0.00	0.0	C45
Kaposi sarcoma	185	1	72	4	35	83	43	17	2	-	8.7	11.8	0.75	9.4	C46
Peripheral nerves	2	0	100	1	-	-	1	-	-	1	0.1	0.1	0.01	0.1	C47
Connective and soft tissue	21	2	90	3	6	5	2	-	2	1	1.0	1.3	0.11	1.6	C49
Breast	171	3	85	-	2	27	65	37	23	14	8.0	10.9	1.55	20.3	C50
Vulva	9	0	89	1	-	-	-	4	3	1	0.4	0.6	0.15	1.7	C51
Vagina	2	1	100	-	-	-	-	-	-	1	0.1	0.1	0.00	0.7	C52
Cervix uteri	410	7	78	-	10	48	100	102	78	65	19.2	26.2	4.30	62.6	C53
Uterus	33	0	67	-	1	2	6	10	7	7	1.5	2.1	0.39	5.9	C54-55
Ovary	52	0	65	2	3	7	7	9	19	5	2.4	3.3	0.75	8.3	C56
Placenta	20	0	85	-	10	8	1	1	-	-	0.9	1.3	0.05	0.8	C58
Kidney	15	0	100	13	-	-	1	1	-	-	0.7	1.0	0.04	0.7	C64
Renal pelvis, ureter and other urinary	0	0	-	-	-	-	-	-	-	-	0.0	0.0	0.00	0.0	C65-66,C68
Bladder	54	0	61	1	-	5	8	12	13	15	2.5	3.5	0.62	10.5	C67
Eye	17	3	94	8	1	4	-	1	1	-	0.8	1.1	0.07	0.9	C69
Brain, nervous system	18	0	33	8	1	2	5	1	1	-	0.8	1.2	0.09	1.1	C70-72
Thyroid	31	0	65	-	3	5	4	3	9	7	1.5	2.0	0.35	5.4	C73
Hodgkin disease	6	0	100	1	1	1	1	2	-	-	0.3	0.4	0.04	0.4	C81
Non-Hodgkin lymphoma	38	0	95	3	5	11	5	5	3	6	1.8	2.4	0.22	4.3	C82-85,C96
Multiple myeloma	18	0	94	-	-	-	1	4	8	5	0.8	1.2	0.29	4.1	C90
Lymphoid leukaemia	16	0	100	8	1	1	1	2	2	1	0.7	1.0	0.14	1.7	C91
Myeloid leukaemia	26	0	96	8	4	3	5	1	2	3	1.2	1.7	0.12	2.4	C92-94
Leukaemia, unspecified	0	0	-	-	-	-	-	-	-	-	0.0	0.0	0.00	0.0	C95
Other and unspecified	60	1	47	5	6	9	8	8	8	15	2.8	3.8	0.43	9.2	O&U
All sites	1586	19	70	71	111	249	312	283	281	260	74.2	100.0	14.73	227.3	ALL
All sites but C44	1565	19	70	71	108	248	309	282	277	251	73.2		14.57	222.9	ALLbC44
Average annual population				200988	153846	97159	47293	21069	8621	5369					

Table 4. Zimbabwe, Harare: African (1994-1997)

NUMBER OF CASES BY AGE GROUP AND SUMMARY RATES OF INCIDENCE - MALE

SITE	ALL AGES	AGE UNK	MV (%)	0-	15-	25-	35-	45-	55-	65+	CRUDE RATE	%	CR 64	ASR (W)	ICD (10th)
Mouth	23	0	74	-	1	-	4	11	2	5	0.8	0.8	0.10	1.9	C00-06
Salivary gland	13	0	69	-	-	3	1	3	4	2	0.5	0.4	0.07	1.0	C07-08
Nasopharynx	12	0	75	3	1	-	3	3	2	-	0.4	0.4	0.05	0.6	C11
Other pharynx	15	0	73	-	-	2	-	2	9	2	0.5	0.5	0.11	1.3	C09-10,C12-14
Oesophagus	169	3	41	-	2	8	10	38	53	55	6.1	5.5	0.89	17.2	C15
Stomach	105	4	64	-	-	8	8	15	37	33	3.8	3.4	0.57	10.6	C16
Colon, rectum and anus	82	1	62	-	3	10	9	14	20	25	2.9	2.7	0.34	7.4	C18-21
Liver	281	1	16	3	13	24	36	46	70	88	10.1	9.2	1.22	26.0	C22
Gallbladder etc.	6	0	33	-	-	1	1	1	-	3	0.2	0.2	0.01	0.6	C23-24
Pancreas	40	0	20	-	-	3	4	7	18	8	1.4	1.3	0.25	3.6	C25
Larynx	40	0	65	-	-	3	4	7	11	15	1.4	1.3	0.19	4.2	C32
Trachea, bronchus and lung	120	0	42	-	-	3	17	19	43	38	4.3	3.9	0.66	12.1	C33-34
Bone	24	0	67	5	6	7	1	1	-	4	0.9	0.8	0.04	1.3	C40-41
Melanoma of skin	24	0	75	-	-	3	3	5	8	5	0.9	0.8	0.12	2.0	C43
Other skin	50	3	88	5	4	7	9	7	8	7	1.8	1.6	0.20	3.3	C44
Mesothelioma	3	0	67	-	-	1	-	1	1	-	0.1	0.1	0.02	0.2	C45
Kaposi sarcoma	1278	17	60	15	51	523	407	170	75	20	45.8	41.8	4.15	50.9	C46
Peripheral nerves	1	0	100	-	-	-	-	1	-	-	0.0	0.0	0.00	0.2	C47
Connective and soft tissue	24	2	71	2	7	4	3	-	4	2	0.9	0.8	0.09	1.2	C49
Breast	4	0	75	-	-	-	-	-	2	2	0.1	0.1	0.02	0.5	C50
Penis	17	0	82	-	-	3	2	1	5	6	0.6	0.6	0.07	1.6	C60
Prostate	209	6	55	-	-	-	2	12	59	130	7.5	6.8	0.78	28.5	C61
Testis	10	0	70	-	3	2	3	2	-	-	0.4	0.3	0.03	0.5	C62
Kidney	23	1	74	12	3	1	-	2	3	1	0.8	0.8	0.07	1.1	C64
Renal pelvis, ureter and other urinary	0	0	-	-	-	-	-	-	-	-	0.0	0.0	0.00	0.0	C65-66,C68
Bladder	71	0	48	-	2	4	4	15	24	22	2.5	2.3	0.40	7.1	C67
Eye	67	7	90	16	3	20	15	3	1	2	2.4	2.2	0.16	2.6	C69
Brain, nervous system	44	1	59	13	7	5	4	4	5	5	1.6	1.4	0.15	2.5	C70-72
Thyroid	12	0	75	-	3	-	3	4	-	2	0.4	0.4	0.04	0.8	C73
Hodgkin disease	18	0	94	5	5	4	4	-	-	-	0.6	0.6	0.04	0.6	C81
Non-Hodgkin lymphoma	120	3	81	9	6	27	36	17	15	7	4.3	3.9	0.46	6.2	C82-85,C96
Multiple myeloma	27	1	85	-	-	-	2	7	8	9	1.0	0.9	0.15	2.9	C90
Lymphoid leukaemia	25	0	100	15	4	-	1	1	2	2	0.9	0.8	0.06	1.2	C91
Myeloid leukaemia	35	0	97	4	6	12	7	3	1	2	1.3	1.1	0.09	1.4	C92-94
Leukaemia, unspecified	6	0	50	1	1	-	1	1	-	2	0.2	0.2	0.01	0.5	C95
Other and unspecified	108	2	47	10	10	12	16	16	16	26	3.9	3.5	0.39	8.4	O&U
All sites	3106	52	57	118	142	703	617	436	507	531	111.3	100.0	12.02	211.9	ALL
All sites but C44	3056	49	56	113	138	696	608	429	499	524	109.5		11.81	208.6	ALLbC44
Average annual population				229844	163096	148372	80020	41879	24090	10644					

Table 4. Zimbabwe, Harare: African (1994-1997)

NUMBER OF CASES BY AGE GROUP AND SUMMARY RATES OF INCIDENCE - FEMALE

SITE	ALL AGES	AGE UNK	MV (%)	0-	15-	25-	35-	45-	55-	65+	CRUDE RATE	%	CR 64	ASR (W)	ICD (10th)
Mouth	10	0	40	2	2	-	1	1	1	4	0.4	0.4	0.03	1.2	C00-06
Salivary gland	14	0	50	2	4	5	1	1	-	1	0.5	0.6	0.04	0.7	C07-08
Nasopharynx	7	0	71	1	2	1	1	-	2	1	0.3	0.3	0.04	0.6	C11
Other pharynx	2	0	50	-	-	-	-	1	-	1	0.1	0.1	0.01	0.1	C09-10,C12-14
Oesophagus	51	0	51	-	-	1	5	11	12	22	1.9	2.3	0.37	8.4	C15
Stomach	70	1	54	1	1	4	11	13	19	21	2.7	3.1	0.61	10.3	C16
Colon, rectum and anus	52	1	58	-	1	4	10	13	11	12	2.0	2.3	0.42	6.7	C18-21
Liver	84	0	21	3	4	8	17	16	12	24	3.2	3.7	0.51	10.6	C22
Gallbladder etc.	9	0	33	-	-	-	2	2	2	3	0.3	0.4	0.07	1.3	C23-24
Pancreas	23	0	35	1	-	3	2	3	7	7	0.9	1.0	0.20	3.4	C25
Larynx	5	0	60	-	-	-	-	-	1	3	0.2	0.2	0.03	0.9	C32
Trachea, bronchus and lung	40	1	43	-	2	4	3	6	9	15	1.5	1.8	0.25	5.9	C33-34
Bone	21	0	71	3	7	7	1	1	1	1	0.8	0.9	0.06	1.0	C40-41
Melanoma of skin	34	2	76	2	1	1	3	14	7	6	1.3	1.5	0.31	4.4	C43
Other skin	33	0	97	-	5	8	7	1	8	2	1.3		0.22	2.5	C44
Mesothelioma	1	0	100	-	-	1	-	-	-	-	0.0	0.0	0.00	0.0	C45
Kaposi sarcoma	482	7	58	6	71	227	117	32	16	6	18.3	21.4	1.70	21.6	C46
Peripheral nerves	1	0	100	-	-	-	-	-	-	1	0.0	0.0	0.00	0.2	C47
Connective and soft tissue	27	1	81	5	4	5	5	1	-	4	1.0	1.2	0.09	2.0	C49
Breast	186	4	72	-	7	12	49	56	36	22	7.0	8.2	1.50	19.8	C50
Vulva	7	1	71	-	-	1	1	-	2	2	0.3	0.3	0.06	1.0	C51
Vagina	3	0	67	-	-	-	-	-	-	2	0.1	0.1	0.02	0.5	C52
Cervix uteri	510	8	69	-	8	80	129	128	87	70	19.3	22.6	3.73	53.1	C53
Uterus	56	1	66	-	-	5	5	11	18	16	2.1	2.5	0.49	8.1	C54-55
Ovary	76	0	47	3	9	16	9	15	14	10	2.9	3.4	0.53	7.4	C56
Placenta	8	0	75	-	2	5	1	-	-	-	0.3	0.4	0.02	0.2	C58
Kidney	25	0	80	15	2	-	-	2	2	3	0.9	1.1	0.09	1.8	C64
Renal pelvis, ureter and other urinary	0	0	-	-	-	-	-	-	-	-	0.0	0.0	0.00	0.0	C65-66,C68
Bladder	62	1	47	1	4	4	9	12	19	15	2.3	2.7	0.56	8.5	C67
Eye	73	13	90	10	4	23	14	6	2	1	2.8	3.2	0.27	3.6	C69
Brain, nervous system	26	0	50	11	2	4	1	3	2	1	1.0	1.2	0.09	1.4	C70-72
Thyroid	21	1	57	-	1	2	1	4	3	9	0.8	0.9	0.11	3.2	C73
Hodgkin disease	15	0	87	3	4	5	7	-	-	-	0.6	0.7	0.04	0.6	C81
Non-Hodgkin lymphoma	77	1	84	8	6	26	15	9	6	6	2.9	3.4	0.34	5.2	C82-85,C96
Multiple myeloma	25	0	96	-	-	-	2	9	7	6	0.9	1.1	0.25	3.7	C90
Lymphoid leukaemia	15	0	93	7	1	-	1	2	1	3	0.6	0.7	0.06	1.3	C91
Myeloid leukaemia	35	0	91	10	1	7	8	2	-	1	1.3	1.6	0.10	1.6	C92-94
Leukaemia, unspecified	5	0	60	-	1	-	1	1	-	-	0.2	0.2	0.03	0.4	C95
Other and unspecified	97	3	40	6	6	17	13	14	21	17	3.7	4.3	0.69	10.6	O&U
All sites	2288	45	63	100	161	490	454	391	331	316	86.7	100.0	13.95	214.4	ALL
All sites but C44	2255	45	62	98	156	482	447	390	323	314	85.4		13.74	211.9	ALLbC44
Average annual population				244515	185833	119978	61553	27504	12768	7635					

Table 5. Zimbabwe, Harare: European (1990-1997)

NUMBER OF CASES BY AGE GROUP AND SUMMARY RATES OF INCIDENCE - MALE

SITE	ALL AGES	AGE UNK	MV (%)	0-	15-	25-	35-	45-	55-	65+	CRUDE RATE	%	CR 64	ASR (W)	ICD (10th)
Mouth	24	0	96	-	-	-	1	6	5	12	15.7	2.4	0.58	9.4	C00-06
Salivary gland	2	0	100	-	-	-	-	-	1	1	1.3	0.2	0.05	0.7	C07-08
Nasopharynx	0	0	-	-	-	-	-	-	-	-	0.0	0.0	0.00	0.0	C11
Other pharynx	5	0	80	-	-	-	-	1	1	3	3.3	0.5	0.10	1.8	C09-10,C12-14
Oesophagus	18	0	50	-	-	-	4	-	-	14	11.8	1.8	0.19	6.3	C15
Stomach	41	0	78	-	-	1	6	1	14	19	26.8	4.1	1.06	15.8	C16
Colon, rectum and anus	133	3	70	-	1	1	6	16	26	80	87.0	13.4	2.48	49.8	C18-21
Liver	23	0	39	-	-	-	-	3	7	13	15.1	2.3	0.48	8.4	C22
Gallbladder etc.	1	0	0	-	-	-	-	-	-	1	0.7	0.1	0.00	0.3	C23-24
Pancreas	23	0	26	-	-	-	1	1	1	20	15.1	2.3	0.15	7.8	C25
Larynx	35	0	86	-	-	-	-	3	8	24	22.9	3.5	0.53	12.2	C32
Trachea, bronchus and lung	112	0	47	-	-	-	-	3	32	77	73.3	11.2	1.70	38.4	C33-34
Bone	5	0	100	-	-	-	-	-	1	4	3.3	0.5	0.05	1.7	C40-41
Melanoma of skin	91	0	96	1	3	6	9	20	21	31	59.5	9.1	2.91	40.5	C43
Other skin	1584	51	99	2	9	42	130	242	424	684	1036.5		42.34	635.3	C44
Mesothelioma	4	0	50	-	-	1	1	-	-	2	2.6	0.4	0.10	1.4	C45
Kaposi sarcoma	2	0	50	-	-	1	-	1	-	-	1.3	0.2	0.09	1.3	C46
Peripheral nerves	0	0	-	-	-	-	-	-	-	-	0.0	0.0	0.00	0.0	C47
Connective and soft tissue	16	1	100	-	1	1	1	4	4	4	10.5	1.6	0.56	7.3	C49
Breast	2	0	100	-	-	-	-	-	-	2	1.3	0.2	0.00	0.6	C50
Penis	1	0	100	-	-	-	-	-	-	1	0.7	0.1	0.00	0.3	C60
Prostate	210	10	84	-	-	-	1	5	33	161	137.4	21.1	1.99	70.1	C61
Testis	5	0	100	-	2	1	1	1	-	-	3.3	0.5	0.24	3.5	C62
Kidney	14	0	100	-	-	-	-	2	5	7	9.2	1.4	0.34	5.2	C64
Renal pelvis, ureter and other urinary	0	0	-	-	-	-	-	-	-	-	0.0	0.0	0.00	0.0	C65-66,C68
Bladder	74	0	88	-	-	-	2	2	18	52	48.4	7.4	1.06	25.6	C67
Eye	6	0	100	-	1	-	-	1	1	3	3.9	0.6	0.15	2.7	C69
Brain, nervous system	24	0	67	-	4	1	2	5	6	6	15.7	2.4	0.87	11.9	C70-72
Thyroid	1	0	100	-	1	-	-	-	-	-	0.7	0.1	0.05	0.9	C73
Hodgkin disease	2	0	100	1	1	-	-	-	-	-	1.3	0.2	0.11	2.0	C81
Non-Hodgkin lymphoma	15	1	80	-	-	1	-	4	4	5	9.8	1.5	0.46	6.1	C82-85,C96
Multiple myeloma	12	0	75	-	-	-	-	-	2	10	7.9	1.2	0.10	3.9	C90
Lymphoid leukaemia	11	0	55	2	-	-	-	-	3	6	7.2	1.1	0.27	5.4	C91
Myeloid leukaemia	14	1	50	-	-	-	1	1	4	7	9.2	1.4	0.31	5.3	C92-94
Leukaemia, unspecified	5	0	20	-	-	-	-	-	2	3	3.3	0.5	0.10	1.7	C95
Other and unspecified	65	0	54	-	-	2	-	9	14	40	42.5	6.5	1.21	23.9	O&U
All sites	2580	67	89	6	23	58	160	332	642	1292	1688.3	100.0	60.61	1007.6	ALL
All sites but C44	996	16	73	4	14	16	30	90	218	608	651.8		18.36	372.6	ALLbC44
Average annual population				3200	2476	2854	2619	2624	2556	2773					

Warning, percentages will be distored because of the high rates for 'Other skin cancer'

Table 5. Zimbabwe, Harare: European (1990-1997)

NUMBER OF CASES BY AGE GROUP AND SUMMARY RATES OF INCIDENCE - FEMALE

SITE	ALL AGES	AGE UNK	MV (%)	0-	15-	25-	35-	45-	55-	65+	CRUDE RATE	%	CR 64	ASR (W)	ICD (10th)
Mouth	17	1	76	-	-	1	-	1	6	8	10.1	1.7	0.38	5.4	C00-06
Salivary gland	2	0	50	-	-	-	-	-	1	1	1.2	0.2	0.09	0.8	C07-08
Nasopharynx	2	0	100	-	-	1	1	-	-	-	1.2	0.2	0.09	1.2	C11
Other pharynx	5	0	60	-	-	-	1	-	-	3	3.0	0.5	0.09	1.6	C09-10,C12-14
Oesophagus	8	0	25	-	-	-	-	-	3	5	4.7	0.8	0.14	2.3	C15
Stomach	18	0	78	-	-	-	1	-	4	13	10.7	1.8	0.23	5.0	C16
Colon, rectum and anus	118	0	76	-	1	3	1	12	25	76	70.0	11.6	1.90	35.5	C18-21
Liver	15	0	13	-	-	-	-	1	3	11	8.9	1.5	0.18	4.1	C22
Gallbladder etc.	3	0	67	-	-	-	-	-	3	-	1.8	0.3	0.14	1.1	C23-24
Pancreas	28	0	21	-	-	-	-	2	5	21	16.6	2.7	0.32	7.5	C25
Larynx	8	1	75	-	-	-	-	-	1	6	4.7	0.8	0.09	2.3	C32
Trachea, bronchus and lung	86	1	51	-	-	-	1	8	18	58	51.0	8.4	1.24	24.5	C33-34
Bone	3	0	100	-	-	1	-	1	-	1	1.8	0.3	0.09	1.2	C40-41
Melanoma of skin	78	2	97	-	1	3	15	13	19	25	46.2	7.6	2.34	30.2	C43
Other skin	1036	27	100	2	5	36	96	173	246	451	614.2	-	25.68	363.3	C44
Mesothelioma	1	0	100	-	-	-	-	-	-	1	0.6	0.1	0.00	0.2	C45
Kaposi sarcoma	0	0	-	-	-	-	-	-	-	-	0.0	0.0	0.00	0.0	C46
Peripheral nerves	1	0	100	-	-	1	-	-	-	-	0.6	0.1	0.04	0.6	C47
Connective and soft tissue	7	0	100	-	2	-	1	-	1	2	4.1	0.7	0.22	3.3	C49
Breast	347	5	85	-	-	4	38	74	73	153	205.7	34.0	8.55	121.2	C50
Vulva	2	0	100	-	-	-	-	1	-	1	1.2	0.2	0.04	0.7	C51
Vagina	1	0	100	-	-	-	-	-	-	1	0.6	0.1	0.00	0.2	C52
Cervix uteri	32	0	91	-	1	4	4	6	5	11	19.0	3.1	0.91	12.7	C53
Uterus	40	2	85	-	-	1	2	4	12	19	23.7	3.9	0.91	12.8	C54-55
Ovary	28	0	86	-	-	1	4	5	7	11	16.6	2.7	0.76	10.3	C56
Placenta	1	0	100	-	-	1	-	-	-	-	0.6	0.1	0.04	0.5	C58
Kidney	6	0	83	-	-	-	1	1	-	4	3.6	0.6	0.09	2.0	C64
Renal pelvis, ureter and other urinary	2	0	100	-	-	-	-	-	-	2	1.2	0.2	0.00	0.5	C65-66,C68
Bladder	32	0	78	-	-	-	-	1	7	22	19.0	3.1	0.45	9.1	C67
Eye	0	0	-	-	-	-	-	-	-	-	0.0	0.0	0.00	0.0	C69
Brain, nervous system	24	0	50	2	1	-	1	5	4	11	14.2	2.4	0.62	10.2	C70-72
Thyroid	7	0	71	-	-	1	-	2	-	4	4.1	0.7	0.13	2.5	C73
Hodgkin disease	5	0	100	-	-	-	1	1	-	1	3.0	0.5	0.18	2.8	C81
Non-Hodgkin lymphoma	19	0	79	-	-	-	2	-	4	12	11.3	1.9	0.32	5.7	C82-85,C96
Multiple myeloma	8	1	63	-	-	-	-	-	-	6	4.7	0.8	0.05	2.0	C90
Lymphoid leukaemia	5	0	100	1	-	-	-	-	-	4	3.0	0.5	0.05	2.2	C91
Myeloid leukaemia	7	0	86	-	-	-	1	1	1	4	4.1	0.7	0.13	2.3	C92-94
Leukaemia, unspecified	0	0	-	-	-	-	-	-	-	-	0.0	0.0	0.00	0.0	C95
Other and unspecified	55	1	38	-	1	-	1	5	13	35	32.6	5.4	0.88	16.0	O&U
All sites	2057	41	87	5	12	62	173	319	463	982	1219.4	100.0	47.33	703.5	ALL
All sites but C44	1021	14	75	3	7	26	77	146	217	531	605.3	-	21.68	340.3	ALLbC44
Average annual population				3275	2558	3024	2785	2925	2687	3832					

Warning, percentages will be distored because of the high rates for 'Other skin cancer'

Table 6. Zimbabwe, Bulawayo: childhood cancer (Skinner, 1988)

Cancer	Bulawayo, 1963–77 (all cases)		Bulawayo, 1963–77 (residents only)		
	No.	%	No.	%	ASR (per million)
Leukaemia	78	14.4%	15	19.2%	16.1
Acute lymphocytic leukaemia	30	5.5%			
Lymphoma	83	15.3%	14	17.9%	14.6
Burkitt lymphoma	19	3.5%			
Hodgkin disease					
Brain and spinal neoplasms	38	7.0%	14	17.9%	14.8
Neuroblastoma	19	3.5%	7	9.0%	8.0
Retinoblastoma	77	14.2%	5	6.4%	5.9
Wilms tumour	69	12.7%	7	9.0%	8.3
Bone tumours	22	4.1%	2	2.6%	2.0
Soft-tissue sarcomas	75	13.8%	8	10.3%	8.6
Kaposi sarcoma					
Other	82	15.1%	6	7.7%	6.8
Total	543	100.0%	78	100.0%	85.1

Table 7. Childhood cancer, Zimbabwe, Harare: African (1990-1997)

	NUMBER OF CASES					REL. FREQ.(%)	RATES PER MILLION					
	0-4	5-9	10-14	All	M/F	Overall	0-4	5-9	10-14	Crude	ASR	%MV
Leukaemia	17	31	27	75	1.2	19.4	12.6	27.0	27.5	21.6	21.6	94.1
Acute lymphoid leukaemia	11	20	10	41	1.7	10.6	8.2	17.4	10.2	11.8	11.8	95.1
Lymphoma	13	21	14	48	2.2	12.4	9.7	18.3	14.3	13.8	13.8	86.2
Hodgkin disease	2	4	7	13	2.3	3.4	1.5	3.5	7.1	3.7	3.8	92.3
Burkitt lymphoma	2	4	0	6	1.0	1.6	1.5	3.5	-	1.7	1.7	100.0
Brain and spinal neoplasms	12	10	19	41	1.2	10.6	8.9	8.7	19.4	11.8	11.9	53.7
Neuroblastoma	8	3	1	12	1.4	3.1	5.9	2.6	1.0	3.5	3.4	75.0
Retinoblastoma	31	5	1	37	1.8	9.6	23.0	4.4	1.0	10.7	10.6	89.2
Wilms tumour	34	13	2	49	0.8	12.7	25.3	11.3	2.0	14.1	14.0	95.9
Bone tumours	2	1	11	14	1.8	3.6	1.5	0.9	11.2	4.0	4.1	85.7
Soft tissue sarcomas	27	16	6	49	1.7	12.7	20.1	14.0	6.1	14.1	14.0	100.0
Kaposi sarcoma	21	11	4	36	2.6	9.3	15.6	9.6	4.1	10.4	10.3	75.0
Germ cell tumours	2	4	1	7	0.2	1.8	1.5	3.5	1.0	2.0	2.0	100.0
Other	8	13	33	54	0.9	14.0	5.9	11.3	33.7	15.5	15.7	57.4
All	154	117	115	386	1.3	100.0	114.4	102.1	117.3	111.1	111.3	81.6

3.5 Southern Africa

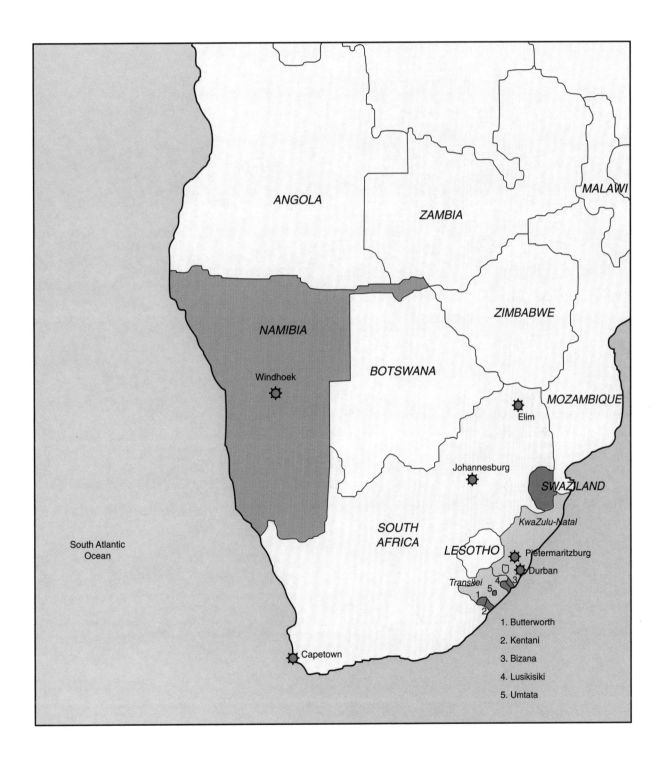

3.5.1 Botswana

Background

Climate: Semi-arid with rainfall ranging from 63 cm in the north-east to 13 cm per year in the south-west.

Terrain: Predominantly flat to gently rolling. The Kalahari desert in the south-west is the largest land area. The lowest altitude is 513 m and the highest 1489 m.

Ethnic groups: Batswana (Bantu) 95%, Khoisan and other 4%, white 1%

Religions: Indigenous beliefs 50%, Christian 50%

Economy—overview: Agriculture provides a livelihood for more than 80% of the population and subsistence farming and cattle-raising predominate. Agriculture is hindered by erratic rainfall and poor soils. The proportion of arable land is 1%. Agriculture supplies about 50% of food needs and accounts for 4% of GDP.

Substantial diamond deposits were found in the 1970s and the mining sector grew to 35% of GDP in 1997. Other industries contribute 10% of GDP. Additional minerals include copper, nickel, salt, soda ash, potash, coal, iron ore and silver. Tourism and other services account for 51% of the GDP (1997 est.).

Industries: Diamonds, copper, nickel, coal, salt, soda ash, potash; livestock processing

Agriculture—products: Sorghum, corn, millet, pulses, groundnuts (peanuts), beans, cowpeas, sunflower seed; livestock

Cancer registration

No formal cancer registry existed in Botswana until 1999. There has been some recent interest in establishing population-based cancer registration in Botswana, but to date no data have been forthcoming.

Review of data

Macrae and Cook (1975) reviewed about 330 000 records of all 10 hospitals in Botswana between 1960 and 1972 and recorded 1445 patients admitted with a cancer. About 40% of the cases were confirmed by microscopy (Table 1). In men, the leading cancers were liver (comprising 16.5% of all male cancers), oesophagus (10.3%), non-melanoma skin cancers (8.1%) and prostate cancer (7.4%). In women, cervix cancer (35.4%) and breast cancer (11.4%) were dominant. Kaposi sarcoma was rare.

Numbers are small but certain contrasting patterns by area and ethnic group were observed; for instance oesophageal cancer was common in the Barolong tribe (5/9 cancers) but rare (1/45) in the Bamangwato tribe. Skin cancer appears more common in people from the Kalahari desert and penile cancers more common in Ngamiland. By contrast, cancer of the cervix appears less common in the same disrtict. The authors noted a decline in connective tissue cancers in males, but not in females between the periods 1964–66 and 1970–72.

Mohapatra and Vyas (1982) reviewed the records of the public pathology laboratory in Gaborone from 1978–82 and documented the distribution of 703 cancers. No breakdown by sex was given. The most common cancers reported were cervix uteri (26.7%), skin (21.6%), breast (8.1%), liver (5.5%) and oesophagus (5.5%). No cases of Kaposi sarcoma were mentioned; they were probably included under connective tissue cancers. Notably, 13/15 eye cancers were of the conjunctiva, and three were retinoblastomas.

References

Macrae, S.M. & Cook, B.V. (1975) A retrospective study of the cancer patterns among hospital in-patients in Botswana 1960-1972. *Br. J. Cancer*, **32**, 121–133

Mohapatra, K.C. & Vyas, P.R. (1982) Incidence of malignant tumours in Botswana. (Paper read at the A.G.M. of the Medical and Dental Association of Botswana 30 July 1982). Botshelo, **13**(4), 48–50

Table 1. Botswana: case series

Site	10 Hospitals 1960–72 (Macrae & Cook, 1975)					Pathology laboratory, Gaborone, 1978–82 (Mohapatra & Vyas,1982)		
	Male		Female		%HV	Both sexes		%HV
	No.	%	No.	%		No.	%	
Oral cavity[1]	16	2.5%	11	1.4%	63	27	3.8	
Nasopharynx	5	0.8%	3	0.4%	50			
Other pharynx	10	1.5%	3	0.4%	69.2			
Oesophagus	67	10.3%	11	1.4%	29.5	39	5.5%	
Stomach	36	5.5%	18	2.3%	5.6	2	0.3%	
Colon/rectum	17	2.6%	12	1.5%	34.5	16	2.3%	
Liver	108	16.5%	35	4.5%	14	39	5.5%	
Pancreas	7	1.1%	5	0.6%	0	2	0.3%	
Lung	17	2.6%	4	0.5%	38.1	26	3.7%	
Melanoma	23	3.5%	24	3.1%	61.7			
Other skin	53	8.1%	32	4.1%	69.4	152	21.6%	
Kaposi sarcoma	6	0.9%	2	0.3%	75			
Breast	7	1.1%	89	11.4%	46.9	57	8.1%	
Cervix uteri			277	35.4%	6.1	188	26.7%	
Corpus uteri			49	6.3%	34.7	9	1.3%	
Ovary etc.			37	4.7%	45.9	12	1.7%	
Prostate	48	7.4%			35.4	6	0.9%	
Penis	26	4.0%			65.4	4	0.6%	
Bladder	14	2.1%	6	0.8%	25	3	0.4%	
Kidney etc.	7	1.1%	6	0.8%	53.8	12	1.7%	
Eye	15	2.3%	16	2.0%	54.8	15	2.1%	
Brain, nervous system	2	0.3%	0	0.0%	100			
Thyroid	2	0.3%	7	0.9%	55.6			
Non-Hodgkin lymphoma	17	2.6%	10	1.3%	63	16	2.3%	
Hodgkin disease			-			13	1.8%	
Myeloma	1	0.2%	1	0.1%	50	0	0.0%	
Leukaemia	27	4.1%	22	2.8%	32.7	30	4.3%	
ALL SITES	653	100.0%	783	100.0%	39.6	703	100.0%	

[1] Includes salivary gland

3.5.2 Lesotho

Background

Climate: Temperate; cool to cold dry winters; hot, wet summers

Terrain: Mostly highland with plateau, hills and mountains, the lowest point being 1400 m and the highest 3482 m.

Ethnic groups: Sotho 99.7%, Europeans 1600, Asians 800

Religions: Christian 80%, rest indigenous beliefs

Economy—overview: Small, landlocked and mountainous, Lesotho has no important natural resources other than water. Its economy is based on agriculture, light manufacturing, and remittances from miners employed in South Africa. The number of such mine workers has declined steadily in recent years; in 1996 their remittances added about 33% to GDP compared with about 67% in 1990. Manufacturing depends largely on farm products which support the milling, canning, leather, and jute industries. Sale of water to South Africa generates some income. Civil disorder and a South African incursion to restore order in 1998 destroyed 80% of the commercial infrastructure in Maseru and two other major towns.

Industries: Food, beverages, textiles, handicrafts construction and tourism.

Agriculture—products: corn, wheat, pulses, sorghum, barley; livestock.

Cancer registration

There has been no systematic cancer registration in Lesotho.

Review of data

Martin *et al.* (1976) described cancer patterns in Lesotho between 1950 and 1969, by scrutinizing the record books of 16 hospitals and one clinic. A total of 586 males and 1281 females with cancer were recorded (Table 1). The proportion of histologically verified cancers was 10%. The leading five cancers in males were: liver (24.6%), stomach (9.0%), oesophagus (7.3%), unspecified sarcomas (6.1%) and lung cancer (5.6%). In females the five leading cancers were cervix (54.9%), breast (14.3%), liver (5.5%), stomach (2.8%) and unspecified sarcomas (2.7%).

MacCormick (1989) attempted to measure the occurrence of oesophageal cancer in Lesotho, after gastroscopy was introduced in the main hospital of the capital city, Maseru. Forty-two carcinomas of the oesophagus were diagnosed in a year, versus 52 cases reported by Martin *et al.* over a 20-year period (1950–69, see Table 1).

References

MacCormick, R.E. (1989) The changing incidence of cancer of the oesophagus in Lesotho. Real, or improved diagnostic ability. *E. Afr. Med. J.*, **65**, 27–30

Martin, P.M.D., Perry, J.W.B. & Keen, P. (1976) The cancer spectrum in Lesotho. *S. Afr. J. Sci.*, **72**, 168–175

Table 1. Lesotho: case series

Site	Hospital records 1950–69 (Martin *et al.*, 1976)				%HV
	Male		Female		
	No.	%	No.	%	
Oral cavity					
Nasopharynx					
Other pharynx					
Oesophagus	43	7.3%	9	0.7%	
Stomach	53	9.0%	36	2.8%	
Colon/rectum	17	2.9%	22	1.7%	
Liver	144	24.6%	71	5.5%	
Pancreas					
Lung	33	5.6%	9	0.7%	
Melanoma	14	2.4%	14	1.1%	
Other skin	15	2.6%	6	0.5%	
Kaposi sarcoma					
Breast	6	1.0%	183	14.3%	
Cervix uteri			703	54.9%	
Corpus uteri			0	0.0%	
Ovary etc.			0	0.0%	
Prostate				0.0%	
Penis	20	3.4%		0.0%	
Bladder	11	1.9%	5	0.4%	
Kidney etc.	5	0.9%	5	0.4%	
Eye					
Brain, nervous system					
Thyroid					
Non-Hodgkin lymphoma					
Hodgkin disease					
Myeloma					
Leukaemia	11	1.9%	5	0.4%	
ALL SITES	586	100.0%	1281	100.0%	10%

3.5.3 Namibia

Background

Climate: Hot and dry with sparse and erratic rainfall.

Terrain: Mainly high plateau with the Namib Desert along the entire Atlantic coast and the Kalahari Desert bordering Botswana and South Africa in the east. The highest point is 2606 m. There are no significant water bodies.

Ethnic groups: Black 86%, white 6.6% and mixed race 7.4%. About 50% of the black population belong to the Ovambo and 9% to the Kavango tribe; other ethnic groups are: Herero 7%, Damara 7%, Nama 5%, Caprivian 4%, Bushmen (San) 3%, Baster 2% and Tswana 0.5%

Religions: Christian (80–90%), about half Lutheran. Other indigenous beliefs comprise 10–20%.

Economy—overview: closely linked to South Africa. Extraction and processing of minerals account for 20% of GDP. Namibia is the fourth largest exporter of non-fuel minerals in Africa and the world's fifth-largest producer of uranium. Half of the population depends on agriculture (largely subsistence agriculture) for its livelihood. Services comprise 55% of GDP. The majority of the people live in poverty because of the inequality of income distribution, with foreigners taking a large share.

Industries: Meat packing, fish processing, dairy products; mining (diamonds, lead, zinc, tin, silver, tungsten, uranium, copper)

Agriculture—products: millet, sorghum, peanuts; livestock; fish

Cancer registration

In 1994, concern about potential cancer risks in a uranium mine led to the registration of all cancers diagnosed by the only central pathology service in Namibia. Cancers diagnosed between 1978 and 1995 were recorded. Data quality was poor and most records had no information on race or ethnic origin. The data are now maintained by the National Cancer Registry in Windhoek, under the auspices of the Cancer Society. In addition to some cases diagnosed in the pathology service, cases attending the oncology services (radiotherapy) in Windhoek are registered.

Review of data

Data from the National Cancer Registry for the period 1995–98 are shown (Table 1). Because the registry is situated in Windhoek, it is likely that registration is most complete for the central districts of the country. However, it has proved difficult to accurately record place of residence of cancer cases, so that data for the whole country are shown. In addition, the registry relies heavily upon histologically diagnosed cases (96% of the cases were registered with a diagnosis confirmed by histology or cytology), so that the more affluent white population is likely to be over-represented. Calculated incidence rates therefore represent minimum, and possibly somewhat biased, estimates of the true values.

The age-adjusted incidence rate was 141.9 per 100 000 in males and 120.2 per 100 000 in females (including skin cancer). Overall, the most commonly diagnosed malignancy was non-melanoma skin cancer and these basal and squamous cell skin cancers are disproportionately found among whites. Excluding these, the most common cancers in men are prostate (17.6%, ASR 21.8), mouth, including lip (13.3%, ASR 15.4), Kaposi sarcoma (7.9%, ASR 6.8), larynx (5.7%, ASR 6.8), oesophagus (5.4%, ASR 6.3) and lung (5.2%, ASR 6.1). In females, the leading cancers (excluding non-melanoma skin cancers) were breast (25.1%, ASR 25.6) (again probably distorted by greater access of whites to histopathology), cervix uteri (22.1%, ASR 22.2), and mouth (6.2%, ASR 6.5). Kaposi sarcoma is rather less frequent in women than in men (sex ratio 3:1); it accounted for 2.6% of cancers, with an ASR of 1.9.

Childhood cancer

Wessels and Hesseling (1996) reported data on the frequency of childhood cancers in Namibia from 1983 to 1988. Data were drawn from Tygerberg Hospital's Tumour Registry in the Western Cape, South Africa (the hospital of choice for most Namibian public sector patients), and from scrutiny of the records of all Namibian District, central and referral hospitals and death certificates. Of these tumours, 91% were histologically verified. Wessels *et al.* (1998) updated these results with a further four years' data, collected for Windhoek Central Hospital, where all children with cancer in Namibia have been treated since 1989. 93.4% of the 241 cases were histologically verified. The pattern is similar to that for the earlier period (Table 2). Incidence rates for the 10-year period 1983–92 were calculated, but they are low, suggesting a fair degree of underdiagnosis of childhood cancer in this widely dispersed population.

The results from the cancer registry for the period 1995–98 are shown in Table 3. The cases are virtually all histologically confirmed and rates are very low. Clearly childhood cancer diagnoses are not being found by the registry.

The results in Table 3, where brain cancer in children comprises only 1% of childhood cancers, contrast with those from the histopathology register (Table 2), with over 16%. Notably, four cases of Kaposi sarcoma and ten of Burkitt lymphoma were recorded in the later pathology series (versus none mentioned in the first).

References

Wessels, G. & Hesseling, P.B. (1996) Unusual distribution of childhood cancer in Namibia. *Pediat. Hematol. Oncol.*, **13**, 9–20

Wessels, G., Hesseling, P.B. & Kuit, S.B. (1998) Namibia. The Namibian Children's Tumour Registry, 1983–1992. In: Parkin, D.M., Kramárová, E., Draper, G.J., Masuyer, E., Michaelis, J., Neglia, J, Qureshi, S. & Stiller, C.A., eds, *International Incidence of Childhood Cancer*, vol. II (IARC Scientific Publications No. 144), Lyon, IARC, pp. 39–41

Table 1. Namibia (1995-1998)

NUMBER OF CASES BY AGE GROUP AND SUMMARY RATES OF INCIDENCE - MALE

SITE	ALL AGES	AGE UNK	MV (%)	0-	15-	25-	35-	45-	55-	65+	CRUDE RATE	%	CR 64	ASR (W)	ICD (10th)
Mouth	265	0	93	-	2	1	19	68	76	99	8.3	13.3	0.97	15.4	C00-06
Salivary gland	18	0	94	-	1	2	1	2	7	5	0.6	0.9	0.07	0.9	C07-08
Nasopharynx	22	0	100	1	2	-	5	4	2	8	0.7	1.1	0.06	1.1	C11
Other pharynx	74	0	99	-	-	-	4	19	23	28	2.3	3.7	0.28	4.4	C09-10,C12-14
Oesophagus	107	0	98	-	-	-	6	21	32	48	3.4	5.4	0.36	6.3	C15
Stomach	49	0	96	-	-	2	9	8	11	19	1.5	2.5	0.15	2.7	C16
Colon, rectum and anus	85	0	96	-	9	3	14	16	21	22	2.7	4.3	0.30	4.4	C18-21
Liver	59	0	85	-	1	3	9	11	16	19	1.9	3.0	0.21	3.2	C22
Gallbladder etc.	6	0	67	-	-	-	2	1	2	1	0.2	0.3	0.02	0.3	C23-24
Pancreas	21	0	76	-	-	-	1	5	7	8	0.7	1.1	0.09	1.3	C25
Larynx	114	0	99	-	-	-	3	32	34	45	3.6	5.7	0.43	6.8	C32
Trachea, bronchus and lung	104	0	87	-	-	-	6	20	38	40	3.3	5.2	0.40	6.1	C33-34
Bone	26	0	100	4	10	-	2	2	3	5	0.8	1.3	0.06	1.0	C40-41
Melanoma of skin	65	0	98	-	-	7	10	6	23	19	2.0	3.3	0.24	3.5	C43
Other skin	588	0	100	4	14	23	80	107	159	201	18.5		2.05	32.5	C44
Mesothelioma	4	0	100	-	-	-	-	1	1	2	0.1	0.2	0.01	0.2	C45
Kaposi sarcoma	158	0	94	6	6	43	42	25	21	15	5.0	7.9	0.53	6.8	C46
Peripheral nerves	2	0	100	1	-	1	-	-	-	-	0.1	0.1	0.00	0.1	C47
Connective and soft tissue	42	0	98	5	6	7	4	4	12	4	1.3	2.1	0.15	1.8	C49
Breast	20	0	95	-	1	-	2	1	4	11	0.6	1.0	0.05	1.1	C50
Penis	14	0	100	-	-	-	-	6	4	4	0.4	0.7	0.06	0.8	C60
Prostate	352	0	97	1	1	-	5	31	90	224	11.1	17.6	0.87	21.8	C61
Testis	23	0	91	-	7	6	3	4	2	1	0.7	1.2	0.07	0.9	C62
Kidney	32	0	94	3	-	4	5	3	11	6	1.0	1.6	0.12	1.6	C64
Renal pelvis, ureter and other urinary		0	-	-	-	-	-	-	-	-	0.0	0.0	0.00	0.0	C65-66,C68
Bladder	60	0	98	-	1	3	5	9	16	26	1.9	3.0	0.18	3.4	C67
Eye	45	0	98	5	3	14	9	3	7	4	1.4	2.3	0.14	1.8	C69
Brain, nervous system	3	0	67	1	1	-	-	1	-	-	0.1	0.2	0.01	0.1	C70-72
Thyroid	9	0	100	1	1	-	2	3	-	2	0.3	0.5	0.02	0.4	C73
Hodgkin disease	15	0	100	2	5	2	-	2	2	2	0.5	0.8	0.04	0.6	C81
Non-Hodgkin lymphoma	54	0	96	7	4	10	8	3	9	9	1.7	2.7	0.17	2.4	C82-85,C96
Multiple myeloma	12	0	92	-	-	-	1	3	2	6	0.4	0.6	0.03	0.7	C90
Lymphoid leukaemia	20	0	100	3	1	2	3	4	3	7	0.6	1.0	0.06	1.0	C91
Myeloid leukaemia	21	0	100	1	3	4	-	3	4	4	0.7	1.1	0.06	0.9	C92-94
Leukaemia, unspecified	1	0	100	-	-	-	-	-	-	-	0.0	0.1	0.00	0.0	C95
Other and unspecified	95	0	97	3	7	3	6	13	23	40	3.0	4.8	0.28	5.3	O&U
All sites	2585	0	96	47	85	141	267	445	666	934	81.3	100.0	8.56	141.9	ALL
All sites but C44	1997	0	95	43	71	118	187	338	507	733	62.8	100.0	6.51	109.4	ALLbC44

| Average annual population | | | | 338924 | 155556 | 110514 | 76641 | 51770 | 34199 | 27161 | | | | | |

Table 1. Namibia (1995-1998)

NUMBER OF CASES BY AGE GROUP AND SUMMARY RATES OF INCIDENCE - FEMALE

SITE	ALL AGES	AGE UNK	MV (%)	0-	15-	25-	35-	45-	55-	65+	CRUDE RATE	%	CR 64	ASR (W)	ICD (10th)
Mouth	130	0	96	-	1	5	7	21	44	52	4.1	6.2	0.42	6.5	C00-06
Salivary gland	16	0	94	-	-	2	1	3	5	4	0.5	0.8	0.06	0.8	C07-08
Nasopharynx	14	0	100	-	6	1	1	1	2	3	0.4	0.7	0.03	0.5	C11
Other pharynx	26	0	96	-	-	1	1	5	10	9	0.8	1.2	0.10	1.3	C09-10,C12-14
Oesophagus	33	0	100	-	-	-	2	2	7	21	1.0	1.6	0.07	1.7	C15
Stomach	37	0	97	-	-	3	2	4	5	18	1.2	1.8	0.08	1.8	C16
Colon, rectum and anus	67	0	99	2	1	2	7	11	19	25	2.1	3.2	0.21	3.3	C18-21
Liver	37	0	89	-	1	1	6	5	9	15	1.2	1.8	0.11	1.8	C22
Gallbladder etc.	15	0	93	-	-	-	3	1	6	5	0.5	0.7	0.05	0.7	C23-24
Pancreas	19	0	79	-	-	2	2	3	5	7	0.6	0.9	0.06	0.9	C25
Larynx	22	0	100	-	-	1	2	7	10	5	0.7	1.0	0.10	1.1	C32
Trachea, bronchus and lung	45	0	96	-	1	3	2	13	18	10	1.4	2.1	0.19	2.3	C33-34
Bone	17	0	88	3	7	3	-	1	3	1	0.5	0.8	0.04	0.6	C40-41
Melanoma of skin	53	0	100	-	-	5	9	12	12	14	1.7	2.5	0.17	2.4	C43
Other skin	438	0	100	5	13	33	43	57	116	171	13.7		1.27	21.1	C44
Mesothelioma	0	0	-	-	-	-	-	-	-	-	0.0	0.0	0.00	0.0	C45
Kaposi sarcoma	54	0	98	4	8	23	10	3	2	4	1.7	2.6	0.13	1.9	C46
Peripheral nerves	2	0	100	-	-	-	1	-	-	1	0.1	0.1	0.00	0.1	C47
Connective and soft tissue	42	0	100	4	8	6	10	5	6	3	1.3	2.0	0.13	1.6	C49
Breast	531	0	95	-	3	31	97	119	119	162	16.6	25.1	1.73	25.6	C50
Vulva	19	0	100	-	-	3	7	-	5	4	0.6	0.9	0.06	0.8	C51
Vagina	5	0	100	-	1	-	2	-	-	1	0.2	0.2	0.01	0.2	C52
Cervix uteri	468	0	98	-	2	26	96	121	106	117	14.6	22.1	1.60	22.2	C53
Uterus	67	0	96	-	3	4	5	13	23	19	2.1	3.2	0.25	3.3	C54-55
Ovary	74	0	86	1	5	7	8	10	22	21	2.3	3.5	0.25	3.5	C56
Placenta	11	0	91	-	4	5	1	1	-	-	0.3	0.5	0.03	0.4	C58
Kidney	26	0	88	4	-	3	5	4	5	5	0.8	1.2	0.08	1.1	C64
Renal pelvis, ureter and other urinary	3	0	100	1	-	-	1	-	-	-	0.1	0.1	0.01	0.1	C65-66,C68
Bladder	20	0	100	1	2	2	1	3	4	7	0.6	0.9	0.05	0.9	C67
Eye	42	0	98	8	1	13	9	5	5	1	1.3	2.0	0.13	1.6	C69
Brain, nervous system	7	0	43	1	-	2	2	2	2	-	0.2	0.3	0.03	0.3	C70-72
Thyroid	37	0	95	-	-	5	11	1	7	13	1.2	1.8	0.10	1.7	C73
Hodgkin disease	9	0	100	-	-	2	2	5	-	-	0.3	0.4	0.03	0.4	C81
Non-Hodgkin lymphoma	36	0	100	1	-	7	4	5	6	13	1.1	1.7	0.09	1.7	C82-85,C96
Multiple myeloma	16	0	94	-	1	-	1	2	6	6	0.5	0.8	0.05	0.8	C90
Lymphoid leukaemia	9	0	100	-	1	1	2	-	2	2	0.3	0.4	0.03	0.4	C91
Myeloid leukaemia	19	0	95	1	3	1	5	3	5	1	0.6	0.9	0.07	0.8	C92-94
Leukaemia, unspecified	1	0	100	-	-	-	-	-	-	1	0.0	0.0	0.00	0.1	C95
Other and unspecified	84	0	98	1	1	6	7	15	23	31	2.6	4.0	0.26	4.1	O&U
All sites	2551	0	97	36	76	207	377	464	619	772	79.6	100.0	8.08	120.2	ALL
All sites but C44	2113	0	96	31	63	174	334	407	503	601	65.9	100.0	6.80	99.1	ALLbC44
Average annual population				332033	153823	110578	77794	55746	38289	33379					

Table 2. Namibia: childhood cancer

Cancer	1983–88 (Wessels & Hesseling,1996)		1983–92 (Wessels *et al.*, 1998)		
	No.	%	No.	%	ASR per 10⁵
Leukaemia	19	11.5%	33	13.7%	6.2
Acute lymphocytic leukaemia			24	10.0%	4.5
Lymphoma	19	11.5%	31	12.9%	5.8
Burkitt lymphoma			10	4.1%	1.9
Hodgkin disease			11	4.6%	2
Brain and spinal neoplasms	28	17.0%	39	16.2%	7.3
Neuroblastoma	14	8.5%	18	7.5%	3.6
Retinoblastoma	16	9.7%	22	9.1%	4.5
Wilms tumour	21	12.7%	30	12.4%	6
Bone tumours	15	9.1%	19	7.9%	3.4
Soft-tissue sarcomas	16	9.7%	25	10.4%	4.6
Kaposi sarcoma	0	0.0%	4	1.7%	0.7
Other	17	10.3%	24	10.0%	4.5
Total	165	100.0%	241	100.0%	45.9

Table 3. Childhood cancer, Namibia (1995-1998)

	NUMBER OF CASES					REL. FREQ.(%)	RATES PER MILLION					
	0-4	5-9	10-14	**All**	*M/F*	Overall	0-4	5-9	10-14	Crude	**ASR**	%MV
Leukaemia	1	0	4	**5**	*4.0*	6.0	1.0	-	5.2	1.9	**1.9**	100.0
Acute lymphoid leukaemia	0	0	0	**0**	-	-	-	-	-	-	**-**	-
Lymphoma	0	1	9	**10**	*9.0*	12.0	-	1.1	11.6	3.7	**3.7**	80.0
Hodgkin disease	0	0	2	**2**	-	2.4	-	-	2.6	0.7	**0.7**	100.0
Burkitt lymphoma	0	1	2	**3**	*2.0*	3.6	-	1.1	2.6	1.1	**1.1**	100.0
Brain and spinal neoplasms	0	1	0	**1**	-	1.2	-	1.1	-	0.4	**0.4**	100.0
Neuroblastoma	1	0	0	**1**	-	1.2	1.0	-	-	0.4	**0.4**	100.0
Retinoblastoma	8	2	1	**11**	*0.6*	13.3	7.9	2.2	1.3	4.1	**4.1**	100.0
Wilms tumour	6	0	1	**7**	*0.8*	8.4	5.9	-	1.3	2.6	**2.7**	100.0
Bone tumours	0	1	6	**7**	*1.3*	8.4	-	1.1	7.7	2.6	**2.6**	85.7
Soft tissue sarcomas	8	5	5	**18**	*1.6*	21.7	7.9	5.6	6.4	6.7	**6.7**	100.0
Kaposi sarcoma	7	2	1	**10**	*1.5*	12.0	6.9	2.2	1.3	3.7	**3.8**	100.0
Germ cell tumours	1	0	2	**3**	-	3.6	1.0	-	2.6	1.1	**1.1**	100.0
Other	6	5	9	**20**	*1.2*	24.1	5.9	5.6	11.6	7.5	**7.5**	100.0
All	31	15	37	**83**	*1.3*	100.0	30.5	16.8	47.7	30.9	**31.1**	97.6

3.5.4 South Africa

South Africa has nine provinces: Northern Province, Mpumalanga, Gauteng, North West Province, KwaZulu-Natal, Free State, Eastern Cape (comprising the former Transkei 'homeland', an area of high oesophageal cancer rates) and the Western Cape. Provinces are divided into magisterial districts.

Climate: Mostly semi-arid; subtropical along the east coast and Mediterranean along the south-western coast

Terrain: An interior plateau, rugged hills and a narrow coastal plain

Ethnic groups: Black (African) 75.2%, white (mainly of European descent) 13.6%, coloured (mixed race) 8.6%, and of Indian/East Asian descent, 2.6%

Religions: Christian 68% (includes most whites and coloureds, about 60% of blacks and about 40% of Indians), Muslim 2%, Hindu 1.5% (60% of Indians), indigenous beliefs and animist 28.5%

Economy—overview: A middle-income developing country with abundant resources, South Africa has well developed financial, legal, information technology, communications, energy and transport sectors.

Industries: Mining of gold, chromium, antimony, coal, iron ore, manganese, nickel, phosphates, tin, uranium, gem diamonds, platinum, copper and vanadium. South Africa was a main producer of all the main types of asbestos, but most operations have now ceased.

Cancer registration
Early attempts to describe the occurrence of cancer in the then Natal and Zululand were made by Watkins Pitchford (1925). These early attempts were reviewed by Oettlé (1960).

Population-based cancer registries using standardized methodology were established in Johannesburg in 1953–55 (Higginson & Oettlé, 1966), in the Cape Peninsula 1956–58 (Muir Grieve, 1967) and in Natal (Schonland & Bradshaw, 1968).

Johannesburg
The Johannesburg Cancer Survey was conducted in 1953–55 by the South African Institute for Medical Research. Cases were registered by medical staff from hospital inpatients, and all case histories were reviewed by the survey directors. Records from radiotherapy and pathology departments and death certificates were also screened. Hospital outpatients were not registered except at a single large clinic at Alexandra Township, where registrations were made by doctors. Doctors attending cases at home were paid for each registration made. Pathologists in medico-legal departments also registered cases.

The Registry covered the metropolitan area of Johannesburg, consisting of the municipal area, and the peri-urban townships, notably Alexandra township in the north-east and a cluster of townships in the south-west. (total populated area 280 km²); the population at the time was 800 000.

Cape Province
The Registry was a project of the Cancer Research Unit of Groote Schuur Hospital Observatory, and was mainly supported by the National Cancer Association of South Africa. The records of major hospitals were scrutinized at weekly intervals and those of minor hospitals every fourth week. Liaison was continuously maintained with all health centres, dispensaries, old-age homes and allied institutions. Every medical practitioner was approached by personal visit or by post, and all pathology slides from cancer cases were made available for review. Very strict criteria of diagnosis were established and maintained.

The records of the Registrars of Death were routinely abstracted, a particularly useful source of information, since burial was not permitted without a death certificate issued by a registered medical practitioner. It was estimated that at least 95% of all cases were registered.

The registration area was Cape Division, a small and relatively narrow tract of land some 1887 km² in extent. The urban area, in which over 95% of the population resided, occupied the middle third of this area. The estimated population in 1956–59 was 741 000 (293 000 white, 378 000 mixed race ("coloured") and 70 000 black ("Bantu"). For the calculation of rates, the age/sex/race breakdown was based on the censuses of 1951 and 1960; for the latter, age was available only for a 10% sample. It was considered that the estimated population at risk for the black population was uncertain, because of internal migrations and uncertainty as to the age of older persons.

Natal
The Natal Cancer Morbidity Survey registered all new cases of cancer occurring between 1 January 1964 and 31 December 1966. African and Indian cases were filed separately. The populations covered were the Indian community of the Metropolitan Area of Durban, and Africans resident in the same area and in the Magisterial District of Pietermaritzburg. Some 28% of the Indian population were Muslim, the remainder Hindu. Over 90% of Africans in Durban and Pietermaritzburg were Zulus. Residential criteria for inclusion in the survey area were strictly applied.

Histology, haematology, cytology and post mortem reports, case-notes, radiotherapy records and death certificates were scrutinized and used as sources. Some cases were notified by private practitioners. Histological confirmation of the diagnosis was obtained in 68.5% of all Indian cases and in 82.2% of all African cases. No cases were followed up.

Metropolitan Durban covers an area of 1402 km² and the District of Pietermaritzburg 1078 km². Both had good hospital and diagnostic facilities. Population at risk was estimated from the 1960 census. For the African population, an annual growth rate of 2.65% was assumed for Pietermaritzburg, while an estimate prepared by the Institute of Social Research, incorporating some data on migration, was used for Durban. It was considered that the population at risk for Durban Indians was probably correct, while the 1965 urban African population was "a knowledgeable guess".

Transkei
Ad hoc cancer surveys were also conducted in areas where there was some suspicion of unusual cancer patterns. For example, Burrell (1957, 1962) and Oettlé (1963) described a high occurrence of oesophageal cancer in the Transkei (Eastern Cape), Transkei became the focus of cancer registration and study since these early reports (Rose 1973), and numerous results from cancer registration efforts have been published since then. Between 1964 and 1969, all hospitals in the Transkei and three major referral hospitals in the Natal (now KwaZulu-Natal) Province and from East London, the major radiotherapy centre just outside the Transkei in the Eastern Cape provided cancer data (Rose and Fellingham 1981). A total of 4247 cases of cancer were recorded.

Umtata Cancer Registry: The cancer registry is operated by the department of oncology/thoracic surgery, and is located in Umtata General Hospital, the main referral hospital for the Transkei region of Eastern Cape Province. Oncology nurses are responsible for recording information on all cancer cases diagnosed or treated in the hospital, using ward registers, the department of pathology register, and diagnostic ultrasound as sources of information. Cases resident in Umtata district have been entered into a computerized database (using CANREG-3) since 1996. Case-finding does not include, therefore, those residents of the district who go elsewhere for diagnosis and treatment (e.g., to East London or Durban), although the follow-up of all local patients treated in the radiotherapy service in East London is carried out in Umtata General Hospital.

The PROMEC registry: Cancer registration was established by the Medical Research Council in the Transkei in two low-risk (Bizana and Lusikisiki) and two high-risk districts (Butterworth and Kentani) in 1981. Case-finding is based upon notifications by a designated nurse in each of the major hospitals in the districts. This is supplemented by active case-finding by the cancer registrar. This component involves annual visits to eight hospitals located in the four districts and in certain neighbouring districts, including Umtata Hospital (the regional referral centre). During these visits, ward registers are scrutinized to check completeness of notification, and missing or incomplete records are updated. Case-finding also extends to hospitals outside Transkei, to which cases may have been referred (or presented themselves). These include the regional radiotherapy referral centre in East London and (since 2000) three referral hospitals for surgery, gynaecology and radiotherapy cases in Durban (Kwa-Zulu Natal Province). Details on malignant cancers (excluding cases for which primary site is uncertain or unknown) are abstracted and data entered into a computerized database, using CANREG-3.

National Cancer Registry

In 1986, a national pathology-based cancer registry was established at the South African Institute for Medical Research (now the National Health Laboratory Service) as a collaborative venture with the Cancer Association of South Africa and the Department of Health. All pathology laboratories began submitting data in 1986. Since 1988, all cytology laboratories were included and all of about 85 private and public laboratories submit data (approximately 50 000 new cases per annum) to the NCR. Laboratories are reminded on a monthly basis to submit data or a 'null' return. Pathology reports are screened manually upon receipt and queries about missing information are sent (once) to the referring doctor. Data once coded and entered are checked automatically for further inconsistencies and unlikely combinations. From 1993 onwards, the proportion of cases with unknown race characteristics increased dramatically, making it difficult to establish minimal incidence rates by these groups.

Review of data

Johannesburg, 1953–55
The results are shown in Table 1. In black males, there were moderately elevated rates of liver cancer (ASR 19.3 per 100 000) and oesophageal cancer (ASR 12.4), while the incidence of lung cancer was low (ASR 7.5). In females, the most striking feature is the very high incidence of cervix cancer (ASR 51.0). The rate for breast cancer is much lower (ASR 14.9) and oesophageal cancer is much less frequent than in males (sex ratio, M:F, 10:1).

Cape Province, 1956–59
The results for the black population are shown in Table 2, for the coloured (mixed race) population in Table 3, and for the white population in Table 4.

The numbers of cases registered in the black population are few, but the incidence of cancers of the oesophagus (ASR 35.6), stomach (ASR 26.9), liver (ASR 26.5) and lung (ASR 25.6) appear quite high. In females, the cervix (15 cases, ASR 24.8) is the principal cancer site.

In the coloured (mixed race) population, there are high rates for cancers of the oesophagus (ASR 53.4) and lung (ASR 42.7) in men and for cancers of the cervix (ASR 34.4), breast (ASR 25.8) and oesophagus (ASR 25.5) in women.

In the white population, excluding the very common non-melanoma skin cancers, the highest rates in men are for lung (ASR 44.8), stomach (ASR 32.9) and prostate cancers (ASR 24.2). Oesophageal cancer is not common, the incidence of large bowel cancer being three times higher. In women, breast cancer ranks first (ASR 57.6), followed by stomach (ASR 22.9) and cervix cancers (ASR 22.6).

Natal, 1964–66
The data for 1964–66 are shown in Tables 5 and 6. For the Indian community, this period was considered to be not long enough, as only 496 new cancer cases were registered. The case-finding programme for the Indian group was extended for a further two years (Schonland and Bradshaw, 1970).

With respect to the black population (mainly Zulu) of the Pietermaritzburg District (Table 6), a bias towards cases with histological confirmation of diagnosis was considered probable, as case-finding was mainly based on pathology records, and scrutiny of death certificates of Africans was not possible there. In men, there was very high incidence of lung cancer (ASR 43.4), oesophageal cancer (ASR 40.1), liver cancer (ASR 27.6) and prostate cancer (ASR 21.8). In Black females, the highest incidence rate was for cervix cancer (ASR 48.5); the rates for oesophageal cancer (ASR 12.0) and lung cancer (ASR 10.1) were about one quarter those in men.

In the Durban Indian group (Table 5), 7.3% of male cancers and 13.8% of female cancers were found by scrutiny of death certificates only. The low overall cancer incidence in Indian males was possibly due in part to mis-certification of cause of death (as non-cancerous conditions) by private practitioners. However, it was noted that in Durban, Indian males did not smoke heavily and chewed betel nut only occasionally. Nevertheless, it is remarkable that, for all cancers of the gastrointestinal tract (oral cavity and pharynx, oesophagus, stomach, colon, rectum), incidence in Indian females exceeded that in males. In males, only gastric cancer (ASR 20.9) occurred at all frequently, while in women, the highest rates were for cervix uteri (ASR 34.7) stomach (ASR 29.1), breast (ASR 19.4), oesophagus (ASR 12.7) and corpus uteri (ASR 12.8).

Transkei
Several publications have described the results of past cancer registration efforts in the Transkei, mainly the Xhosa population, in particular with respect to geographical variation and temporal trends in the incidence of oesophageal cancer (see chapter on Oesophagus cancer). Here we present recent data from the two cancer registries in the Transkei district, Umtata registry and the PROMEC rural districts registry.

Umtata: Results for the period 1996–98 are shown (Table 7). Since the registry almost certainly includes a large majority of cases diagnosed among the residents of Umtata district (see above), incidence rates have been calculated using the census data for 1996. 593 cases are included. The overall (all sites) incidence is 141.3 in men and 105.8 in women. In men the principal cancers are oesophagus (ASR 62.5), lung (ASR 15.7) and liver (ASR 16.0); in women, the main cancers are oesophagus (ASR 34.5), cervix uteri (ASR 26.3) and breast (ASR 14.9). Kaposi sarcoma was clearly rare at this time (only one case in a male); the lack of haematological malignancies suggests some under-diagnosis or under-registration.

PROMEC (Bizana, Butterworth, Kentani and Lusikisiki districts): Results for the period 1996–98 are shown (Table 8). The incidence rates have been calculated using an estimate of the population, based upon the census data for 1996. Because of incomplete registration, cases (and population at risk) from Butterworth are omitted for two years (1996, 1997) and from Kentani for one year (1996). 663 cases are included. The overall (all sites) incidence is low – 68.5 in men and 65.4 in women. In men the principal cancers are oesophagus (ASR 37.5), liver (ASR 5.5), lung (ASR 4.9) and prostate (ASR 2.9); in women, the main cancers are oesophagus (ASR 26.5), cervix uteri (ASR 21.7) and breast (ASR 6.1). Only three cases of Kaposi sarcoma were recorded and three cases of leukaemia. The low overall rates and some irregularity in numbers of cases registered by year and district suggest some under-diagnosis and/or under-registration at this time; the small numbers of 'other & unspecified' cancers may partly reflect the exclusion of metastatic cancers from the database.

Early data: Between 1964 and 1969, a total of 4247 cases of cancer were recorded from all hospitals in the Transkei, and three major referral hospitals in the Natal (now KwaZulu-Natal) Province and East London (Rose, 1973).

Overall, the age-standardized cancer incidence rate per 100 000 using the world population standard in males was 102 in the high-risk districts, 59.5 in the moderate-risk districts and 22.4 in the low-risk districts. The rates in moderate-risk districts were similar to those observed in Durban in 1964–66 (ASR 40.7) (Schonland & Bradshaw, 1968) and in Cape Town (ASR 37.5) (Muir Grieve, 1967). Rates for oesophageal cancer in Johannesburg black males were lower (ASR 12.9). Records from Umtata hospital also show a dramatic increase in the relative frequency of oesophageal cancer over all other major cancer types (liver, cervix and breast); in 1925 oesophageal cancer comprised less than 10% of all these cancers, but by 1969 this proportion had increased to just under 60% (Rose & Fellingham, 1981).

In subsequent reports from the Transkei concerning cases diagnosed in 1981–84 (Jaskiewicz *et al.*, 1987) and 1985–90 (Makaula *et al.*, 1996), it appears that the incidence of oesophageal cancer has been declining in the high-risk districts and increasing in the low-risk districts. The reasons for this 'equalization' of oesophageal cancer rates in the Transkei are unclear.

Johannesburg/Soweto
In a study at Baragwanath Hospital, which serves the black population of Johannesburg and Soweto, Robertson (1969) abstracted all the clinical records of 4093 male and 3724 female patients clinically diagnosed with a cancer during 1948–64. Of these cancers, 84% were confirmed by microscopy. An increase in the relative frequency of oesophageal cancer was observed, from 4.8% of all cancers in 1948 to 14.8% in 1964. In females there was little change in relative frequency, which ranged from 2.4% in 1948 to 1.9% in 1964. Between 1966 and 1975, all histologically diagnosed cancers diagnosed at Baragwanath Hospital were recorded but all haematological, eye and pancreatic cancers were omitted (Isaacson *et al.*, 1978). Attempts were made to estimate minimal incidence rates by using the population at risk of Johannesburg and Soweto (Isaacson *et al.*, 1978) or the whole of the Transvaal (Robertson, 1969), but in both studies there was no clear definition of residential status. These differences in methodology limit the comparability of the two studies.

Northern and Eastern Transvaal (Northern Province, Mpumalanga)
Higginson and Oettlé (1960) reported the cancer patterns of 174 black male and 250 female cancer patients attending four rural

hospitals in the North-Eastern Transvaal (now the Northern Province and Mpumalanga): Jane Furse, Elim, Pietersburg and Groothoek. The leading cancers in males were liver (primary), comprising 20.7% of all cancers, lung (7.5%), colon/rectum (7.5%) and prostate (4.6%). In females, the leading cancers were cervix (27.2%), breast (11.2%), liver (6.0%) and melanoma (5.6%). Kaposi sarcoma comprised 2.9% of male and 0.4% of female cancers.

Table 9 shows data collected at Elim Hospital in Northern Province during 1991–94. 567 cases were recorded. In males, the leading cancers were oesophagus (17.7%), mouth (16.5%) and liver (15.6%), while in females, the principal cancers were cervix (39.8%) and breast (12.9%), while oesophagus cancers comprised just 5% of the total. One case of Kaposi sarcoma was recorded among the males (0.4%) and two in females (0.6%).

Sutherland (1968) described high occurrences of cervical, liver and bladder cancers between 1957 and 1966 in Acornhoek, Eastern Transvaal (Mpumalanga Province, near Mozambique) and Berman (1935) described the unusually high occurrence of liver cancer among the black residents of Johannesburg and gold miners.

Studies among miners
Information on patterns of cancer in young black males coming from several areas of the country was derived from studies on a large cohort of miners (5.8 million person-years) in two eight-year periods, 1964–71 (Harington *et al.*, 1975) and 1972–79 (Bradshaw *et al.*, 1982). Overall, the most common cancer in this population was liver cancer, with, among miners from South Africa, the highest incidence in those from Natal. A decline in incidence over time was observed for most groups. Oesophageal cancer was second in importance. The highest rates were in miners from Transkei and Ciskei. In the first period (1964–71), there were wide variations in incidence between miners from different districts in the Transkei (based on a crude person-years calculation of expected values), concurring with the observations of Rose and McGlashan (1975). In the second period, these differences were much less marked, in agreement with the observations of Jaskiewicz *et al.* (1987) and Makaula *et al.* (1996). It also appears that the crude incidence rate of oesophageal cancer was declining gradually among miners from Transkei.

National data
Various publications have presented the results of the National Cancer Registry, including estimates of 'minimum incidence', based on histopathologically diagnosed cancers alone. (National Cancer Registry, 1987, 1988; Sitas *et al.*, 1992, 1994, 1996, 1998). Data from 1989–92 are presented in this report (Tables 10–13).

In blacks, 38 115 in males and 41 691 cancers in females were reported. The ASR per 100 000 for all cancers was 123.7 in males and 109.8 in females. In black males, the leading cancers were oesophagus (ASR 23.1, 19.1%), prostate (ASR 14.3, 9.4%), lung (ASR 11.2, 9.1%), mouth (ASR 8.7, 6.9%) and liver (ASR 5.6, 5.1%); since liver cancer is not often histologically confirmed, many cases are missed. In black females, the leading cancers were cervix (ASR 40.3, 38.1%), breast (ASR 13.6, 12.6%), oesophagus (ASR 9.1, 7.9%) and colorectal and lung cancers (both ASR 2.3, 2.1%).

In whites, 50 815 cancers were recorded in males and 42 767 in females (Table 11). The large number of squamous and basal-cell skin cancers (24 620 in males and 16 448 in females) dominated the picture. Excluding non-melanoma skin cancers, the leading cancers in males were prostate (ASR 41.1, 17% of all cancers), bladder (ASR 25.8, 10.7%), colorectal (ASR 22.0, 9.2%) and lung (ASR 20.3, 8.3%). In white females, the leading cancers were breast (ASR 62.8, 29.6%), colorectal (ASR 17.1, 8.7%), melanoma (ASR 14.2, 6.7%) and cervix (ASR 11.9, 5.6%).

In the mixed race ('coloured'), 5984 cancers in males and 6304 in females were reported (Table 12). Age-standardized incidence rates for all cancer per 100 000 were 177.9 for males and 136.7 for females. In males, the leading sites were prostate (ASR 25.4, 11.8%), lung (ASR 19.2, 10.9%), stomach (ASR 16.1, 9.3%) and oesophagus (ASR 16.0, 9.0%). In females, the leading cancer sites were the cervix (ASR 31.6, 25.5% of all cancers), breast (ASR 28.1, 21.2%), colorectum (ASR 6.4, 4.6%) and stomach (ASR 6.4, 4.6%).

In the Asian (Indian) population (Table 13), 2185 male cancers and 2542 female cancers were reported. The overall age-standardized cancer incidence rates per 100 000 were 172.5 for males and 164.3 for females. In males, the leading cancers were lung (ASR 22.5, 13.6%), colorectum (ASR 14.2, 7.6%), oesophagus (ASR 13.1, 8.4%) and prostate (ASR 13.0, 5.7%). In females the leading cancers were breast (ASR 42.5, 27.9% of all cancers), cervix (ASR 20.2, 13.3%), colorectum (ASR 9.4, 5.3%) and stomach (ASR 6.4, 3.7%).

Mortality studies

Before the 1992 elections, there was almost complete national ascertainment of deaths for the white, coloured and Indian populations (about 98% of the events of death recorded), with less than 10% of deaths recorded with an 'ill-defined' underlying cause of death. Among the black population, about 50% of deaths were recorded, but, of these, 25% were classified as 'ill-defined'. There was, however, wide variation in the proportion of ill-defined conditions and especially in some black urban magisterial districts, the data were of better quality than in the rest of the country (McGlashan, 1985). However valuable these data may be, they tell little of the mortality patterns in the poorer rural areas. Bourne (1995) compiled a list of all available mortality statistics.

In 1990, the former government removed racial categorization from the death notification forms. A new death notification form was introduced in 1998 which again includes the racial category of the deceased, as well as their 'usual' address, main occupation and smoking and pregnancy status, to allow better epidemiological use of death statistics. With the re-incorporation of the former 'homelands' back into South Africa, ascertainment of the event of death has now risen to over 98% in adults, but only about 60% of death notifications have information on the race/population group of the deceased individual.

Bradshaw and Harington (1985) reviewed the available mortality data for South Africa from 1949–79 for whites, coloureds

and Asians and from 1968–77 for blacks residing in 33 selected magisterial areas where mortality statistics were considered more reliable. In the black population, the proportions of deaths in 1977 were 21% due to infectious and parasitic diseases, 14% circulatory disorders and 12% respiratory disease. In contrast, among whites in 1979, only 2% were due to infectious and parasitic diseases, with circulatory disorders accounting for 48% and cancer 17%. In black males, the leading causes of cancer death were oesophageal cancer (29%), lung and liver cancers (both 15%), stomach (7%) and prostate and oral cancer (both 4%). In black females, cancer of the cervix was the leading cancer death (24%), followed by oesophageal (16%), breast (9%) and liver cancer (8%). The main causes of cancer death in white males were lung (29%), prostate, stomach and colorectal (each 9%) and urinary tract cancers (6%). In white females they were breast (20%), colorectal (14%), lung (12%) and stomach cancer (10%).

Over the period 1968–77, age-standardized mortality rates per 100 000 (world standard) for all cancers among males increased in blacks from about 90 to 125, in whites from 120 to 160, in coloureds from 130 to 220 and in Asian/Indians from 105 to 95 (these figures have been read off graphs; actual data were not published). In females, the rates among blacks remained stable at about 100 per 100 000, in whites declined from 118 to 105, in coloureds stable at 110, and in Asian/Indians stable at 80.

Figures 1–5 (from Bradshaw & Harington, 1985) show time trends in mortality rates (cumulative rate, per cent) for five cancer sites.

In black males, there were increases in oesophageal and lung cancer mortality between 1967 and 1977. In females there was a small increase mortality from cancer of the cervix, breast and lung, while stomach cancer mortality declined slightly.

In coloured males, there were dramatic increases in mortality from lung cancer and oesophageal cancer over the period 1949–79, while stomach cancer mortality declined after 1969. In females, mortality from stomach cancer declined throughout the 30-year period, while the rates for both cervix and breast cancer increased.

In white males, lung cancer mortality increased markedly (almost three-fold), while there was a decrease of about the same magnitude in stomach cancer. Mortality from prostate and colorectal

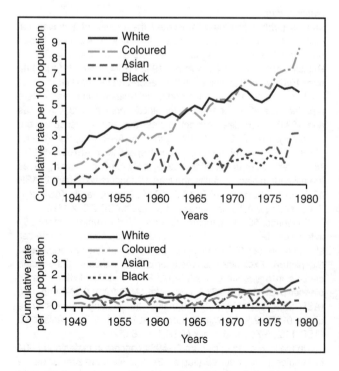

Figure 1. Lung cancer, males (above) and females (below).

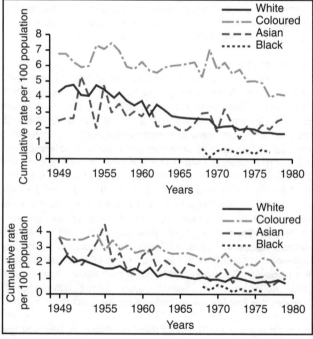

Figure 2. Stomach cancer, males (above) and females (below).

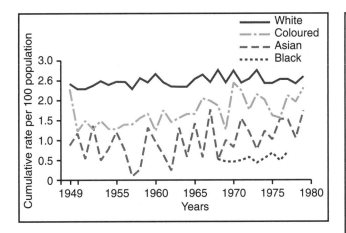

Figure 3. Cancer of the female breast.

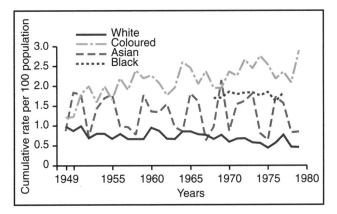

Figure 4. Cancer of the uterine cervix.

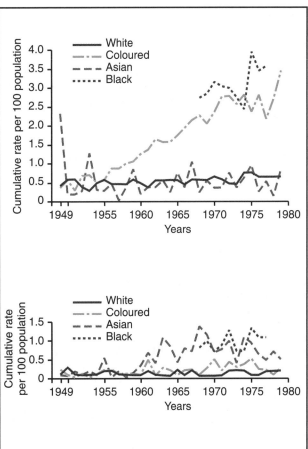

Figure 5. Cancer of the oesophagus, males (above) and females (below).

cancers remained stable. In white females, breast cancer mortality increased slightly, while mortality from lung cancer, although low, more than doubled. Mortality from stomach cancer and from cervix cancer declined. Colorectal cancer mortality remained stable.

The mortality rates in the Asian population show a lot of fluctuation from year to year, because of small numbers of deaths, but there has been an increase in lung cancer mortality in males and breast cancer in females, and decreases in stomach cancer mortality in both sexes.

Other studies
South Africa has one of the highest rates of mesothelioma in the world, because of its long involvement in asbestos mining and processing. A nationwide survey conducted for the period 1976–84 (Zwi *et al.*, 1989) identified 1347 histologically confirmed cases, corresponding to incidence rates per million in those aged 15 years and over for white, coloured, and black males 32.9, 24.8 and 7.6 per million, and in females 8.9, 13.9 and 3.0 respectively. The reasons for the low rates among blacks were thought to be underreporting in this group due to lack of access to diagnostic services. By comparison, mortality for pleural mesothelioma in the United Kingdom was 5 per million in men and 2 per million in women (Gardner *et al.*, 1982). In the Northern Cape, the incidence of mesothelioma among 'white' residents in one town (Prieska), where death certification was relatively complete, was high: 348 and 172 per million for males and females, respectively, and similar to rates in the the Wittenboom district in Australia (267 per million) where asbestos was also mined (Kielkowski *et al.*, 2000).

Kaposi sarcoma (reviewed in Chapter 4.6) was also a relatively rare cancer, although in the northern Transvaal in the 1950s and 1960s it comprised about 2% of all cancers. In the National Cancer Registry data, Kaposi sarcoma comprised only 0.6% of all cancers in black males and 0.2% in black females in 1989-92 (Table 10), suggesting some reduction in its occurrence between the 1960s and the 1980s. However, increases in incidence have been noted since 1992, in keeping with the development of the HIV epidemic (Sitas *et al.*, 1998, Sitas & Newton, 2000).

Summary
In summary, in South Africa a number of attempts have been made to estimate the burden of cancer and its heterogeneity. The methodologies used in these different attempts have differed significantly (for example, haematological and eye cancers in the Johannesburg survey of 1966–75 were excluded; the National Cancer Registry is only pathology-based) and with regard to the methods of analyses employed. Some of the Transkei age-standardized rates have been published using the 'African' population standard. While fashionable at the time, most registries have now moved to using the World standard in order to promote international comparability. Unfortunately, the raw data from some of the earlier surveys are not available, making it difficult to use these data for comparative purposes.

Despite these limitations, it is clear that South Africa experienced an enormous increase in the incidence of oesophageal cancer, and since the mid-1980s a decrease, as shown in the declining proportion of oesophageal cancers over time in the National Cancer Registry. Similar increases have occurred in oral cancers. Some of the contrasts in oesophageal cancer noted in the Transkei have become less significant over time. The reasons for these secular trends with regard to oesophageal cancer remain elusive. Data from over a decade ago suggest that liver cancer is also declining, but lung cancer appears to be slowly increasing.

Colorectal cancer is one of the leading cancers among whites, but 10 times rarer in the black than the white population. However, although there is an eight-fold difference in incidence in the older groups (e.g., males 55–64 years: 276.3 vs 33/100 000), there is no difference in incidence in the younger age groups (e.g., 15–24 years: 1.6 vs 1.6 per 100 000), suggesting that the lifestyle of the younger black generation is coming to resemble that of the younger white generation.

The incidence of melanoma and non-melanoma skin cancers in whites is high and similar to that observed in Caucasians in Australia. Incidence rates for mesothelioma (at least in whites) are similar to those in other countries where asbestos was formerly mined, such as Australia. Cancer of the cervix is the leading cancer in black females, and the rates are similar to those observed in the rest of Africa.

Childhood cancers

The data on childhood cancer from the National Cancer Registry are shown in Tables 14–17. The cases are histologically diagnosed cancers, recorded in 1989-1992; the rates therefore represent minimum incidence and cannot be compared directly with those from population-based series.

In black children (Table 14), 2295 cancers were recorded, with an overall incidence (ASR) of 53.5 per million and sex ratio (boys:girls) of 1.3. Burkitt lymphoma is relatively rare (10% of lymphomas, 1.3% of all cancers). Neuroblastomas comprised 4.1% of childhood cancers, considerably less than Wilms tumour (9.7%) and retinoblastoma (5.3%).

In white children (Table 15), a total of 819 cases were recorded with an estimated ASR of 192.2 per million. The leading cancers were leukaemias (23.8%, ASR 46.5 per million) and lymphomas (12.3%, ASR 22.2 per million). Neuroblastoma (6%, ASR 12.2 per million) was the most common solid tumour.

297 cases were recorded in mixed race children (Table 16), an overall ASR of 70.5 per million, while there were 157 cases among Indian children (Table 17), an ASR of 131.8 per million.

References

Berman, C. (1935) Malignant diseases in the Bantu of Johannesburg and the Witwatersrand gold mines. *S. Afr. J. Med. Sci.*, pp. 12–30

Bourne, D. (1995) Sources of South African mortality data 1910-1992. *S. Afr. Med. J.*, **85**, 1020–1022

Bradshaw, E. & Harington, J.S. (1985) The changing pattern of cancer mortality in South Africa 1949-1979. *S. Afr. Med. J.*, **68**, 455–465

Bradshaw, E., McGlashan, N.D., Fitzgerald, D. & Harington, J.S. (1982) Analyses of cancer incidence in black gold miners from Southern Africa (1964-1979). *Br. J. Cancer*, **46**, 737–748

Burrell, R.J.W. (1957) Oesophageal cancer in the Bantu. *S. Afr. Med. J.*, **31**, 401–409

Burrell, R.J. (1962) Esophageal cancer among Bantu in the Transkei. *J. Natl Cancer Inst.*, **29**, 495–514

Gardner, M.J., Acheson, E.D. & Winter, P.D. (1982) Mortality from mesothelioma during 1968-78 England and Wales. *Br. J. Cancer*, **46**, 81–88

Harington, J.S., McGlashan, N.D., Bradshaw, E., Geddes, E.W. & Purves, L.R. (1975) A spatial and temporal analysis of four cancers in African gold miners from Southern Africa. *Br. J. Cancer*, **31**, 665–678

Higginson, J. & Oettlé, A.G. (1960). Cancer Incidence in the Bantu and "Cape Colored" races of South Africa: report of a cancer survey in the Travaal (1953-1955). *J. Natl Cancer Inst.*, **24**, 589–671

Higginson, J. & Oettlé, A.G. (1966) South Africa, Johannesburg (Bantu). In: Doll, R., Payne, P. & Waterhouse, J., eds, *Cancer Incidence in Five Continents,* Vol. I, Geneva, UICC; Berlin,

Springer Verlag, pp.38-43

Isaacson, C., Selzer, G., Kaye, V., Greenberg, M., Woodruff, D., Davies, J., Ninin, D., Vetten, D. & Andrew, M. (1978) Cancer in the urban blacks of South Africa. *S. Afr. Cancer Bull.*, **22**, 49–84

Jaskiewicz, K., Marasas, W.F.O. & Van der Walt, F.E. (1987) Oesophageal and other main cancer patterns in four districts of Transkei 1981-1984. *S. Afr. Med. J.*, **72**, 27–30

Kielkowski, D., Nelson, G. & Rees, D. (2000) Risk of mesothelioma from exposure to crocidolite asbestos: a 1995 update of a South African mortality study. *Occup. Environ. Med.*, **57**, 563–567

Makaula, A.N., Marasas, W.F., Venter, F.S., Badenhorst, C., Bradshaw, D. & Swanevelder, S. (1996) Oesophageal and other cancer patterns in four selected districts of Transkei, South Africa. 1985-1990. *Afr. J. Health Sci.*, **3**, 11–15

McGlashan, N.D. (1985) Death certifications of blacks in South Africa as a data source for geographical epidemiology. *S. Afr. Med. J.*, **61**, 571–578

Muir Grieve, J. (1967) *Cancer in the Cape Division of South Africa. A Demographic and Medical Survey, Oxford*, Oxford University Press

Muir Grieve, J. (1970) South Africa, Cape Province. In: Doll, R., Muir, C. & Waterhouse, J., eds, *Cancer Incidence in Five Continents,* Vol. II, Berlin, Springer Verlag, pp.98–109

National Cancer Registry (1987) *Cancer in South Africa 1986*. Johannesburg, SAIMR

National Cancer Registry (1988) *Cancer in South Africa 1987*, Johannesburg, SAIMR

Oettlé, A.G. (1960) Cancer in the South African Bantu. In: Raven R.W., Cancer Prog., London, Butterworth (ed.), pp.232-340

Oettlé, A.G. (1962) A historical review of past histopathological material at the South African Institute for Medical Research between 1911 and 1927. *S. Afr. Med. J.*, **36**, 628–631

Oettlé, A.G. (1963) Regional variations in the frequency of Bantu oesophageal cancer cases admitted to hospitals in South Africa. *S.Afr. Med. J.*, **37**, 434–439

Oettlé, A.G. & Higginson, J. (1966) Age specific cancer incidence rates in the South African Bantu: Johannesburg (1953-1955). *S. Afr. J. Med. Sci.*, **31**, 21–41

Robertson, M.A. (1969) Clinical observations on cancer patterns at the non-white hospital, Baragwanath, Johannesburg 1948-1964. *S. Afr. Med. J.*, **26**, 915–931

Rose, E.F. (1973) Esophageal cancer in the Transkei 1955-1969. *J. Natl Cancer Inst*, **51**, 7–16

Rose, E.F. & McGlashan, N.D. (1975) The spatial distribution of oesophageal carcinomas in the Transkei, South Africa. *Br. J. Cancer*, **31**, 197–206

Rose, E.F. & Fellingham, S.A. (1981) Cancer patterns in Transkei. *S. Afr. J. Sci.*, **77**, 555–561

Schonland, M. & Bradshaw, R. (1968) Cancer in the Natal African and Indian 1964-1966. *Int. J. Cancer*, **3**, 304–316

Schonland, M. & Bradshaw, E. (1970) South Africa, Natal. In: Doll, R., Muir, C. & Waterhouse, J., eds, *Cancer Incidence in Five Continents*, Vol. II, Berlin, Springer Verlag, pp. 110–117

Sitas, F. (1992) *Histologically Diagnosed Cancer in South Africa 1988*, Johannesburg, South African Institute of Medical Research

Sitas, F. & Newton, R. (2000) Kaposi's sarcoma in South Africa. *J. Natl Cancer Inst.* Monographs, **28**, 1–4

Sitas, F. & Pacella, R. (1994) *Histologically Diagnosed Cancer in South Africa 1989*, Johannesburg, South African Institute of Medical Research

Sitas, F., Terblanche, M. & Madhoo, J. (1996) *Incidence and Geographical Distribution of Histologically Diagnosed Cancer in South Africa, 1990 and 1991*, Johannesburg, South African Institute of Medical Research

Sitas, F., Blaauw, D., Terblanche, M. & Madhoo, J. (1998) *Incidence of Histologically Diagnosed Cancer in South Africa 1992*, Johannesburg, South African Institute of Medical Research

Sutherland, J.C. (1968) Cancer in a mission hospital in South Africa. *Cancer*, **22**, 372-378

Watkins Pitchford, W. (1925) The prevalence of cancer amongst the native races of Natal and Zululand during the years 1906-1909. *Med. J. S. Afr.*, **25**, 257–260

Zwi, A.B., Reid, G., Landan, S.P., Sitas, P. & Bechlake, M.R. (1989) Mesothelioma in South Africa, 1976-84: incidence and case characteristics. *Int. J. Epidemiol.*, **18**, 320–329

Table 1. South Africa, Johannesburg: Bantu (1953-1955)

NUMBER OF CASES BY AGE GROUP AND SUMMARY RATES OF INCIDENCE - MALE

SITE	ICD (10th)	ALL AGES	AGE UNK	0-	15-	25-	35-	45-	55-	65+	CRUDE RATE	%	ASR (W)
Mouth	C00-C08	21	0	1	-	1	5	5	4	5	2.6	4.3	5.6
Nasopharynx	C11	6	0	-	2	2	1	1	1	-	0.8	1.2	0.8
Other pharynx	C09-C10,C12-C14	1	0	-	-	1	-	-	-	-	0.1	0.2	0.1
Oesophagus	C15	54	1	-	-	-	12	25	6	10	6.8	11.0	12.4
Stomach	C16	41	0	-	1	1	9	14	9	7	5.1	8.4	10.0
Colon, rectum and anus	C18-C21	12	0	1	-	1	1	3	4	3	1.5	2.5	3.7
Liver	C22	113	0	1	3	22	34	31	10	12	14.2	23.1	19.3
Pancreas	C25	10	0	-	-	3	-	3	3	1	1.3	2.0	2.3
Larynx	C32	8	0	-	-	-	-	5	1	2	1.0	1.6	2.2
Trachea, bronchus and lung	C33-C34	40	0	-	-	2	7	22	6	3	5.0	8.2	7.5
Melanoma of skin	C43	5	1	-	-	1	1	1	-	-	0.6		1.1
Other skin	C44	9	0	-	-	3	2	2	1	1	1.1	1.0	1.6
Kaposi sarcoma	C46												
Breast	C50	3	0	-	-	-	1	1	-	1	0.4	0.6	0.8
Penis	C60	8	0	-	-	1	3	2	1	1	1.0	1.6	1.5
Prostate	C61	21	0	-	-	-	-	3	7	11	2.6	4.3	9.3
Kidney etc.	C64-C66,C68	5	0	-	1	-	1	2	2	-	0.6	1.0	1.1
Bladder	C67	17	0	-	-	2	3	6	3	2	2.1	3.5	3.5
Eye	C69	5	0	2	-	-	1	2	-	-	0.6	1.0	0.7
Brain, nervous system	C70-C72	14	0	3	3	4	4	-	-	-	1.8	2.9	1.5
Thyroid	C73	1	0	-	-	-	1	-	-	-	0.1	0.2	0.1
Hodgkin disease	C81	10	0	1	3	2	3	1	-	-	1.3	2.0	1.0
Non-Hodgkin lymphoma	C82-C85,C96	11	0	2	1	3	3	1	1	-	1.4	2.2	1.4
Multiple myeloma	C90	6	0	-	1	-	1	3	1	-	0.8	1.2	1.0
Leukaemia	C91-C95	18	0	4	2	4	5	1	1	1	2.3	3.7	2.7
Other and unspecified	O&U	50	0	2	4	7	8	12	8	9	6.3	10.2	11.6
All sites	ALL	489	2	16	21	60	106	145	69	70	61.3	100.0	102.6
All sites but C44	ALLbC44	480	2	16	21	57	104	143	68	69	60.2	98.2	101.0
Average annual population				56160	48060	69690	52880	27710	7400	4020			

Source: Cancer Incidence in Five Continents volume 1

Table 1. South Africa, Johannesburg: Bantu (1953-1955)

NUMBER OF CASES BY AGE GROUP AND SUMMARY RATES OF INCIDENCE - FEMALE

SITE	ALL AGES	AGE UNK	0-	15-	25-	35-	45-	55-	65+	CRUDE RATE	%	ASR (W)	ICD (10th)
Mouth	5	0	-	-	1	1	1	-	2	0.8	1.1	1.7	C00-C08
Nasopharynx	2	0	-	-	-	-	-	1	1	0.3	0.4	1.1	C11
Other pharynx	0	0	-	-	-	-	-	-	-	0.0	0.0	0.0	C09-C10,C12-C14
Oesophagus	2	0	-	-	-	-	-	1	1	0.3	0.4	1.1	C15
Stomach	18	0	-	-	2	3	5	6	2	2.8	4.0	6.4	C16
Colon, rectum and anus	15	0	-	-	2	3	-	9	1	2.4	3.3	6.1	C18-C21
Liver	25	0	-	-	4	2	3	10	5	3.9	5.5	9.9	C22
Pancreas	4	0	-	-	-	1	-	1	2	0.6	0.9	1.8	C25
Larynx	2	0	-	-	1	1	-	-	-	0.3	0.4	0.2	C32
Trachea, bronchus and lung	8	0	-	-	3	-	-	2	3	1.3	1.8	3.1	C33-C34
Melanoma of skin	6	0	-	-	-	2	2	1	1	0.9	1.3	1.9	C43
Other skin	7	0	-	-	2	-	1	3	1	1.1	1.6	2.7	C44
Kaposi sarcoma													C46
Breast	49	0	-	2	8	8	16	4	11	7.7	10.9	14.9	C50
Cervix uteri	189	0	-	2	29	59	53	24	22	29.8	41.9	51.0	C53
Uterus	1	0	-	-	-	1	-	-	-	0.2	0.2	0.1	C54-C55
Ovary etc.	19	0	-	3	5	6	3	1	1	3.0	4.2	3.6	C56-C57
Kidney etc.	3	0	2	-	-	1	-	-	-	0.5	0.7	0.5	C64-C66,C68
Bladder	3	0	-	-	-	1	1	-	1	0.5	0.7	1.0	C67
Eye	2	0	1	1	-	-	-	-	-	0.3	0.4	0.3	C69
Brain, nervous system	10	0	2	1	-	1	2	3	1	1.6	2.2	3.3	C70-C72
Thyroid	7	0	-	-	3	2	-	1	1	1.1	1.6	1.7	C73
Hodgkin disease	5	0	-	1	2	-	-	2	-	0.8	1.1	1.4	C81
Non-Hodgkin lymphoma	7	0	2	1	-	1	1	1	1	1.1	1.6	2.0	C82-C85,C96
Multiple myeloma	4	0	-	-	-	-	-	1	3	0.6	0.9	2.3	C90
Leukaemia	16	0	5	1	3	3	-	3	1	2.5	3.5	3.9	C91-C95
Other and unspecified	42	0	1	5	5	8	8	8	7	6.6	9.3	12.9	O&U
All sites	451	0	13	17	70	105	96	82	68	71.2	100.0	134.9	ALL
All sites but C44	444	0	13	17	68	105	95	79	67	70.0	98.4	132.3	ALLbC44
Average annual population			62930	44630	52070	28950	13810	4860	4030				

Source: Cancer Incidence in Five Continents volume 1

Table 2. South Africa, Cape Province: Bantu (1956-1959)

NUMBER OF CASES BY AGE GROUP AND SUMMARY RATES OF INCIDENCE - MALE

SITE	ALL AGES	AGE UNK	0-	10-	20-	30-	40-	50-	60+	CRUDE RATE	%	ASR (W)	ICD (10th)
Mouth	14	0	-	-	-	3	4	5	2	7.6	7.0	12.3	C00-C08
Nasopharynx	0	0	-	-	-	-	-	-	-	0.0	0.0	0.0	C11
Other pharynx	6	0	-	-	-	-	1	2	3	3.3	3.0	10.3	C09-C10,C12-C14
Oesophagus	35	1	-	-	-	3	10	15	6	19.0	17.6	35.6	C15
Stomach	19	0	-	-	2	2	4	3	8	10.3	9.5	26.9	C16
Colon, rectum and anus	8	0	-	-	3	2	2	-	1	4.3	4.0	5.0	C18-C21
Liver	38	0	-	-	6	14	8	5	5	20.6	19.1	26.5	C22
Pancreas	3	0	-	-	-	2	-	-	1	1.6	1.5	3.1	C25
Larynx	1	0	-	-	-	-	1	-	-	0.5	0.5	0.4	C32
Trachea, bronchus and lung	19	0	-	-	-	3	4	5	7	10.3	9.5	25.6	C33-C34
Melanoma of skin	3	0	-	-	-	3	-	-	-	1.6	1.5	0.7	C43
Other skin	1	0	-	-	-	-	-	1	-	0.5	0.5	0.9	C44
Kaposi sarcoma			-	-	-	-	-	-	-				C46
Breast	1	0	-	-	-	-	1	-	-	0.5	0.5	0.4	C50
Penis	1	0	-	-	-	-	-	-	1	0.5	0.5	2.7	C60
Prostate	8	0	-	-	-	-	-	2	6	4.3	4.0	17.4	C61
Kidney etc.	2	0	1	-	-	-	1	-	-	1.1	1.0	1.3	C64-C66,C68
Bladder	4	0	-	-	-	-	-	2	2	2.2	2.0	7.2	C67
Eye	0	0	-	-	-	-	-	-	-	0.0	0.0	0.0	C69
Brain, nervous system	1	0	-	-	-	1	-	-	-	0.5	0.5	0.2	C70-C72
Thyroid	0	0	-	-	-	-	-	-	-	0.0	0.0	0.0	C73
Hodgkin disease	2	0	-	-	-	-	2	-	-	1.1	1.0	0.9	C81
Non-Hodgkin lymphoma	5	0	-	1	-	1	-	3	-	2.7	2.5	4.1	C82-C85,C96
Multiple myeloma	2	0	-	-	-	-	1	-	1	1.1	1.0	3.6	C90
Leukaemia	6	0	2	-	-	1	1	1	1	3.3	3.0	6.0	C91-C95
Other and unspecified	20	1	-	-	5	3	3	6	2	10.9	10.1	15.1	O&U
All sites	199	2	3	1	16	38	43	50	46	108.0	100.0	206.4	ALL
All sites but C44	198	2	3	1	16	38	43	49	46	107.5	99.5	205.5	ALLbC44
Average annual population			6262	3785	12343	13189	6978	2477	1030				

Source: Cancer Incidence in Five Continents volume 2

Table 2. South Africa, Cape Province: Bantu (1956-1959)

NUMBER OF CASES BY AGE GROUP AND SUMMARY RATES OF INCIDENCE - FEMALE

SITE	ALL AGES	AGE UNK	0-	10-	20-	30-	40-	50-	60+	CRUDE RATE	%	ASR (W)	ICD (10th)
Mouth	4	0	–	–	1	2	1	–	–	4.2	4.4	3.5	C00-C08
Nasopharynx	0	0	–	–	–	–	–	–	–	0.0	0.0	0.0	C11
Other pharynx	1	0	–	–	–	–	1	–	–	1.0	1.1	1.3	C09-C10,C12-C14
Oesophagus	6	0	–	–	–	–	3	1	2	6.3	6.6	14.1	C15
Stomach	8	0	–	–	–	–	3	3	2	8.3	8.8	18.2	C16
Colon, rectum and anus	3	0	–	–	–	1	–	–	2	3.1	3.3	8.9	C18-C21
Liver	2	0	–	–	–	–	–	–	2	2.1	2.2	8.1	C22
Pancreas	1	0	–	–	–	–	–	–	1	1.0	1.1	4.1	C25
Larynx	0	0	–	–	–	–	–	–	–	0.0	0.0	0.0	C32
Trachea, bronchus and lung	2	0	–	–	–	1	–	–	1	2.1	2.2	4.8	C33-C34
Melanoma of skin	2	0	–	–	1	–	1	–	–	2.1	2.2	3.3	C43
Other skin	1	0	–	–	1	–	–	–	–	1.0	–	0.8	C44
Kaposi sarcoma	11	0	–	–	–	5	3	3	–	11.5	12.1	13.6	C46
Breast	15	0	–	–	–	2	7	5	1	15.7	16.5	24.8	C50
Cervix uteri	4	0	–	–	–	2	–	1	1	4.2	4.4	5.5	C53
Uterus	7	1	–	–	–	–	5	1	1	7.3	7.7	8.4	C54-C55
Ovary etc.	2	0	1	–	1	–	–	–	–	2.1	2.2	2.8	C56-C57
Kidney etc.	2	0	–	–	–	–	–	2	–	2.1	2.2	2.0	C64-C66,C68
Bladder	2	0	–	–	–	1	–	–	1	2.1	2.2	1.5	C67
Eye	2	0	1	–	–	1	–	–	–	2.1	2.2	3.3	C69
Brain, nervous system	3	0	–	–	–	2	1	–	–	3.1	3.3	2.7	C70-C72
Thyroid	0	0	–	–	–	–	–	–	–	0.0	0.0	0.0	C73
Hodgkin disease	0	0	–	–	–	–	–	–	–	0.0	0.0	0.0	C81
Non-Hodgkin lymphoma	1	0	–	–	1	–	–	–	–	1.0	1.1	0.8	C82-C85,C96
Multiple myeloma	2	0	–	–	–	–	–	1	1	2.1	2.2	3.3	C90
Leukaemia	1	0	–	–	–	1	–	–	–	1.0	1.1	0.7	C91-C95
Other and unspecified	9	0	2	–	1	–	2	2	2	9.4	9.9	18.5	O&U
All sites	91	1	4	–	6	18	27	22	13	95.0	100.0	155.5	ALL
All sites but C44	90	1	4	–	5	18	27	22	13	93.9	98.9	154.7	ALLbC44
Average annual population			6824	3779	5084	4171	2324	1099	675				

Source: Cancer Incidence in Five Continents volume 2

Table 3. South Africa, Cape Province: Coloured (1956-1959)

NUMBER OF CASES BY AGE GROUP AND SUMMARY RATES OF INCIDENCE - MALE

SITE	ALL AGES	AGE UNK	0-	15-	25-	35-	45-	55-	65+	CRUDE RATE	%	ASR (W)	ICD (10th)
Mouth	35	0	-	1	2	9	7	4	12	4.8	4.8	10.2	C00-C08
Nasopharynx	4	0	1	2	-	-	1	-	-	0.6	0.5	0.6	C11
Other pharynx	17	0	-	-	-	3	4	4	6	2.3	2.3	5.4	C09-C10,C12-C14
Oesophagus	34	0	-	-	2	2	9	14	7	4.7	4.7	10.1	C15
Stomach	176	0	-	-	6	23	39	62	46	24.3	24.2	53.4	C16
Colon, rectum and anus	28	0	-	2	2	5	8	2	9	3.9	3.8	7.9	C18-C21
Liver	6	0	-	-	-	-	4	2	-	0.8	0.8	1.5	C22
Pancreas	19	0	-	-	1	3	2	6	7	2.6	2.6	6.1	C25
Larynx	8	0	-	-	-	1	3	2	2	1.1	1.1	2.4	C32
Trachea, bronchus and lung	129	0	-	-	-	12	27	43	47	17.8	17.7	42.7	C33-C34
Melanoma of skin	1	0	-	-	-	-	-	-	1	0.1	0.1	0.2	C43
Other skin	12	0	-	1	-	2	1	1	7	1.7		4.2	C44
Kaposi sarcoma		0	-	-	-	-	-	-	-				C46
Breast	3	0	-	-	-	2	1	-	-	0.4	0.4	0.9	C50
Penis	8	0	-	-	-	-	3	3	2	1.1	1.1	2.5	C60
Prostate	51	0	-	-	-	-	-	19	32	7.0	7.0	20.5	C61
Kidney etc.	15	0	2	-	-	2	3	5	3	2.1	2.1	4.1	C64-C66,C68
Bladder	19	0	-	-	-	3	3	4	9	2.6	2.6	6.5	C67
Eye	2	0	2	-	-	-	-	-	-	0.3	0.3	0.2	C69
Brain, nervous system	9	1	2	2	1	-	-	1	2	1.2	1.2	2.0	C70-C72
Thyroid	2	0	-	1	-	-	-	-	1	0.3	0.3	0.6	C73
Hodgkin disease	14	0	2	3	2	2	2	1	2	1.9	1.9	2.8	C81
Non-Hodgkin lymphoma	24	0	8	3	3	2	5	1	2	3.3	3.3	4.2	C82-C85,C96
Multiple myeloma	7	0	-	1	-	3	-	2	1	1.0	1.0	1.7	C90
Leukaemia	31	0	12	6	2	3	3	2	3	4.3	4.3	5.3	C91-C95
Other and unspecified	74	0	2	4	9	8	11	20	20	10.2	10.2	21.0	O&U
All sites	728	1	31	26	30	85	136	198	221	100.6	100.0	217.1	ALL
All sites but C44	716	1	31	25	30	83	135	197	214	99.0	98.4	212.9	ALLbC44
Average annual population			78195	36190	26230	17686	12145	6615	3808				

Source: Cancer Incidence in Five Continents volume 2

Table 3. South Africa, Cape Province: Coloured (1956-1959)

NUMBER OF CASES BY AGE GROUP AND SUMMARY RATES OF INCIDENCE - FEMALE

SITE	ALL AGES	AGE UNK	0-	15-	25-	35-	45-	55-	65+	CRUDE RATE	%	ASR (W)	ICD (10th)
Mouth	22	0	-	3	3	7	6	1	2	2.8	2.8	3.8	C00-C08
Nasopharynx	1	0	-	-	1	-	-	-	-	0.1	0.1	0.1	C11
Other pharynx	1	0	-	-	-	-	1	-	-	0.1	0.1	0.2	C09-C10,C12-C14
Oesophagus	0	0	-	-	-	-	-	-	-	0.0	0.0	0.0	C15
Stomach	104	1	-	-	4	12	16	24	47	13.2	13.4	25.5	C16
Colon, rectum and anus	48	0	-	-	5	5	10	8	20	6.1	6.2	11.2	C18-C21
Liver	4	0	1	-	1	-	-	2	-	0.5	0.5	0.7	C22
Pancreas	9	0	-	-	-	2	-	3	4	1.1	1.2	2.2	C25
Larynx	0	0	-	-	-	-	-	-	-	0.0	0.0	0.0	C32
Trachea, bronchus and lung	19	0	-	-	2	3	5	3	6	2.4	2.4	4.2	C33-C34
Melanoma of skin	6	0	1	1	-	2	1	1	-	0.8	0.8	1.0	C43
Other skin	13	0	-	-	-	5	2	3	3	1.6		2.8	C44
Kaposi sarcoma													C46
Breast	117	0	-	-	5	26	28	31	27	14.8	15.1	25.8	C50
Cervix uteri	173	0	-	2	21	51	37	39	23	21.9	22.3	34.4	C53
Uterus	48	0	-	-	-	7	12	15	13	6.1	6.2	11.1	C54-C55
Ovary etc.	45	0	-	2	8	11	11	8	5	5.7	5.8	8.5	C56-C57
Kidney etc.	9	0	2	-	1	-	3	1	2	1.1	1.2	1.7	C64-C66,C68
Bladder	10	0	-	-	-	-	2	2	6	1.3	1.3	2.7	C67
Eye	4	0	1	-	1	1	-	1	-	0.5	0.5	0.6	C69
Brain, nervous system	13	0	4	1	-	-	3	4	1	1.6	1.7	2.4	C70-C72
Thyroid	7	0	-	2	1	2	1	-	1	0.9	0.9	1.1	C73
Hodgkin disease	7	0	2	3	1	1	-	-	-	0.9	0.9	0.8	C81
Non-Hodgkin lymphoma	15	0	1	2	1	2	3	5	1	1.9	1.9	2.9	C82-C85,C96
Multiple myeloma	3	0	-	-	-	-	1	1	1	0.4	0.4	0.7	C90
Leukaemia	23	0	6	4	5	2	2	3	1	2.9	3.0	3.3	C91-C95
Other and unspecified	76	1	4	3	4	10	14	12	28	9.6	9.8	16.9	O&U
All sites	777	2	22	23	65	149	158	167	191	98.6	100.0	164.7	ALL
All sites but C44	764	2	22	23	65	144	156	164	188	96.9	98.3	161.9	ALLbC44
Average annual population			79305	40879	29445	19431	14166	7865	5987				

Source: Cancer Incidence in Five Continents volume 2

219

Table 4. South Africa, Cape Province: White (1956-1959)

NUMBER OF CASES BY AGE GROUP AND SUMMARY RATES OF INCIDENCE - MALE

SITE	ALL AGES	AGE UNK	0-	15-	25-	35-	45-	55-	65+	CRUDE RATE	%	ASR (W)	ICD (10th)
Mouth	173	31	-	1	11	25	37	29	39	30.6	8.6	30.8	C00-C08
Nasopharynx	2	0	-	-	-	-	-	1	1	0.4	0.1	0.4	C11
Other pharynx	37	0	-	-	-	-	10	18	9	6.6	1.8	6.9	C09-C10,C12-C14
Oesophagus	33	0	-	-	-	-	3	12	18	5.8	1.6	6.4	C15
Stomach	174	0	-	-	3	9	27	42	93	30.8	8.6	32.9	C16
Colon, rectum and anus	98	4	-	3	1	2	14	27	47	17.4	4.9	18.6	C18-C21
Liver	6	0	-	-	-	-	-	5	1	1.1	0.3	1.2	C22
Pancreas	33	1	-	-	-	2	6	11	13	5.8	1.6	6.2	C25
Larynx	19	0	-	-	-	2	5	5	7	3.4	0.9	3.5	C32
Trachea, bronchus and lung	237	2	-	1	1	7	40	86	100	42.0	11.8	44.8	C33-C34
Melanoma of skin	18	2	-	-	2	5	5	2	2	3.2	0.9	3.1	C43
Other skin	730	165	-	-	7	55	145	111	247	129.2		134.1	C44
Kaposi sarcoma	8	0	-	-	-	1	-	2	5	1.4	0.4	1.5	C46
Breast		0	-	-	-	-	-	-	-				C50
Penis	4	0	-	-	-	-	1	-	3	0.7	0.2	0.8	C60
Prostate	122	2	-	-	-	-	1	14	105	21.6	6.1	24.2	C61
Kidney etc.	24	0	2	-	-	3	2	9	8	4.2	1.2	4.5	C64-C66,C68
Bladder	51	1	-	-	-	1	8	16	25	9.0	2.5	9.7	C67
Eye	8	0	-	1	-	-	1	3	3	1.4	0.4	1.5	C69
Brain, nervous system	20	0	4	-	3	3	3	5	2	3.5	1.0	3.6	C70-C72
Thyroid	6	1	-	-	-	1	1	-	4	1.1	0.3	1.2	C73
Hodgkin disease	15	1	-	-	2	3	3	2	4	2.7	0.7	2.7	C81
Non-Hodgkin lymphoma	39	1	-	-	1	5	12	12	8	6.9	1.9	7.0	C82-C85,C96
Multiple myeloma	12	0	-	-	-	-	3	4	5	2.1	0.6	2.2	C90
Leukaemia	34	1	8	1	-	1	4	7	12	6.0	1.7	6.4	C91-C95
Other and unspecified	109	4	6	2	5	12	20	21	39	19.3	5.4	20.0	O&U
All sites	2012	216	20	9	36	137	350	444	800	356.2	100.0	374.7	ALL
All sites but C44	1282	51	20	9	29	82	205	333	553	227.0	63.7	240.2	ALLbC44
Average annual population			41369	24335	20070	19109	17175	10395	8757				

Source: Cancer Incidence in Five Continents volume 2

Table 4. South Africa, Cape Province: White (1956-1959)

NUMBER OF CASES BY AGE GROUP AND SUMMARY RATES OF INCIDENCE - FEMALE

SITE	ALL AGES	AGE UNK	0-	15-	25-	35-	45-	55-	65+	CRUDE RATE	%	ASR (W)	ICD (10th)
Mouth	51	2	1	2	5	4	10	7	20	8.4	2.6	7.5	C00-C08
Nasopharynx	3	0	-	-	-	-	1	-	2	0.5	0.2	0.4	C11
Other pharynx	6	0	-	-	-	-	-	3	3	1.0	0.3	0.9	C09-C10,C12-C14
Oesophagus	7	0	-	-	-	-	-	3	4	1.2	0.4	1.0	C15
Stomach	103	3	1	3	-	-	8	19	73	17.0	5.3	14.4	C16
Colon, rectum and anus	160	5	1	3	5	8	15	33	90	26.4	8.3	22.9	C18-C21
Liver	4	0	1	-	-	-	-	-	3	0.7	0.2	0.6	C22
Pancreas	24	0	-	-	-	2	4	4	14	4.0	1.2	3.4	C25
Larynx	3	0	-	-	-	-	-	1	2	0.5	0.2	0.4	C32
Trachea, bronchus and lung	37	0	-	-	-	2	8	8	19	6.1	1.9	5.3	C33-C34
Melanoma of skin	34	1	1	3	3	9	5	3	9	5.6	1.8	5.1	C43
Other skin	511	106	-	4	12	29	78	87	195	84.4		73.2	C44
Kaposi sarcoma													C46
Breast	398	24	-	1	10	55	106	83	119	65.8	20.6	57.6	C50
Cervix uteri	154	2	-	1	7	34	41	44	25	25.4	8.0	22.6	C53
Uterus	99	1	-	3	1	6	25	33	30	16.4	5.1	14.4	C54-C55
Ovary etc.	71	1	-	2	1	11	23	12	21	11.7	3.7	10.3	C56-C57
Kidney etc.	16	1	1	-	-	1	1	5	8	2.6	0.8	2.3	C64-C66,C68
Bladder	22	0	-	-	-	3	3	2	17	3.6	1.1	3.1	C67
Eye	4	0	-	-	1	1	1	1	-	0.7	0.2	0.6	C69
Brain, nervous system	19	0	2	1	1	4	3	6	2	3.1	1.0	2.9	C70-C72
Thyroid	20	1	-	1	4	3	2	5	4	3.3	1.0	3.0	C73
Hodgkin disease	8	0	-	3	1	-	1	2	1	1.3	0.4	1.2	C81
Non-Hodgkin lymphoma	34	1	3	1	-	5	4	6	14	5.6	1.8	5.0	C82-C85,C96
Multiple myeloma	4	0	-	1	-	-	-	2	2	0.7	0.2	0.6	C90
Leukaemia	33	0	7	1	-	4	9	4	8	5.5	1.7	5.1	C91-C95
Other and unspecified	109	3	3	-	6	4	10	21	62	18.0	5.6	15.7	O&U
All sites	1934	151	20	26	56	181	358	394	748	319.5	100.0	279.6	ALL
All sites but C44	1423	45	20	22	44	152	280	307	553	235.1	73.6	206.3	ALLbC44
Average annual population			39699	25336	21129	20038	18842	13515	12759				

Source: Cancer Incidence in Five Continents volume 2

Table 5. South Africa, Natal: Indian (1964-1966)

NUMBER OF CASES BY AGE GROUP AND SUMMARY RATES OF INCIDENCE - MALE

SITE	ALL AGES	AGE UNK	0-	15-	25-	35-	45-	55-	65+	CRUDE RATE	%	ASR (W)	ICD (10th)
Mouth	10	0	-	-	1	-	-	4	5	2.4	4.5	7.5	C00-C08
Nasopharynx	0	0	-	-	-	-	-	-	-	0.0	0.0	0.0	C11
Other pharynx	2	0	-	-	-	-	-	2	-	0.5	0.9	1.2	C09-C10,C12-C14
Oesophagus	8	0	-	-	-	-	1	6	1	1.9	3.6	5.0	C15
Stomach	32	0	-	1	1	4	6	7	13	7.7	14.5	20.9	C16
Colon, rectum and anus	9	0	-	-	-	1	3	1	4	2.2	4.1	6.0	C18-C21
Liver	13	0	-	-	-	1	3	3	6	3.1	5.9	9.1	C22
Pancreas	6	0	-	-	1	3	1	1	-	1.5	2.7	2.2	C25
Larynx	4	0	-	-	-	-	-	2	2	1.0	1.8	3.1	C32
Trachea, bronchus and lung	30	0	-	-	-	4	9	5	12	7.3	13.6	19.5	C33-C34
Melanoma of skin	1	0	-	-	-	-	-	-	1	0.2	0.5	1.0	C43
Other skin	5	0	-	-	-	2	2	-	1	1.2	2.3	2.4	C44
Kaposi sarcoma													C46
Breast	2	0	-	-	-	-	-	1	1	0.5	0.9	1.6	C50
Penis	4	0	-	-	-	-	1	1	2	1.0	1.8	2.8	C60
Prostate	10	0	-	-	-	-	-	1	9	2.4	4.5	9.2	C61
Kidney etc.	3	0	-	-	-	-	3	-	-	0.7	1.4	1.3	C64-C66,C68
Bladder	12	0	-	-	1	1	4	2	4	2.9	5.5	7.3	C67
Eye	3	0	2	-	-	-	-	-	1	0.7	1.4	1.3	C69
Brain, nervous system	9	0	6	-	-	2	-	-	1	2.2	4.1	2.6	C70-C72
Thyroid	1	0	-	-	-	-	-	-	1	0.2	0.5	1.0	C73
Hodgkin disease	4	0	3	-	1	-	-	-	-	1.0	1.8	0.8	C81
Non-Hodgkin lymphoma	5	0	1	1	1	1	-	-	1	1.2	2.3	1.9	C82-C85,C96
Multiple myeloma	2	0	-	-	-	1	-	1	-	0.5	0.9	1.0	C90
Leukaemia	17	0	11	1	1	1	-	3	-	4.1	7.7	4.4	C91-C95
Other and unspecified	28	0	2	6	5	2	4	5	4	6.8	12.7	11.9	O&U
All sites	220	0	25	9	12	23	37	45	69	53.2	100.0	124.9	ALL
All sites but C44	215	0	25	9	12	21	35	45	68	52.0	97.7	122.5	ALLbC44
Average annual population			60415	29148	19499	13343	8708	4360	2439				

Source: Cancer Incidence in Five Continents volume 2

Table 5. South Africa, Natal: Indian (1964-1966)

NUMBER OF CASES BY AGE GROUP AND SUMMARY RATES OF INCIDENCE - FEMALE

SITE	ALL AGES	AGE UNK	0-	15-	25-	35-	45-	55-	65+	CRUDE RATE	%	ASR (W)	ICD (10th)
Mouth	14	0	–	–	1	1	3	6	3	3.5	5.1	11.4	*C00-C08*
Nasopharynx	0	0	–	–	–	–	–	–	–	0.0	0.0	0.0	*C11*
Other pharynx	2	0	–	–	–	–	–	1	1	0.5	0.7	2.3	*C09-C10,C12-C14*
Oesophagus	17	0	–	–	1	4	2	7	3	4.2	6.2	12.7	*C15*
Stomach	32	0	–	–	2	7	5	5	13	7.9	11.6	29.1	*C16*
Colon, rectum and anus	20	0	–	–	–	4	4	6	6	4.9	7.2	17.2	*C18-C21*
Liver	5	0	–	–	–	–	3	1	1	1.2	1.8	3.8	*C22*
Pancreas	2	0	–	–	–	–	–	1	1	0.5	0.7	2.3	*C25*
Larynx	0	0	–	–	–	–	–	–	–	0.0	0.0	0.0	*C32*
Trachea, bronchus and lung	4	0	–	–	–	1	–	2	1	1.0	1.4	3.4	*C33-C34*
Melanoma of skin	0	0	–	–	–	–	–	–	–	0.0	0.0	0.0	*C43*
Other skin	6	0	–	1	–	2	2	–	1	1.5	2.2	3.4	*C44*
Kaposi sarcoma		0	–	–	–	–	–	–	–				*C46*
Breast	31	0	–	–	5	7	7	8	4	7.6	11.2	19.4	*C50*
Cervix uteri	62	0	–	–	8	18	18	13	5	15.3	22.5	34.7	*C53*
Uterus	19	0	–	1	–	5	7	4	3	4.7	6.9	12.8	*C54-C55*
Ovary etc.	6	0	–	–	1	1	3	–	1	1.5	2.2	3.4	*C56-C57*
Kidney etc.	2	0	1	–	–	–	1	–	–	0.5	0.7	0.7	*C64-C66,C68*
Bladder	5	0	–	–	–	–	1	2	2	1.2	1.8	5.1	*C67*
Eye	0	0	–	–	–	–	–	–	–	0.0	0.0	0.0	*C69*
Brain, nervous system	2	0	2	–	–	–	–	–	–	0.5	0.7	0.3	*C70-C72*
Thyroid	7	0	–	2	2	–	1	2	–	1.7	2.5	2.9	*C73*
Hodgkin disease	2	0	–	–	2	–	–	–	–	0.5	0.7	0.5	*C81*
Non-Hodgkin lymphoma	3	0	–	1	1	–	1	–	–	0.7	1.1	0.8	*C82-C85,C96*
Multiple myeloma	1	0	–	1	–	–	–	–	–	0.2	0.4	1.5	*C90*
Leukaemia	8	0	3	–	1	1	1	1	1	2.0	2.9	3.8	*C91-C95*
Other and unspecified	26	0	1	5	–	4	8	5	3	6.4	9.4	14.9	*O&U*
All sites	276	0	7	11	23	55	66	64	50	68.0	100.0	186.8	*ALL*
All sites but C44	270	0	7	10	23	53	64	64	49	66.5	97.8	183.4	*ALLbC44*
Average annual population			61919	29854	19013	12101	7489	3365	1522				

Source: Cancer Incidence in Five Continents volume 2

Table 6. South Africa, Natal: African (1964-1966)

NUMBER OF CASES BY AGE GROUP AND SUMMARY RATES OF INCIDENCE - MALE

SITE	ALL AGES	AGE UNK	0-	15-	25-	35-	45-	55-	65+	CRUDE RATE	%	ASR (W)	ICD (10th)
Mouth	26	0	-	-	1	6	7	8	4	3.7	2.9	6.4	C00-C08
Nasopharynx	0	0	-	-	-	-	-	-	-	0.0	0.0	0.0	C11
Other pharynx	15	0	-	-	-	1	7	5	2	2.2	1.7	3.9	C09-C10,C12-C14
Oesophagus	169	0	-	2	9	30	54	57	19	24.3	19.2	40.1	C15
Stomach	46	0	-	2	3	13	10	9	9	6.6	5.2	11.1	C16
Colon, rectum and anus	14	0	-	-	-	4	4	5	1	2.0	1.6	3.1	C18-C21
Liver	140	0	-	9	20	26	49	25	11	20.1	15.9	27.6	C22
Pancreas	10	0	-	-	1	1	2	5	1	1.4	1.1	2.5	C25
Larynx	19	0	-	-	1	5	5	5	3	2.7	2.2	4.6	C32
Trachea, bronchus and lung	183	0	-	2	5	49	61	36	30	26.3	20.7	43.4	C33-C34
Melanoma of skin	6	0	-	1	1	3	-	1	-	0.9	0.7	0.8	C43
Other skin	16	0	-	1	5	2	5	2	1	2.3		2.8	C44
Kaposi sarcoma													C46
Breast	0	0	-	-	-	-	-	-	-	0.0	0.0	0.0	C50
Penis	27	0	-	-	2	5	9	7	4	3.9	3.1	6.5	C60
Prostate	54	0	-	-	-	1	11	12	30	7.8	6.1	21.8	C61
Kidney etc.	8	0	1	-	-	-	2	5	-	1.1	0.9	1.9	C64-C66,C68
Bladder	15	0	-	-	2	3	5	1	4	2.2	1.7	3.9	C67
Eye	4	0	3	-	-	-	-	1	-	0.6	0.5	0.8	C69
Brain, nervous system	10	0	5	-	-	-	4	1	-	1.4	1.1	1.8	C70-C72
Thyroid	1	0	-	-	-	-	1	-	-	0.1	0.1	0.2	C73
Hodgkin disease	17	0	-	6	2	3	4	1	1	2.4	1.9	2.7	C81
Non-Hodgkin lymphoma	17	0	3	2	2	4	3	1	2	2.4	1.9	3.3	C82-C85,C96
Multiple myeloma	11	0	-	-	1	3	2	4	1	1.6	1.2	2.5	C90
Leukaemia	25	0	10	2	5	4	1	2	1	3.6	2.8	4.1	C91-C95
Other and unspecified	49	0	2	5	5	12	11	9	5	7.0	5.6	9.9	O&U
All sites	882	0	24	30	65	175	257	202	129	126.8	100.0	205.7	ALL
All sites but C44	866	0	24	29	60	173	252	200	128	124.5	98.2	202.9	ALLbC44
Average annual population			61713	52635	46291	36899	20562	9515	4271				

Source: Cancer Incidence in Five Continents volume 2

Table 6. South Africa, Natal: African (1964-1966)

NUMBER OF CASES BY AGE GROUP AND SUMMARY RATES OF INCIDENCE - FEMALE

SITE	ALL AGES	AGE UNK	0-	15-	25-	35-	45-	55-	65+	CRUDE RATE	%	ASR (W)	ICD (10th)
Mouth	6	0	-	1	1	-	1	1	2	1.2	1.2	2.3	C00-C08
Nasopharynx	1	0	-	-	-	1	-	-	-	0.2	0.2	0.2	C11
Other pharynx	0	0	-	-	-	-	-	-	-	0.0	0.0	0.0	C09-C10,C12-C14
Oesophagus	32	0	-	1	-	6	10	8	7	6.4	6.3	12.0	C15
Stomach	18	0	-	-	-	3	2	6	7	3.6	3.5	7.9	C16
Colon, rectum and anus	15	0	-	-	-	4	4	2	5	3.0	3.0	5.7	C18-C21
Liver	21	0	-	1	6	2	3	6	3	4.2	4.1	6.8	C22
Pancreas	10	0	-	-	-	3	2	4	1	2.0	2.0	3.5	C25
Larynx	1	0	-	-	-	-	-	-	1	0.2	0.2	0.6	C32
Trachea, bronchus and lung	25	0	-	-	1	3	8	3	10	5.0	4.9	10.1	C33-C34
Melanoma of skin	6	0	-	1	1	1	-	2	2	1.2	1.2	2.4	C43
Other skin	6	0	-	1	2	1	2	-	-	1.2		1.3	C44
Kaposi sarcoma													C46
Breast	36	0	-	2	6	6	7	9	6	7.2	7.1	12.0	C50
Cervix uteri	176	0	-	3	32	63	35	24	19	35.2	34.6	48.5	C53
Uterus	14	0	-	-	4	4	5	2	3	2.8	2.8	4.8	C54-C55
Ovary etc.	23	0	2	1	4	6	5	1	4	4.6	4.5	6.4	C56-C57
Kidney etc.	7	0	5	-	-	-	1	1	-	1.4	1.4	1.6	C64-C66,C68
Bladder	7	0	-	1	2	2	1	-	3	1.4	1.4	2.6	C67
Eye	3	0	1	1	-	-	-	-	1	0.6	0.6	1.0	C69
Brain, nervous system	6	0	2	1	1	-	2	-	-	1.2	1.2	1.3	C70-C72
Thyroid	9	0	-	1	1	2	1	1	3	1.8	1.8	3.2	C73
Hodgkin disease	3	0	-	-	1	1	-	-	-	0.6	0.6	0.5	C81
Non-Hodgkin lymphoma	8	0	1	2	-	-	1	-	1	1.6	1.6	1.9	C82-C85,C96
Multiple myeloma	8	0	-	-	-	-	-	4	4	1.6	1.6	4.2	C90
Leukaemia	12	0	3	1	4	2	1	1	-	2.4	2.4	2.4	C91-C95
Other and unspecified	55	0	2	5	12	7	11	11	7	11.0	10.8	16.7	O&U
All sites	508	0	16	22	76	117	102	86	89	101.7	100.0	159.7	ALL
All sites but C44	502	0	16	21	74	116	100	86	89	100.5	98.8	158.5	ALLbC44
Average annual population			63322	23995	34274	22498	12561	5765	4055				

Source: Cancer Incidence in Five Continents volume 2

Table 7. South Africa, Transkei, Umtata District (1996-1998)

NUMBER OF CASES BY AGE GROUP AND SUMMARY RATES OF INCIDENCE - MALE

SITE	ALL AGES	AGE UNK	MV (%)	0-	15-	25-	35-	45-	55-	65+	CRUDE RATE	%	CR 64	ASR (W)	ICD (10th)
Mouth	14	0	93	-	-	-	-	6	3	5	3.9	5.0	0.64	7.9	C00-06
Salivary gland	0	0	-	-	-	-	-	-	-	-	0.0	0.0	0.00	0.0	C07-08
Nasopharynx	4	0	25	-	-	-	1	-	2	1	1.1	1.4	0.20	2.1	C11
Other pharynx	10	0	80	1	-	-	1	1	3	4	2.8	3.5	0.36	4.6	C09-10,C12-14
Oesophagus	117	0	38	-	1	2	10	31	35	38	32.7	41.5	5.30	62.5	C15
Stomach	5	0	40	-	-	-	-	-	1	4	1.4	1.8	0.05	2.0	C16
Colon, rectum and anus	10	0	50	-	-	2	-	2	2	4	2.8	3.5	0.37	4.9	C18-21
Liver	35	0	20	-	3	2	3	4	8	15	9.8	12.4	1.16	16.0	C22
Gallbladder etc.	4	0	25	-	-	-	-	1	1	2	1.1	1.4	0.16	2.1	C23-24
Pancreas	3	0	0	-	-	-	-	-	2	1	0.8	1.1	0.15	1.5	C25
Larynx	6	0	67	-	-	-	-	1	3	2	1.7	2.1	0.33	3.5	C32
Trachea, bronchus and lung	33	0	45	-	-	-	1	7	7	18	9.2	11.7	1.03	15.7	C33-34
Bone	1	0	100	1	-	-	-	-	-	-	0.3	0.4	0.01	0.2	C40-41
Melanoma of skin	0	0	-	-	-	-	-	-	-	-	0.0	0.0	0.00	0.0	C43
Other skin	4	0	100	-	-	-	3	1	-	-	1.1		0.16	1.9	C44
Mesothelioma	0	0	-	-	-	-	-	-	-	-	0.0	0.0	0.00	0.0	C45
Kaposi sarcoma	1	0	100	-	-	1	-	-	-	-	0.3	0.4	0.02	0.3	C46
Peripheral nerves	0	0	-	-	-	-	-	-	-	-	0.0	0.0	0.00	0.0	C47
Connective and soft tissue	0	0	-	-	-	-	-	-	-	-	0.0	0.0	0.00	0.0	C49
Breast	4	0	25	-	-	-	-	1	1	2	1.1	1.4	0.10	1.6	C50
Penis	1	0	100	-	-	-	-	1	-	-	0.3	0.4	0.07	0.7	C60
Prostate	11	0	0	-	-	-	-	-	-	11	3.1	3.9	0.00	3.7	C61
Testis	1	0	100	-	1	-	-	-	-	-	0.3	0.4	0.01	0.2	C62
Kidney	0	0	-	-	-	-	-	-	-	-	0.0	0.0	0.00	0.0	C64
Renal pelvis, ureter and other urinary	0	0	-	-	-	-	-	-	-	-	0.0	0.0	0.00	0.0	C65-66,C68
Bladder	2	0	0	-	-	-	-	-	1	1	0.6	0.7	0.07	0.9	C67
Eye	0	0	-	-	-	-	-	-	-	-	0.0	0.0	0.00	0.0	C69
Brain, nervous system	1	0	100	-	-	-	-	1	-	-	0.3	0.4	0.05	0.6	C70-72
Thyroid	0	0	-	-	-	-	-	-	-	-	0.0	0.0	0.00	0.0	C73
Hodgkin disease	1	0	100	-	1	-	-	-	-	-	0.3	0.4	0.01	0.2	C81
Non-Hodgkin lymphoma	6	0	17	-	2	1	-	1	-	2	1.7	2.1	0.09	1.9	C82-85,C96
Multiple myeloma	5	0	60	-	-	-	-	3	1	1	1.4	1.8	0.28	3.1	C90
Lymphoid leukaemia	1	0	100	1	-	-	-	-	-	-	0.3	0.4	0.01	0.2	C91
Myeloid leukaemia	1	0	0	-	-	-	-	-	-	1	0.3	0.4	0.00	0.3	C92-94
Leukaemia, unspecified	1	0	0	-	-	-	-	-	-	1	0.3	0.4	0.00	0.3	C95
Other and unspecified	4	0	25	1	-	-	-	2	-	1	1.1	1.4	0.18	2.2	O&U
All sites	286	0	41	4	8	8	19	63	70	114	79.9	100.0	10.82	141.3	ALL
All sites but C44	282	0	40	4	8	8	16	62	70	114	78.8		10.66	139.3	ALLbC44
Average annual population				53610	24958	14315	9871	5558	4119	6894					

Table 7. South Africa, Transkei, Umtata District (1996-1998)

NUMBER OF CASES BY AGE GROUP AND SUMMARY RATES OF INCIDENCE - FEMALE

SITE	ALL AGES	AGE UNK	MV (%)	0-	15-	25-	35-	45-	55-	65+	CRUDE RATE	%	CR 64	ASR (W)	ICD (10th)
Mouth	2	0	100	-	-	-	-	-	-	2	0.5	0.7	0.00	0.6	C00-06
Salivary gland	0	0	-	-	-	-	-	-	-	-	0.0	0.0	0.00	0.0	C07-08
Nasopharynx	0	0	-	-	-	-	-	-	-	-	0.0	0.0	0.00	0.0	C11
Other pharynx	5	0	40	-	-	-	-	1	2	2	1.2	1.6	0.14	1.8	C09-10,C12-14
Oesophagus	97	0	21	-	-	4	13	16	30	34	22.9	31.9	2.57	34.5	C15
Stomach	4	0	50	-	-	-	-	-	1	3	0.9	1.3	0.05	1.3	C16
Colon, rectum and anus	5	0	60	-	-	-	2	-	-	3	1.2	1.6	0.05	1.5	C18-21
Liver	15	0	40	-	3	3	2	2	3	2	3.5	4.9	0.35	4.5	C22
Gallbladder etc.	0	0	-	-	-	-	-	-	-	-	0.0	0.0	0.00	0.0	C23-24
Pancreas	3	0	33	-	-	-	-	1	1	1	0.7	1.0	0.10	1.2	C25
Larynx	0	0	-	-	-	-	-	-	-	-	0.0	0.0	0.00	0.0	C32
Trachea, bronchus and lung	10	0	30	-	-	-	1	2	4	3	2.4	3.3	0.30	3.6	C33-34
Bone	0	0	-	-	-	-	-	-	-	-	0.0	0.0	0.00	0.0	C40-41
Melanoma of skin	0	0	-	-	-	-	-	-	-	-	0.0	0.0	0.00	0.0	C43
Other skin	3	0	33	1	-	-	1	1	-	-	0.7	1.0	0.08	1.0	C44
Mesothelioma	0	0	-	-	-	-	-	-	-	-	0.0	0.0	0.00	0.0	C45
Kaposi sarcoma	0	0	-	-	-	-	-	-	-	-	0.0	0.0	0.00	0.0	C46
Peripheral nerves	0	0	-	-	-	-	-	-	-	-	0.0	0.0	0.00	0.0	C47
Connective and soft tissue	3	0	67	-	-	1	1	-	1	-	0.7	1.0	0.06	0.9	C49
Breast	42	0	76	-	-	4	9	9	13	7	9.9	13.8	1.30	14.9	C50
Vulva	4	0	75	-	-	-	-	-	1	3	0.9	1.3	0.05	1.3	C51
Vagina	2	0	50	-	-	-	-	-	1	1	0.5	0.7	0.00	0.6	C52
Cervix uteri	75	0	79	-	-	11	10	13	28	13	17.7	24.7	2.35	26.3	C53
Uterus	2	0	100	-	-	-	-	1	-	1	0.5	0.7	0.04	0.8	C54-55
Ovary	9	0	56	-	-	-	2	1	4	2	2.1	3.0	0.30	3.3	C56
Placenta	2	0	100	-	-	-	2	-	-	-	0.5	0.7	0.05	0.6	C58
Kidney	6	0	50	2	-	1	-	1	-	2	1.4	2.0	0.08	1.6	C64
Renal pelvis, ureter and other urinary	0	0	-	-	-	-	-	-	-	-	0.0	0.0	0.00	0.0	C65-66,C68
Bladder	0	0	-	-	-	-	-	-	-	-	0.0	0.0	0.00	0.0	C67
Eye	0	0	-	-	-	-	-	-	-	-	0.0	0.0	0.00	0.0	C69
Brain, nervous system	0	0	-	-	-	-	-	-	-	-	0.0	0.0	0.00	0.0	C70-72
Thyroid	2	0	100	-	-	-	-	-	2	-	0.5	0.7	0.10	0.8	C73
Hodgkin disease	1	0	100	-	1	-	-	-	-	-	0.2	0.3	0.01	0.2	C81
Non-Hodgkin lymphoma	4	0	75	-	1	-	-	1	1	1	0.9	1.3	0.08	1.1	C82-85,C96
Multiple myeloma	3	0	67	-	-	-	-	1	-	2	0.7	1.0	0.02	0.9	C90
Lymphoid leukaemia	0	0	-	-	-	-	-	-	-	-	0.0	0.0	0.00	0.0	C91
Myeloid leukaemia	1	0	100	-	-	-	-	-	-	1	0.2	0.3	0.00	0.3	C92-94
Leukaemia, unspecified	1	0	0	-	1	-	-	-	-	-	0.2	0.3	0.00	0.3	C95
Other and unspecified	6	0	33	-	2	-	2	1	-	1	1.4	2.0	0.12	1.8	O&U
All sites	307	0	52	3	7	25	45	49	91	87	72.3	100.0	8.20	105.8	ALL
All sites but C44	304	0	52	2	7	25	44	48	91	87	71.6	100.0	8.13	104.8	ALLbC44
Average annual population				52866	31754	20797	13880	7686	6867	7646					

Table 8. South Africa, Transkei, 4 Districts (1996-1998)

NUMBER OF CASES BY AGE GROUP AND SUMMARY RATES OF INCIDENCE - MALE

SITE	ALL AGES	AGE UNK	MV (%)	0-	15-	25-	35-	45-	55-	65+	CRUDE RATE	%	CR 64	ASR (W)	ICD (10th)
Mouth	11	0	73	-	-	-	-	-	6	4	1.5	4.5	0.25	2.9	C00-06
Salivary gland	1	0	100	-	-	-	-	-	1	-	0.1	0.4	0.04	0.3	C07-08
Nasopharynx	1	0	0	-	-	-	-	-	1	-	0.1	0.4	0.04	0.3	C11
Other pharynx	2	0	100	-	-	-	-	-	1	1	0.3	0.8	0.04	0.5	C09-10,C12-14
Oesophagus	134	0	10	-	-	1	13	31	38	51	18.5	54.5	2.83	37.5	C15
Stomach	7	0	14	-	-	2	1	1	1	2	1.0	2.8	0.13	1.8	C16
Colon, rectum and anus	6	0	50	-	-	2	1	-	2	1	0.8	2.4	0.14	1.6	C18-21
Liver	19	0	58	1	-	1	2	8	2	5	2.6	7.7	0.42	5.5	C22
Gallbladder etc.	0	0		-	-	-	-	-	-	-	0.0	0.0	0.00	0.0	C23-24
Pancreas	3	0	33	-	-	1	1	-	2	-	0.4	1.2	0.09	0.8	C25
Larynx	5	0	60	-	-	-	-	2	1	2	0.7	2.0	0.10	1.4	C32
Trachea, bronchus and lung	15	0	33	-	-	-	2	7	4	2	2.1	6.1	0.46	4.9	C33-34
Bone	3	0	67	-	1	-	-	-	1	1	0.4	1.2	0.05	0.5	C40-41
Melanoma of skin	3	0	67	-	-	-	1	1	1	1	0.4	1.2	0.08	0.9	C43
Other skin	3	0	67	-	-	-	1	-	-	-	0.4		0.10	1.0	C44
Mesothelioma	2	0	50	-	-	-	-	2	-	-	0.3	0.8	0.08	0.8	C45
Kaposi sarcoma	2	0	100	-	-	-	1	1	-	-	0.3	0.8	0.07	0.7	C46
Peripheral nerves	0	0		-	-	-	-	-	-	-	0.0	0.0	0.00	0.0	C47
Connective and soft tissue	2	0	100	-	-	-	-	-	-	1	0.3	0.8	0.04	0.4	C49
Breast	1	0	100	-	1	-	-	-	-	-	0.1	0.4	0.00	0.2	C50
Penis	0	0		-	-	-	-	-	-	-	0.0	0.0	0.00	0.0	C60
Prostate	12	0	42	-	-	-	-	1	3	8	1.7	4.9	0.15	2.9	C61
Testis	0	0		-	-	-	-	-	-	-	0.0	0.0	0.00	0.0	C62
Kidney	3	0	33	2	-	-	-	-	1	-	0.4	1.2	0.03	0.5	C64
Renal pelvis, ureter and other urinary	0	0		-	-	-	-	-	-	-	0.0	0.0	0.00	0.0	C65-66,C68
Bladder	2	0	50	-	-	-	-	-	-	2	0.3	0.8	0.00	0.4	C67
Eye	1	0	100	1	-	-	-	-	-	-	0.1	0.4	0.00	0.1	C69
Brain, nervous system	1	0	0	1	-	-	-	-	-	-	0.1	0.4	0.00	0.1	C70-72
Thyroid	0	0		-	-	-	-	-	-	-	0.0	0.0	0.00	0.0	C73
Hodgkin disease	0	0		-	-	-	-	-	-	-	0.0	0.0	0.00	0.0	C81
Non-Hodgkin lymphoma	1	0	100	-	-	-	1	-	-	-	0.1	0.4	0.03	0.3	C82-85,C96
Multiple myeloma	1	0	0	-	-	-	-	1	-	-	0.1	0.4	0.03	0.4	C90
Lymphoid leukaemia	0	0		-	-	-	-	-	-	-	0.0	0.0	0.00	0.0	C91
Myeloid leukaemia	0	0		-	-	-	-	-	-	-	0.0	0.0	0.00	0.0	C92-94
Leukaemia, unspecified	1	0	0	-	-	-	1	-	-	-	0.1	0.4	0.04	0.4	C95
Other and unspecified	7	0	86	1	1	2	-	-	2	1	1.0	2.8	0.12	1.5	O&U
All sites	249	0	31	7	3	8	24	57	69	81	34.4		5.35	68.5	ALL
All sites but C44	246	0	30	7	3	8	23	56	68	81	33.9	100.0	5.25	67.5	ALLbC44

Average annual population   127729   48959   19366   15381   9782   9125   11263

Table 8. South Africa, Transkei, 4 Districts (1996-1998)

NUMBER OF CASES BY AGE GROUP AND SUMMARY RATES OF INCIDENCE - FEMALE

SITE	ALL AGES	AGE UNK	MV (%)	0-	15-	25-	35-	45-	55-	65+	CRUDE RATE	%	CR 64	ASR (W)	ICD (10th)
Mouth	2	0	100	-	-	-	1	-	-	1	0.2	0.5	0.02	0.3	C00-06
Salivary gland	0	0	-	-	-	-	-	-	-	-	0.0	0.0	0.00	0.0	C07-08
Nasopharynx	1	0	0	-	-	-	-	-	-	1	0.1	0.2	0.00	0.1	C11
Other pharynx	0	0	-	-	-	-	-	-	-	-	0.0	0.0	0.00	0.0	C09-10,C12-14
Oesophagus	173	0	6	-	-	2	14	25	67	65	19.2	41.9	2.01	26.5	C15
Stomach	2	0	0	-	-	-	-	-	1	1	0.2	0.5	0.01	0.3	C16
Colon, rectum and anus	6	0	33	-	-	-	1	1	-	4	0.7	1.5	0.03	0.9	C18-21
Liver	7	0	71	-	-	-	1	2	2	2	0.8	1.7	0.09	1.2	C22
Gallbladder etc.	0	0	-	-	-	-	-	-	-	-	0.0	0.0	0.00	0.0	C23-24
Pancreas	2	0	0	-	-	-	-	1	1	-	0.2	0.5	0.04	0.4	C25
Larynx	1	0	100	-	-	-	-	1	-	-	0.1	0.2	0.02	0.2	C32
Trachea, bronchus and lung	4	0	100	-	-	-	-	2	1	1	0.4	1.0	0.06	0.7	C33-34
Bone	5	0	60	1	-	-	1	1	2	-	0.6	1.2	0.08	0.8	C40-41
Melanoma of skin	1	0	100	-	-	-	1	-	-	-	0.1	0.2	0.02	0.2	C43
Other skin	1	0	0	-	-	-	-	-	-	1	0.1	0.2	0.00	0.1	C44
Mesothelioma	0	0	-	-	-	-	-	-	-	-	0.0	0.0	0.00	0.0	C45
Kaposi sarcoma	1	0	0	-	-	1	-	-	-	-	0.1	0.2	0.01	0.1	C46
Peripheral nerves	0	0	-	-	-	-	-	-	-	-	0.0	0.0	0.00	0.0	C47
Connective and soft tissue	2	0	100	1	-	1	-	-	-	-	0.2	0.5	0.01	0.2	C49
Breast	36	0	64	-	-	2	6	13	6	9	4.0	8.7	0.48	6.1	C50
Vulva	0	0	-	-	-	-	-	-	-	-	0.0	0.0	0.00	0.0	C51
Vagina	1	0	100	-	-	-	-	-	1	-	0.1	0.2	0.02	0.2	C52
Cervix uteri	134	0	78	-	-	9	28	22	45	30	14.9	32.4	1.83	21.7	C53
Uterus	8	0	88	-	-	-	3	-	3	2	0.9	1.9	0.10	1.3	C54-55
Ovary	5	0	80	-	-	-	-	-	4	1	0.6	1.2	0.08	0.8	C56
Placenta	2	0	100	-	-	-	1	1	-	-	0.2	0.5	0.02	0.3	C58
Kidney	0	0	-	-	-	-	-	-	-	-	0.0	0.0	0.00	0.0	C64
Renal pelvis, ureter and other urinary	0	0	-	-	-	-	-	-	-	-	0.0	0.0	0.00	0.0	C65-66,C68
Bladder	1	0	0	-	-	-	-	-	-	1	0.1	0.2	0.02	0.1	C67
Eye	4	0	100	1	-	-	1	-	-	2	0.4	1.0	0.02	0.5	C69
Brain, nervous system	2	0	100	1	-	-	1	-	-	-	0.2	0.5	0.02	0.3	C70-72
Thyroid	3	0	100	-	-	-	-	1	1	1	0.3	0.7	0.04	0.5	C73
Hodgkin disease	0	0	-	-	-	-	-	-	-	-	0.0	0.0	0.00	0.0	C81
Non-Hodgkin lymphoma	2	0	0	-	-	1	1	-	-	-	0.2	0.5	0.02	0.3	C82-85,C96
Multiple myeloma	1	0	0	-	-	-	-	-	-	1	0.1	0.2	0.00	0.1	C90
Lymphoid leukaemia	0	0	-	-	-	-	-	-	-	-	0.0	0.0	0.00	0.0	C91
Myeloid leukaemia	2	0	100	-	-	1	-	1	-	-	0.2	0.5	0.03	0.3	C92-94
Leukaemia, unspecified	0	0	-	-	-	-	-	-	-	-	0.0	0.0	0.00	0.0	C95
Other and unspecified	5	0	20	-	-	-	-	2	2	1	0.6	1.2	0.08	0.9	O&U
All sites	414	0	44	4	-	18	60	73	136	123	46.0	100.0	5.19	65.4	ALL
All sites but C44	413	0	45	4	-	18	60	73	136	122	45.9	100.0	5.19	65.3	ALLbC44
Average annual population				126832	60421	34832	25946	16179	17322	18410					

Table 9. South Africa, Elim (1991-1994)

NUMBER OF CASES BY AGE GROUP - MALE

SITE	ICD (10th)	ALL AGES	AGE UNK	MV (%)	0-	15-	25-	35-	45-	55-	65+	%
Mouth	C00-06	38	1	82	-	-	1	4	2	10	20	16.5
Salivary gland	C07-08	19	2	53	-	-	2	1	2	2	9	8.2
Nasopharynx	C11	2	0	100	-	-	-	-	1	-	1	0.9
Other pharynx	C09-10,C12-14	4	0	100	-	-	-	-	-	2	2	1.7
Oesophagus	C15	41	0	78	-	1	2	5	9	8	16	17.7
Stomach	C16	3	0	100	-	-	1	-	1	1	1	1.3
Colon, rectum and anus	C18-21	4	0	100	-	-	2	-	2	-	-	1.7
Liver	C22	36	1	100	-	-	4	7	7	5	12	15.6
Gallbladder etc.	C23-24	0	0	-	-	-	-	-	-	-	-	0.0
Pancreas	C25	4	0	50	-	-	-	1	1	1	2	1.7
Larynx	C32	9	0	100	-	-	-	1	-	3	6	3.9
Trachea, bronchus and lung	C33-34	16	0	81	-	1	-	1	7	4	3	6.9
Bone	C40-41	2	0	100	-	-	1	-	-	1	-	0.9
Melanoma of skin	C43	2	0	100	-	-	1	-	-	1	1	0.9
Other skin	C44	10	0	100	-	1	-	2	2	-	5	-
Mesothelioma	C45	1	0	100	-	-	-	-	-	1	-	0.4
Kaposi sarcoma	C46	1	0	100	-	-	-	-	-	-	1	0.4
Peripheral nerves	C47	0	0	-	-	-	-	-	-	-	-	0.0
Connective and soft tissue	C49	4	0	100	-	-	1	1	-	1	1	1.7
Breast	C50	2	0	50	-	-	-	1	-	-	1	0.9
Penis	C60	0	0	-	-	-	-	-	-	-	-	0.0
Prostate	C61	0	0	-	-	-	-	-	-	-	-	0.0
Testis	C62	0	0	-	-	-	-	-	-	-	-	0.0
Kidney	C64	0	0	-	-	-	-	-	-	-	-	0.0
Renal pelvis, ureter and other urinary	C65-66,C68	0	0	-	-	-	-	-	-	-	-	0.0
Bladder	C67	6	0	83	-	-	-	-	1	-	5	2.6
Eye	C69	5	0	80	2	1	1	-	1	-	-	2.2
Brain, nervous system	C70-72	2	0	50	-	-	-	-	-	-	2	0.9
Thyroid	C73	0	0	-	-	-	-	-	-	-	-	0.0
Hodgkin disease	C81	4	1	100	-	1	-	-	1	1	-	1.7
Non-Hodgkin lymphoma	C82-85,C96	6	0	100	-	-	-	-	1	2	3	2.6
Multiple myeloma	C90	1	0	100	-	-	-	-	1	-	-	0.4
Lymphoid leukaemia	C91	2	0	100	-	-	-	1	-	1	-	0.9
Myeloid leukaemia	C92-94	1	0	100	-	-	-	-	-	-	1	0.4
Leukaemia, unspecified	C95	1	0	100	1	-	-	-	-	-	-	0.4
Other and unspecified	O&U	15	1	73	-	-	1	-	2	7	4	6.5
All sites	ALL	241	6	84	5	5	17	22	39	50	97	100.0
All sites but C44	ALLbC44	231	6	84	5	4	17	20	37	50	92	

Table 9. South Africa, Elim (1991-1994)

NUMBER OF CASES BY AGE GROUP - FEMALE

SITE	ICD (10th)	ALL AGES	AGE UNK	MV (%)	0-	15-	25-	35-	45-	55-	65+	%
Mouth	C00-06	14	0	79	1	-	-	2	2	4	5	4.4
Salivary gland	C07-08	18	0	72	-	-	-	4	2	4	8	5.6
Nasopharynx	C11	0	0	-	-	-	-	-	-	-	-	0.0
Other pharynx	C09-10,C12-14	0	0	-	-	-	-	-	-	-	-	0.0
Oesophagus	C15	16	0	63	-	-	2	3	-	3	8	5.0
Stomach	C16	1	0	100	-	-	-	-	1	-	-	0.3
Colon, rectum and anus	C18-21	2	0	100	-	-	-	-	-	1	1	0.6
Liver	C22	12	0	92	-	1	1	1	1	4	4	3.8
Gallbladder etc.	C23-24	1	0	100	-	-	-	-	-	-	1	0.3
Pancreas	C25	1	0	0	-	-	-	-	-	-	1	0.3
Larynx	C32	2	0	50	-	-	-	-	-	1	1	0.6
Trachea, bronchus and lung	C33-34	1	0	100	-	-	-	-	-	1	-	0.3
Bone	C40-41	0	0	-	-	-	-	-	-	-	-	0.0
Melanoma of skin	C43	11	0	100	-	1	-	-	2	-	8	3.4
Other skin	C44	7	0	100	-	1	-	-	1	3	2	
Mesothelioma	C45	1	0	100	-	-	-	-	-	-	1	0.3
Kaposi sarcoma	C46	2	0	100	-	1	-	1	-	-	-	0.6
Peripheral nerves	C47	0	0	-	-	-	-	-	-	-	-	0.0
Connective and soft tissue	C49	3	1	100	1	-	-	-	-	-	1	0.9
Breast	C50	41	2	83	-	-	3	7	2	17	10	12.9
Vulva	C51	2	0	100	-	-	-	-	1	-	1	0.6
Vagina	C52	0	0	-	-	-	-	-	-	-	-	0.0
Cervix uteri	C53	127	1	88	-	1	7	12	34	39	33	39.8
Uterus	C54-55	15	1	100	-	-	2	-	1	2	9	4.7
Ovary	C56	0	0	-	-	-	-	-	-	-	-	0.0
Placenta	C58	0	0	-	-	-	-	-	-	-	-	0.0
Kidney	C64	0	0	-	-	-	-	-	-	-	-	0.0
Renal pelvis, ureter and other urinary	C65-66,C68	1	0	100	-	-	-	-	-	-	1	0.3
Bladder	C67	11	0	45	-	1	1	1	1	3	4	3.4
Eye	C69	16	0	94	7	-	-	-	4	1	4	5.0
Brain, nervous system	C70-72	1	0	0	1	-	-	-	-	-	-	0.3
Thyroid	C73	0	0	-	-	-	-	-	-	-	-	0.0
Hodgkin disease	C81	1	0	100	-	-	-	1	-	-	-	0.3
Non-Hodgkin lymphoma	C82-85,C96	4	0	100	-	1	-	-	1	1	1	1.3
Multiple myeloma	C90	2	0	100	-	1	-	-	1	-	-	0.6
Lymphoid leukaemia	C91	0	0	-	-	-	-	-	-	-	-	0.0
Myeloid leukaemia	C92-94	0	0	-	-	-	-	-	-	-	-	0.0
Leukaemia, unspecified	C95	2	0	100	1	-	-	-	-	-	1	0.6
Other and unspecified	O&U	11	2	82	-	-	-	2	-	2	5	3.4
All sites	ALL	326	7	85	11	8	16	34	54	86	110	100.0
All sites but C44	ALLbC44	319	7	85	11	7	16	34	53	83	108	

Table 10. South Africa: Black (1989-1992)

NUMBER OF CASES BY AGE GROUP AND SUMMARY RATES OF INCIDENCE - MALE

SITE	ALL AGES	AGE UNK	MV (%)	0-	15-	25-	35-	45-	55-	65+	CRUDE RATE	%	CR 64	ASR (W)	ICD (10th)
Mouth	2545	194	100	21	25	52	256	562	742	693	4.5	6.9	0.58	8.7	C00-06
Salivary gland	149	10	100	5	10	13	26	24	32	29	0.3	0.4	0.03	0.4	C07-08
Nasopharynx	445	25	100	6	21	16	53	102	117	105	0.8	1.2	0.10	1.4	C11
Other pharynx	361	27	100	2	7	7	35	94	111	78	0.6	1.0	0.09	1.2	C09-10,C12-14
Oesophagus	7009	402	100	15	33	211	879	1785	1993	1691	12.3	19.1	1.61	23.1	C15
Stomach	1085	72	100	6	9	43	123	246	269	317	1.9	3.0	0.22	3.6	C16
Colon, rectum and anus	981	72	100	9	47	114	143	170	194	232	1.7	2.7	0.18	3.0	C18-21
Liver	1863	155	100	32	63	168	292	343	411	399	3.3	5.1	0.38	5.6	C22
Gallbladder etc.	89	7	100	–	1	2	8	17	16	34	0.2	0.2	0.01	0.3	C23-24
Pancreas	189	15	100	1	2	2	12	41	57	59	0.3	0.5	0.04	0.7	C25
Larynx	1516	120	100	7	11	26	132	380	475	365	2.7	4.1	0.37	5.1	C32
Trachea, bronchus and lung	3347	298	100	8	19	60	371	854	969	768	5.9	9.1	0.79	11.2	C33-34
Bone	577	51	100	55	112	45	63	93	83	75	1.0	1.6	0.10	1.5	C40-41
Melanoma of skin	349	26	100	3	9	22	39	64	87	99	0.6	1.0	0.07	1.2	C43
Other skin	1446	115	100	21	50	117	173	247	271	452	2.5		0.25	4.7	C44
Mesothelioma	205	16	100	2	1	6	28	58	54	40	0.4	0.6	0.05	0.6	C45
Kaposi sarcoma	232	19	100	3	7	32	40	39	32	60	0.4	0.6	0.04	0.7	C46
Peripheral nerves	39	6	100	5	5	9	9	2	3	–	0.1	0.1	0.01	0.1	C47
Connective and soft tissue	843	69	100	81	57	76	100	136	168	156	1.5	2.3	0.16	2.4	C49
Breast	299	26	100	2	5	10	20	72	82	82	0.5	0.8	0.07	1.0	C50
Penis	404	27	100	5	5	21	77	94	81	94	0.7	1.1	0.08	1.3	C60
Prostate	3432	236	100	16	9	19	47	213	714	2178	6.0	9.4	0.44	14.3	C61
Testis	111	10	100	15	22	15	14	15	8	12	0.2	0.3	0.02	0.3	C62
Kidney	327	34	100	140	10	5	27	31	41	39	0.6	0.9	0.05	0.8	C64
Renal pelvis, ureter and other urinary	54	4	100	1	1	–	7	7	10	24	0.1	0.1	0.01	0.2	C65-66,C68
Bladder	545	39	100	13	6	28	63	89	116	191	1.0	1.5	0.10	1.8	C67
Eye	271	30	100	98	12	21	20	29	27	34	0.5	0.7	0.04	0.6	C69
Brain, nervous system	298	16	100	116	33	32	25	38	24	14	0.5	0.8	0.04	0.6	C70-72
Thyroid	171	17	100	4	11	15	22	37	26	39	0.3	0.5	0.03	0.5	C73
Hodgkin disease	390	52	100	86	57	66	45	42	27	15	0.7	1.1	0.05	0.8	C81
Non-Hodgkin lymphoma	974	79	100	109	110	100	122	168	145	141	1.7	2.7	0.17	2.5	C82-85,C96
Multiple myeloma	450	52	100	5	2	13	51	106	118	103	0.8	1.2	0.10	1.5	C90
Lymphoid leukaemia	449	23	100	129	55	16	20	47	67	92	0.8	1.2	0.07	1.2	C91
Myeloid leukaemia	504	31	100	90	87	85	67	61	42	41	0.9	1.4	0.07	1.1	C92-94
Leukaemia, unspecified	319	74	100	38	30	40	41	38	29	29	0.6	0.9	0.05	0.8	C95
Other and unspecified	5847	541	100	136	127	231	605	1278	1498	1431	10.3	15.9	1.26	19.0	O&U
All sites	38115	2990	100	1285	1071	1742	4055	7622	9139	10211	67.0	100.0	7.72	123.7	ALL
All sites but C44	36669	2875	100	1264	1021	1625	3882	7375	8868	9759	64.5		7.47	119.1	ALLbC44
Average annual population				5404020	2848118	2382196	1608623	995154	586000	387310					

Table 10. South Africa: Black (1989-1992)

NUMBER OF CASES BY AGE GROUP AND SUMMARY RATES OF INCIDENCE - FEMALE

SITE	ALL AGES	AGE UNK	MV (%)	0-	15-	25-	35-	45-	55-	65+	CRUDE RATE	%	CR 64	ASR (W)	ICD (10th)
Mouth	598	46	100	11	12	22	55	118	141	193	1.1	1.5	0.11	1.7	C00-06
Salivary gland	124	11	100	8	11	7	15	26	19	27	0.2	0.3	0.02	0.3	C07-08
Nasopharynx	111	6	100	5	15	9	15	22	19	20	0.2	0.3	0.02	0.3	C11
Other pharynx	64	2	100	5	3	2	9	8	20	15	0.1	0.2	0.01	0.2	C09-10,C12-14
Oesophagus	3220	220	100	10	24	142	400	692	926	806	5.7	7.9	0.68	9.1	C15
Stomach	702	55	100	6	15	48	90	107	166	215	1.2	1.7	0.13	2.0	C16
Colon, rectum and anus	870	53	100	8	29	70	144	161	165	240	1.5	2.1	0.15	2.3	C18-21
Liver	736	55	100	24	42	66	97	123	153	176	1.3	1.8	0.13	1.9	C22
Gallbladder etc.	122	10	100	-	1	2	11	27	38	33	0.2	0.3	0.03	0.4	C23-24
Pancreas	161	17	100	3	5	2	15	31	28	60	0.3	0.4	0.03	0.5	C25
Larynx	182	14	100	2	2	1	26	46	46	45	0.3	0.4	0.04	0.5	C32
Trachea, bronchus and lung	841	72	100	6	9	44	109	160	215	226	1.5	2.1	0.16	2.3	C33-34
Bone	397	31	100	61	94	43	31	44	36	57	0.7	1.0	0.05	0.8	C40-41
Melanoma of skin	475	38	100	3	12	21	33	78	106	184	0.8	1.2	0.08	1.4	C43
Other skin	1174	93	100	17	55	86	168	183	229	343	2.1		0.20	3.2	C44
Mesothelioma	86	6	100	-	2	3	18	25	20	12	0.2	0.2	0.02	0.2	C45
Kaposi sarcoma	69	5	100	6	9	10	3	14	10	12	0.1	0.2	0.01	0.2	C46
Peripheral nerves	31	4	100	3	6	7	1	6	2	2	0.1	0.1	0.00	0.1	C47
Connective and soft tissue	721	68	100	69	74	99	101	98	95	117	1.3	1.8	0.11	1.7	C49
Breast	5117	392	100	12	51	413	1015	1096	1093	1045	9.1	12.6	1.00	13.6	C50
Vulva	0	0		-	-	-	-	-	-	-	0.0	0.0	0.00	0.0	C51
Vagina	166	25	100	2	4	16	31	34	35	19	0.3	0.4	0.04	0.4	C52
Cervix uteri	15450	1193	100	29	164	1348	3423	3514	3243	2536	27.4	38.1	3.15	40.3	C53
Uterus	1349	97	100	3	26	41	106	196	381	499	2.4	3.3	0.24	4.0	C54-55
Ovary	892	88	100	29	46	105	133	144	206	141	1.6	2.2	0.18	2.3	C56
Placenta	92	15	100	1	13	32	13	14	-	4	0.2	0.2	0.01	0.2	C58
Kidney	320	20	100	137	10	19	35	30	39	30	0.6	0.8	0.04	0.7	C64
Renal pelvis, ureter and other urinary	92	7	100	-	1	7	18	18	26	15	0.2	0.2	0.02	0.3	C65-66,C68
Bladder	509	54	100	6	18	32	93	101	106	99	0.9	1.3	0.10	1.3	C67
Eye	206	24	100	79	8	28	12	13	13	29	0.4	0.5	0.02	0.4	C69
Brain, nervous system	213	16	100	76	31	25	23	19	16	7	0.4	0.5	0.03	0.4	C70-72
Thyroid	476	43	100	6	25	79	72	79	110	62	0.8	1.2	0.10	1.2	C73
Hodgkin disease	213	17	100	24	41	47	40	17	14	13	0.4	0.5	0.03	0.4	C81
Non-Hodgkin lymphoma	635	60	100	66	58	69	66	92	101	123	1.1	1.6	0.10	1.5	C82-85,C96
Multiple myeloma	418	53	100	-	3	15	43	97	103	104	0.7	1.0	0.09	1.2	C90
Lymphoid leukaemia	302	15	100	108	35	15	14	26	46	43	0.5	0.7	0.04	0.7	C91
Myeloid leukaemia	388	14	100	57	57	79	54	51	45	31	0.7	1.0	0.06	0.8	C92-94
Leukaemia, unspecified	263	62	100	26	29	31	22	34	31	28	0.5	0.6	0.04	0.6	C95
Other and unspecified	3906	335	100	102	116	249	505	747	881	971	6.9	9.6	0.73	10.6	O&U
All sites	41691	3336	100	1010	1156	3334	7059	8291	8923	8582	73.9		7.99	109.8	ALL
All sites but C44	40517	3243	100	993	1101	3248	6891	8108	8694	8239	71.8	100.0	7.80	106.7	ALLbC44

| Average annual population | | | | 5331163 | 2810970 | 2236349 | 1515883 | 1004179 | 660820 | 542967 | | | | | |

Table 11. South Africa: White (1989-1992)

NUMBER OF CASES BY AGE GROUP AND SUMMARY RATES OF INCIDENCE - MALE

SITE	ALL AGES	AGE UNK	MV (%)	0-	15-	25-	35-	45-	55-	65+	CRUDE RATE	%	CR 64	ASR (W)	ICD (10th)
Mouth	1294	56	100	3	9	38	110	288	318	472	12.9	4.9	0.77	11.8	C00-06
Salivary gland	132	7	100	1	5	5	6	24	29	55	1.3	0.5	0.07	1.2	C07-08
Nasopharynx	123	6	100	-	-	2	12	31	37	35	1.2	0.5	0.08	1.1	C11
Other pharynx	84	2	100	-	-	1	3	19	26	33	0.8	0.3	0.05	0.8	C09-10,C12-14
Oesophagus	597	23	100	2	2	8	30	101	177	254	5.9	2.3	0.35	5.5	C15
Stomach	1110	49	100	3	4	18	72	150	254	560	11.0	4.2	0.53	10.1	C16
Colon, rectum and anus	2414	69	100	8	7	37	104	267	563	1359	24.0	9.2	1.06	22.2	C18-21
Liver	353	15	100	5	3	25	36	58	93	118	3.5	1.3	0.22	3.2	C22
Gallbladder etc.	67	1	100	-	-	-	2	9	14	41	0.7	0.3	0.03	0.6	C23-24
Pancreas	201	6	100	-	-	2	10	27	63	93	2.0	0.8	0.11	1.9	C25
Larynx	641	18	100	-	4	2	28	105	220	264	6.4	2.4	0.39	5.9	C32
Trachea, bronchus and lung	2187	63	100	5	15	16	80	278	714	1016	21.7	8.3	1.23	20.3	C33-34
Bone	224	9	100	15	40	21	18	36	46	39	2.2	0.9	0.15	2.1	C40-41
Melanoma of skin	1718	150	100	8	57	156	272	296	328	451	17.1	6.6	1.05	15.3	C43
Other skin	24620	2175	100	64	147	524	1834	3887	5277	10712	244.6		12.58	224.3	C44
Mesothelioma	299	12	100	1	1	9	22	53	82	120	3.0	1.1	0.17	2.7	C45
Kaposi sarcoma	68	12	100	1	3	14	10	4	3	21	0.7	0.3	0.03	0.6	C46
Peripheral nerves	14	2	100	2	2	-	3	2		3	0.1	0.1	0.01	0.1	C47
Connective and soft tissue	543	27	100	18	31	35	50	77	109	196	5.4	2.1	0.30	5.0	C49
Breast	206	17	100	1	1	7	13	40	50	77	2.0	0.8	0.12	1.9	C50
Penis	75	5	100	-	-	4	3	8	24	31	0.7	0.3	0.04	0.7	C60
Prostate	4455	114	100	10	7	13	27	150	890	3244	44.3	17.0	1.33	41.1	C61
Testis	292	11	100	5	54	101	73	25	12	11	2.9	1.1	0.19	2.5	C62
Kidney	378	15	100	20	1	7	21	77	108	129	3.8	1.4	0.24	3.6	C64
Renal pelvis, ureter and other urinary	213	9	100	-	1	2	3	20	53	125	2.1	0.8	0.09	2.0	C65-66,C68
Bladder	2810	57	100	6	12	44	88	313	642	1648	27.9	10.7	1.19	25.8	C67
Eye	102	4	100	7	2	7	14	14	15	39	1.0	0.4	0.05	1.0	C69
Brain, nervous system	328	11	100	42	21	26	51	50	65	62	3.3	1.3	0.22	3.1	C70-72
Thyroid	177	7	100	4	6	14	25	40	28	53	1.8	0.7	0.10	1.6	C73
Hodgkin disease	215	17	100	18	37	38	36	31	21	17	2.1	0.8	0.14	2.0	C81
Non-Hodgkin lymphoma	1143	91	100	49	59	62	104	158	228	392	11.4	4.4	0.64	10.6	C82-85,C96
Multiple myeloma	146	13	100	-	-	4	5	31	31	62	1.5	0.6	0.08	1.3	C90
Lymphoid leukaemia	347	11	100	73	25	14	11	36	60	117	3.4	1.3	0.19	3.6	C91
Myeloid leukaemia	329	21	100	21	25	29	32	51	47	103	3.3	1.3	0.18	3.1	C92-94
Leukaemia, unspecified	126	17	100	17	9	12	8	15	13	35	1.3	0.5	0.07	1.2	C95
Other and unspecified	2784	145	100	37	55	67	162	374	696	1248	27.7	10.6	1.47	25.8	O&U
All sites	50815	3267	100	445	645	1364	3378	7145	11336	23235	504.8		25.48	465.7	ALL
All sites but C44	26195	1092	100	381	498	840	1544	3258	6059	12523	260.2	100.0	12.91	241.3	ALLbC44
Average annual population				572487	444607	413159	378575	308289	203799	195430					

Warning, percentages will be distored because of the high rates for 'Other skin cancer'

Table 11. South Africa: White (1989-1992)

NUMBER OF CASES BY AGE GROUP AND SUMMARY RATES OF INCIDENCE - FEMALE

SITE	ALL AGES	AGE UNK	MV (%)	0-	15-	25-	35-	45-	55-	65+	CRUDE RATE	%	CR 64	ASR (W)	ICD (10th)
Mouth	559	17	100	4	4	17	31	79	128	279	5.5	2.1	0.26	4.3	C00-06
Salivary gland	60	3	100	-	2	4	2	9	10	30	0.6	0.2	0.03	0.5	C07-08
Nasopharynx	42	3	100	-	-	1	6	5	7	20	0.4	0.2	0.02	0.3	C11
Other pharynx	26	1	100	1	-	-	1	5	5	13	0.3	0.1	0.01	0.2	C09-10,C12-14
Oesophagus	208	8	100	-	1	4	9	33	42	112	2.0	0.8	0.09	1.6	C15
Stomach	638	25	100	1	1	19	59	71	116	346	6.3	2.4	0.26	4.8	C16
Colon, rectum and anus	2295	74	100	4	11	37	132	272	441	1324	22.5	8.7	0.91	17.1	C18-21
Liver	210	6	100	4	-	8	12	41	38	101	2.1	0.8	0.10	1.6	C22
Gallbladder etc.	106	2	100	1	-	-	7	9	25	62	1.0	0.4	0.04	0.8	C23-24
Pancreas	211	1	100	-	-	3	14	24	46	123	2.1	0.8	0.09	1.6	C25
Larynx	131	5	100	1	1	1	8	27	40	48	1.3	0.5	0.08	1.1	C32
Trachea, bronchus and lung	1120	32	100	3	6	23	64	170	319	503	11.0	4.3	0.60	8.8	C33-34
Bone	201	3	100	31	23	24	12	26	29	53	2.0	0.8	0.12	1.8	C40-41
Melanoma of skin	1762	130	100	10	72	180	326	280	258	506	17.3	6.7	0.99	14.2	C43
Other skin	16448	1380	100	33	109	465	1453	2389	2759	7860	161.6		7.27	125.1	C44
Mesothelioma	131	9	100	1	2	3	13	27	32	44	1.3	0.5	0.08	1.1	C45
Kaposi sarcoma	17	4	100	-	2	-	1	1	2	7	0.2	0.1	0.01	0.1	C46
Peripheral nerves	15	1	100	5	3	2	1	1	-	1	0.1	0.1	0.01	0.2	C47
Connective and soft tissue	388	28	100	9	13	34	30	65	69	140	3.8	1.5	0.21	3.2	C49
Breast	7801	190	100	6	20	271	1198	1746	1765	2605	76.6	29.6	4.67	62.8	C50
Vulva	0	0	-	-	-	-	-	-	-	-	0.0	0.0	0.00	0.0	C51
Vagina	65	5	100	2	2	-	9	10	12	25	0.6	0.2	0.03	0.5	C52
Cervix uteri	1465	64	100	-	30	182	302	267	258	362	14.4	5.6	0.91	11.9	C53
Uterus	1052	26	100	1	6	13	61	170	281	494	10.3	4.0	0.55	8.2	C54-55
Ovary	893	27	100	6	27	44	98	221	220	250	8.8	3.4	0.58	7.4	C56
Placenta	2	0	100	-	2	-	1	1	-	-	0.0	0.0	0.00	0.0	C58
Kidney	258	8	100	19	4	7	16	40	53	111	2.5	1.0	0.13	2.2	C64
Renal pelvis, ureter and other urinary	98	2	100	-	1	2	3	8	13	69	1.0	0.4	0.03	0.7	C65-66,C68
Bladder	870	21	100	7	4	14	35	101	175	513	8.5	3.3	0.34	6.5	C67
Eye	77	3	100	10	4	5	5	10	10	30	0.8	0.3	0.04	0.7	C69
Brain, nervous system	287	7	100	53	31	22	29	48	44	53	2.8	1.1	0.18	2.7	C70-72
Thyroid	560	9	100	6	38	110	132	92	69	100	5.5	2.1	0.35	4.7	C73
Hodgkin disease	181	13	100	6	37	41	19	18	12	35	1.8	0.7	0.10	1.6	C81
Non-Hodgkin lymphoma	1023	70	100	28	27	45	72	168	208	405	10.0	3.9	0.54	8.2	C82-85,C96
Multiple myeloma	103	1	100	-	-	-	3	23	18	58	1.0	0.4	0.04	0.8	C90
Lymphoid leukaemia	225	9	100	55	19	7	17	18	29	71	2.2	0.9	0.12	2.2	C91
Myeloid leukaemia	275	12	100	16	14	22	31	51	45	84	2.7	1.0	0.16	2.3	C92-94
Leukaemia, unspecified	124	16	100	13	10	10	16	21	16	22	1.2	0.5	0.08	1.2	C95
Other and unspecified	2840	114	100	34	36	88	244	415	609	1300	27.9	10.8	1.40	22.2	O&U
All sites	42767	2329	100	374	561	1708	4471	6961	8204	18159	420.1		21.47	335.3	ALL
All sites but C44	26319	949	100	341	452	1243	3018	4572	5445	10299	258.5	100.0	14.15	210.0	ALLbC44
Average annual population				548928	429377	406348	369657	298402	212906	279288					

Warning, percentages will be distored because of the high rates for 'Other skin cancer'

Table 12. South Africa: Mixed Race (1989-1992)

NUMBER OF CASES BY AGE GROUP AND SUMMARY RATES OF INCIDENCE - MALE

SITE	ALL AGES	AGE UNK	MV (%)	0-	15-	25-	35-	45-	55-	65+	CRUDE RATE	%	CR 64	ASR (W)	ICD (10th)
Mouth	449	6	100	2	4	9	43	115	135	135	7.0	7.8	0.87	13.5	C00-06
Salivary gland	19	0	100	-	-	2	3	2	4	8	0.3	0.3	0.02	0.5	C07-08
Nasopharynx	97	2	100	4	3	3	18	25	25	17	1.5	1.7	0.18	2.5	C11
Other pharynx	64	1	100	-	1	3	8	14	22	15	1.0	1.1	0.13	1.8	C09-10,C12-14
Oesophagus	520	11	100	1	1	6	34	134	190	143	8.1	9.0	1.13	16.0	C15
Stomach	534	21	100	1	2	22	55	111	146	176	8.3	9.3	0.95	16.1	C16
Colon, rectum and anus	252	1	100	-	10	15	25	45	75	81	3.9	4.4	0.46	7.5	C18-21
Liver	124	1	100	6	8	8	12	23	36	30	1.9	2.2	0.24	3.5	C22
Gallbladder etc.	19	0	100	1	-	-	2	6	3	8	0.3	0.3	0.03	0.6	C23-24
Pancreas	46	1	100	1	3	-	4	7	19	11	0.7	0.8	0.10	1.4	C25
Larynx	311	8	100	-	-	13	24	82	125	72	4.9	5.4	0.73	9.4	C32
Trachea, bronchus and lung	627	14	100	-	-	13	47	143	251	159	9.8	10.9	1.43	19.2	C33-34
Bone	51	2	100	2	19	5	6	7	5	5	0.8	0.9	0.06	1.0	C40-41
Melanoma of skin	27	0	100	-	-	1	7	5	6	8	0.4	0.5	0.05	0.8	C43
Other skin	227	7	100	4	7	9	31	40	44	85	3.5		0.34	6.8	C44
Mesothelioma	39	2	100	-	-	-	6	11	11	9	0.6	0.7	0.08	1.2	C45
Kaposi sarcoma	23	0	100	2	1	3	3	3	3	8	0.4	0.4	0.03	0.6	C46
Peripheral nerves	4	0	100	2	-	1	1	-	-	-	0.1	0.1	0.00	0.1	C47
Connective and soft tissue	97	5	100	6	6	9	12	25	20	14	1.5	1.7	0.17	2.4	C49
Breast	30	-	100	-	-	-	3	4	5	16	0.5	0.5	0.03	1.0	C50
Penis	43	1	100	-	1	4	5	4	13	15	0.7	0.7	0.07	1.2	C60
Prostate	681	15	100	3	2	4	5	35	133	486	10.6	11.8	0.67	25.4	C61
Testis	21	0	100	1	7	4	2	4	3	-	0.3	0.4	0.03	0.4	C62
Kidney	62	0	100	11	3	4	7	8	15	14	1.0	1.1	0.10	1.6	C64
Renal pelvis, ureter and other urinary	18	0	100	-	-	-	1	5	5	7	0.3	0.3	0.03	0.6	C65-66,C68
Bladder	245	2	100	-	1	4	19	40	59	120	3.8	4.3	0.37	8.1	C67
Eye	12	0	100	9	-	1	-	1	-	-	0.2	0.2	0.01	0.2	C69
Brain, nervous system	67	0	100	19	10	8	8	13	7	2	1.0	1.2	0.10	1.3	C70-72
Thyroid	19	0	100	2	1	-	4	4	2	6	0.3	0.3	0.03	0.5	C73
Hodgkin disease	74	1	100	17	14	18	11	8	7	-	1.2	1.3	0.09	1.2	C81
Non-Hodgkin lymphoma	180	1	100	12	23	36	23	33	25	27	2.8	3.1	0.26	4.0	C82-85,C96
Multiple myeloma	53	0	100	-	-	7	7	10	17	19	0.8	0.9	0.10	1.7	C90
Lymphoid leukaemia	70	1	100	29	13	6	4	5	3	9	1.1	1.2	0.07	1.3	C91
Myeloid leukaemia	86	1	100	9	17	9	14	13	10	13	1.3	1.5	0.11	1.8	C92-94
Leukaemia, unspecified	12	1	100	2	2	3	1	2	-	1	0.2	0.2	0.01	0.2	C95
Other and unspecified	781	35	100	19	11	36	67	165	244	204	12.2	13.6	1.56	22.9	O&U
All sites	5984	141	100	164	170	244	524	1150	1666	1925	93.4	100.0	10.65	177.9	ALL
All sites but C44	5757	134	100	160	163	235	493	1110	1622	1840	89.9	100.0	10.32	171.2	ALLbC44
Average annual population				548187	360858	287096	183680	110196	67033	44040					

Table 12. South Africa: Mixed Race (1989-1992)

NUMBER OF CASES BY AGE GROUP AND SUMMARY RATES OF INCIDENCE - FEMALE

SITE	ALL AGES	AGE UNK	MV (%)	0-	15-	25-	35-	45-	55-	65+	CRUDE RATE	%	CR 64	ASR (W)	ICD (10th)
Mouth	143	9	100	-	-	7	17	35	32	43	2.1	2.4	0.22	3.3	C00-06
Salivary gland	12	2	100	-	-	1	2	5	2	3	0.2	0.2	0.02	0.3	C07-08
Nasopharynx	24	0	100	1	2	2	2	5	8	4	0.4	0.4	0.04	0.5	C11
Other pharynx	18	3	100	-	-	-	3	7	4	1	0.3	0.3	0.04	0.4	C09-10,C12-14
Oesophagus	178	6	100	-	-	2	20	38	59	53	2.7	2.9	0.31	4.2	C15
Stomach	281	7	100	3	3	17	39	49	69	94	4.2	4.6	0.40	6.4	C16
Colon, rectum and anus	280	7	100	2	5	21	33	36	55	121	4.2	4.6	0.33	6.4	C18-21
Liver	52	0	100	2	4	5	3	8	13	17	0.8	0.9	0.07	1.1	C22
Gallbladder etc.	30	2	100	-	-	-	2	5	9	12	0.4	0.5	0.05	0.8	C23-24
Pancreas	33	0	100	-	-	-	4	8	10	11	0.5	0.5	0.05	0.8	C25
Larynx	81	1	100	-	-	3	13	20	34	10	1.2	1.3	0.17	1.8	C32
Trachea, bronchus and lung	220	5	100	-	4	9	25	68	62	47	3.3	3.6	0.40	5.1	C33-34
Bone	47	1	100	5	11	2	7	3	11	7	0.7	0.8	0.06	0.9	C40-41
Melanoma of skin	45	3	100	1	2	-	4	7	13	15	0.7	0.7	0.07	1.1	C43
Other skin	256	8	100	4	3	16	23	51	46	105	3.8		0.31	5.9	C44
Mesothelioma	18	0	100	-	-	1	3	1	4	9	0.3	0.3	0.02	0.4	C45
Kaposi sarcoma	5	0	100	-	2	-	1	1	-	1	0.1	0.1	0.00	0.1	C46
Peripheral nerves	0	0	-	-	-	-	-	-	-	-	0.0	0.0	0.00	0.0	C47
Connective and soft tissue	88	7	100	8	5	13	12	18	15	10	1.3	1.5	0.13	1.7	C49
Breast	1285	15	100	7	2	87	253	344	288	289	19.2	21.2	2.07	28.1	C50
Vulva	0	0	-	-	-	-	-	-	-	-	0.0	0.0	0.00	0.0	C51
Vagina	10	1	100	-	-	1	3	2	1	2	0.1	0.2	0.01	0.2	C52
Cervix uteri	1541	35	100	4	14	150	421	404	287	226	23.0	25.5	2.50	31.6	C53
Uterus	200	5	100	1	1	3	20	32	56	83	3.0	3.3	0.28	4.8	C54-55
Ovary	196	3	100	6	13	13	38	38	48	37	2.9	3.2	0.31	4.0	C56
Placenta	9	0	100	-	2	4	2	1	-	-	0.1	0.1	0.01	0.1	C58
Kidney	30	0	100	9	3	2	2	5	7	2	0.4	0.5	0.04	0.6	C64
Renal pelvis, ureter and other urinary	17	0	100	-	-	3	2	3	7	2	0.3	0.3	0.04	0.4	C65-66,C68
Bladder	69	0	100	-	2	-	6	8	23	30	1.0	1.1	0.10	1.7	C67
Eye	23	1	100	9	1	5	1	3	-	3	0.3	0.4	0.02	0.4	C69
Brain, nervous system	56	2	100	21	7	5	8	5	10	3	0.8	0.9	0.07	1.0	C70-72
Thyroid	38	0	100	-	2	11	8	7	4	5	0.6	0.6	0.05	0.7	C73
Hodgkin disease	38	1	100	2	2	10	11	3	6	3	0.6	0.6	0.05	0.7	C81
Non-Hodgkin lymphoma	158	5	100	8	7	18	21	24	35	40	2.4	2.6	0.22	3.3	C82-85,C96
Multiple myeloma	44	0	100	-	-	-	4	7	16	17	0.7	0.7	0.07	1.1	C90
Lymphoid leukaemia	39	0	100	15	4	2	2	6	5	5	0.6	0.6	0.04	0.7	C91
Myeloid leukaemia	71	0	100	7	9	14	6	6	14	15	1.1	1.2	0.09	1.3	C92-94
Leukaemia, unspecified	10	0	100	3	2	1	-	-	-	3	0.1	0.2	0.01	0.2	C95
Other and unspecified	659	21	100	16	11	37	110	106	165	193	9.8	10.9	0.98	14.7	O&U
All sites	6304	151	100	133	123	465	1127	1365	1418	1522	94.1	100.0	9.68	136.7	ALL
All sites but C44	6048	143	100	129	120	449	1104	1314	1372	1417	90.3	100.0	9.37	130.8	ALLbC44
Average annual population				544737	363740	299908	198008	122021	79656	66843					

Table 13. South Africa: Indian (1989-1992)

NUMBER OF CASES BY AGE GROUP AND SUMMARY RATES OF INCIDENCE - MALE

SITE	ALL AGES	AGE UNK	MV (%)	0-	15-	25-	35-	45-	55-	65+	CRUDE RATE	%	CR 64	ASR (W)	ICD (10th)
Mouth	65	0	100	-	1	2	2	26	23	11	3.3	3.1	0.38	4.8	C00-06
Salivary gland	10	0	100	-	-	1	-	2	4	3	0.5	0.5	0.05	0.8	C07-08
Nasopharynx	7	0	100	-	1	-	-	3	-	3	0.4	0.3	0.02	0.6	C11
Other pharynx	14	2	100	-	-	-	2	1	4	5	0.7	0.7	0.06	1.2	C09-10,C12-14
Oesophagus	179	16	100	-	1	7	26	50	52	27	9.2	8.4	1.04	13.1	C15
Stomach	140	9	100	3	-	2	16	32	36	42	7.2	6.6	0.68	11.7	C16
Colon, rectum and anus	161	9	100	1	-	8	12	25	41	65	8.3	7.6	0.66	14.2	C18-21
Liver	47	2	100	1	2	-	5	13	9	15	2.4	2.2	0.20	3.8	C22
Gallbladder etc.	6	0	100	-	-	-	3	1	2	4	0.3	0.3	0.03	0.6	C23-24
Pancreas	16	0	100	-	-	3	3	1	5	4	0.8	0.8	0.07	1.2	C25
Larynx	52	3	100	-	-	1	4	12	18	14	2.7	2.5	0.30	4.4	C32
Trachea, bronchus and lung	288	7	100	1	2	9	25	82	104	58	14.8	13.6	1.69	22.5	C33-34
Bone	35	4	100	5	9	1	-	6	7	2	1.8	1.7	0.16	2.1	C40-41
Melanoma of skin	13	2	100	-	-	2	2	5	2	-	0.7	0.6	0.07	0.7	C43
Other skin	65	3	100	-	2	5	7	11	13	24	3.3	3.0	0.25	5.4	C44
Mesothelioma	4	0	100	-	-	-	-	1	-	4	0.2	0.2	0.00	0.5	C45
Kaposi sarcoma	2	0	100	-	-	-	-	1	-	1	0.1	0.1	0.00	0.2	C46
Peripheral nerves	0	0	-	-	-	-	-	-	-	-	0.0	0.0	0.00	0.0	C47
Connective and soft tissue	47	2	100	8	5	3	3	10	8	8	2.4	2.2	0.21	3.3	C49
Breast	20	3	100	1	-	-	4	4	4	4	1.0	0.9	0.10	1.6	C50
Penis	23	1	100	-	-	1	1	5	5	10	1.2	1.1	0.09	2.1	C60
Prostate	121	3	100	-	2	-	-	8	23	85	6.2	5.7	0.31	13.0	C61
Testis	30	1	100	9	6	8	4	-	-	1	1.5	1.4	0.08	1.5	C62
Kidney	26	0	100	5	1	2	1	5	6	6	1.3	1.2	0.11	1.9	C64
Renal pelvis, ureter and other urinary	11	0	100	-	-	-	1	2	5	3	0.6	0.5	0.07	0.9	C65-66,C68
Bladder	88	4	100	-	1	2	6	18	27	30	4.5	4.2	0.44	7.7	C67
Eye	7	0	100	5	-	-	-	-	1	1	0.4	0.3	0.02	0.5	C69
Brain, nervous system	24	2	100	7	-	1	3	3	4	4	1.2	1.1	0.09	1.6	C70-72
Thyroid	21	4	100	-	2	1	3	2	5	4	1.1	1.0	0.10	1.5	C73
Hodgkin disease	22	4	100	3	3	6	4	4	-	1	1.1	1.0	0.08	1.1	C81
Non-Hodgkin lymphoma	106	4	100	7	5	9	22	17	20	22	5.4	5.0	0.45	7.4	C82-85,C96
Multiple myeloma	22	0	100	-	-	-	-	5	-	9	1.1	1.0	0.09	1.9	C90
Lymphoid leukaemia	37	2	100	24	3	-	1	1	4	2	1.9	1.7	0.13	2.2	C91
Myeloid leukaemia	28	0	100	9	4	3	7	5	-	-	1.4	1.3	0.09	1.4	C92-94
Leukaemia, unspecified	30	3	100	8	5	3	5	5	-	1	1.5	1.4	0.11	1.6	C95
Other and unspecified	418	20	100	9	8	14	41	99	125	102	21.4	19.7	2.21	33.3	O&U
All sites	2185	106	100	106	63	95	210	465	566	574	112.1		10.44	172.5	ALL
All sites but C44	2120	103	100	106	61	90	203	454	553	550	108.7	100.0	10.18	167.1	ALLbC44

| Average annual population | | | | 151764 | 98737 | 81849 | 68799 | 46298 | 25173 | 14765 | | | | | |

Table 13. South Africa: Indian (1989-1992)

NUMBER OF CASES BY AGE GROUP AND SUMMARY RATES OF INCIDENCE - FEMALE

SITE	ALL AGES	AGE UNK	MV (%)	0-	15-	25-	35-	45-	55-	65+	CRUDE RATE	%	CR 64	ASR (W)	ICD (10th)
Mouth	83	5	100	-	2	2	8	20	32	14	4.2	3.3	0.45	5.5	C00-06
Salivary gland	8	0	100	-	-	-	-	3	4	1	0.4	0.3	0.05	0.5	C07-08
Nasopharynx	6	0	100	-	-	1	2	-	-	1	0.3	0.2	0.02	0.4	C11
Other pharynx	7	0	100	1	-	1	1	2	-	2	0.4	0.3	0.02	0.4	C09-10,C12-14
Oesophagus	102	7	100	1	1	-	10	16	34	32	5.1	4.1	0.46	7.3	C15
Stomach	91	6	100	-	-	6	14	15	16	34	4.6	3.7	0.31	6.4	C16
Colon, rectum and anus	132	5	100	-	-	5	15	25	38	44	6.7	5.3	0.56	9.4	C18-21
Liver	16	0	100	-	1	-	-	2	7	6	0.8	0.6	0.07	1.2	C22
Gallbladder etc.	12	0	100	-	-	-	-	1	4	7	0.6	0.5	0.04	1.0	C23-24
Pancreas	17	1	100	-	-	-	-	2	5	9	0.9	0.7	0.06	1.4	C25
Larynx	9	3	100	-	1	1	1	1	1	1	0.5	0.4	0.04	0.5	C32
Trachea, bronchus and lung	50	0	100	-	-	2	8	13	15	11	2.5	2.0	0.24	3.3	C33-34
Bone	26	0	100	3	-	-	4	5	6	8	1.3	1.0	0.10	1.8	C40-41
Melanoma of skin	13	1	100	-	-	-	-	4	4	3	0.7	0.5	0.06	0.9	C43
Other skin	60	2	100	-	7	4	6	8	9	24	3.0		0.19	4.2	C44
Mesothelioma	1	0	100	-	-	-	-	-	1	-	0.1	0.0	0.01	0.1	C45
Kaposi sarcoma	2	0	100	-	-	-	-	-	-	1	0.1	0.1	0.00	0.1	C46
Peripheral nerves	0	0	-	-	-	-	-	-	-	-	0.0	0.0	0.00	0.0	C47
Connective and soft tissue	32	3	100	2	-	-	2	6	11	6	1.6	1.3	0.16	2.1	C49
Breast	693	46	100	1	3	36	150	182	167	108	34.9	27.9	3.24	42.5	C50
Vulva	0	0	-	-	-	-	-	-	-	-	0.0	0.0	0.00	0.0	C51
Vagina	8	2	100	-	-	-	1	1	3	1	0.4	0.3	0.05	0.5	C52
Cervix uteri	330	25	100	1	-	21	69	88	68	58	16.6	13.3	1.45	20.2	C53
Uterus	127	6	100	-	-	2	13	30	43	33	6.4	5.1	0.62	8.9	C54-55
Ovary	94	11	100	1	1	4	18	15	26	18	4.7	3.8	0.44	6.1	C56
Placenta	2	0	100	-	-	1	-	-	-	-	0.1	0.1	0.01	0.1	C58
Kidney	12	1	100	2	-	1	2	2	2	2	0.6	0.5	0.05	0.7	C64
Renal pelvis, ureter and other urinary	8	0	100	-	-	-	2	2	2	3	0.4	0.3	0.03	0.6	C65-66,C68
Bladder	37	1	100	1	-	-	3	7	14	11	1.9	1.5	0.18	2.7	C67
Eye	3	0	100	1	-	-	-	1	-	-	0.2	0.1	0.01	0.2	C69
Brain, nervous system	10	0	100	4	-	-	2	4	-	-	0.5	0.4	0.04	0.5	C70-72
Thyroid	53	1	100	1	6	9	14	8	9	5	2.7	2.1	0.22	2.9	C73
Hodgkin disease	9	0	100	1	1	3	3	3	1	-	0.5	0.4	0.04	0.4	C81
Non-Hodgkin lymphoma	66	5	100	5	4	4	3	13	19	13	3.3	2.7	0.31	4.4	C82-85,C96
Multiple myeloma	19	3	100	-	-	-	2	6	6	2	1.0	0.8	0.11	1.2	C90
Lymphoid leukaemia	21	0	100	13	1	-	2	4	1	2	1.1	0.8	0.06	1.1	C91
Myeloid leukaemia	21	2	100	3	2	3	2	4	2	3	1.1	0.8	0.07	1.2	C92-94
Leukaemia, unspecified	23	2	100	5	3	3	2	5	1	2	1.2	0.9	0.08	1.2	C95
Other and unspecified	339	20	100	4	5	22	35	88	93	72	17.1	13.7	1.57	22.1	O&U
All sites	2542	160	100	51	41	133	392	584	644	537	128.1		11.42	164.3	ALL
All sites but C44	2482	158	100	51	34	129	386	576	635	513	125.1	100.0	11.23	160.1	ALLbC44
Average annual population				148195	98169	82547	70205	48651	29350	19001					

Table 14. Childhood cancer, South Africa: Black (1989-1992)

	NUMBER OF CASES					REL. FREQ.(%)	RATES PER MILLION					
	0-4	5-9	10-14	All	M/F	Overall	0-4	5-9	10-14	Crude	ASR	%MV
Leukaemia	112	190	148	**450**	1.4	19.6	7.1	13.4	11.3	10.5	**10.4**	100.0
Acute lymphoid leukaemia	62	104	65	**231**	1.2	10.1	3.9	7.3	5.0	5.4	**5.3**	100.0
Lymphoma	42	123	123	**288**	2.2	12.5	2.7	8.7	9.4	6.7	**6.6**	100.0
Hodgkin disease	7	51	52	**110**	3.6	4.8	0.4	3.6	4.0	2.6	**2.5**	100.0
Burkitt lymphoma	12	13	4	**29**	1.6	1.3	0.8	0.9	0.3	0.7	**0.7**	100.0
Brain and spinal neoplasms	43	75	64	**182**	1.6	7.9	2.7	5.3	4.9	4.2	**4.2**	100.0
Neuroblastoma	49	26	19	**94**	1.6	4.1	3.1	1.8	1.5	2.2	**2.2**	100.0
Retinoblastoma	109	12	1	**122**	1.2	5.3	6.9	0.8	0.1	2.8	**3.0**	100.0
Wilms tumour	132	70	20	**222**	1.0	9.7	8.4	4.9	1.5	5.2	**5.3**	100.0
Bone tumours	7	22	78	**107**	0.9	4.7	0.4	1.6	6.0	2.5	**2.4**	100.0
Soft tissue sarcomas	59	41	45	**145**	1.1	6.3	3.8	2.9	3.4	3.4	**3.4**	100.0
Kaposi sarcoma	2	3	4	**9**	0.5	0.4	0.1	0.2	0.3	0.2	**0.2**	100.0
Germ cell tumours	36	10	10	**56**	0.3	2.4	2.3	0.7	0.8	1.3	**1.3**	100.0
Other	259	181	189	**629**	1.2	27.4	16.5	12.8	14.5	14.6	**14.7**	100.0
All	848	750	697	**2295**	1.3	100.0	54.0	52.9	53.4	53.4	**53.5**	100.0

Table 15. Childhood cancer, South Africa: White (1989-1992)

	NUMBER OF CASES					REL. FREQ.(%)	RATES PER MILLION					
	0-4	5-9	10-14	All	M/F	Overall	0-4	5-9	10-14	Crude	ASR	%MV
Leukaemia	97	60	38	**195**	1.3	23.8	69.9	37.5	25.4	43.5	**46.5**	100.0
Acute lymphoid leukaemia	62	42	21	**125**	1.3	15.3	44.7	26.3	14.0	27.9	**29.8**	100.0
Lymphoma	28	33	40	**101**	2.0	12.3	20.2	20.6	26.7	22.5	**22.2**	100.0
Hodgkin disease	3	10	11	**24**	3.0	2.9	2.2	6.3	7.3	5.4	**5.0**	100.0
Burkitt lymphoma	3	6	1	**10**	4.0	1.2	2.2	3.8	0.7	2.2	**2.2**	100.0
Brain and spinal neoplasms	24	32	32	**88**	0.8	10.7	17.3	20.0	21.3	19.6	**19.3**	100.0
Neuroblastoma	31	14	4	**49**	1.1	6.0	22.3	8.8	2.7	10.9	**12.2**	100.0
Retinoblastoma	11	1	0	**12**	1.0	1.5	7.9	0.6	-	2.7	**3.3**	100.0
Wilms tumour	22	14	1	**37**	1.2	4.5	15.9	8.8	0.7	8.2	**9.2**	100.0
Bone tumours	5	13	28	**46**	0.5	5.6	3.6	8.1	18.7	10.3	**9.4**	100.0
Soft tissue sarcomas	9	8	7	**24**	2.0	2.9	6.5	5.0	4.7	5.4	**5.5**	100.0
Kaposi sarcoma	0	0	1	**1**	-	0.1	-	-	0.7	0.2	**0.2**	100.0
Germ cell tumours	5	3	5	**13**	0.6	1.6	3.6	1.9	3.3	2.9	**3.0**	100.0
Other	139	58	57	**254**	1.2	31.0	100.2	36.3	38.0	56.6	**61.5**	100.0
All	371	236	212	**819**	1.2	100.0	267.4	147.6	141.4	182.6	**192.2**	100.0

Table 16. Childhood cancer, South Africa: Mixed Race (1989-1992)

	NUMBER OF CASES					REL. FREQ.(%)	RATES PER MILLION					
	0-4	5-9	10-14	**All**	*M/F*	Overall	0-4	5-9	10-14	Crude	**ASR**	%MV
Leukaemia	28	20	17	**65**	*1.6*	21.9	19.0	13.0	12.5	14.9	**15.2**	100.0
Acute lymphoid leukaemia	21	12	11	**44**	*1.9*	14.8	14.3	7.8	8.1	10.1	**10.4**	100.0
Lymphoma	12	14	13	**39**	*2.9*	13.1	8.1	9.1	9.5	8.9	**8.9**	100.0
Hodgkin disease	2	7	10	**19**	*8.5*	6.4	1.4	4.6	7.3	4.3	**4.1**	100.0
Burkitt lymphoma	5	1	0	**6**	*5.0*	2.0	3.4	0.7	-	1.4	**1.5**	100.0
Brain and spinal neoplasms	15	7	15	**37**	*0.9*	12.5	10.2	4.6	11.0	8.5	**8.6**	100.0
Neuroblastoma	20	3	2	**25**	*1.1*	8.4	13.6	2.0	1.5	5.7	**6.3**	100.0
Retinoblastoma	15	2	0	**17**	*0.9*	5.7	10.2	1.3	-	3.9	**4.4**	100.0
Wilms tumour	14	4	0	**18**	*1.3*	6.1	9.5	2.6	-	4.1	**4.5**	100.0
Bone tumours	1	4	1	**6**	*0.5*	2.0	0.7	2.6	0.7	1.4	**1.3**	100.0
Soft tissue sarcomas	6	3	5	**14**	*1.0*	4.7	4.1	2.0	3.7	3.2	**3.3**	100.0
Kaposi sarcoma	1	0	1	**2**	-	0.7	0.7	-	0.7	0.5	**0.5**	100.0
Germ cell tumours	5	1	5	**11**	*0.4*	3.7	3.4	0.7	3.7	2.5	**2.6**	100.0
Other	34	16	15	**65**	*1.1*	21.9	23.1	10.4	11.0	14.9	**15.5**	100.0
All	150	74	73	**297**	*1.2*	100.0	101.8	48.2	53.6	67.9	**70.5**	100.0

Table 17. Childhood cancer, South Africa: Indian (1989-1992)

	NUMBER OF CASES					REL. FREQ.(%)	RATES PER MILLION					
	0-4	5-9	10-14	**All**	*M/F*	Overall	0-4	5-9	10-14	Crude	**ASR**	%MV
Leukaemia	17	28	17	**62**	*2.0*	39.5	43.4	66.6	43.9	51.7	**51.0**	100.0
Acute lymphoid leukaemia	8	15	13	**36**	*2.0*	22.9	20.4	35.7	33.6	30.0	**29.1**	100.0
Lymphoma	2	6	8	**16**	*1.7*	10.2	5.1	14.3	20.6	13.3	**12.6**	100.0
Hodgkin disease	0	3	1	**4**	*3.0*	2.5	-	7.1	2.6	3.3	**3.1**	100.0
Burkitt lymphoma	0	0	0	**0**	-	-	-	-	-	-	**-**	-
Brain and spinal neoplasms	2	4	5	**11**	*1.8*	7.0	5.1	9.5	12.9	9.2	**8.8**	100.0
Neuroblastoma	0	0	0	**0**	-	-	-	-	-	-	**-**	-
Retinoblastoma	3	2	0	**5**	*4.0*	3.2	7.7	4.8	-	4.2	**4.5**	100.0
Wilms tumour	3	1	0	**4**	*3.0*	2.5	7.7	2.4	-	3.3	**3.7**	100.0
Bone tumours	1	3	4	**8**	*1.7*	5.1	2.6	7.1	10.3	6.7	**6.3**	100.0
Soft tissue sarcomas	5	1	3	**9**	*3.5*	5.7	12.8	2.4	7.7	7.5	**8.0**	100.0
Kaposi sarcoma	0	0	0	**0**	-	-	-	-	-	-	**-**	-
Germ cell tumours	6	1	1	**8**	-	5.1	15.3	2.4	2.6	6.7	**7.4**	100.0
Other	16	11	7	**34**	*1.6*	21.7	40.8	26.2	18.1	28.3	**29.5**	100.0
All	55	57	45	**157**	*2.1*	100.0	140.4	135.5	116.1	130.9	**131.8**	100.0

241

3.5.5 Swaziland

Background

Climate: Varies from subtropical in the plains to near temperate in the mountains and hills.

Terrain: A high-veld region along the western border with South Africa, a middle-veld a low-veld region and the Lubombo mountain range (the end of the Rift Valley) to the east along the border with Mozambique. The lowest point is the Great Usutu River, 21 m, and the highest Emlembe Mountain, 1862 m.

Ethnic groups: African 97%, European 3%

Religions: Christian 60%, indigenous beliefs 40%

Economy—overview: Subsistence agriculture occupies more than 60% of the population, but overgrazing, soil depletion, drought and sometimes floods are recurrent problems. Manufacturing features a number of agro-processing factories. Despite its deposits of minerals, there is little mining activity at present. Nearly 90% of imports come from South Africa. Remittances from Swazi workers in South African mines contribute significantly to the economy.

Industries: Mining (coal and asbestos), wood pulp, sugar, soft drink concentrates

Agriculture—products: Sugar-cane, cotton, maize, tobacco, rice, citrus, pineapples, corn, sorghum, peanuts; cattle, goats, sheep

Cancer registration

A cancer registry operated during 1979–83, as part of a research project to investigate the relationships between aflatoxin contamination of foodstuffs, hepatitis B virus and primary liver cancer. The registry attempted to collect information on all cases of clinical cancer that were diagnosed within the country. Initially, this was done by regular visits of clerical workers to all of the main cancer referral centres. For the final two years, this system was replaced by scrutiny of all hospital discharge abstracts for cases in which a diagnosis of cancer had been recorded, followed by letters or visits to the hospitals concerned to collect detailed data for registration. All of the 13 hospitals in Swaziland contributed cases. At the same time (1982), a local histopathology service became available for the first time in Swaziland, so that histopathology reports acted as an independent source of notification of cancer cases. Although the completeness of registration increased over the five-year period, it is probable that the system of inpatient discharge returns was incomplete and up to one half of hospital discharges were not so recorded.

Cancer registration recommenced in 1995. The registry is located in the Department of Pathology of the Central Laboratory Service, Ministry of Health (Manzini). It has access to all cancer diagnoses based on pathology or cytology, since there is only one laboratory in the country. In addition, a schedule of visits is carried out twice yearly to all hospitals and clinics in the country. There are about 20, including government referral hospitals in each of the four regions, as well as hospitals belonging to missionary groups, mining companies, or privately owned. The main sources of information are the hospital admission and discharge registers; case notes may be consulted for supplementary information. The registry also has access to death certificates from the seven civil registrars' offices throughout the country. Death certification is fairly universal, although cause of death is not accurate for deaths occurring at home. Place of residence is not well recorded in any of

these data sources; however, few non-residents are likely to be treated within the country. Information on residents treated (or diagnosed) in South Africa is forwarded by the South African National (pathology-based) Cancer Register (see Chapter 3.5.4).

Review of data

The Swaziland Cancer Registry, 1979–83

A total of 308 male and 390 female cases were reported by Peers and Keen (1986) (Table 1); the leading cancers in males were cancers of the liver (20.8% of all cancers), oesophagus (17.5%) and the lung and respiratory organs (4.5%). In females the leading cancers were cervix (51.5%), breast (8.7%) and liver cancer (5.6%). Minimum incidence rates were calculated, based on estimates of the population for mid-1981: for cervix cancer, the estimated ASR was 28.2 per 100 000.

Research on liver cancer in Swaziland contributed to the understanding of the carcinogenic effects of aflatoxin exposure. Substantial differences in the incidence of liver cancer between and within a number of African and other regions – including Swaziland (Keen & Martin, 1971; Peers *et al.*, 1976) have been correlated with differences in the estimated intake of aflatoxin B1 (IARC, 1993).

The most detailed study in Swaziland (Peers *et al.*, 1987) attempted to evaluate differences in liver cancer incidence, as recorded by the cancer registry, in sub-regions of the country in relation to exposure to aflatoxins and hepatitis B infection. Aflatoxin consumption was estimated from a defined sampling of foods in 11 areas, analysed for aflatoxin content, and surveys of locally grown crops between harvesting and consumption. Hepatitis B virus markers were measured in blood donors. A statistical correlation model incorporating daily consumption of total aflatoxins (not just aflatoxin B1) and the proportion of people positive for HBsAg provided the best fit to the variation in liver cancer incidence. Thus, at an area or ecological level, aflatoxin exposure appeared to be more important in explaining the variation in liver cancer incidence. However the prevalence of HBsAg was quite uniform (23–35%) and markers of past infection with HBV over 74–91% in both sexes, so it is unlikely that there was sufficient contrast between regions to demonstrate the true effect of hepatitis B infection on liver cancer. Hepatitis C levels were not measured.

Swaziland Cancer Registry, 1996–99

The cases registered in this period include cancers diagnosed clinically or detected via a death certificate. 1293 males and 1607 females were registered in the four-year period 1996–99 (Table 2). The percentage with diagnosis based on pathology or cytology was 29%. The relatively low rates for haematological malignancies, and the fact that 81% of leukaemia cases were recorded as 'unspecified subtype' reflects the absence of haematology services in the country.

It is difficult to make comparisons with the earlier data because of the differences in case ascertainment. Nevertheless, many of the changes reflect the epidemic of AIDS, which is severe in Swaziland: prevalence of HIV infection in adults was estimated to be 25.3% at the end of 1999 (see chapter on AIDS and Cancer). Thus, the frequency of Kaposi sarcoma has increased enormously, to reach 16.8% of all cancers in males (ASR 17.2 per 100 000) and 10.4% in females (ASR 9.5 per 100 000). In males, the incidence of liver cancer is high (ASR 22.0) and so is that of prostate cancer (ASR 21.5) and cancer of the oesophagus (ASR 14.0). In females, the picture is dominated by the extraordinarily high rate of cervix cancer—41.7% of all cancer (ASR 59.3); breast cancer is much less common (8.9%, ASR 12.9) and liver cancer and oesophageal cancers are considerably less frequent than in males (M:F ratios in the range 3–4:1).

Childhood cancers

Table 3 shows the 93 childhood cancers registered in 1996–99. The incidence is low and the principal cancer recorded was Burkitt lymphoma (ASR 7.6 per million). There were seven cases of Kaposi sarcoma (7.5%, ASR 4.4 per million).

References

IARC (1993) *IARC Monographs on the Evaluation of Carcinogenic Risks to Humans. Volume 56. Some Naturally Occurring Substances: Food Items and Constituents, Heterocyclic Aromatic Amines and Mycotoxins*, Lyon, IARC

Keen, P. & Martin, P. (1971) Is aflatoxin carcinogenic in man? The evidence in Swaziland. *Trop. Geog. Med.*, **23**, 44–53

Peers, F. & Keen, P. (1986) Swaziland. In: Parkin, D.M., ed., *Cancer Occurrence in Developing Countries* (IARC Scientific Publications No. 75), Lyon, IARC, pp. 89–92

Peers, F., Bosch, X., Kaldor, J., Linsell, A. & Pluijmen, M. (1987) Aflatoxin exposure, hepatitis B infection and liver cancer in Swaziland. *Int. J. Cancer*, **39**, 545–553

Peers, F.G., Gilman, G.A. & Linsell, C.A. (1976) Dietary aflatoxins and human liver cancer. A study in Swaziland. *Int. J. Cancer*, **17**, 167–176

Pritchard, D., Sitas, F. & Viljoen, E. (1999) Tobacco consumption among Swaziland high school students, and their parents and teachers. *S. Afr. Med. J.*, **89**, 558–559

Table 1. Swaziland: case series

Site	Swaziland Cancer Registry, 1979–83 (Peers & Keen 1986)				%HV
	Male		Female		
	No.	%	No.	%	
Oral cavity	4	1.3%	9	2.3%	
Nasopharynx	3	1.0%	0	0.0%	
Other pharynx	3	1.0%	1	0.3%	
Oesophagus	54	17.5%	15	3.8%	
Stomach	7	2.3%	1	0.3%	
Colon/rectum	8	2.6%	3	0.8%	
Liver	64	20.8%	22	5.6%	
Pancreas	4	1.3%	1	0.3%	
Lung	14	4.5%	3	0.8%	
Melanoma	3	1.0%	10	2.6%	
Other skin	17	5.5%	6	1.5%	
Kaposi sarcoma	6	1.9%	0	0.0%	
Breast	2	0.6%	34	8.7%	
Cervix uteri		0.0%	201	51.5%	
Corpus uteri		0.0%	2	0.5%	
Ovary etc.		0.0%	0	0.0%	
Prostate	11	3.6%		0.0%	
Penis	0	0.0%		0.0%	
Bladder	11	3.6%	6	1.5%	
Kidney etc.	3	1.0%	5	1.3%	
Eye	0	0.0%	5	1.3%	
Brain, nervous system	2	0.6%	0	0.0%	
Thyroid	5	1.6%	3	0.8%	
Non-Hodgkin lymphoma	13	4.2%	5	1.3%	
Hodgkin disease	6	1.9%	3	0.8%	
Myeloma	1	0.3%	0	0.0%	
Leukaemia	4	1.3%	8	2.1%	
ALL SITES	308	100.0%	390	100.0%	

Table 2. Swaziland (1996-1999)

NUMBER OF CASES BY AGE GROUP AND SUMMARY RATES OF INCIDENCE - MALE

SITE	ALL AGES	AGE UNK	MV (%)	0-	15-	25-	35-	45-	55-	65+	CRUDE RATE	%	CR 64	ASR (W)	ICD (10th)
Mouth	18	3	56	1	-	-	1	3	5	5	1.0	1.4	0.15	2.2	C00-06
Salivary gland	2	0	50	-	-	-	-	1	1	-	0.1	0.2	0.03	0.3	C07-08
Nasopharynx	2	0	50	-	-	-	-	2	-	-	0.1	0.2	0.02	0.2	C11
Other pharynx	24	1	25	-	-	1	1	5	11	5	1.4	1.9	0.26	3.0	C09-10,C12-14
Oesophagus	113	7	7	-	-	2	5	39	30	30	6.4	9.1	1.01	14.0	C15
Stomach	36	2	11	-	-	2	4	6	10	12	2.0	2.9	0.29	4.5	C16
Colon, rectum and anus	39	3	41	-	3	5	6	8	3	11	2.2	3.1	0.22	4.2	C18-21
Liver	193	36	7	2	7	11	28	35	40	34	11.0	15.5	1.65	22.0	C22
Gallbladder etc.	2	0	50	-	-	-	-	-	-	1	0.1	0.2	0.02	0.2	C23-24
Pancreas	9	0	11	-	-	2	-	3	3	1	0.5	0.7	0.10	1.1	C25
Larynx	37	2	38	-	-	-	5	8	10	12	2.1	3.0	0.29	4.5	C32
Trachea, bronchus and lung	81	9	10	-	-	4	8	16	20	24	4.6	6.5	0.68	10.1	C33-34
Bone	20	0	40	3	3	1	1	3	4	5	1.1	1.6	0.13	2.0	C40-41
Melanoma of skin	6	1	83	-	-	-	2	2	-	1	0.3	0.5	0.04	0.6	C43
Other skin	46	5	63	2	1	2	5	5	14	12	2.6	3.7	0.39	5.5	C44
Mesothelioma	2	0	50	-	-	-	-	-	-	2	0.1	0.2	0.00	0.3	C45
Kaposi sarcoma	209	37	19	5	9	69	46	30	8	5	11.9	16.8	1.37	17.2	C46
Peripheral nerves	1	0	100	-	-	-	-	1	-	-	0.1	0.1	0.01	0.1	C47
Connective and soft tissue	15	4	73	4	-	2	2	-	-	2	0.9	1.2	0.07	1.2	C49
Breast	5	1	40	-	-	-	-	2	1	-	0.3	0.4	0.05	0.7	C50
Penis	31	5	32	-	4	4	7	6	4	5	1.8	2.5	0.22	3.2	C60
Prostate	153	13	24	-	2	2	4	9	45	80	8.7	12.3	1.07	21.5	C61
Testis	6	0	17	-	1	1	1	-	-	2	0.3	0.5	0.04	0.7	C62
Kidney	14	0	21	3	-	1	1	4	4	-	0.8	1.1	0.13	1.5	C64
Renal pelvis, ureter and other urinary	0	2	-	-	-	-	-	-	-	-	0.0	0.0	0.00	0.0	C65-66,C68
Bladder	44	2	16	1	1	-	5	4	10	21	2.5	3.5	0.28	5.7	C67
Eye	16	3	100	1	-	3	5	2	-	-	0.9	1.3	0.11	1.4	C69
Brain, nervous system	9	0	11	-	3	1	1	1	1	2	0.5	0.7	0.05	0.8	C70-72
Thyroid	9	0	44	-	1	-	3	3	2	-	0.5	0.7	0.09	0.9	C73
Hodgkin disease	8	0	75	4	2	1	1	-	-	-	0.5	0.6	0.03	0.4	C81
Non-Hodgkin lymphoma	40	5	73	8	1	6	9	6	1	2	2.3	3.2	0.25	3.3	C82-85,C96
Multiple myeloma	3	1	33	-	-	-	-	-	1	-	0.2	0.2	0.05	0.4	C90
Lymphoid leukaemia	5	1	80	2	1	1	-	-	-	-	0.3	0.4	0.02	0.2	C91
Myeloid leukaemia	0	0	-	-	-	-	-	-	-	-	0.0	0.0	0.00	0.0	C92-94
Leukaemia, unspecified	19	1	53	4	4	2	1	1	-	6	1.1	1.5	0.05	1.6	C95
Other and unspecified	76	6	26	4	1	5	3	18	14	25	4.3	6.1	0.52	9.0	O&U
All sites	1293	148	25	44	37	129	154	227	247	307	73.4		9.67	145.3	ALL
All sites but C44	1247	143	24	42	36	127	149	222	233	295	70.8	100.0	9.29	139.9	ALLbC44
Average annual population				204705	93582	52135	35810	25260	15083	12247					

Table 2. Swaziland (1996-1999)

NUMBER OF CASES BY AGE GROUP AND SUMMARY RATES OF INCIDENCE - FEMALE

SITE	ALL AGES	AGE UNK	MV (%)	0-	15-	25-	35-	45-	55-	65+	CRUDE RATE	%	CR 64	ASR (W)	ICD (10th)
Mouth	12	1	17	1	-	-	1	1	3	5	0.6	0.8	0.07	1.2	C00-06
Salivary gland	4	0	75	-	2	-	1	-	-	-	0.2	0.3	0.02	0.3	C07-08
Nasopharynx	0	0	-	-	-	-	-	-	-	-	0.0	0.0	0.00	0.0	C11
Other pharynx	5	0	60	-	-	1	3	1	-	1	0.3	0.3	0.03	0.4	C09-10,C12-14
Oesophagus	41	3	15	-	1	-	6	12	9	10	2.1	2.6	0.32	4.1	C15
Stomach	24	3	17	-	-	4	5	3	7	4	1.2	1.5	0.19	2.2	C16
Colon, rectum and anus	26	3	31	-	2	2	2	7	6	4	1.3	1.7	0.20	2.4	C18-21
Liver	63	8	6	2	6	6	10	14	7	10	3.2	4.0	0.37	5.2	C22
Gallbladder etc.	1	0	0	-	-	-	1	-	-	-	0.1	0.1	0.02	0.1	C23-24
Pancreas	7	3	14	-	-	-	1	1	2	-	0.4	0.4	0.08	0.7	C25
Larynx	8	0	63	-	2	1	1	2	2	2	0.4	0.5	0.03	0.6	C32
Trachea, bronchus and lung	15	2	20	-	-	1	1	5	2	4	0.8	1.0	0.10	1.4	C33-34
Bone	33	0	33	9	7	3	1	2	2	9	1.7	2.1	0.09	2.2	C40-41
Melanoma of skin	10	2	50	-	1	-	1	3	1	1	0.5	0.6	0.07	0.9	C43
Other skin	37	3	65	-	3	8	3	7	8	5	1.9	2.3	0.27	3.2	C44
Mesothelioma	0	0	-	-	-	-	-	-	-	-	0.0	0.0	0.00	0.0	C45
Kaposi sarcoma	164	24	18	2	37	51	34	8	4	4	8.4	10.4	0.70	9.5	C46
Peripheral nerves	0	0	-	-	-	-	-	-	-	-	0.0	0.0	0.00	0.0	C47
Connective and soft tissue	17	4	65	3	2	2	-	3	3	-	0.9	1.1	0.12	1.2	C49
Breast	139	21	35	-	5	11	23	27	31	21	7.1	8.9	1.07	12.9	C50
Vulva	10	2	80	-	1	2	1	3	1	-	0.5	0.6	0.08	0.8	C51
Vagina	5	0	60	3	-	-	1	-	1	-	0.3	0.3	0.03	0.3	C52
Cervix uteri	655	107	33	-	7	63	122	163	115	78	33.4	41.7	4.96	59.3	C53
Uterus	58	10	38	-	-	3	9	13	12	11	3.0	3.7	0.44	5.6	C54-55
Ovary	43	7	44	2	6	8	6	-	7	5	2.2	2.7	0.25	3.2	C56
Placenta	9	0	89	-	1	7	1	-	-	-	0.5	0.6	0.03	0.5	C58
Kidney	14	2	43	6	1	1	-	3	-	1	0.7	0.9	0.05	0.9	C64
Renal pelvis, ureter and other urinary	1	0	100	1	-	-	-	-	-	-	0.1	0.1	0.00	0.0	C65-66,C68
Bladder	18	2	11	-	1	3	4	4	-	2	0.9	1.1	0.12	1.5	C67
Eye	13	2	77	2	-	4	2	1	1	1	0.7	0.8	0.06	0.9	C69
Brain, nervous system	6	0	33	-	2	2	1	-	4	-	0.3	0.4	0.07	0.6	C70-72
Thyroid	17	3	53	-	2	4	1	2	1	4	0.9	1.1	0.07	1.3	C73
Hodgkin disease	8	1	75	1	1	2	1	1	1	1	0.4	0.5	0.03	0.5	C81
Non-Hodgkin lymphoma	30	2	70	9	5	6	2	3	1	2	1.5	1.9	0.11	1.7	C82-85,C96
Multiple myeloma	0	0	-	-	-	-	-	-	-	-	0.0	0.0	0.00	0.0	C90
Lymphoid leukaemia	2	0	100	2	-	-	-	-	-	-	0.1	0.1	0.00	0.1	C91
Myeloid leukaemia	4	2	50	-	1	-	-	1	-	-	0.2	0.3	0.02	0.3	C92-94
Leukaemia, unspecified	15	2	60	3	2	-	2	-	2	2	0.8	1.0	0.07	1.1	C95
Other and unspecified	93	10	10	3	3	14	15	13	16	19	4.7	5.9	0.56	7.9	O&U
All sites	1607	226	33	49	99	211	260	307	249	206	82.1		10.66	134.8	ALL
All sites but C44	1570	223	32	49	96	203	257	300	241	201	80.2	100.0	10.39	131.6	ALLbC44
Average annual population				208424	103868	68064	45497	28427	16703	17015					

Table 3. Childhood cancer, Swaziland (1989-1999)

	NUMBER OF CASES					REL. FREQ.(%)	RATES PER MILLION					
	0-4	5-9	10-14	All	M/F	Overall	0-4	5-9	10-14	Crude	ASR	%MV
Leukaemia	3	5	3	11	1.2	11.8	5.5	9.0	5.5	6.7	6.6	75.0
Acute lymphoid leukaemia	1	2	0	3	0.5	3.2	1.8	3.6	-	1.8	1.9	100.0
Lymphoma	12	4	6	22	1.2	23.7	22.0	7.2	10.9	13.3	14.0	80.0
Hodgkin disease	1	0	4	5	4.0	5.4	1.8	-	7.3	3.0	2.8	80.0
Burkitt lymphoma	6	4	2	12	1.0	12.9	11.0	7.2	3.6	7.3	7.6	83.3
Brain and spinal neoplasms	0	0	0	0	-	-	-	-	-	-	-	-
Neuroblastoma	2	0	0	2	1.0	2.2	3.7	-	-	1.2	1.4	100.0
Retinoblastoma	2	1	0	3	0.5	3.2	3.7	1.8	-	1.8	2.0	66.7
Wilms tumour	9	0	0	9	0.5	9.7	16.5	-	-	5.4	6.4	44.4
Bone tumours	1	4	7	12	0.3	12.9	1.8	7.2	12.7	7.3	6.7	50.0
Soft tissue sarcomas	5	7	1	13	2.3	14.0	9.2	12.6	1.8	7.9	8.1	100.0
Kaposi sarcoma	3	4	0	7	2.5	7.5	5.5	7.2	-	4.2	4.4	28.6
Germ cell tumours	1	0	1	2	-	2.2	1.8	-	1.8	1.2	1.2	100.0
Other	6	10	3	19	0.9	20.4	11.0	18.0	5.5	11.5	11.6	42.1
All	41	31	21	93	0.9	100.0	75.1	55.7	38.2	56.3	58.1	63.4

4. Cancer by site

MALES: 283,000 cases

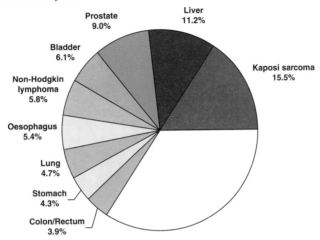

FEMALES: 299,000 cases

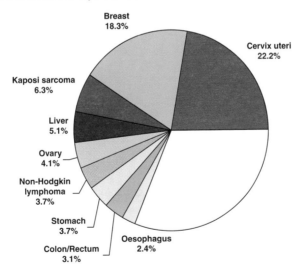

Estimated incident cases in 2002
(GLOBOCAN 2002, in preparation)

4.1 Bladder cancer

Introduction

Worldwide, an estimated 336 000 cancers of the urinary bladder occur each year (about 3.3% of all new cancers). More than one third of these occur in the populations of Europe and North America. In Africa, there were an estimated 26 000 new cases in 2000 (4.1% of cancers), with a considerable predominance in men (20 000 cases, 6.7%) over women (6000 cases, 1.9%).

Descriptive epidemiology in Africa

Table 1 shows age-standardized incidence rates from different centres, as reported in this volume, with data from Europe and North America for comparison. Table 2 shows incidence data from time periods in the 1960s and 1970s. The area of the world with the highest rates of bladder cancer mortality (in both sexes) and incidence (in men) is north Africa. Although the rates are relatively high in most countries of that region, they are particularly striking in Egypt, where, in men, the estimated rates of incidence (ASR 37.1 per 100 000) and mortality (ASR 20.8 per 100 000) are extremely high (Figure 1). Though rates are high in women too (incidence 8.6 per 100 000; mortality 4.7 per 100 000), they are similar to those in some countries of east Africa (Malawi, Zambia, Zimbabwe). Moderately raised rates are observed also in west Africa (Mali, Niger).

Comparability of statistics on the incidence of bladder cancer between populations is limited due to different practices concerning cystoscopy, biopsy of lesions, the extent of histological examination of biopsy material, and the classification of malignant, non-invasive tumours. These problems are likely to be less important in most of Africa, since an incident case almost always implies a frankly invasive, relatively advanced tumour.

In the United States, the incidence in the white population is higher than in blacks – about double among men and 50% greater among women (Table 1). It is unlikely that this is due to differences in exposure to environmental carcinogens, and explanations based upon differential susceptibility have been proposed (see Genetic Polymorphisms, below).

The most common histological type of bladder cancer in western countries is transitional cell carcinoma (TCC), which comprises 89.6% of cancers in England and Wales, 95.2% in the Netherlands and 94.6% in France (Parkin *et al.*, 2002). In the United States, the differences in histology by race are small, with, whites having 94.5% TCCs and 1.3% squamous cell carcinomas (SCCs), while the proportions are 87.8% and 3.2%, respectively, in blacks. In Africa, the majority of bladder cancers in Algeria and Tunisia (high-risk countries; see Table 1) are TCCs, with SCCs comprising less than 5% (Table 3). In some west African countries (Mali, Niger), and in east and south-east Africa (Zimbabwe, Malawi, Tanzania), SCCs predominate, as they do in Egypt (see Chapter 3.1.2). In South Africa, there are marked differences in histology between blacks (36% SCC, 41% TCC) and whites (2% SCC, 94% TCC). Similar findings with respect to black–white differences in proportions of the different histological types of bladder cancer have been reported from clinical series, for example in the Durban hospitals (Groeneveld *et al.*, 1996). These observations (as well as clinical features such as sex ratio, mean age at diagnosis and stage) relate to the prevalence of infection with *Schistosoma haematobium* (see below).

Migrants to France from Algeria and from west Africa (both areas of relatively high incidence of bladder cancer) appear to retain rates higher than the local-born population of France (Bouchardy *et al.*, 1995, 1996).

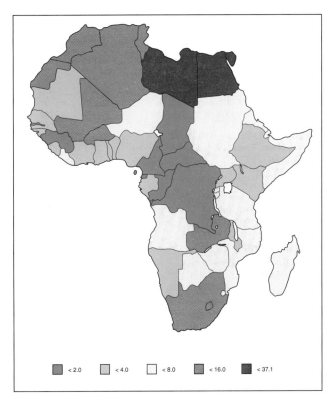

Figure 1. Incidence of bladder cancer: ASR (world) – Males

Thomas & Onyemenen (1995) reviewed cases of bladder cancer in Ibadan, Nigeria, over an 11-year period (1979–89) and noted an overall increase in the frequency of TCC (50%) relative to SCC of the bladder (although SCC remained the most common histological type under age 50 years). They speculated upon the roles of increasing urbanization, tobacco smoking and industrial exposures in the apparent increase in TCC.

Risk factors

Tobacco smoking

In 1986, IARC concluded, on the basis of many cohort and case–control studies, conducted in various parts of the world, that tobacco smoking (particularly of cigarettes) is an important cause of bladder cancer. The relationships of risk with duration and intensity of smoking are similar to those for lung cancer, although the risks are lower. Pipe and/or cigar smoking probably also increase the risk of bladder cancer, but at lower levels than the risk due to cigarette smoking. There have been relatively few studies in Africa, however.

Makhyoun (1974) studied 365 men with bladder cancer and age-matched hospital controls without cancer in Egypt (1966–71). 278 of the cases had previous urinary bilharziasis, and so the controls for these cases were matched for bilharziasis also. The odds ratio (OR) associated with cigarette smoking can be calculated as 3.3 (95% CI 1.2–9.3) for heavy smokers without bilharziasis, and 1.4 (95% CI 0.7–3.1) for those with bilharziasis.

In a study based upon data from the Bulawayo cancer registry (1963–72), Vizcaino *et al.* (1994) compared smoking history of 697 bladder cancer cases (71.2% of which were SCC) with cases of cancer not associated with tobacco smoking (i.e., excluding oesophagus, larynx and lung). A smoking history was available for 57% of cases, 55% controls. Adjusted for infection with *S. haematobium* (and other variables), there was only a

Table 1. Age-standardized (world) and cumulative (0-64) incidence
Bladder (C67)

	MALE				FEMALE			
	Cases	CRUDE	ASR(W) (per 100,000)	Cumulative (%)	Cases	CRUDE	ASR(W) (per 100,000)	Cumulative (%)
Africa, North								
Algeria, Algiers (1993-1997)	402	7.3	**10.8**	0.61	86	1.6	**2.3**	0.12
Algeria, Constantine (1994-1997)	37	2.4	**4.6**	0.23	6	0.4	**0.7**	0.05
Algeria, Oran (1996-1998)	148	8.4	**13.6**	0.70	15	0.9	**1.3**	0.07
Algeria, Setif (1993-1997)	62	2.1	**4.0**	0.29	2	0.1	**0.1**	0.02
Tunisia, Centre, Sousse (1993-1997)	146	12.7	**17.4**	0.83	12	1.1	**1.4**	0.05
Tunisia, North, Tunis (1994)	204	9.4	**12.3**	0.64	15	0.7	**1.0**	0.05
Tunisia, Sfax (1997)	47	12.0	**14.9**	0.89	13	3.4	**4.6**	0.41
Africa, West								
The Gambia (1997-1998)	6	0.6	**1.2**	0.09	3	0.3	**0.5**	0.01
Guinea, Conakry (1996-1999)	12	0.5	**1.5**	0.10	13	0.6	**1.9**	0.13
Mali, Bamako (1988-1997)	160	4.1	**9.6**	0.57	61	1.7	**3.8**	0.31
Niger, Niamey (1993-1999)	30	1.6	**4.8**	0.35	25	1.4	**3.7**	0.23
Nigeria, Ibadan (1998-1999)	16	1.1	**2.3**	0.17	3	0.2	**0.3**	0.03
Africa, Central								
Congo, Brazzaville (1996-1999)	3	0.2	**0.4**	0.04	3	0.2	**0.3**	0.03
Africa, East								
France, La Reunion (1988-1994)	154	7.3	**10.2**	0.48	35	1.6	**1.7**	0.05
Kenya, Eldoret (1998-2000)	10	1.1	**2.9**	0.19	5	0.5	**1.4**	0.04
Malawi, Blantyre (2000-2001)	16	1.8	**3.4**	0.26	16	1.8	**4.1**	0.35
Uganda, Kyadondo County (1993-1997)	17	0.6	**2.9**	0.09	8	0.3	**1.1**	0.05
Zimbabwe, Harare: African (1990-1993)	95	4.0	**12.5**	0.53	54	2.5	**10.5**	0.62
Zimbabwe, Harare: African (1994-1997)	71	2.5	**7.1**	0.40	62	2.3	**8.5**	0.56
Zimbabwe, Harare: European (1990-1997)	74	48.4	**25.6**	1.06	32	19.0	**9.1**	0.45
Africa, South								
Namibia (1995-1998)	60	1.9	**3.4**	0.18	20	0.6	**0.9**	0.05
South Africa: Black (1989-1992)	545	1.0	**1.8**	0.10	509	0.9	**1.3**	0.10
South Africa: Indian (1989-1992)	88	4.5	**7.7**	0.44	37	1.9	**2.7**	0.18
South Africa: Mixed race (1989-1992)	245	3.8	**8.1**	0.37	69	1.0	**1.7**	0.10
South Africa: White (1989-1992)	2810	27.9	**25.8**	1.19	870	8.5	**6.5**	0.34
South Africa, Transkei, Umtata (1996-1998)	2	0.6	**0.9**	0.07	-	-	**-**	-
South Africa, Transkei, 4 districts (1996-1998)	2	0.3	**0.4**	-	1	0.1	**0.1**	0.02
Swaziland (1996-1999)	44	2.5	**5.7**	0.28	18	0.9	**1.5**	0.12
Europe/USA								
USA, SEER: White (1993-1997)	16059	33.0	**24.3**	1.01	5688	11.3	**6.7**	0.31
USA, SEER: Black (1993-1997)	683	10.2	**11.7**	0.50	377	5.1	**4.6**	0.17
France, 8 registries (1993-1997)	3638	26.5	**18.0**	0.78	792	5.5	**2.7**	0.09
The Netherlands (1993-1997)	8606	22.5	**15.8**	0.57	2500	6.4	**3.4**	0.14
UK, England (1993-1997)	39077	32.6	**19.8**	0.76	15519	12.1	**5.7**	0.22

In italics: histopathology-based registries

Table 2. Incidence of bladder cancer in Africa, 1953–74

Registry	Period	ASR (per 100 000)		Source
		Male	Female	(see Chap. 1)
Senegal, Dakar	1969–74	1.2	1.3	4
Mozambique, Lourenço Marques	1956–60	17.5	14.2	1
Nigeria, Ibadan	1960–69	3.9	2.0	3
SA, Cape Province: Bantu	1956–59	*8.6*	*2.0*	2
SA, Cape Province: Coloured	1956–59	6.5	2.6	2
SA, Cape Province: White	1956–59	9.6	3.0	2
SA, Johannesburg, Bantu	1953–55	19.2	*9.9*	1
SA, Natal province: African	1964–66	3.6	*2.6*	2
SA, Natal province: Indian	1964–66	7.3	*5.1*	2
Uganda, Kyadondo	1954–60	7.0	1.5	1
Uganda, Kyadondo	1960–71	5.6	*0.9*	5
Zimbabwe, Bulawayo	1963–72	17.9	9.5	6

Italics: Rate based on less than 10 cases

Table 3. Percentage distribution of microscopically verified cases by histological type
Bladder (C67) - Both sexes

| | | Carcinoma | | | | Sarcoma | Other | Unspecified | Number of cases | |
	Squamous	Transl.	Adeno	Other	Unspec.				MV	Total
Algeria, Algiers	2.9	64.8	17.6	-	14.2	0.2	-	0.2	**415**	488
Algeria, Batna	7.7	46.2	23.1	-	-	-	-	23.1	**13**	19
Algeria, Constantine	18.2	66.7	3.0	-	9.1	-	-	3.0	**33**	43
Algeria, Oran	1.3	86.6	0.7	-	10.1	-	-	1.3	**149**	163
Algeria, Setif	3.6	12.7	78.2	-	1.8	-	-	3.6	**55**	64
Burkina Faso, Ouagadougou	20.0	40.0	20.0	-	-	-	-	20.0	**5**	23
Congo, Brazzaville	-	-	-	-	100.0	-	-	-	**1**	6
France, La Reunion	2.7	87.2	3.7	-	5.3	-	-	1.1	**187**	189
The Gambia	33.3	-	-	-	66.7	-	-	-	**3**	9
Guinea, Conakry	41.7	58.3	-	-	-	-	-	-	**12**	25
Kenya, Eldoret	14.3	71.4	-	-	14.3	-	-	-	**7**	15
Malawi, Blantyre	71.4	14.3	7.1	-	7.1	-	-	-	**14**	32
Mali, Bamako	71.0	22.6	3.2	-	3.2	-	-	-	**31**	221
Namibia	6.3	73.4	10.1	1.3	2.5	3.8	-	2.5	**79**	80
Niger, Niamey	46.2	38.5	-	-	15.4	-	-	-	**13**	55
Nigeria, Ibadan	14.3	64.3	14.3	-	-	7.1	-	-	**14**	19
Rwanda, Butare	-	80.0	-	-	-	-	-	20.0	**5**	7
South Africa: Black	36.3	40.5	3.5	0.3	6.3	2.2	0.4	10.5	**1054**	1054
South Africa: White	2.0	93.6	1.2	0.0	2.3	0.4	0.2	0.2	**3680**	3680
South Africa: Indian	4.0	80.8	-	-	7.2	0.8	-	7.2	**125**	125
South Africa: Mixed race	7.3	83.8	1.3	0.6	5.1	1.6	0.3	-	**314**	314
South Africa, Elim	40.0	40.0	10.0	-	10.0	-	-	-	**10**	17
South Africa, Transkei, Umtata	-	-	-	-	-	-	-	-	**-**	2
South Africa, Transkei, 4 districts	-	100.0	-	-	-	-	-	-	**1**	3
Swaziland	11.1	77.8	11.1	-	-	-	-	-	**9**	62
Tanzania, Dar Es Salaam	45.3	28.3	3.8	-	9.4	5.7	-	7.5	**53**	53
Tanzania, Kilimanjaro	10.0	60.0	25.0	-	-	5.0	-	-	**20**	26
Tunisia, Centre, Sousse	3.2	93.6	1.3	-	1.9	-	-	-	**157**	158
Tunisia, North, Tunis	3.2	90.8	0.9	0.5	3.2	0.5	-	0.9	**217**	219
Tunisia, Sfax	3.4	96.6	-	-	-	-	-	-	**59**	60
Uganda, Mbarara	-	-	-	-	-	-	-	-	**-**	2
Uganda, Kyadondo County	27.3	45.5	-	-	27.3	-	-	-	**11**	25
Zimbabwe, Harare: African	47.4	28.6	8.4	-	12.3	1.3	1.3	0.6	**154**	282
Zimbabwe, Harare: European	6.7	86.7	3.3	1.1	-	-	2.2	-	**90**	106

weak association (OR in males smoking 15 g tobacco per day relative to never-smokers was 1.4 (95% CI 0.9–2.3). For transitional cell/adenocarcinomas, the OR for this smoking category was 2.0 (95% CI 0.8–.3).

Bedwani *et al.* (1997) compared 151 male bladder cancer cases hospitalized in Alexandria, Egypt (67% TCC) with 157 male controls (hospitalized for diseases not related to smoking). After adjustment for various confounders (including age), the risk of bladder cancer in current smokers (relative to non-smokers) was 6.6 (95% CI 3.1–13.9) and in ex-smokers 4.4 (95% CI 1.7–11.3). There was a significant trend in risk with intensity and duration of smoking. The risk was greater for TCC (9.1) than for other histologies (4.4). There was a significant interaction with a history of schistosomiasis (obtained by questionnaire), but it appeared that risk of tobacco smoking was *lower* in subjects with such a history.

Occupational exposures

Various occupational categories are associated with increased risk of bladder cancer. These include workers with dyestuffs, aromatic amine manufacturing, rubber workers, leather workers, and painters. There do not appear to have been any studies of such factors in Africa (other than of agricultural workers in relation to exposure to schistosomiasis; see below).

Genetic susceptibility

Genetic polymorphism of metabolic enzymes seems to influence the risk of bladder cancer. These enzymes are involved in bio-activation of carcinogens or in their detoxification and excretion.

N-Acetyltransferase (NAT) is involved in detoxification of some of the aromatic amines that are carcinogenic to the bladder. The NAT2 genotype is characterized by the rate of acetylation of certain marker drugs such as isoniazid or caffeine (the phenotypic distinction by acetylator status preceded identification of the genotype). Several studies have suggested a link between slow acetylator status (NAT2 slow polymorphisms) and bladder cancer (with a meta-analysis of 16 studies giving an overall OR of 1.4 (Vineis *et al.*, 1999)).It is possible that different prevalences of this polymorphism might explain some of the difference in bladder cancer risk between ethnic groups. In Los Angeles, (Yu *et al.*, 1994) noted that prevalence of tobacco smoking did not differ much between whites, Asians, and blacks, though bladder cancer incidence certainly does. The prevalence of the slow-acetylator phenotype followed the risk of bladder cancer. Similarly, the levels of haemoglobin adducts of 3-aminobiphenyl were higher in white, than black, than Asians, at all levels of smoking. This difference is a consequence of the different prevalence of slow acetylators.

Glutathione S-transferase 1 (GSTM1) is involved in conjugation of several reactive chemicals, including arylamines and nitrosamines. The null polymorphism has been associated with risk of bladder cancer in several studies. In Egypt, Anwar *et al.* (1996) compared 22 bladder cancer cases (19 with a history of schistosomiasis) and 21 control subjects, matched for age and smoking history. The OR associated with the null genotype of GSTM1 was 6.97 (95% CI 1.34–45.69). Lafuente *et al.* (1996) conducted a case–control study comparing 80 hospitalized cases of bladder SCC with 70 controls drawn from the hospital staff in Assiut, Egypt. Among the male subjects, they found a risk for the null genotype of GSTM1 of 4.80 (95% CI 1.06–21.77) among smokers, but not for all subjects (OR = 0.72; 95% CI 0.26–1.97). Abdel-Rahman *et al.* (1998) investigated the role of GSTM1 and GSTT1 as potential risk factors for bladder cancer among 37 Egyptian cases (26 TCC and 11 SCC), compared with 34 matched controls. Eighteen of the cases were infected with *Schistosoma*. The GSTM1 null genotype was associated with increased risk of bladder cancer (OR = 2.99; 95% CI 1.0–9.0). The GSTT1 polymorphism was also associated with risk of bladder cancer, and the risk for individuals with a null genotype for both GSTM1 and GSTT1 was 9.9 (95% CI 1.8–46.9), with a significantly higher risk for SCC (OR = 14.6) than TCC (OR = 8.5).

The IARC meta-analysis of 11 studies (Vineis *et al.*, 1999) gave an OR of 1.57. Yu *et al.* (1995) found that the null genotype of GSTM1 combined with the slow acetylator phenotype of NAT2 resulted in higher levels of 3- and 4-aminobiphenyl-haemoglobin adducts than did lower-risk profiles (rapid acelylator and/or at least one functional GSTM1 gene allele). The highest risk profile was seen in 27% of whites, 15% of blacks and 3% of Asians.

CYP2D6 polymorphism has been shown to be associated with bladder cancer in some studies, although the overall OR in the IARC meta-analysis (Vineis *et al.*, 1999) was 1.12 (95%CI 0.77–1.64). The case–control study of Anwar *et al.* (1996) in Egypt found an OR of 2.36 (95% CI 0.68–9.90) for extensive metabolizers (EM), relative to poor metabolizer (PM) genotypes. There was a significant interaction between CYP2D6 EM and GSTM1 null polymorphisms, with the OR for this combination (relative to PM/GSTM1+/+ genotypes) being 8.4 (95% CI 1.26–56.03).

Schistosomiasis and bladder cancer

Schistosomes are trematode worms that live in the bloodstream of human beings and animals. Three species (*Schistosoma haematobium*, *S. mansoni* and *S. japonicum*) account for the majority of human infections. People are infected by exposure to water containing the infective larvae (cercariae). The worms mature in the veins that drain the bladder (*S. haematobium*) or in the intestine (other species). The adults do not multiply in the body but live there for several years, producing eggs. Some eggs leave the body in the urine or faeces and hatch in water to liberate the miracidium larva, which infects certain types of freshwater snail. Within the snail, the parasites multiply asexually to produce free-swimming cercaria larvae, which infect people by skin penetration. Eggs remaining in the human body are trapped in the tissues, where they elicit hypersensitivity granulomas that cause disease in the urogenital system (*S. haematobium*) or in the liver and intestines (other species).

The diagnosis of infection with *S. haematobium* infection is based on a history of haematuria, observation of gross haematuria, detection of haematuria by chemical reagent strips or detection of eggs in urine by microscopy. Infections can be quantified by egg counts in urine.The available immunodiagnostic tests are useful for detecting light infections.

The geographical distribution of the schistosomiasis roughly corresponds to the distribution of susceptible snail hosts, which are present in many tropical and subtropical regions of Africa (Figure 2, Table 4).

Within endemic areas, transmission may be focal and can be localized to specific water sources. The intensity and frequency of exposure to contaminated fresh water determine the occurrence of the heavy infection that leads to disease. Prevalence and intensity of infection are usually correlated in endemic areas and especially among children. Sex differences in intensity of infection have been linked to differences in exposure.

Treatment with safe, effective antischistosomal drugs (i) results in a high rate of resolution of infection, (ii) prevents development of disease in people with heavy infection, (iii) arrests progression of existing severe disease and (iv) reverses some disease manifestations, particularly in children. Control of schistosomiasis has been achieved in some countries through combined approaches to intervention, including health education, improved water supplies and sanitation, environmental management, snail control and treatment.

The evidence linking infection with *S. haematobium* with bladder cancer has been extensively reviewed (Cheever, 1978; IARC, 1994; Mostafa *et al.*, 1999). There are essentially three lines of evidence:

- Clinical observations that the two diseases appear to frequently co-exist in the same individual, and that the bladder cancers tend to be of squamous cell origin, rather than transitional cell carcinomas.
- Descriptive studies showing a correlation between the two diseases in different populations.
- Case–control studies, comparing infection with *S. haematobium* in bladder cancer cases and control subjects.

Clinical series

The first suggestion of a link between schistosomiasis and cancer came from careful assessment of clinical and pathological observations (Goebel, 1905; Ferguson, 1911). Subsequent large series of cases of urinary bladder cancer in African countries have been reported in association with evidence of *S. haematobium* infection:

- Angola (da Silva Lopes, 1984)
- Egypt (Mohamed, 1954; Mustacchi & Shimkin, 1958; El-Gazayerli & Khalil, 1959; Hashem *et al.*, 1961; Aboul Nasr *et al.*, 1962; Makhyoun *et al.*, 1971; El-Bolkainy *et al.*, 1972; Khafagy *et al.*,1972; El-Sebai, 1980; El-Bolkainy *et al.*,1981; Christie *et al.*, 1986; Tawfik, 1988; Fukushima *et al.*,1989)
- Kenya (Anjarwalla, 1971; Bowry, 1975)
- Malawi (Lucas, 1982b)
- Mozambique (Prates & Gillman, 1959; Gillman & Prates, 1962; Ebert, 1987)
- Nigeria (Attah & Nkposong, 1976),
- Senegal (Quenum, 1967)
- South Africa (Transvaal) (Higginson & Oettlé, 1962; Hinder & Schmaman, 1969; Kisner, 1973); (Natal) (Cooppan *et al.* 1984; Groenveld *et al.* 1996)
- Sudan (Malik *et al.*, 1975; Sharfi *et al.*, 1992)
- Tanzania (Kitinya *et al.*, 1986)
- Uganda (Dodge, 1962)
- Zambia (Bhagwandeen, 1976; Elem & Purohit, 1983, Elem & Patil, 1991)
- Zimbabwe (Houston, 1964; Gelfand *et al.*, 1967; Thomas *et al.*, 1990)

The case descriptions have repeatedly emphasized the preponderance of squamous-cell urinary bladder tumours among cases with evidence of schistosomal infection, their rather different distribution within the bladder (notably the rarity of occurrence in the trigone) in comparison with bladder tumours in developed countries, and the prevalence of metaplastic changes in conjunction with evidence of infection (da Silva Lopes, 1984). Cases with evidence of a link to *S. haematobium* infection are consistently described as being younger than other cases.

Correlation studies

Some studies have attempted to correlated the presence or intensity of infection with *S. haematobium* with the geographical occurrence of bladder cancer, and squamous cell tumours in particular (Table 5).

The table also draws attention to other associations, for example, between the proportion of bladder cancers in the population that are squamous-cell tumours and the proportion of cancerous bladder specimens from that population which contain evidence of past schistosomal infection in the form of eggs or egg remnants (Lucas, 1982a). In the Nile delta, 99% of the bladder cancers occurring in high-risk male agricultural workers (*fellahin*) were associated with histological evidence of *S. haematobium* infection, whereas only 52% of the cases occurring in men with lower-risk occupations showed such evidence (Makhyoun *et al.*, 1971). Men do most of the agricultural work in the Nile Delta, and the ratio of male to female cases of urinary bladder cancer with histological evidence of past infection reached as high as 12:1 (Makhyoun *et al.*, 1971), while the sex ratio among those without such evidence approximated the 4:1 ratio seen in the United Kingdom (Prates & Gillman, 1959). In contrast, in Mozambique (Prates, 1963) and adjacent regions of the Transvaal in South Africa (Keen & Fripp, 1980), where women do most of the agricultural labour and are therefore more commonly infected, the sex ratios were reversed to 1:1.1 or even 1:2, even though ratios of 2:1 prevailed among cases referred from nearby areas. The sex ratio of bladder cancer cases has also been linked to the histologically measured intensity of infection in tumour specimens, and ranged from 8.7:1 in heavily infected people, to 4:1 in those who were lightly infected, to 2:1 in those without eggs in Egypt (Tawfik, 1988).

El-Bolkainy *et al.* (1982) described 10 cases of bladder cancer, detected during cytological screening of urinary bladder cancer conducted from 1976 to 1979 in the Nile Delta area, where *S. haematobium* infection is highly endemic. All the 10 cases of histologically confirmed bladder cancer appeared among the 4769 agricultural workers screened, who were presumed to have a higher prevalence of infection than the 1112 persons with other occupations.

In a community in Angola, where both males and females work in agriculture, the minimal age of infection with *S. haematobium* was 11 years. The mean age of patients with urinary bladder carcinomas associated with schistosomiasis was 44 years. The sex ratio was 1.6:1 for bladder carcinoma associated with schistosomiasis and 3.2:1 for bladder carcinoma not associated with schistosomal disease (p ~ 0.05) (da Silva Lopes, 1984).

It should be noted that in Uganda, although squamous-cell carcinomas of the urinary bladder are commoner than in Europe or North America, there is no evident association with prevalence of *S. haematobium* (Anthony, 1974).

Because of the lack of population-based cancer registration, the secular trends in incidence of SCC- or TCC of the urinary bladder have not been formally evaluated. In an area of the Nile Delta where the prevalence of *S. haematobium* infection was brought from a level of 60% in 1968 to 10% in 1988, no impact upon the rate of bladder cancer was clinically evident at the end of that period, although the mean age at diagnosis had increased (Tawfik, 1988). Some case series suggest that TCC has become more common relative to SCC in Egypt (Koraitim *et al.*, 1995) and elsewhere (Thomas & Onyemenen, 1995).

Case–control studies

Five case–control studies have been reported in which controls were properly matched to the cases with respect to age and sex. Table 6 summarizes these studies.

Mustacchi and Shimkin (1958) identified 48 male and 7 female hospitalized patients with urinary bladder cancer in the Egyptian Nile Delta city of Tanta among 1472 consecutive admissions to the

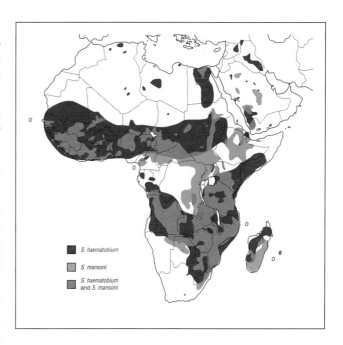

Figure 2. Geographical distribution of schistosomiasis in Africa

hospital. All patients were evaluated for the presence of *S. haematobium* eggs in a urine sample taken at admission, and any subsequent evidence of *S. haematobium* infection. After adjustment for age, sex and urban or rural origin, ORs of 2.1 (p = 0.04) were seen for the finding of eggs at the time of admission and 2.2 (p < 0.01) for any subsequent evidence of schistosomal infection.

In Harare, Zimbabwe, Gelfand *et al.* (1967) compared 33 patients with urinary bladder cancer with other hospital patients who had been 'submitted to similar investigation' and were matched on age, sex and race. Comparisons were made on the basis of the results of pelvic X-rays (33 pairs) and rectal biopsies (31 pairs). Among the 16 pairs discordant for calcified eggs identified by X-ray, the case was positive in 15, giving an OR of 15 (95% CI 2.0–114); among the 15 pairs discordant for the results of rectal biopsy, the case was positive in 13, giving an OR of 6.5 (95% CI 1.5–29). The diagnoses of disease in the controls were not described, and no adjustment was made for differences in smoking habits or place of origin.

In Zambia, Elem and Purohit (1983) compared the bladders of 50 patients who had died of urinary bladder cancer with bladders from age- and sex-matched cadavers (mostly trauma victims matched on age and sex to the decedent) by means of X-ray examination and digestion of tissues away from the eggs they contained. The bladders of the cases were 3.8 (95% CI 1.4–10) times as likely to show schistosomiasis by X-ray and 14 (95% CI 4.6–43) times as likely to contain *S. haematobium* eggs.

In the Bulawayo region of Zimbabwe, the cancer registrar interviewed cancer cases between 1963 and 1977, obtaining information on past history of clinical schistosomiasis ('bilharzia' or 'blood in the urine'), as well as other exposures (Vizcaino *et al.*, 1994). Some difference in the availability of information about past schistosomiasis is evident between cases of urinary bladder cancer (61%) and cases of cancer of other types (50%). The exposures of 412 patients with bladder cancer were compared with those of 4483 other cancer patients, excluding those with cancers known to be linked to smoking. The occurrence of bladder cancer was associated with place of origin and a lower level of education. For a history of schistosomiasis in men, the OR (relative to no such history and adjusted for age, tobacco use, province of origin, education and occupation) was 3.9 (95% CI 2.9–5.2), and 5.7 (95% CI 3.7–8.7) in women. The association was rather stronger for squamous-cell carcinomas than transitional-cell/adenocarcinomas, especially in women.

Table 4. Geographical distribution of schistosomiasis by species

Country	S. haematobium	S. mansoni	S. intercalatum
Algeria	+		
Angola	+	+	
Benin	+	+	
Botswana	+	+	
Burkina Faso	+	+	
Burundi		+	
Cameroon	+	+	+
Central African Republic	+	+	+[a]
Chad	+	+	+[a]
Congo	+	+	+[a]
Côte d'Ivoire	+	+	
Equatorial Guinea			+
Ethiopia	+	+	
Gabon	+	+	+
Gambia	+	+	
Ghana	+	+	
Guinea	+	+	
Guinea-Bissau	+	+	
Kenya	+	+	
Liberia	+	+	
Madagascar	+	+	
Malawi	+	+	
Mali	+	+	+[a]
Mauritania	+		
Mauritius	+		
Mozambique	+	+	
Namibia	+	+	
Niger	+	+	
Nigeria	+	+	+[a]
Rwanda	+		
Sao Tome and Principe	+[a]		+
Senegal	+	+	
Sierra Leone	+	+	
South Africa	+	+	
Swaziland	+	+	
Togo	+	+	
Uganda	+	+	
United Republic of Tanzania	+	+	
Zaire	+	+	+
Zambia	+	+	
Zimbabwe	+	+	

Source: IARC (1994)

[a] Confirmation required

Table 5. Descriptive studies of infection with *Schistosoma haematobium* and urinary bladder cancer

Reference	Location	Outcome index	Exposure index	Geographical correlations	Secular or occupational correlations	Correlated sex ratios or age distributions
Anjarwalla (1971)	Kenya, referral pathology service	Proportional frequencies	Frequency of schistosomiasis diagnoses and school surveys	Patients from coastal area, where schistosomiasis is common	–	–
Makhyoun et al. (1971)[a]	Egypt, Nile Delta University hospital	Proportional frequencies	Common knowledge	–	Cases in male fellahin: 99% histologically *S. haematobium* egg-positive Cases in men in other occupations: 52% positive	Exceptionally higher sex ratio for bilharzial cases (11.8:1) than for non-bilharzial cases (4.8:1).
Anthony (1974)	Uganda, referral hospital –	Proportional frequencies	Frequency of schistosomiasis diagnoses	Bladder cancer, including squamous-cell cancers, unrelated to small foci of schistosomiasis	–	–
Bowry (1975)[a]	Kenya, referral pathology service	Proportional frequencies	Frequency of schistosomiasis diagnoses and school surveys	Cancer foci on coast and near Lake Victoria. both known foci of schistosomiasis	–	–
Malik et al. (1975)[a]	Sudan, referral hospital	Proportional frequencies	Ministry of Health records of 'highest endemicity'	Correspondence between frequency of bladder cancer and endemicity by province	–	–
Keen & Fripp (1980)[a]	South Africa (Transvaal)	Frequencies identified in regional surveys	None explicit	–	–	Wide variations in sex ratio (from 2:1 to 1:2) according to region and tribe
Lucas (1982a)[a]	Africa	Proportional frequencies	Histological identification of *et al.* eggs in bladder specimens	Geographical distribution of percentage of histologically *S. haematobium* egg-positive tumours correlated directly with percentage of all bladder cancers that are squamous-cell and inversely with the percentage that are transitional-cell tumours		
Kitinya et al. (1986)a	Tanzania referral hospital	Proportional frequencies	Known distribution - of snail vectors in relation to altitude	Low proportion of squamous-cell tumours and low prevalence of *S. haematobium* at high elevations near Mt Kilimanjaro	–	
Tawfik (1988)a	Egypt, referral hospital	Proportional frequencies	Histological identification of *et al.* eggs n bladder ispecimens; records of control programme	–	High bladder cancer proportional frequency despite 20 years of successful control efforts (prevalence reduced from 60 to 10% in one province)	High sex ratio correlated with documented intensity of infection. As period of successful control efforts lengthens, mean age of bladder cancer cases increases.
Thomas et al. (1990)	Zimbabwe, referral hospital	Proportional frequencies	National prevalence surveys among schoolchildren	Estimated bladder cancer incidence correlated with prevalence of *S. haematobium* infection (r = 0.87; p < 0.01). Ratio of squamous-cell to transitional-cell tumours linked to *S. haematobium* prevalence: 12:1 where prevalence was 67%, 2:1 where prevalence was 17%	–	Sex ratio for squamous-cell tumours, 1.0; for transitional-cell tumours, 2.9:1.

[a] Correlation not formally tested

Bedwani *et al.* (1998) reported on a case–control study in Alexandria, Egypt, of 190 bladder cancer cases and 186 hospitalized controls (with non-neoplastic, non-urinary tract conditions). Information on infection (and other exposures) was obtained by questionnaire. The OR, adjusted for age and sex, associated with a history of schistosomiasis was 1.8 (95% CI 1.2–2.9), or 1.7 (95% CI 1.0–2.9) after adjustment for other variables (including smoking and a history of other urinary infections). The OR increased with younger age at first infection, or with increasing time since first diagnosis. The paper gave no information on the histological type of bladder tumours included, although from another report of the same study (Bedwani *et al.*, 1997), only 18% of the 151 male cases were SCC.

Other comparative studies

Prates and Gillman (1959) compared 100 urinary bladder cancer cases in Maputo, Mozambique, with 185 "control" cases found at autopsy in people over 40 years of age (causes of death not described) with respect to the frequency of identification of *S. haematobium* eggs in relation to the histological type of bladder cancer. Eggs were found in 33 of the cases found at autopsy and in 61% of controls. Eggs were found in 56% of the 59 SCC patients but in none of the TCC patients. It is not possible to reconcile the figures of 61% infection rate in controls with the 0% (0/41) figure for non-SCC cases. In addition, the methods used to examine the biopsy and autopsy specimens were dissimilar.

Hinder and Schmaman (1969) compared the prevalence of histologically identified eggs in punch biopsy specimens from 79 patients with urinary bladder carcinoma in Johannesburg, South Africa, with the prevalence in two or more full-thickness biopsy specimens from 101 people over the age of 15 years who came to autopsy. Eggs were identified in 34.2% of the cases but in only 9.0% of the autopsied patients. The causes of death of the controls were not reported, and no adjustment was made for differences in specific age or place of origin. When cases were analysed by histological type, 19% of TCC and 68% of SCC contained eggs.

Mechanisms of carcinogenesis

Numerous explanations have been offered for the proposed association between schistosomiasis and human cancers.

Chronic irritation and inflammation with increased cell turnover provide opportunities for mutagenic events, genotoxic effects and activation of carcinogens through several mechanisms, including the production of nitric oxide by inflammatory cells (activated macrophages and neutrophils) (Rosin *et al.*, 1994a, b).

Alterered metabolism of mutagens may be responsible for genotoxic effects (Gentile, 1985, 1991; Gentile *et al.*, 1985). Quantitatively altered tryptophan metabolism in *S. haematobium*-infected patients results in higher concentrations of certain metabolites (e.g., indican, anthranilic acid glucuronide, 3-hydroxyanthranilic acid, L-kynurenine, 3-hydroxy-L-kynurenine and acetyl-L-kynurenine) in pooled urine (Abdel-Tawab *et al.*, 1966a, 1968b; Fripp & Keen, 1980). Some of these metabolites have been reported to be carcinogenic to the urinary bladder (Bryan, 1969).

Immunological changes have been suggested as playing a role (Raziuddin *et al.*, 1991, 1992, 1993; Gentile & Gentile, 1994).

Secondary bacterial infection may result in a variety of metabolic effects, and therefore may play an intermediary role in the genesis of squamous-cell carcinoma. Secondary bacterial infection of *Schistosoma*-infected bladders is a well documented event (Lehman et al, 1973; Laughlin *et al.*, 1978; Hill, 1979; El-Aaser *et al.*, 1982; Hicks *et al.*, 1982).

Nitrate, nitrite and N-nitroso compounds are detected in the urine of *S. haematobium*-infected patients (Hicks *et al.*, 1977, 1978, 1982;

Tricker *et al.*, 1989, 1991; Abdel Mohsen *et al.*, 1999). Nitrosamines are formed by nitrosation of secondary amines with nitrites by bacterial catalysis (or via urinary phenol catalysis); they may be carcinogenic to bladder mucosa. Mostafa *et al.* (1994) also demonstrated the presence of nitrates and nitrites in the saliva and increased concentrations of *N*-nitroso compounds in the urine of *et al.*-infected people who were not on controlled diets. The high levels of urinary nitrosamines may also be explained by macrophage accumulation as a consequence of chronic inflammation, as noted above. The etiological significance of these findings is, however, unclear in the light of the finding that urine from schistosomiasis patients is not mutagenic (Everson *et al.*, 1983).

Nitrosamines have been detected in the urine of paraplegic patients with urinary tract infections due to urinary stasis (Hicks *et al.*, 1977, 1978). On follow-up of 6744 paraplegic patients in the United Kingdom, 25 urinary bladder cancers were identified (El Masri & Fellows, 1981). On the basis of information for an otherwise comparable population, 1.6% of these would have been expected to be of squamous origin, whereas 44% actually were (estimated relative risk = 49; 95% CI 20–119). In Uganda, squamous-cell bladder cancers are commonly seen in the absence of *S. haematobium* infection but in the presence of other urinary tract abnormalities (Anthony, 1974).

The findings with respect to enhanced risk in subjects with schistosomiasis-associated cancers and the null genotype of GSTM1 (see above) suggest that this enzyme may play a role either by preventing formation or in detoxication of *N*-nitroso compounds.

Viruses: Cooper *et al.* (1997) found no evidence of infection with human papillomavirus types 6, 11, 16, 18, 31 or 33 in specimens of 25 squamous-cell carcinomas associated with schistosomiasis in South Africa.

Elevated β-glucuronidase levels in schistosome-infected subjects could increase the release of carcinogenic metabolites from their glucuronides. No data are available at present to confirm this association, although schistosome-infected humans are known to have elevated β-glucuronidase activity in urine (Fripp, 1960; Abdul-Fadl & Metwalli, 1963; Fripp, 1965; Abdel-Tawab *et al.*, 1966b, 1968a; Norden & Gelfand, 1972; El-Sewedy *et al.*, 1978; El-Aaser *et al.*, 1979), for reasons that are unknown.

Genetic damage in the form of slightly increased sister chromatid exchange and micronucleus frequencies were seen in peripheral blood lymphocytes harvested from schistosomiasis patients (Shubber, 1987; Anwar, 1994), and micronuclei were more frequent in urothelial cells from chronic schistosomiasis patients than in controls (Rosin & Anwar, 1992). The mean frequency of micronuclei was reduced significantly after treatment with praziquantel, which may indicate that infection is involved in chromosomal breakage in epithelial cells (Anwar & Rosin, 1993). Some chromosomal abnormalities appear to be more frequent in SCCs associated with schistosomiasis than in TCCs; for example, loss of heterozygosity of 9p, in the region of the CDKN2 tumour-suppressor gene (Gonzalez-Zulueta *et al.*, 1995; Shaw *et al.*, 1999).

Several studies have investigated *H-ras* oncogene mutations in bladder cancers. Their frequency, and the expression of the corresponding protein, are similar for schistosomiasis-associated cancers and other cases (Badawi, 1996). However, Ramchurren *et al.* (1995) found point mutations in codon 13 of this gene in 2/21 schistosomiasis-related tumours. No mutation was detected at codon 12 of the *H-ras* oncogene in nine SCCs associated with schistosomiasis (Fujita *et al.*, 1987).

Mutations of the p53 tumour-suppressor gene are more frequent in schistosomiasis-associated tumours than in other cases. Habuchi *et al.* (1993) found p53 mutations in six of seven SCCs associated with *S. haematobium*; no specific pattern of mutation emerged, in contrast to the pattern seen in TCCs related

Table 6. Case–control studies of infection with *Schistosoma haematobium* and urinary bladder cancer

Reference	Location	Source of cases	Source of controls	Measure of exposure	No. of cases/ no. of controls	Cases/controls exposed (%)	Odds ratio	95% CI (or p)	Cases with squamous-cell tumours (%)
Mustacchi & Shimkin (1958)	Tanta, Nile Delta, Egypt	Hospital	Other admissions to hospital	Eggs in first urine sample	55/1417	14.5/7.6	2.1[a]	0.04	Not specified
				All clinical evidence, including history and cystoscopy	55/1417	49.0/23.3	2.2[a]	< 0.01	
Gelfand *et al.* (1967)	Harare, Zimbabwe	Hospital	Matched patients[b] of same age, sex, race, on different hospital ward	Pelvic X-ray	33/33	45.5/3.03	[15	2.0–114]	62 (62 with past exposure)
				Rectal biopsy	31/31	54.8/19.4 (discordant matched pairs) 1)15/1 2)13/2)	[6.5	1.5–29]	
Elem & Purohit (1983)	Lusaka, Zambia	Autopsies	Cadavers without malignancy (mostly traumatic death)	Digestion and centri-fugation of bladder	50/50	94.0/40.0	[14	4.6–43]	72
				Pelvic X-ray	50/50	38/14	[3.8	1.4–10]	
Vizcaino *et al.* (1994)	Bulawayo, Zimbabwe	Cancer registry cases	Registry cases with other cancers	Self-reported history of bilharzia or blood in urine	300/2078 M 112/2405 F	33.7/12.6 M 34.8/4.7 F	3.9[c] 5.7[c]	2.9–5.2 3.7–8.7	71. No change when tobacco-related cancers excluded from controls
Bedwani *et al.* (1998)	Alexandria, Egypt	Hospital cases	Hospital without cancer or urinary tract disease	Self-reported history of schistosomiasis	190/187	45.3/36.9	1.7[d]	1.0–2.9	18[e]

[a] Adjusted for age, sex and urban or rural residence
[b] Who were 'submitted to same procedure'
[c] Adjusted for age, period, province, drinking and smoking
[d] Adjusted for age, sex, education, smoking, history of urinary infection, occupation
[e] For males, from Bedwani *et al.* (1997).

to tobacco smoking. p53 mutations limited to exons 7 and 8 were reported for 21 individuals with schistosomiasis-associated bladder cancer in South Africa (Ramchurren et al., 1995). Warren et al. (1995) described p53 mutations in 90 bladder cancers from Egyptian patients with a history of schistosomiasis. Mutations in exons 5-8 were present in 17/53 SCCs and 8/23 TCCs, and molecular changes were consistent with nitric oxide production by inflammatory cells.

Tamimi et al. (1996) found deletion of the cyclin-dependent kinase inhibitor p16^{INK4} in 23/47 samples from schistosomiasis-associated bladder cancer patients (more frequent than in other bladder tumours).

The Bcl-2 gene was found to be over-expressed in 32% schistosomiasis-associated bladder cancers, and this seemed to occur only in SCCs and adenocarcinomas, but not significantly in TCCs. Altered p53 expression was also found in the majority of tumours (Chaudhary et al., 1997).

Methylation of DNA as shown by detection of O^6-methyldeoxyguanosine has been found in a high percentage of patients with schistosomiasis-associated cancers in Egypt (Badawi et al., 1992, 1994).

References

Abdel Mohsen, M.A., Hassan, A.A., El-Sewedy, S.M., Aboul-Azm, T., Magagnotti, C., Fanelli, R. & Airoldi, L. (1999) Biomonitoring on n-nitroso compounds, nitrite and nitrate in the urine of Egyptian bladder cancer patients with or without *Schistosoma haematobium* infection. *Int. J. Cancer*, **82**,: 789–794

Abdel-Rahman, S.Z., Anwar, W.A., Abdel-Aal, W.E., Mostafa, H.M. & Au, W.W. (1998) GSTM1 and GSTT1 genes are potential risk modifiers for bladder cancer. *Cancer Detect. Prev.*, **22**, 129–138

Abdel-Tawab, G.A., Kelada, ES., Kelada, N.L., Abdel-Daim, M.H. & Makhyoun. N. (1966a) Studies on the aetiology of bilharzial carcinoma of the urinary bladder. V Excretion of tryptophan metabolites in urine. *Int. J. Cancer*, **1**, 377–382

Abdel-Tawab, G.A., El-Zoghby, S.M., Abdel-Samie, Y.M., Zaki, A. & Saad. A.A. (1966b) Studies on the aetiology of bilharzial carcinoma of the urinary bladder. VI. Beta-glucuronidases in urine. *Int. J. Cancer*, **1**, 383–389

Abdel-Tawab, G.A., El-Zoghby, S.M., Abdel-Samie, Y.M., Zaki, A.M., Kholef, I.S. & El-Sewedy, S.H.M. (1968a) Urinary beta-glucuronidase enzyme activity in some bilharzial urinary tract diseases. *Trans. R. Soc. Trop. Med. Hyg.*, **62**, 501–505

Abdel-Tawab, G.A., Ibrahim, E.K., El-Masri, A., Al-Ghorab, M. & Makhyoun, N. (1968b) Studies on tryptophan metabolism in bilharzial bladder cancer patients. *Invest. Urol.*, **5**, 591–601

Abdul-Fadl, M.A.M. & Metwalli, O.M. (1963) Studies on certain urinary blood serum enzymes in bilharziasis and their possible relation to bladder cancer in Egypt. *Br. J. Cancer*, **15**, 137–141

Aboul Nasr, A.L., Gazayerli, M.E., Fawzi, R.M. & El-Sibai, I. (1962) Epidemiology and pathology of cancer of the bladder in Egypt. *Acta Union Int. Contra Cancrum*, **18**, 528–537

Anjarwalla, K.A. (1971) Carcinoma of the bladder in the coast province of Kenya. *E. Afr. Med. J.*, **48**, 502–509

Anthony, P.P. (1974) Carcinoma of the urinary tract and urinary retention in Uganda. *Br. J. Urol.*, **46**, 201–208

Anwar, WA. (1994) Praziquantel (antischistosomal drug): is it clastogenic, co-clastogenic or anticlastogenic? *Mutat. Res.*, **305**, 165–173

Anwar, WA. & Rosin, M.P (1993) Reduction in chromosomal damage in schistosomiasis patients after treatment with praziquantel. *Mutat. Res.*, **298**, 179–185

Anwar, W.A., Abdel-Rahman, S.Z., El-Zein, R.A., Mostafa, H.M. & Au, W.W. (1996) Genetic polymorphism of GSTM1, CYP2E1 and CYP2D6 in Egyptian bladder cancer patients. *Carcinogenesis*, **17**, 1923–1929

Attah, E.D.'B. & Nkposong, E.O. (1976) Schistosomiasis and carcinoma of the bladder: a critical appraisal of causal relationship. *Trop. Geogr. Med.*, **28**, 268–272

Badawi, A.F, Mostafa, M.H., Ahoul-Azm, I, Haboubi, N.Y., O'Connor, P.J. & Cooper. D.P. (1992) Promutagenic methylation damage in bladder DNA from patients with bladder cancer associated with schistosomiasis and from normal individuals. *Carcinogenesis*, **13**, 877–881

Badawi, A.F, Cooper, D.P., Mostafa, M.H., Aboul-Asm, T., Barnard, R., Margison, G.P. & O'Connor, P.J. (1994) O^6-Alkylguanine-DNA-alkyl transferase activity in schistosomiasis-associated human bladder cancer. *Eur. J. Cancer*, **30**, 1314–1319

Badawi, AF. (1996) Molecular and genetic events in schistosomiasis-associated human bladder cancer: role of oncogenes and tumor suppressor genes. *Cancer Lett.*, **105**, 123–138

Bedwani, R. el-Khwsky, F., Renganathan, E., Braga, C., Abu Seif, H.H., Abul Azm, T., Zaki, A., Franceschi, S., Boffetta, P. & La Vecchia, C. (1997) Epidemiology of bladder cancer in Alexandria, Egypt: tobacco smoking. *Int. J. Cancer*, **73**, 64–67

Bedwani, R., Renganathan, E., El Kwhsky, F., Braga, C., Abu Seif, H.H., Abul Azm, T., Zaki, A., Franceschi, S., Boffetta, P. & La Vecchia, C. (1998) Schistosomiasis and the risk of bladder cancer in Alexandria, Egypt. *Br. J. Cancer*, **77**, 1186–1189

Bhagwandeen, S.B. (1976) Schistosomiasis and carcinoma of the bladder in Zambia. *S. Afr. Med. J.*, **50**, 1616–1620.

Bouchardy C., Wanner P. & Parkin D.M. (1995) Cancer mortality among sub-Saharan African migrants in France. *Cancer Causes Control*, **6**, 539–544

Bouchardy C., Parkin D.M., Wanner P. & Khlat M. (1996) Cancer mortality among north African migrants in France. *Int. J. Epidemiol.* **25**, 5–13

Bowry, I.R. (1975) Carcinoma of bladder in Kenya. *E. Afr. Med. J.*, **52**, 356–364

Bryan, G.T (1969) Role of tryptophan metabolites in urinary bladder cancer. *Am. Ind. Hyg Assoc. J.*, **30**, 27–34

Chaudhary, K.S., Lu, Q.-L., Abel, P.D., Khandan-Nia, N., Shoma, A.M., El-Baz M., Stamp, G.W., & Lalani E.N. (1997) Expression on bcl-2 and p53 oncoproteins in schistosomiasis-related transitional and squamous cell carcinoma of the urinary bladder. *Br. J. Urol.*, **79**, 78–84

Cheever, A.W. (1978) Schistosomiasis and neoplasia. *J. natl. Cancer Inst.*, **61**, 13–18

Christie, J.D., Crouse, D., Kelada, A.S., Anis-Ishak, E., Smith, J.H. & Kamel, I.A. (1986) Patterns of *Schistosoma haematobium* egg distribution in the human lower urinary tract. III. Cancerous lower urinary tracts. *Am. J. Trop. Med. Hyg.*, **35**, 759–764

Cooper, K., Haffajee, Z. & Taylor, L. (1997) Human papillomavirus and schistosomiasis-associated bladder cancer. *Mol. Pathol.*, **50**, 145–148

Cooppan, R.M., Bhoola, K.D.N. & Mayet, F.G.H. (1984) Schistosomiasis and bladder carcinoma in Natal. *S. Afr. Med. J.*, **66**, 841–843

Dodge, O.G. (1962) Tumours of the bladder in Uganda Africans. *Acta Unio Int. Contra Cancrum*, **18**, 548–559

Ebert, W. (1987) Studies on the frequency and significance of bilharziasis in the People's Republic of Mozambique. *Z. Urol. Nephrol.*, **80**, 625–628 (in German)

El-Aaser, A.A., El-Merzabani, M.M., Higgy, N.A. & Kader, M.M.A. (1979) A study on the aetiological factors of bilharzial bladder cancer in Egypt. 3. Urinary ß-glucuronidase. *Eur. J. Cancer*, **15**, 573–583

El-Aaser, A.A., El-Merzabani, M.M., Higgy, N.A. & El-Habet, A.E. (1982) A study on the etiological factors of bilharzial bladder cancer in Egypt. 6. The possible role of urinary bacteria. *Tumori*, **68**, 23–28

El-Bolkainy, M.N., Ghoneim, M.A. & Mansour, M.A. (1972) Carcinoma of bilharzial bladder in Egypt: clinical and pathological features. *Br J. Cancer*, **44**, 561–570

El-Bolkainy, M.N., Mokhtar, N.M., Ghoneim, M.A. & Hussein, M.H. (1981) The impact of schistosomiasis on the pathology of bladder carcinoma. *Cancer*, **48**, 2643–2648

El-Bolkainy, M.N., Chu, E.W, Ghoneim, M.A. & Ibrahim, A.S. (1982) Cytologic detection of bladder cancer in a rural Egyptian population infested with schistosomiasis. *Acta Cytol.*, **26**, 303–310

Elem, B. & Purohit, R. (1983) Carcinoma of the urinary bladder in Zambia. A quantitative estimation of *Schistosoma haematobium* infection. *Br. J. Urol.*, **55**, 275–278

Elem, B. & Patil, P.S. (1991) Pattern of urological malignancy in Zambia. A hospital-based histopathological study. *Br. J. Urol.*, **67**, 37–39

El-Gazayerli, M. & Khalil, H.A. (1959) Bilharziasis and cancer of the urinary tract. Some observations. *Alexandria Med. J.*, **5**, 31–36

El-Masri, W.S. & Fellows, G. (1981) Bladder cancer after spinal cord injury. *Paraplegia*, **19**, 265–270

El-Sebai, I. (1980) Carcinoma of the urinary bladder in Egypt: current clinical experience. In: El Bolkainy, M.N. & Chu, E.W, eds, *Detection of Bladder Cancer Associated with Schistosomiasis*, Cairo, Al-Ahram Press, pp. 9–18

El-Sewedy, S.M., Arafa, A., Abdel-Aal, G. & Mostafa, M.H. (1978) The activities of urinary a-esterases in bilharziasis and their possible role in the diagnosis of bilharzial bladder cancer in Egypt. *Trans. R. Soc. Trop. Med. Hyg.*, **72**, 525–528

Everson, R.B., Gad-el-Mawla, N.M., Attia, M.A.M., Chevlen,. E.M., Thorgeirsson, S.S., Alexander, L.A., Flack, P.M., Staiano, N. & Ziegler, J.L. (1983) Analysis of human urine for mutagens associated with carcinoma of the bilharzial bladder by the Ames Salmonella plate assay. Interpretation employing quantitation of viable lawn bacteria. *Cancer*, **51**, 371–377

Ferguson, A.R. (1911) Associated bilharziosis and primary malignant disease of the urinary bladder with observations on a series of forty cases. *J. Pathol. Bacteriol.*, **16**, 76–98

Fripp, P.J. (1960) Schistosomiasis and urinary ß-glucuronidase activity. *Nature*, **189**, 507–508

Fripp, P.J. (1965) The origin of urinary ß-glucuronidase. *Br. J. Cancer*, **19**, 330–335

Fripp, P.J. & Keen, P. (1980) Bladder cancer in an endemic *Schistosoma haematobium* area. The excretion patterns of 3-hydroxyanthranilic acid and kynurenine. *S. Afr. J. Sci.*, **76**, 212–215

Fujita, J., Nakayama, H., Onoue, H., Rhim, J.S., El-Bolkainy, M.N., El-Aaser, A.A. & Kitamura, Y. (1987) Frequency of active *ras* oncogene in human bladder cancers associated with schistosomiasis. *Jpn. J. Cancer Res. (Gann)*, **78**, 915–920

Fukushima, S., Asamoto, M., Imaida, K., El-Bolkainy, M.N., Tawfik, H.N. & Ito, N. (1989) Comparative study of urinary bladder carcinomas in Japanese and Egyptians. *Acta Pathol. Jpn*, **39**, 176–179

Gelfand, M., Weinberg, R.W & Castle, W.M. (1967) Relation between carcinoma of the bladder and infestation with *Schistosoma haematobium*. *Lancet*, **i**, 1249–1251

Gentile, J.M. (1985) Schistosome related cancers: a possible role for genotoxins. *Environ. Mutag.*, 7, 775–785

Gentile, J.M. (1991) A possible role for genotoxins in parasite-associated cancers. *Rev. Latinoam. Genet.*, **1**, 239–248

Gentile, J.M. & Gentile, G.J. (1994) Implications for the involvement of the immune system in parasite-associated cancers. *Mutat. Res.*, **305**, 315–320

Gentile, J.M., Brown, S., Aardema, M., Clark, D. & Blankespoor, H. (1985) Modified mutagen metabolism in *Schistosoma hematobium*-infested organisms. *Arch. Environ. Health*, **40**, 5–12

Gillman, J. & Prates, M.D. (1962) Histological types and histogenesis of bladder cancer in the Portuguese East African with special reference to bilharzial cystitis. *Acta Unio Int. Contra Can crum*, **18**, 560–574

Goebel, C. (1905) Occurrence of bladder tumours due to bilharziasis, with particular attention to carcinomas. *Z. Krebsforsch.*, **3**, 369–513 (in German)

Gonzalez-Zulueta, M., Shibata, A., Ohneseit, P.F., Spruck, C.H., Busch, C., Shamaa, M., El-Baz, M., Nichols, P.W., Gonzalgo, M.L., Malmström, P.-U. & Jones, P.A. (1995) High frequency of chromosome 9p allelic loss and CDKN2 tumor suppressor gene alterations in squamous cell carcinoma of the bladder. *J. Natl. Cancer Inst.*, **87**, 1383–1393

Groenveld A.E., Marszalek W.W. & Heyns C.F. (1996) Bladder cancer in various population groups in the greater Durban area of KwaZulu-Natal, South Africa. *Br. J. Urol.*, **78**, 205–208

Habuchi, T., Takahashi, R., Yamada, H., Ogawa, O., Kakehi, Y., Ogura, K., Hamazaki, S., Toguchida, J., Ishizaki, K., Fujita, J., Sugiyama, T. & Yoshida, O. (1993) Influence of cigarette smoking and schistosomiasis on p53 gene mutation in urothelial cancer. *Cancer Res.*, **53**, 3795–3799

Hashem, M., Zaki, S.A. & Hussein, M. (1961) The bilharzial bladder cancer and its relation to schistosomiasis. A statistical study. *J. Egypt. Med. Assoc.*, **44**, 579–597

Hicks, R.M., Walters, C.L., Elsebai, I., El Aasser, A.-B., El Merzabani, M. & Gough, T.A. (1977) Demonstration of nitrosamines in human urine: preliminary observations on a possible etiology for bladder cancer in association with chronic urinary tract infections. *Proc. R. Soc. Med.*, **70**, 413–417

Hicks, R.M., Gough, T.A. & Walters, C.L. (1978) Demonstration of the presence of nitrosamines in human urine: preliminary observations on a possible etiology for bladder cancer in association with chronic urinary tract infection. In: Walker, E.A., Castegnaro, M., Griciute, L. & Lyle, R.E., eds, *Environmental Aspects of N-Nitroso Compounds* (IARC Scientific Publications No. 19), Lyon, IARC, pp. 465–475

Hicks, R.M., Ismail, M.M., Walters, C.L., Beecham, P.T., Rabie, M.F & El Alamy, M.A. (1982) Association of bacteriuria and urinary nitrosamine formation with *Schistosoma haematobium* infection in the Qalyub area of Egypt. *Trans. R. Soc.Trop. Med. Hyg.*, **76**, 519–527

Higginson, J. & Oettlé, A.G. (1962) Cancer of the bladder in the South African Bantu. *Acta Unio Int. Contra Cancrum*, **18**, 579–584

Hill, M.J. (1979) Role of bacteria in human carcinogenesis. *J. Hum. Nutr.*, **33**, 416–426

Hinder, R.A. & Schmaman, A. (1969) Bilharziasis and squamous carcinoma of the bladder. *S. Afr. Med. J.*, **43**, 617–618

Houston, W (1964) Carcinoma of the bladder in Southern Rhodesia. *Br. J. Urol.*, **36**, 71–76

IARC (1986) *IARC Monographs on the Evaluation of Carcinogenic Risks to Humans*, Volume 38, *Tobacco Smoking*, Lyon, IARC

IARC (1994) *IARC Monographs on the Evaluation of Carcinogenic Risks to Humans*, Volume 61, *Schistosomes, Liver Flukes and Helicobacter pylori*, Lyon, IARC

Keen, P. & Fripp, P.J. (1980) Bladder cancer in an endemic schistosomiasis area: geographical and sex distribution. *S. Afr. J. Sci.*, **76**, 228–230

Khafagy, M.M., El-Bolkainy, M.N. & Mansour, M.A. (1972) Carcinoma of the bilharzial urinary bladder. A study of the associated mucosal lesions in 86 cases. *Cancer*, **30**, 150–159

Kisner, C.D. (1973) Vesical bilharziasis, pathological changes and relationship to squamous carcinoma. *S. Afr. J. Surg.*, **11**, 79–87

Kitinya, J.N., Lauren, PA., Eshleman, L.J., Paljärvi, L. & Tanaka, K. (1986) The incidence of squamous and transitional cell carcinomas of the urinary bladder in northern Tanzania in areas of high and low levels of endemic *Schistosoma haematobium* infection. *Trans. R. Soc. Trop. Med. Hyg.*, **80**, 935–939

Koraitim, N.M., Metwalli, N.E., Attah, M.A., & El-Sadr, A.A. (1995) Changing age incidence and pathological typs of *Schistosoma*-associated bladder carcinoma. *J. Urol.*, **154**, 1714–1716

Lafuente, A., Zakahary, M.M., El-Aziz, M.A.A., Ascaso, C., Lafuente, M.J., Trias, M. & Carretro, P. (1996) Influence of smoking in the glutathione-S-transferase M1 deficiency-associated risk for squamous cell carcinoma of the bladder in schistosomiasis patients in Egypt. *Br. J. Cancer*, **74**, 836–838

Laughlin, L.W., Farid, Z., Mansour, N., Edman, D.C. & Higashi, G.I. (1978) Bacteriuria in urinary schistosomiasis in Egypt. A prevalence survey. *Am. J. Trop. Med. Hyg.*, **27**, 916–918

Lehman, J.S., Farid, Z., Smith, Z., Bassily, J.H. & El-Masry, N.A. (1973) Urinary schistosomiasis in Egypt: clinical, radiological, bacteriological and parasitological correlations. *Trans R. Soc. Trop. Med. Hyg.*, **7**, 384–399

Lucas, S.B. (1982a) Squamous cell carcinoma of the bladder and schistosomiasis. *E. Afr Med. J.*, **59**, 345–351

Lucas, S.B. (1982b) Bladder tumours in Malawi. *Br. J. Urol.*, **54**, 275–279

Makhyoun, N.A. (1974) Smoking and bladder cancer in Egypt. *Br J. Cancer*, **30**, 577–581

Makhyoun, N.A., El-Kashlan, K.M., Al-Ghorab, M.M. & Mokhles, A.S. (1971) Aetiological factors in bilharzial bladder cancer. *J. Trop. Med. Hyg.*, **74**, 73–78

Malik, M.O.A., Veress, B., Daoud, E.H. & El Hassan, A.M. (1975) Pattern of bladder cancer in the Sudan and its relation to schistosomiasis: a study of 255 vesical carcinomas. *J. Trop. Med. Hyg.*, **78**, 219–226

Mohamed, A.S. (1954) The association of bilharziasis and malignant disease in the urinary bladder. Pathogenesis of bilharzial cancer in the urinary bladder. *J. Egypt. Med. Assoc.*, **37**, 1066–1085

Mostafa, M.H., Helmi, S., Badawi, A.E, Tricker, A.R., Spiegelhalder, B. & Preussmann, R. (1994) Nitrate, nitrite and volatile N-nitroso compounds in the urine of *Schistosoma haematobium* and *Schistosoma mansoni* infected patients. *Carcinogenesis*, **15**, 619–625

Mustacchi, P & Shimkin, M.S. (1958) Cancer of the bladder and infestation with *Schistosoma haematobium*. *J. Natl Cancer Inst.*, **20**, 825–842

Norden, D.A. & Gelfand, M. (1972) Bilharzia and bladder cancer. An investigation of urinary ß-glucuronidase associated with S. *haematobium* infection. *Trans. R. Soc. Trop. Med. Hyg.*, **66**, 864–866

Parkin, D.M., Whelan, S.L., Ferlay, J., Teppo, L. & Thomas, D.B. (2002) *Cancer Incidence in Five Continents*, Vol. VIII (IARC Scientific Publications No. 155), Lyon, IARCPress

Prates, M.D. (1963) The rates of cancer of the bladder in the Portuguese East Africans of Lourenço Marques. In: Stewart, H. & Clemmensen, J., eds, *Geographical Pathology of Neoplasms of Urinary Bladder*, New York, S. Karger, pp. 125–129

Prates, M.D. & Gillman, J. (1959) Carcinoma of the urinary bladder in the Portuguese East African with special reference to bilharzial cystitis and preneoplastic reactions. *S. Afr. J. Med. Sci.*, **24**, 13–40

Quenum, C. (1967) Cancers of the bladder and bilharzial endemy in Senegal. *Indian Pract.*, **20**, 171–178

Ramchurren, N., Cooper, K. & Summerhays, I.C. (1995) Molecular events underlying schistosomiasis-related bladder cancer. *Int. J. Cancer*, **62**, 237–244

Raziuddin, S., Shetty, S. & Ibrahim, A. (1991) T-Cell abnormality and defective interleukin-2 production in patients with carcinoma of the urinary bladder with schistosomiasis. *J. Clin. Immunol.*, **11**, 103–113

Raziuddin, S., Shetty, S. & Ibrahim, A. (1992) Soluble interleukin-2 receptor levels and immune activation in patients with schistosomiasis and carcinoma of the urinary bladder. *Scand. J. 1mmunol.*, **35**, 637–641

Raziuddin, S., Masihuzzaman, M., Shetty, S. & Ibrahim, A. (1993) Tumor necrosis factor alpha production in schistosomiasis with carcinoma of urinary bladder. *J. Clin. Immunol.*, **13**, 23–29

Rosin, M.P. & Anwar, W (1992) Chromosomal damage in urothelial cells from Egyptians with chronic *Schistosoma haematobium* infections. *Int. J. Cancer*, **51**, 1–5

Rosin, M.P., Anwar W.A. & Ward, A.J. (1994a) Inflammation, chromosomal instability and cancer: the schistosomiasis model. *Cancer Res.*, **54**, 1929–1933

Rosin, M.P., El-Din, S.S., Ward, A.J. & Anwar, W.A. (1994b) Involvement of inflammatory reactions and elevated cell proliferation in the development of bladder cancer in schistosomiasis patients. *Mutat. Res.*, **305**, 283–292

Sharfi, A.R.A., El Sir, S. & Beleil, O. (1992) Squamous cell carcinoma of the urinary bladder. *Br. J. Urol.*, **69**, 369–371

Shaw, M.E., Elder, P.A., Abbas, A. & Knowles, M.A. (1999) Partial allelotype of schistosomiasis-associated bladder cancer. *Int. J. Cancer*, **80**, 656–661

Shubber, E.K. (1987) Sister-chromatid exchanges in lymphocytes from patients with Schistosoma hematobium. *Mutat. Res.*, **180**, 93–99

da Silva Lopes, C.A. (1984) *Cancerizacão Vesical e Schistosomiase* [bladder cancer and schistosomiasis], Porto, Faculty of Medicine (thesis)

Tamimi, Y., Bringuier, P.P., Smit, F., Bokhoven, A., Abbas, A., Debruyne, F.M. & Schalken, J.A. (1996) Homozygous deletions of p16^{INK4} occur frequently in bilharziasis-associated bladder cancer. *Int. J. Cancer*, **68**, 183–187

Tawfik, H.N. (1988) Carcinoma of the urinary bladder associated with schistosomiasis in Egypt: the possible causal relationship. In: Miller, R.W, Watanabe, S., Fraumeni, J.F, Jr, Sugimura, I, Takayama, S. & Sugano, H., eds, *Unusual Occurrences as Clues to Cancer Etiology*, Tokyo, Japan Scientific Societies Press, pp. 197–209

Thomas, J.E., Bassett, M.I, Sigola, L.B. & Taylor, P (1990) Relationship between bladder cancer incidence, *Schistosoma haematobium* infection, and geographical region in Zimbabwe. *Trans. R. Soc. Trop. Med. Hyg.*, **84**, 551–553

Thomas J.O. & Onyemenen, N.Y. (1995) Bladder carcinoma in Ibadan, Nigeria: a changing trend? *East Afr. Med. J.*, **72**, 49–50

Tricker, A.R., Mostafa, M.H., Spiegelhalder, B. & Preussmann, R. (1989) Urinary excretion of nitrate, nitrite, and N-nitroso compounds in schistosomiasis and bilharzia bladder cancer patients. *Carcinogenesis*, **10**, 547–552

Tricker, A.R., Mostafa, M.H., Spiegelhalder, B. & Preussmann, R. (1991) Urinary nitrate, nitrite and N-nitroso compounds in bladder cancer patients with schistosomiasis (bilharzia). In: O'Neill, I.K., Chen, J. & Barsch, H., eds, *Relevance to Human Cancer of N-Nitroso Compounds, Tobacco Smoke and Mycotoxins* (IARC Scientific Publications No. 105), Lyon, IARC, pp. 178–181

Vineis, P, d'Errico, A., Malats, N. & Boffetta, P. (1999) Overall evaluation and research perspectives. In: Vineis, P, Malats, N., Lang, M., d'Errico, A., Caporaso, N., Cuzick, J. & Boffetta, P., *Metabolic Polymorphisms and Susceptibility to Cancer* (IARC Scientific Publications No. 148), Lyon, IARC, pp. 403–408

Vizcaino A.P., Parkin D.M., Boffetta P. & Skinner M.E. (1994) Bladder cancer: epidemiology and risk factors in Bulawayo, Zimbabwe. *Cancer Causes Control*, **5**, 517–522

Wabinga, H.R., Parkin, D.M., Wabire-Mangen, F. & Nambooze, S. (2000) Trends in incidence in Kyadondo County, Uganda, 1960–1997. *Br. J. Cancer*, **82**, 1585–1592

Warren, W., Biggs, P.J., El-Baz, M., Ghoneim, M.A., Stratton, M.R. & Venitt, R. (1995) Mutations in the p53 gene in schistosomal bladder cancer: a study of 92 tumours from Egyptian patients and a comparison between mutation spectra from schistosomal and non-schistosomal urothelial tumours. *Carcinogenesis*, **16**, 1181–1189

Yu, M.C., Skipper, P.L., Taghizadek, K., Tannenbaum, S.R., Chan, K.K., Henderson, B.E. & Ross, R.K. (1994) Acetylator phenotype, aminobiphenyl haemoglobin adduct levels and bladder cancer in white black and Asian men in Los Angeles, California. *J. Natl Cancer Inst.*, **86**, 712–716

4.2 Breast cancer

Introduction

Worldwide, cancer of the breast is by far the most common cancer of women, with an estimated 1.05 million new cases in the year 2000, comprising 22% of all new cancers in women. In Africa, however, it is relatively less common, with an estimated 59 000 new cases (18% of cancers in women). There is a fair amount of regional variation, however, and in north Africa, breast cancer is considerably more common than cervical cancer, accounting for 27% of cancers, compared with 15.7% in sub-Saharan Africa.

Descriptive epidemiology in Africa

Table 1 shows age-standardized incidence rates from different centres, as reported in this volume, with comparison data from Europe and North America. Table 2 shows incidence data from time periods in the 1960s and 1970s. Figure 1 shows estimated incidence rates by country, based on these data, and other information reported in this volume.

Incidence is highest in populations of north Africa and, in sub-Saharan Africa, in urban rather than rural settings. Thus, current incidence rates are highest in cities such as Abidjan (Côte d'Ivoire) and Harare (Zimbabwe). It also seems that incidence rates in the more recent registry series are higher than those reported in the past.

Robertson *et al.* (1971) calculated incidence rates of 3.7 per 100 000 (crude) and 4.5 (age-adjusted, African standard) in the rural low-veld area of South Africa for the period 1962–67. Rose and Fellingham (1981) reported a rate of 3.2 per 100 000 (age-adjusted, African standard) in women of rural Transkei in 1965–69. Isaacson *et al.* (1978) noted that rates in urban populations such as Soweto were higher than in rural populations, but that they were still low.

The incidence in white women living in Africa is much higher than in black Africans. This is clear in the old data in Table 2. Recent data (1993–95) from the National Cancer Registry of South Africa (Sitas *et al.*, 1998) indicate age-standardized rates of 70.2 per 100 000 in white females, and 11.3 per 10^5 in blacks (although some of this variation may represent differences in rates of treatment or biopsy, since the data are based on histologically diagnosed cases only). In Harare, Zimbabwe, in 1990–92, age-standardized incidence was 127.7 per 100 000 in white females and 20.4 per 100 000 in blacks. These large differences probably reflect the prevalence of risk factors (e.g., reproductive, body mass, etc.); in the United States, Brinton *et al.* (1997) found that the 20% difference in incidence between black and white women (at least at ages 40–54 years) was fully explicable in terms of difference in prevalence of reproductive variables (number of births, age at first birth, age at menarche) and lifestyle factors (oral contraceptive use, body mass, alcohol).

The risk of breast cancer increases with age, but the rate of increase slows down after the menopause, the lowering of risk coinciding with a decrease in circulating estrogens (Henderson *et al.*, 1988). In low-incidence countries, the slope of the age–incidence curve after the menopause may be very flat, or even negative. Almost certainly, this reflects increasing risks in successive generations of women, rather than a true decline in risk with age (Moolgavkar *et al.*, 1979). The young age structure of African populations, coupled with this rather flat age–incidence curve, means that the average age at diagnosis of cases in Africa is lower than in European and American populations. This is often remarked upon in clinical series from Africa (e.g., Ihekwaba, 1992; Muguti, 1993; Maalej *et al.*, 1999), but it has no etiological or prognostic significance.

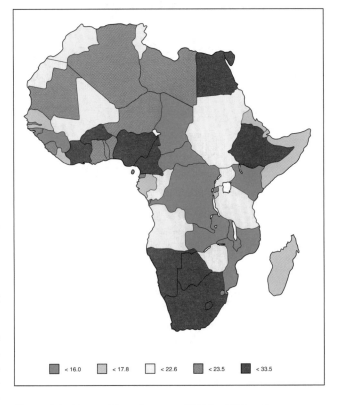

Figure 1. Incidence of breast cancer - ASR (world) females

Legend: < 16.0 | < 17.8 | < 22.6 | < 23.5 | < 33.5

Figure 2 shows age-specific incidence rates from four of the registry series in this volume (Oran, Algeria; Tunisia, Tunis; Kampala, Uganda; and Harare, Zimbabwe), in comparison with the black population covered by the SEER program of the United States.

Migrant studies suggest that migrants from north and east Africa to France retain their relatively low breast cancer mortality rates on migration to France (Bouchardy *et al.*, 1995, 1996), although African migrants to England and Wales do not have a significantly low mortality (Grulich *et al.*, 1992). Jewish migrants from North Africa to Israel also have low incidence rates (except for Jews born in Egypt (Steinitz *et al.*, 1989)).

Stage at presentation of tumours in African women is generally very advanced, with correspondingly poor prognosis (Walker *et al.*, 1984; Dansey *et al.*, 1988).

Time trends

In almost all developing countries with relatively low rates of incidence of breast cancer, the risk appears to be increasing (Parkin, 1994). There are very few data from Africa. As noted, rates appear to be rather higher in more recent data than in older series. In Ibadan, Nigeria, incidence in 1998–99 was 24.7 per 100 000, compared with 13.7 per 100 000 in 1960–69. In Kampala, Uganda, there has been a significant increase in incidence since the 1960s (Figure 3) (Wabinga *et al.*, 2000). Mortality rates in Mauritius have also been increasing since the 1960s (Figure 4).

Risk factors

The risk of breast cancer is clearly associated with socioeconomic status, with women of higher social class (as measured by education, income, housing, etc.) being at higher risk (Kogevinas *et al.*, 1997). In Bulawayo, women registered with breast cancer during 1963-1977 had a higher level of literacy than women with other types of cancer

Table 1. Age-standardized (world) and cumulative (0-64) incidence
Breast (C50)

| | MALE | | | | FEMALE | | | |
	Cases	CRUDE (per 100,000)	ASR(W)	Cumulative (%)	Cases	CRUDE (per 100,000)	ASR(W)	Cumulative (%)
Africa, North								
Algeria, Algiers (1993-1997)	26	0.5	**0.7**	0.05	906	16.6	**21.2**	1.73
Algeria, Constantine (1994-1997)	6	0.4	**0.7**	0.01	291	19.1	**28.3**	2.25
Algeria, Oran (1996-1998)	11	0.6	**0.9**	0.05	481	27.3	**34.5**	2.83
Algeria, Setif (1993-1997)	8	0.3	**0.5**	0.05	317	10.5	**17.0**	1.47
Tunisia, Centre, Sousse (1993-1997)	5	0.4	**0.6**	0.04	209	18.6	**22.7**	1.71
Tunisia, North, Tunis (1994)	6	0.3	**0.3**	0.02	409	19.4	**24.1**	1.85
Tunisia, Sfax (1997)	4	1.0	**1.2**	0.04	73	19.3	**22.7**	1.81
Africa, West								
The Gambia (1997-1998)	-	-	**-**	-	41	4.0	**7.0**	0.47
Guinea, Conakry (1996-1999)	-	-	**-**	-	188	8.5	**15.5**	1.33
Mali, Bamako (1988-1997)	10	0.3	**0.6**	0.04	249	6.9	**14.9**	1.23
Niger, Niamey (1993-1999)	7	0.4	**1.1**	0.13	175	9.7	**25.0**	2.05
Nigeria, Ibadan (1998-1999)	7	0.5	**1.3**	0.04	227	15.0	**25.3**	2.19
Africa, Central								
Congo, Brazzaville (1996-1999)	4	0.3	**0.5**	0.03	205	17.0	**22.5**	1.95
Africa, East								
France, La Reunion (1988-1994)	10	0.5	**0.6**	0.05	566	26.2	**29.2**	2.18
Kenya, Eldoret (1998-2000)	3	0.3	**0.8**	0.01	59	6.5	**14.3**	1.30
Malawi, Blantyre (2000-2001)	5	0.6	**1.7**	0.04	48	5.5	**12.0**	1.07
Uganda, Kyadondo County (1993-1997)	10	0.4	**1.1**	0.04	224	7.7	**21.0**	1.62
Zimbabwe, Harare: African (1990-1993)	5	0.2	**0.4**	0.04	171	8.0	**20.3**	1.55
Zimbabwe, Harare: African (1994-1997)	4	0.1	**0.5**	0.02	186	7.0	**19.8**	1.50
Zimbabwe, Harare: European (1990-1997)	2	1.3	**0.6**	-	347	205.7	**121.2**	8.55
Africa, South								
Namibia (1995-1998)	20	0.6	**1.1**	0.05	531	16.6	**25.6**	1.73
South Africa: Black (1989-1992)	299	0.5	**1.0**	0.07	5117	9.1	**13.6**	1.00
South Africa: Indian (1989-1992)	20	1.0	**1.6**	0.10	693	34.9	**42.5**	3.24
South Africa: Mixed race (1989-1992)	30	0.5	**1.0**	0.03	1285	19.2	**28.1**	2.07
South Africa: White (1989-1992)	206	2.0	**1.9**	0.12	7801	76.6	**62.8**	4.67
South Africa, Transkei, Umtata (1996-1998)	4	1.1	**1.6**	0.10	42	9.9	**14.9**	1.30
South Africa, Transkei, 4 districts (1996-1998)	1	0.1	**0.2**	-	36	4.0	**6.1**	0.48
Swaziland (1996-1999)	5	0.3	**0.7**	0.05	139	7.1	**12.9**	1.07
Europe/USA								
USA, SEER: White (1993-1997)	477	1.0	**0.8**	0.04	67272	134.1	**92.4**	6.51
USA, SEER: Black (1993-1997)	63	0.9	**1.1**	0.07	6527	87.9	**83.4**	5.98
France, 8 registries (1993-1997)	164	1.2	**0.8**	0.05	16870	116.8	**81.1**	6.20
The Netherlands (1993-1997)	268	0.7	**0.5**	0.02	49570	126.9	**85.9**	6.37
UK, England (1993-1997)	1036	0.9	**0.5**	0.03	150322	117.6	**75.6**	5.67

In italics: histopathology-based registries

Table 2. Incidence of breast cancer in Africa, 1953–74

| Registry | Period | ASR (per 100 000) | | Source |
		Male	Female	(see Chap. 1)
Senegal, Dakar	1969–74	*0.7*	11.8	4
Mozambique, Lourenço Marques	1956–60	*0.0*	3.2	1
Nigeria, Ibadan	1960–69	*0.1*	15.3	3
SA, Cape Province: Bantu	1956–59	*0.4*	13.6	2
SA, Cape Province: Coloured	1956–59	*0.9*	25.9	2
SA, Cape Province: White	1956–59	*1.6*	57.2	2
SA, Johannesburg, Bantu	1953–55	*0.8*	15.3	1
SA, Natal Province: African	1964–66	*0.0*	11.9	2
SA, Natal Province: Indian	1964–66	*1.8*	19.9	2
Uganda, Kyadondo	1954–60	*0.3*	9.7	1
Uganda, Kyadondo	1960–71	*0.6*	10.8	5
Zimbabwe, Bulawayo	1963–72	*0.3*	13.4	6

Italics: Rate based on less than 10 cases

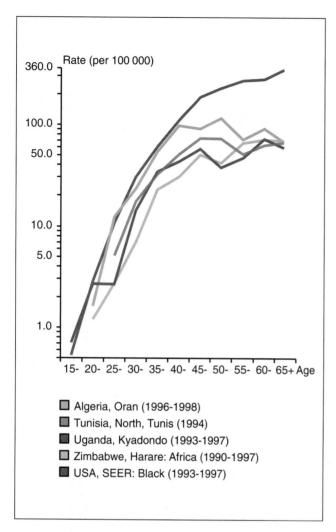

Figure 2. Age-specific incidence rates of breast cancer in Africa, and in black females in the United States

(Skinner *et al.*, 1993). Such differences may be due to the prevalence of risk factors between social classes (such as parity, age at menstruation and menopause, height, weight, alcohol consumption).

The most important risk factors for breast cancer are reproductive and hormonal factors. Thus, the risk is increased by early menarche, late menopause, late age at first birth, and low parity. All of these reflect a hormonal pattern of exposure to high levels of endogenous estrogens, in particular free estradiol (Henderson *et al.*, 1988).

In Kampala, Uganda, Ssali *et al.* (1995) compared 86 histologically diagnosed cases with 86 age-matched hospital controls. Most cases were pre-menopausal (median age 47.2 years); there was a clear association with age at first delivery (OR = 4.3 (95% CI 1.7–10.8) for age 22 years or more) and number of pregnancies (OR 0.21 (95% CI 0.09–0.49) for 4 or more vs 3 or less). There was an increased risk with *late* age at menarche, although this was not independent of the above associations. Adebamowo and Adekunle (1999), in a study of 250 breast cancer cases and age-matched hospital controls in Ibadan, Nigeria, also found a significantly older age at first pregnancy in cases than controls, but no difference in age at menarche. Using the cancer registry data from Bulawayo (1963–77), Parkin *et al.* (1994) found that late age at menarche and early age at menopause were associated with reduced risk of breast cancer, although the effects were small and not statistically significant. Parity and age at first pregnancy affected risk only in women aged 45 years or more at diagnosis. This

observation may relate to the high parity of this African population, as similar observations have been made in other developing countries with high fertility and low age at first birth (e.g., Mirra *et al.*, 1971; Rosero-Bixby *et al.*, 1987). It probably relates to the increase in risk of breast cancer that follows each pregnancy, manifested as an increased risk in relation to age at last birth (Kelsey *et al.*, 1993); in young women with breast cancer, it is quite likely that with multiple pregnancies, the last one had occurred quite recently. This may explain the finding in the Ibadan study (Adebamowo & Adekunle, 1999) of fewer pregnancies (mean =4) in control subjects than in breast cancer patients (mean = 6), since the subjects were very young (mean age 43 years). A similar apparently anomalous finding in a case–control study in Tanzania (Amir *et al.*, 1998) of increasing risk with higher parity was a consequence of failure to adjust for the large age difference between case and control subjects.

In a large case–control study of 446 breast cancers in black and "coloured" women in Capetown, South Africa, Coogan et al (1999) found an association between risk of breast cancer and late age at first birth. Reporting on the same study, Shapiro *et al.* (2000) noted that there were associations between breast cancer risk and family history, low parity, and high socioeconomic status (as measured by medical insurance coverage), though no data were provided. Abdel-Rahman *et al.* (1993) compared 180 breast cancer cases from two hospitals in Egypt with 192 hospital controls (without malignancy). It seems that prevalent cancers were included, and, although the controls were stated to be age-matched, the age distribution of cases and control subjects was not very similar. Breast cancer was associated with the usual reproductive variables (nulliparity, age at first birth, age of menarche, and age of natural menopause), as well as a family history of breast cancer, height and weight (but not with body mass index). In a univariate analysis, there was no association with number of pregnancies (for >5 vs ≤ 5, OR = 1.4; 95% CI 0.9–2.4).

Since the report of Lane-Claypon over 70 years ago (1926), lactation has frequently been examined as being possibly protective against breast cancer, particularly in premenopausal women. The results are quite mixed. In the large case–control study in Capetown, Coogan *et al.* (1999) found no effect of lactation (age at onset, frequency, duration) on risk.

The possible effects of oral contraceptive hormones on risk of breast cancer has been the subject of much research. It seems that there is a small but detectable increase in risk in women taking oral contraceptives, but this diminishes when contraception ceases, and after 10 years, none of the excess risk remains (Reeves, 1996). In the large case–control study of 419 breast cancers in black and "coloured" women in Capetown, South Africa, Shapiro et al (2000) found a weak association in women taking combined estrogen/progesterone contraceptives (OR = 1.2), which was strongest in young women under 35 years of age (OR = 1.7), but no association with recency or duration of use. The same study investigated the risk associated with injectable progestogen contraceptives, especially depot medroxyprogesterone acetate (DMPA). Most studies have suggested that these pose only a small risk, if any, and that it is confined to young women (Skegg, 1996); there was no elevated risk in South African women, even in those aged under 35 years at diagnosis.

In a study of breast cancer cases and controls in Egypt and Britain, no differences in hormonal levels were found between cancer cases and controls (Anglo-Egyptian Health Agreement Collaborative Study, 1988). However, Egyptian women had a rather higher percentage of free estradiol than British women, and it was suggested that this might be associated with the claim that breast cancer presents in a more aggressive form in Egypt.

The role of diet in breast cancer has been controversial. Dietary fat appears as an important determinant of risk in inter-population studies (Prentice & Sheppard, 1990). However, in

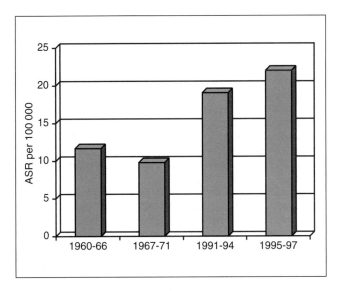

Figure 3. Trends in breast cancer incidence: Kampala, Uganda

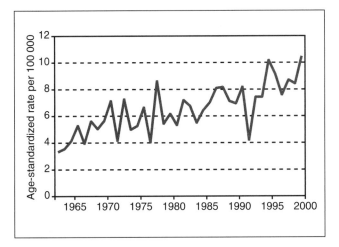

Figure 4. Mortality from breast cancer: Mauritius 1965–97

studies of individuals (case–control or cohort), this association has been difficult to confirm (Hunter *et al.*, 1996). Obesity in postmenopausal women is, however, important, increasing risk by some 2% per unit increase in body mass index (Bergström *et al.*, 2001). In a small hospital-based study in Johannesburg, Walker *et al.* (1989) observed higher nulliparity, obesity (body mass index ≥ 30) and a higher percentage of energy intake from dietary fat in breast cancer cases than in control patients. In their case–control study in Nigeria, Adebamowo and Adekunle (1999) found that breast cancer cases were significantly taller and heavier than (hospital) controls.

No studies of diet and breast cancer in African populations appear to have been reported. Traditional diets in Africa are low in animal products (especially fat) and high in fibre (Manning *et al.*, 1971; Labadarios *et al.*, 1996). This pattern is gradually being modified by urbanization and westernization of lifestyles. It is probable that average body weight in postmenopausal women in urban environments has increased (Steyn *et al.*, 1998). All these changes will tend to favour an increase in breast cancer incidence in African populations.

The role of genetic factors in breast cancer etiology has received much attention. At least part of the obvious family risk of the disease is mediated through the major susceptibility genes

BRCA1 and *BRCA2*. In European populations, around 2% of breast cancers are likely to be due to *BRCA1* mutations, but the proportion is much higher in younger breast cancer cases, for example 10% below the age of 40 years (Ford *et al.*, 1995). Nothing is known of the prevalence of mutations in *BRCA1* and *BRCA2* in African populations.

Inflammatory breast cancer

Inflammatory breast cancer (IBC) is characterized by inflammatory symptoms (erythema, skin oedema or '*peau d'orange*' and ridging of the skin) and invasion of breast dermal lymphatic ducts with tumour emboli (Jaiyesimi *et al.*, 1992). A special code is allocated in ICD-O (8530/3), although the condition does not have specific histological characteristics. It is the most lethal and fulminant form of breast cancer, with rapid growth, short doubling times and rapid systemic dissemination. Inflammatory breast cancer represents 1–6% of breast cancers in the United States, affects younger women disproportionately, and is characterized by extremely poor survival (between 0 and 28% at five years, with a median of 18 months) (Chang *et al.*, 1998a).

In the United States, IBC incidence doubled between 1975–77 and 1990–92, increasing among whites from 0.3 to 0.7 per 100 000 and among blacks from 0.6 to 1.1 per 100 000; this increase was considerably greater than for other forms of breast cancer (Chang *et al.*, 1998a).

Little is known about the causes of inflammatory breast cancer; no studies have investigated the risk factors, thus it is not known whether they differ from those for breast carcinoma in general (Chang *et al.*, 1998a). High body mass index has been found to be significantly associated with increased risk of IBC. This association did not vary by menopausal status, although IBC patients were more likely to be of pre-menopausal status (Chang *et al.*, 1998b).

This form of breast cancer, also known as '*poussée evolutive*' (PEV) has been reported to be particularly frequent in Tunisia, comprising as many as 55% of breast cancer cases in clinical series (Mourali *et al.*, 1980), although some authors are more sceptical of these high figures (Maalej *et al.*, 1999). Breast tumours with inflammatory signs were larger and had more frequent metastases (Tabbane *et al.*, 1989). IBC is particularly frequent among younger patients (under 30 years), though this may be due, in part at least, to the frequent association with pregnancy or lactation; nearly all the cases of breast cancer associated with pregnancy or lactation were rapidly growing inflammatory cancer (Tabbane *et al.*, 1985). There appears to be associations with rural residence and with blood group A (Mourali *et al.*, 1980); although this suggests a genetic predisposition, there was no association with any particular HLA antigen (Levine *et al.*, 1981), and cellular immunity appears to be normal in these patients.

Male breast cancer

Male breast cancer is a rare tumour in all parts of the world. About 1% of all breast cancers occur in men, but the male/female ratio is higher among black than among white populations. The male/female ratio is also relatively high in case series and registry data from Africa, including north Africa (Nectoux & Parkin, 1992; Sasco *et al.*, 1993). It is not clear, however, that this represents a higher incidence in men in these populations; rather it is the result of relatively low rates of breast cancer in women in Africa. Nevertheless, incidence rates in the black population of the United States are significantly higher (about 60%) than those among whites (Parkin *et al.*, 1997). As in females, there appears to be higher risk in Jewish subjects (Sasco *et al.*, 1993). A study in Egypt (El-Gazayerli & Abdel-Aziz, 1963) found that cases of male breast cancer (and of gynaecomastia) frequently had associated bilharziasis, raising the possibility of an etiological link.

References

Abdel-Rahman, H.A., Moustafa, R., Shoulah, A.R., Wassif, O.M., Salih, M.A., el-Gendy, S.D. & Abdo, A.S. (1993) An epidemiological study of cancer breast in greater Cairo. *J. Egypt Public Health Assoc.*, **68**, 119–142

Adebamowo, C.A. & Adekunle, O.O. (1999) Case-controlled study of the epidemiological risk factors for breast cancer in Nigeria. *Br. J. Surg.*, **86**, 665–668

Amir, H., Makwaya, C.K., Aziz, M.R. & Jessani, S. (1998) Breast cancer and risk factors in an African population: a case referent study. *E. Afr. Med. J.*, **75**, 268–270

Anglo-Egyptian Health Agreement Collaborative Study (1988) Serum hormone levels in breast cancer patients and controls in Egypt and Great Britain. *Eur. J. Cancer Clin. Oncol.*, **24**, 1329–1335

Bergström, A., Pisani, P., Tenet, V., Wolk, A. & Adami, H.O. (2001) Overweight as an avoidable cause of cancer in Europe. *Int. J. Cancer*, **91**, 421–430

Bouchardy, C., Wanner, P. & Parkin, D.M. (1995) Cancer mortality among sub-Saharan African migrants in France. *Cancer Causes Control*, **6**, 539–544

Bouchardy, C., Parkin, D.M., Wanner, P. & Khlat, M. (1996) Cancer mortality among North African migrants in France. *Int. J. Epidemiol.*, **25**, 5–13

Brinton, L.A., Benichou, J., Gammon, M.D., Brogan, D.R., Coates, R. & Schoenberg, J.B. (1997) Ethnicity and variation in breast cancer incidence. *Int. J. Cancer*, **73**, 349–355

Chang, S., Parker, S.L., Tuan Pham, Buzdar, A.U. & Stephen, D.H. (1998a) Inflammatory breast cancer incidence and survival. *Cancer*, **82**, 2366–2372

Chang, S., Parker, S.L., Buzdar, A.U., & Stephen, D.H. (1998b) Inflammatory breast cancer and body mass index. *J. Clin. Oncol.*, **16**, 3731–3735

Coogan, P.F., Rosenberg, L., Shapiro, S. & Hoffmann, M. (1999) Lactation and breast carcinoma risk in a South African population. *Cancer*, **86**, 982–989

Dansey, R.D., Hessel, P.A., Browde, S., Lange, M., Derman, D., Nissenbaum, M., Bezwoda, W.R. (1988) Lack of a significant independent effect of race on survival in breast cancer. *Cancer*, **61**, 1908–1912

El-Gazayerli, M.& Abdel-Aziz, A.S. (1963) On bilharziasis and male breast cancer in Egypt, a preliminary report and review of the literature. *Br. J. Cancer*, **17**, 566–571

Ford, D., Easton, D.F. & Peto, J. (1995) Estimates of the gene frequency of BRCA1 and its contribution to breast and ovarian cancer incidence. *Am. J. Hum. Genet.*, **57**, 1457–1462

Grulich, A.E., Swerdlow, A.J., Head, J. & Marmot, M.G. (1992).Cancer mortality in African and Caribbean migrants to England and Wales. *Br. J. Cancer*, **66**, 905–911

Henderson, B.E., Ross, R. & Bernstein, L. (1988) Estrogens as a cause of human cancer: the Richard and Hinda Rosenthal Foundation award lecture. *Cancer Res.*, **48**, 246–253

Hunter, D.J., Spiegelman, D., Adami, H.O., Beeson, L., van den Brandt, P.A., Folsom, A.R., Fraser, G.E., Goldbohm, R.A., Graham, S., Howe, G.R., Kushi, L.H., Marshall, J.R., McDermott, A., Miller, A.B., Speizer, F.E., Wolk, A., Yuan, S. & Willett, W. (1996) Cohort studies of fat intake and the risk of breast cancer – a pooled analysis. *New Engl. J. Med.*, **334**, 356–361

Ihekwaba, F.N. (1992) Breast cancer in Nigerian women. *Br. J. Surg.*, **79**, 771–775

Isaacson, C., Selzer, G., Kaye, V., Greenberg, M., Woodruff, J.D., Davies, J., Ninin, D., Vetten, D. & Andrew, M. (1978) Cancer in the urban blacks of South Africa. *S. Afr. Cancer Bull.*, **22**, 49–84

Jaiyesimi, I.A., Buzdar, A.U. & Hortobagyi, G. (1992) Inflammatory breast cancer: a review. *J. Clin. Oncol.*, **10**, 1014–1024

Kelsey, J.L., Gammon, M.D. & John, E.M. (1993) Reproductive factors and breast cancer. *Epidemiol. Rev.*, **15**, 36–47

Kogevinas, M., Pearce, N., Susser, M. & Boffetta, P. (eds) (1997) *Social Inequalities and Cancer* (IARC Scientific Publications No. 138), Lyon, IARC

Labadarios, D., Walker, A.R., Blaauw, R. & Walker, B.F.(1996) Traditional diets and meal patterns in South Africa. *World Rev. Nutr. Diet*, **79**, 70–108

Lane-Claypon, J.E. (1926) *A Further Report on Cancer of the Breast with Special Reference to its Associate Antecedent Conditions* (Report on Public Health and Medical Subjects No. 32), London, HMSO

Levine, P.H., Mourali, N., Tabbane, F., Loon, J., Terasaki, P. & Bekesi, J.G. (1981) Studies of the role of cellular immunity and genetics in the etiology of rapidly progressing breast cancer in Tunisia. *Int. J. Cancer*, **27**, 611–615

Maalej, M., Frikha, H., Ben Salem, S., Daoud, J., Bouaouina, N., Ben Abdallah, M. & Ben Romdhane, K. (1999) Le cancer du sein en Tunisie: étude clinique et épidémiologie [Breast cancer in Tunisia: clinical and epidemiological study]. *Bull. Cancer*, **86**, 302–306

Manning, E.B., Mann, J.I., Sophangisa, E. & Truswell, A.S. (1971) Dietary patterns in urbanised blacks. A study in Guguletu, Cape Town. *S. Afr. Med. J.*, **48**, 485–498

Mirra, A.P., Cole, P. & MacMahon, B. (1971) Breast cancer in an area of high parity: Sao Paulo, Brazil. *Cancer Res.*, **31**, 77–83

Moolgavkar, S.H., Stevens, R.G., Lee,J.A. (1979) Effect of age on incidence of breast cancer in females. *J. Natl Cancer Inst.*, **62**, 493–501

Mourali, N., Muenz, L.R., Tabbane, F., Belhassen, S., Bahi, J. & Levine, P.H. (1980) Epidemiologic features of rapidly progressing breast cancer in Tunisia. *Cancer*, **46**, 2741–2746

Muguti, G.I. (1993) Experience with breast cancer in Zimbabwe. *J. R. Coll. Surg. Edin.*, **37**, 159–161

Nectoux, J. & Parkin, D.M. (1992) Epidémiologie du cancer du sein chez l'homme. *Bull. Cancer*, **79**, 991–998

Parkin, D.M., Vizcaino, A.P., Skinner, M.E.G. & Ndhlovu, A. (1994) Cancer patterns and risk factors in the African population of southwestern Zimbabwe, 1963–1977. *Cancer Epidemiol. Biomarkers Prev.*, **3**, 537–547

Parkin, D.M., Whelan, S.L., Ferlay, J., Raymond, L., & Young, J. (1997) *Cancer Incidence in Five Continents*, Vol. VII (IARC Scientific Publications No. 143), Lyon, IARC

Prentice, R.L. & Sheppard, L. (1990) Dietary fat and cancer: consistency of the epidemiologic data, and disease prevention that may follow from a practical reduction in fat consumption. *Cancer Causes Control*, **1**, 81–97

Reeves, G. (1996) Breast cancer and oral contraceptives – the evidence so far. *Cancer Causes Control*, **7**, 495–496

Robertson, M.A., Harington, J.S., Bradshaw, E. (1971) The cancer pattern in African gold miners. *Br. J. Cancer*, **25**, 395–402

Rose, E.F. & Fellingham, S.A. (1981) Cancer patterns in the Transkei. *S. Afr. J. Sci.*, **77**, 555–561

Rosero-Bixby, L., Oberle, M.W. & Lee, N.C. (1987) Reproductive history and breast cancer in a population of high fertility, Costa Rica, 1984–85. *Int. J. Cancer*, **40**, 747–754

Sasco, A., Lowels, A.B. & Pasker de Jong, P. (1993) Epidemiology of male breast cancer. A meta-analysis of published case-control studies and discussion of selected etiological factors. *Int. J. Cancer*, **53**, 538–549

Shapiro, S., Rosenberg, L., Hoffman, M.. Truter, H., Cooper, D., Rao, S., Dent, D., Gudgeon, A., van Zyl, J., Katzenellenbogen, J. & Baillie, R. (2000) Risk of breast cancer in relation to the use of injectable progestogen contraceptives and combined estrogen/progestogen contraceptives. *Am. J. Epidemiol.*, **151**, 396–403

Sitas, F., Madhoo, J. & Wessie, J. (1998) *Incidence of histologically diagnosed cancer in South Africa, 1993–1995*. Johannesburg, National Cancer Registry, South African Institute for Medical Research

Skegg, D.C., Paul, C., Spears, G.F. & Williams, S.M. (1996) Progestogen-only oral contraceptives and risk of breast cancer in New Zealand. *Cancer Causes Control*, **7**, 513–519

Skinner, M.E.G., Parkin, D.M., Vizcaino, A.P. & Ndhlovu, A. (1993) *Cancer in the African Population of Bulawayo, Zimbabwe, 1963–1977* (IARC Technical Report No. 15), Lyon, IARC

Ssali, J.C., Gakwaya, A. & Katangole-Mbidde, E. (1995) Risk factors for breast cancer in Ugandan women: a case control study. *E. Cent. Afr. J. Surg.*, **1**, 9–13

Steinitz, R., Parkin, D.M., Young, J.L., Bieber, C.A. & Katz, L. (eds.) (1989) *Cancer Incidence in Jewish migrants to Israel, 1961–1981*. (IARC Scientific Publications, 98), Lyon, IARC

Steyn, K., Bourne, L., Jooste, P., Fourie, J.M., Rossouw, K. & Lombard, C. (1998) Anthropometric profile of a black population of the Cape Peninsula in South Africa. *E. Afr. Med. J.*, **75**, 35–40

Tabbane, F., El May, A., Hachiche, M., Bahi, J., Jaziry, M., Cammoun, M. & Moutali, N. (1985) Breast cancer in women under 30 years of age. *Breast Cancer Res. Treat.*, **6**, 137–144

Tabbane, F., Bahi, J., Rahal, K., el May, A., Riahi, M., Cammoun, M., Hechiche, M., Jaziri, M. & Mourali, N. (1989) Inflammatory symptoms in breast cancer. Correlations with growth rate, clinicopathologic variables, and evolution. *Cancer*, **64**, 2081–2089

Wabinga, H.R., Parkin, D.M., Wabwire-Mangen, F. & Nambooze, S. (2000) Trends in incidence in Kyadondo County, Uganda, 1960–1997. *Br. J. Cancer*, **82**, 1585–1592

Walker, A.R., Walker, B.F., Tshabalala, E.N., Isaacson, C. & Segal, I. (1984) Low survival of South African urban black women with breast cancer. *Br. J. Cancer*, **49**, 241–244

Walker, A.R.P., Walker, B.F., Funani, S. & Walker, A.J. (1989) Characteristics of black women with breast cancer in Soweto, South Africa. *Cancer J.*, **2**, 316–319

4.3 Cervix cancer

Introduction

Cancer of the cervix uteri is the second most common cancer among women worldwide, with an estimated 468 000 new cases and 233 000 deaths in the year 2000. Almost 80% of the cases occur in developing countries, where, in many regions, this is the most common cancer among women.

Descriptive epidemiology in Africa

The incidence is high in sub-Saharan Africa, with an estimated 57 000 cases in 2000, comprising 22% of all cancers in women, equivalent to an age-standardized incidence of 31 per 100 000. In north Africa, the incidence is rather lower. Table 1 shows age-standardized incidence rates from different centres, as reported in this volume, with comparison data from Europe and North America. Table 2 shows incidence data from time periods in the 1960s and 1970s.

Figure 1 shows estimated incidence rates by country, based on these data and other information reported in this volume. The scale has been chosen to be equivalent to quintiles of incidence rates on a global basis, to show the moderate–high incidence throughout the continent, except for the relatively low-incidence rates estimated for Tunisia (based on the data from Table 1) and Egypt (see Chapter 3.1.2). The latter observation is supported by a low prevalence of cervical intraepithelial neoplasia (0.36%) found on cytological evaluation of women attending a gynaecology clinic in Cairo (Mohga *et al.*, 1987).

On the basis of frequency of different cancers in hospital case series, Cook-Mozaffari (1982) hypothesized the existence of a 'belt' of low incidence of cervix cancer along the line of the western Rift Valley in Uganda, Rwanda, Burundi and Zaire. This observation seems not to be confirmed.

The relationship of cervix cancer risk with age is unusual for an epithelial cancer. In most countries, risk rises to a maximum at about age 50 years, and then somewhat declines; the age of maximum incidence may, however, be rather later in African populations – 50–65 years (Gustafsson *et al.*, 1997). The young age structure of African populations, coupled with this rather flat age–incidence curve, means that the average age at diagnosis of cases in Africa is lower than in European and American populations. This is often noted in clinical series from Africa (e.g., Rogo *et al.*, 1990), but has no etiological or prognostic significance.

Figure 2 shows age-specific incidence rates from five of the registry series in this volume (Algiers, Algeria; Bamako, Mali; Conakry, Guinea; Kampala, Uganda; and Harare, Zimbabwe). All show the rapid rise in incidence in young women, and a peak or plateau in older women. However, in several populations (Algeria, Mali, Zimbabwe), the peak incidence appears to occur relatively late.

Migrant studies suggest that migrants to France from north Africa (Algeria, Tunisia) have relatively low mortality rates compared with the local-born population (Bouchardy *et al.*, 1996), although migrants from sub-Saharan Africa to France (Bouchardy *et al.*, 1995) and to England and Wales (Grulich *et al.*, 1992) do not have significantly higher rates than the local populations. On the other hand, Jewish migrants from north Africa to Israel have significantly higher incidence rates, although these are no longer present in the daughters of migrants (Parkin & Iscovich, 1997).

In all large case series, squamous cell carcinomas comprise the large majority of tumours, with adenocarcinomas accounting for 4% (Schonland & Bradshaw, 1969; Rogo *et al.*, 1990) to 7% (Oettlé, 1961).

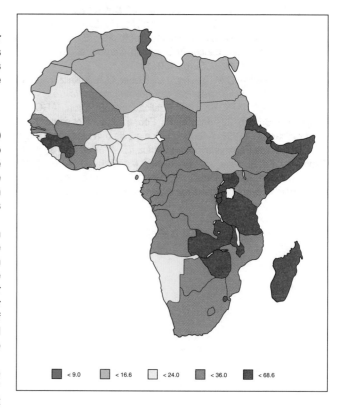

Figure 1. Age-standardized incidence of cervix cancer in Africa

Legend: < 9.0   < 16.6   < 24.0   < 36.0   < 68.6

Stage at presentation of tumours in African women is generally very advanced (Schonland & Bradshaw,1969; Lomalisa *et al.*, 2000), with correspondingly poor prognosis (Rogo *et al.*, 1990).

Time trends

In many developed countries, declining incidence of invasive cervix cancer has been observed, as a consequence of the introduction of screening programmes. There are very few data from Africa. In Bulawayo, Zimbabwe, the frequency of cervix cancer increased significantly during the period 1963–77 (Skinner *et al.*, 1993). Mortality data from South Africa suggested some increase in rates for the 'coloured' population between 1949 and 1979, but little change in the black population from 1964 to 1977 (Bradshaw & Harington, 1985). Updating this study, Bailie *et al.* (1996) observed that, after about 1980, the mortality in the 'coloured' population remained more or less constant, while in the white population, mortality had declined since the mid 1960s. The difference was ascribed to the availability of screening services, particularly for older women.

In some registry series, the more recent rates appear to be higher than the older ones. In Kampala, Uganda, for example, there has been a significant increase in incidence since the 1960s (Figure 3) (Wabinga *et al.*, 2000). On the other hand, there seems to have been little change in the recorded rate in Nigeria; it was 21.6 in 1960–69 (Table 2) and 19.4 in 1998–99 (Table 1).

Risk factors

Early observers noted the very marked differences in risk of cervix cancer according to such classical demographic variables as social status, religion, occupation, marital status and ethnicity. Later, epidemiological studies (mainly case–control studies) showed a consistent association between risk and early age at

Table 1. Age-standardized (world) and cumulative (0-64) incidence
Cervix uteri (C53)

	MALE				FEMALE			
	Cases	CRUDE	ASR(W) (per 100,000)	Cumulative (%)	Cases	CRUDE	ASR(W) (per 100,000)	Cumulative (%)
Africa, North								
Algeria, Algiers (1993-1997)	-	-	·	-	506	9.3	**12.6**	1.07
Algeria, Constantine (1994-1997)	-	-	·	-	113	7.4	**12.1**	0.89
Algeria, Oran (1996-1998)	-	-	·	-	324	18.4	**24.9**	2.14
Algeria, Setif (1993-1997)	-	-	·	-	203	6.7	**11.5**	0.96
Tunisia, Centre, Sousse (1993-1997)	-	-	·	-	70	6.2	**7.9**	0.61
Tunisia, North, Tunis (1994)	-	-	·	-	103	4.9	**6.1**	0.51
Tunisia, Sfax (1997)	-	-	·	-	10	2.6	**3.4**	0.32
Africa, West								
The Gambia (1997-1998)	-	-	·	-	170	16.6	**29.6**	2.53
Guinea, Conakry (1996-1999)	-	-	·	-	659	29.7	**49.6**	4.03
Mali, Bamako (1988-1997)	-	-	·	-	516	14.3	**30.8**	2.50
Niger, Niamey (1993-1999)	-	-	·	-	167	9.3	**19.6**	1.60
Nigeria, Ibadan (1998-1999)	-	-	·	-	157	10.4	**19.9**	1.53
Africa, Central								
Congo, Brazzaville (1996-1999)	-	-	·	-	279	23.1	**31.7**	2.67
Africa, East								
France, La Reunion (1988-1994)	-	-	·	-	447	20.7	**22.3**	1.74
Kenya, Eldoret (1998-2000)	-	-	·	-	93	10.2	**25.9**	2.22
Malawi, Blantyre (2000-2001)	-	-	·	-	222	25.6	**53.1**	4.47
Uganda, Kyadondo County (1993-1997)	-	-	·	-	465	16.1	**40.7**	3.26
Zimbabwe, Harare: African (1990-1993)	-	-	·	-	410	19.2	**62.6**	4.30
Zimbabwe, Harare: African (1994-1997)	-	-	·	-	510	19.3	**53.1**	3.73
Zimbabwe, Harare: European (1990-1997)	-	-	·	-	32	19.0	**12.7**	0.91
Africa, South								
Namibia (1995-1998)	-	-	·	-	468	14.6	**22.2**	1.60
South Africa: Black (1989-1992)	-	-	·	-	15450	27.4	**40.3**	3.15
South Africa: Indian (1989-1992)	-	-	·	-	330	16.6	**20.2**	1.45
South Africa: Mixed race (1989-1992)	-	-	·	-	1541	23.0	**31.6**	2.50
South Africa: White (1989-1992)	-	-	·	-	1465	14.4	**11.9**	0.91
South Africa, Transkei, Umtata (1996-1998)	-	-	·	-	75	17.7	**26.3**	2.35
South Africa, Transkei, 4 districts (1996-1998)	-	-	·	-	134	14.9	**21.7**	1.83
Swaziland (1996-1999)	-	-	·	-	655	33.4	**59.3**	4.96
Europe/USA								
USA, SEER: White (1993-1997)	-	-	·	-	4372	8.7	**6.7**	0.53
USA, SEER: Black (1993-1997)	-	-	·	-	853	11.5	**10.3**	0.75
France, 8 registries (1993-1997)	-	-	·	-	1771	12.3	**8.9**	0.67
The Netherlands (1993-1997)	-	-	·	-	3594	9.2	**6.6**	0.50
UK, England (1993-1997)	-	-	·	-	14294	11.2	**8.2**	0.62

In italics: histopathology-based registries

Table 2. Incidence of cervix cancer in Africa, 1953–74

Registry	Period	ASR (per 100 000)		Source
		Male	Female	(see Chap. 1)
Senegal, Dakar	1969–74		17.2	4
Mozambique, Lourenço Marques	1956–60		28.5	1
Nigeria, Ibadan	1960–69		21.6	3
SA, Cape Province: Bantu	1956–59		24.9*	2
SA, Cape Province: Coloured	1956–59		34.4*	2
SA, Cape Province: White	1956–59		22.7*	2
SA, Johannesburg, Bantu	1953–55		52.0	1
SA, Natal Province: African	1964–66		49.4	2
SA, Natal Province: Indian	1964–66		19.9	2
Uganda, Kyadondo	1954–60		22.2	1
Uganda, Kyadondo	1960–71		19.4	5
Zimbabwe, Bulawayo	1963–72		32.0	6

Italics: Rate based on less than 10 cases

* Includes carcinoma *in situ*

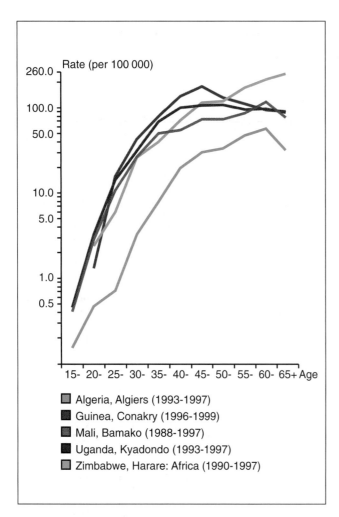

Figure 2. Age-specific incidence of cancer of cervix

Rate (per 100 000)

■ Algeria, Algiers (1993-1997)
■ Guinea, Conakry (1996-1999)
■ Mali, Bamako (1988-1997)
■ Uganda, Kyadondo (1993-1997)
■ Zimbabwe, Harare: Africa (1990-1997)

initiation of sexual activity, increasing number of sexual partners of females or of their sexual partners, and other indicators of sexual behaviour. These findings were strongly suggestive of a causative role for a sexually transmitted agent. Additional factors included an increasing number of pregnancies, smoking, possibly exposure to oral contraceptives, and specific dietary patterns. Within the last 20 years, it has become established that certain sexually transmitted types of human papillomavirus (HPV), notably types 16, 18, 31 and 45, are responsible for the initiation of the disease in the vast majority of cases. The virus is found in almost all cancers and a much smaller proportion of controls, with relative risks reaching several hundreds for certain viral types in the most recent studies. Studies of the natural history of HPV suggest that infection is very common in young women after the onset of sexual activity, but that the prevalence of infection declines with time (or age), possibly reflecting elimination of the virus by immunological mechanisms. Women who remain infected at later ages (30–50 years) are at risk of developing the epithelial abnormalities recognized as precursors of cancer.

Since 1993, cervix cancer has been considered to be an 'AIDS-defining' condition, meaning that if it occurs in someone who is positive for human immunodeficiency virus (HIV), that person is deemed to have AIDS. However, it was only some year later that studies in the United States, Italy, and France, linking cohorts of subjects with HIV/AIDS to cancer registries, demonstrated the increased risk of invasive cancer of the cervix (Goedert et al., 1998; Franceschi et al., 1998; Serraino et al., 1999; Frisch et al., 2000). A similar study in Australia was negative (Grulich et al., 1999). Estimates of the risk in these studies are between 5 and 15. It is not clear how much of the excess risk is due to the confounding effect of HPV infection, which is known to be associated with HIV infection, because of their common mode of transmission. The prevalence of cervical intraepithelial neoplasia (CIN) is clearly higher in HIV-infected women, although most of the early studies failed to adjust for infection by HPV. Careful adjustment for such confounding suggests that there is an independent effect of HIV on risk of CIN, although it is not very large, and that there is an interaction between the effects of HIV and HPV, as might be expected if the role of HIV was indirect, through creation of immune dysfunction (Mandelblatt et al., 1999).

The roles of other infectious agents, especially herpes simplex virus type 2 (HSV-2) and *Chlamydia trachomatis*, independent of HPV infection, in the etiology of cervix cancer remain much less clear.

Social class
An association between lower social status (as measured by literacy) and cervix cancer risk was observed in Bulawayo (Skinner et al., 1993) and a case–control study by Chaouki et al. (1998) in Morocco (see section on HPV below) found a very strong negative association with social status, family income and educational attainment.

Ethnicity
Data on hospital admissions in Moshi, northern Tanzania, indicated a higher incidence of cervix cancer in the Pare tribe, compared to the Chaggas, although, on the grounds of proximity to the hospital, the opposite might have been expected (Kitinya et al., 1988). The difference was ascribed to sexual lifestyles, with multiple partners reportedly more common among the Pare.

Sexual and reproductive variables
Several studies in Africa have investigated effects of sexual and reproductive variables on risk. In an early study of Johannesburg residents, Oettlé (1961) compared cervix cancer cases with other cancers (excluding breast and female genital sites) as controls (age-matched). There was almost no difference between the two groups in age at menarche or in parity (slightly fewer pregnancies or births to cervix cancer cases), but age at marriage and age at birth of first child were lower for cervix cancer cases (though not significantly). In a later study in Africans in Durban, South Africa (Schonland & Bradshaw, 1969), cervix cancer cases had a significantly earlier age at first intercourse (18.2 years), age at first pregnancy and higher parity than controls. There was no difference in age at menarche. Freedman et al. (1974) compared 48 cervix cancers patients from Baragwanath Hospital (Johannesburg) with age-matched (± 10 years) controls from the same hospital. Although the results are not clearly presented, there appears to be no significant difference between cases and controls in education level, mean age at first coitus (16.2 years in both groups), average number of sexual partners (2.4 in cases; 2.8 in controls) or age at menarche. There was a suggestion of higher parity in the cases than the controls. In a study in Kampala, Uganda, comparing 62 cases of cervix cancer with a group of age-matched controls, Adam et al. (1972) noted earlier age at first intercourse (and of marriage and first pregnancy) in cases versus controls, but no difference with respect to parity or history of venereal disease. Adelusi (1977) compared cervix cancer patients and healthy women attending a family planning clinic in Ibadan, Nigeria; although the latter were considerably younger, they reported a significantly later age at first intercourse than the cervix cancer patients

In a registry-based case–control study in Bulawayo (Parkin et al., 1994), age at first intercourse had little effect on risk, although the range of ages given was narrow, with half of the cases reporting age 17 or 18 years. The median age (18.3 years) was relatively high, as in the earlier studies summarized above. The number of

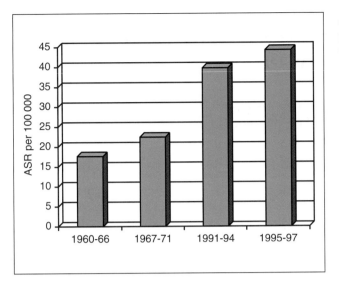

Figure 3. Trends in incidence of cervix cancer, Kampala, Uganda (Wabinga *et al.* 2000)

sexual partners was not investigated, but high parity appeared to confer an increased risk, with ORs of 1.3 (95% CI 1.0–1.7) for 3–6 full-term pregnancies, and 1.8 (95% CI 1.3–2.3) for more than six pregnancies, relative to less than three.

The results of a hospital-based case–control study in Nairobi, Kenya, with 112 cases and 749 controls, conducted as part of the WHO collaborative study on neoplasia and steroid contraceptives, were reported by Williams *et al.* (1994). Age at first intercourse, number of lifetime sexual partners, parity and a history of abnormal vaginal discharge were independently significantly associated with risk.

In a study in Bamako, Mali, Bayo *et al.* (2002) compared 82 cases of cervix cancer with 92 hospital controls. There were almost no differences between the two groups with respect to age at first intercourse (or marriage) and number of sexual partners (one quarter of cases and controls reported at least one casual partner). Having a husband with more than one wife was associated with an increase in risk (OR = 2.2, 95% CI 1.0–5.0). There was a clearly increased risk with increasing parity (OR for >10 versus <5 children = 4.8, 95% CI 1.5–4.7).

It has been suggested that trauma to the cervix through multiple childbearing, particularly at young ages, in some way increases the risk of neoplastic change, or that hormonal or nutritional influences of pregnancy are responsible. If so, high fertility may provide part of the explanation for the elevated incidence of cervix cancer in sub-Saharan Africa.

Male circumcision
Because of the previously observed high rates of penile cancer in Uganda and the geographical correlations in the frequency of penile and cervical cancer, the importance of non-circumcision of the male partners has been raised (Dodge *et al.*, 1973). However, the evidence that circumcision status really plays a role in the etiology of cervix cancer is weak, and probably is related simply to the degree of penile hygiene (Schmauz & Owor, 1984).

Smoking
The prevalence of smoking in women in Bulawayo was very low, and there was no apparent excess risk for cervix cancer in smokers (Parkin *et al.*, 1994).

Alcohol
Alcohol drinking has rarely been reported as an independent risk factor for cervix cancer. In a survey in Johannesburg residents with

cancer, undertaken in 1953–55, Oettlé (1961) found a higher proportion of cervix cancer cases reporting a history of local beer drinking; compared with age-matched other cancers (excluding breast and genital sites), the relative risk was 3.0. In a study in Lesotho (Martin & Hill, 1984), comparing 257 cervix cancer cases with controls (matched for age, parity and residence), there was a significantly increased risk (RR = 3.2) for consumption of indigenous alcohol (frequent versus never) and European alcohols (RR = 1.9) (each adjusted for the other, and for tobacco consumption). In the case–control study using data from the Bulawayo cancer registry (Parkin *et al.*, 1994), an excess risk (OR = 1.6, 95% CI 1.3–1.9) was observed for frequent alcohol drinkers, relative to abstainers.

Oral contraceptives
Long-term use of oral contraceptives was found to be associated with risk of cervix cancer in HPV-positive women in the case–control study of Chaouki *et al.* (1998) in Rabat, Morocco (see section on HPV below). In the case–control study in Nairobi, Kenya, which was part of the WHO collaborative study on neoplasia and steroid contraceptives (Williams *et al.*, 1994), the association with use of oral contraceptives was weak and non-significant.

Genital hygiene
The case–control study of Bayo *et al.* (2002) in Bamako, Mali, found that vaginal douching decreased the risk of cervical cancer [OR ever versus never = 0.06 (95% CI 0.01–0.24)] while use of home-made sanitary napkins and re-use of such napkins were strong predictors of risk. The study in Morocco by Chaouki *et al.* (1998) had made similar observations: a decreased risk (adjusted for age, income and HPV status) associated with washing the genital area during menstruation (OR ever versus never = 0.26, 95% CI 0.10–0.72), and use of commercial (rather than home-made) sanitary pads (OR = 0.36, 95% CI 0.13–0.95).

HPV
The evidence for the causative role of certain types of human papilloma virus, especially HPV16 and HPV 18 in cervical cancer etiology is now accepted (Walboomers *et al.*, 1999). In east Africa HPV 18 infection may be particularly important (Schmauz *et al.*, 1989; Ter Meulen *et al.*, 1992).

Chaouki *et al.* (1998) carried out a case–control study, with 214 cases of invasive cancer and 203 control subjects recruited in the National Cancer Institute, Rabat, Morocco as part of an IARC-coordinated multinational study. Testing for 30 HPV types was carried out by PCR using cellular material from biopsies (cases) or scrapes (controls). The OR for any HPV was 61.6 (95% CI 29.2–130), with HPV 16 the most common type (present in 68% of cases), followed by HPV 18. In addition to the strong effect of HPV, low socioeconomic status, multiple partners before age 20 years, use of oral contraceptives, and parity emerged as independent risk factors.

La Ruche *et al.* (1998b) compared 13 cases of cervix cancer, from among gynaecology outpatients in Abidjan, Côte d'Ivoire, with 65 age-matched controls with normal cytology; HPV infection, present in 10 cases, was strongly associated with risk (OR = 13.3; 95% CI 3.2–55.5).

In the case–control study in Bamako, Mali (Bayo *et al.*, 2002), HPV infection in cases and controls was evaluated by the presence of antibodies to HPV virus-like particles (VLPs). At an optical density cut-off point of 0.4, antibodies to HPV 16, 18 and 31 were detected in 60.4% of cases and 45.4% of controls (OR = 1.8, 95% CI 1.0–2.2). HPV DNA was present in 63/65 (96.9%) of the tumours tested. As described above, high parity, a polygamous husband and poor genital hygiene were independent risk factors.

Several studies in Africa have examined the association between HPV infection and precursor lesions (CIN and squamous intra-epithelial lesions (SIL)), the latter usually diagnosed on the basis of cytology (Table 3). In a study of 198 prostitutes in Nairobi,

Table 3. Percentage distribution of microscopically verified cases by histological type
Cervix uteri (C53)

	Squamous	Carcinoma Adeno	Carcinoma Other	Carcinoma Unspecified	Sarcoma	Other	Unspecified	Number of cases MV	Number of cases Total
Algeria, Algiers	69.3	11.6	-	18.5	0.6	-	-	475	506
Algeria, Batna	90.3	5.6	-	1.4	1.4	1.4	-	72	72
Algeria, Constantine	86.6	5.4	-	6.3	-	-	1.8	112	113
Algeria, Oran	75.2	4.4	0.3	3.5	0.3	-	16.4	318	324
Algeria, Setif	94.9	2.1	-	2.6	0.5	-	-	195	203
Burkina Faso, Ouagadougou	36.7	20.0	13.3	16.7	3.3	6.7	3.3	30	41
Congo, Brazzaville	71.3	1.3	0.6	26.1	-	-	0.6	157	279
France, La Reunion	86.7	5.4	2.7	4.7	-	0.5	-	444	447
The Gambia	78.3	4.3	-	6.5	-	-	10.9	46	170
Guinea, Conakry	81.1	3.1	-	15.6	-	-	0.3	359	659
Kenya, Eldoret	81.8	4.5	-	10.6	1.5	1.5	-	66	93
Malawi, Blantyre	86.9	5.6	-	5.6	-	-	1.9	107	222
Mali, Bamako	90.6	3.0	0.6	4.5	0.3	-	0.9	330	516
Namibia	87.2	10.2	0.2	2.0	-	0.2	0.2	460	468
Niger, Niamey	82.1	7.7	-	6.4	-	1.3	2.6	78	167
Nigeria, Ibadan	87.2	7.7	0.9	3.4	0.9	-	-	117	157
Rwanda, Butare	15.2	2.2	-	-	-	-	82.6	46	46
South Africa: Black	72.5	8.1	0.5	4.1	0.3	0.3	14.2	15450	15450
South Africa: White	79.5	13.9	0.5	4.5	0.5	0.3	0.8	1465	1465
South Africa: Indian	67.6	10.3	0.6	4.8	1.2	0.6	14.8	330	330
South Africa: Mixed race	86.0	11.0	0.5	1.9	0.1	0.1	0.4	1541	1541
South Africa, Elim	78.6	12.5	-	8.9	-	-	-	112	127
South Africa, Transkei, Umtata	86.4	1.7	-	6.8	-	-	5.1	59	75
South Africa, Transkei, 4 districts	90.5	1.9	-	7.6	-	-	-	105	134
Swaziland	94.5	4.6	-	0.9	-	-	-	219	655
Tanzania, Dar Es Salaam	90.4	7.0	-	2.1	0.4	0.2	-	530	530
Tanzania, Kilimanjaro	72.0	10.0	-	17.3	-	0.7	-	150	168
Tunisia, Centre, Sousse	94.3	4.3	-	-	1.4	-	-	70	70
Tunisia, North, Tunis	88.2	7.8	-	1.0	1.0	1.0	1.0	102	103
Tunisia, Sfax	80.0	10.0	10.0	-	-	-	-	10	10
Uganda, Mbarara	91.5	3.4	-	5.1	-	-	-	59	143
Uganda, Kyadondo County	82.2	8.4	0.3	7.7	-	-	1.3	297	465
Zimbabwe, Harare: African	83.3	6.5	0.1	9.7	0.1	0.1	-	672	920
Zimbabwe, Harare: European	62.1	17.2	-	13.8	6.9	-	-	29	32

Kreiss et al. (1992) found HPV in 81% of Pap smears showing CIN, compared with 28% without (adjusted OR = 7.2, 95% CI 1.6–32.1). HPV was present in 19/25 cases of SIL and 59/204 normal smears (OR = 7.4, p < 0.001) from post-partum women in Malawi (Miotti et al., 1996). Among attenders at a family planning clinic in Nairobi, HSIL was strongly associated with presence of HPV (OR = 14.9, 95% CI 6.8–32.8) (Temmerman et al., 1999). In the study of La Ruche et al. (1998b), comparison of HPV prevalence in 60 cases of high-grade SIL (HSIL) (half of them defined by colposcopy or biopsy) and controls, gave an OR of 14.3 (6.6–30.9) and in 151 cases of cytologically diagnosed low-grade SIL (LSIL) and 151 controls, an OR of 4.4 (2.6–7.4). These ORs were adjusted for HIV status (see below). A strong association with a cytological diagnosis of SIL and presence of DNA from high-risk HPV types was also observed in a study of two groups of women in Abidjan, Côte d'Ivoire (Vernon et al., 1999). The ORs (adjusted for age, HIV, and various variables related to sexual behaviour) were 5.4 (95% CI 1.5–19.8) in a group of 258 women participating in a study of mother–child HIV transmission, and 23.7 (95% CI 4.4–126.0) among 278 prostitutes. In a study of 612 women attending an antenatal clinic in Mwanza, Tanzania (Mayaud et al., 2001), SIL was significantly more prevalent among HPV-positive women (14% vs 4%, OR = 3.7, 95% CI 1.9–7.0, especially among women with high-risk HPV (17%, OR =4.8, 95% CI 2.3–9.8).

The prevalence of HPV in the general population has not been carefully studied in Africa, most investigations being of women attending screening or other clinics, and with the information on prevalence not stratified by age. In Chitungwiza (a satellite of Harare), Zimbabwe, 2206 women aged 25–55 years attending primary care clinics were recruited and cervical cells, obtained by cytobrush, were tested for HPV by hybrid capture II test (HC II) (Womack et al., 2000a). In this population at high risk for cervix cancer, HPV prevalence was very high (42.7%) but declined with age: 48.5% at 25–34, 34.9% at 35–44, 25.6% at 45–55 years. HSIL lesions (biopsy-proved) were five times more common in HPV-positive women than in those who were HPV-negative. In a random sample of 960 women aged 15–59 years in rural Uganda, HPV prevalence (evaluated by hybrid capture II assay) in self-collected vaginal swabs, was 16.7% overall (Serwadda et al., 1999). Prevalence was strongly associated with infection with HIV (age-adjusted OR = 5.4, 95% CI 3.8–7.5). In HIV-negative women, prevalence was highest in the 15–19 years age group (23.7%), and was only 4% over 30 years of age. In pregnant women in Mwanza, Tanzania, HPV prevalence was much higher (34%), with little difference by age (Mayaud et al., 2001).

The prevalence of HPV infection, in relation to other genital infections, and lifestyle variables, has been studied in several different African populations, as in a myriad of similar investigations elsewhere.

Table 4. Case–control studies of CIN in relation to infection with HPV in Africa

Reference	Area, subjects	Cases, controls	HPV test	HPV prevalence (%)		Odds ratios (95% CI)	Comments/adjustments
Kreiss et al., 1992	Nairobi, Kenya Prostitutes	16 CIN 47 normal cytology	Dot filter Southern transfer hybridization	Cases: 81.3 Controls: 27.7		7.2 (1.6–32.1)	OR adjusted for age and duration of prostitution HPV types 6, 11, 16, 18, 31, 33, 35
Miotti et al., 1996	Malawi Post-natal clinic	28 SIL 268 normal cytology	PCR. L1 primer	Cases: 76.0 Controls: 28.9		7.4 (p<0.001)	High-grade SIL was associated with HPV only in HIV-seronegative subjects
Langley et al., 1996	Dakar, Senegal Prostitutes	48 SIL 485 normal cytology	PCR	Cases: Any HPV: 66.7 HPV 16,18,45: 12.5 Controls: Any HPV: 39.0 HPV 16,18,45: 8.3		3.6 (1.8–7.3) any HPV 4.8(1.8–12.7) HPV 16, 18, 45 LSIL: 4.4 (2.6–7.4) HSIL:14.3 (6.6–30.9)	ORs adjusted for HIV status
La Ruche et al., 1998b	Abidjan, Côte d'Ivoire Gynaecology clinic	151 LSIL; 60 HSIL 151 and 240 age-matched subjects, normal cytology	PCR. L1 primer GP 5/6 primers	Cases: LSIL all HPV : 68.2 HPV 16/18: 16.8 HSIL all HPV: 81.7 HPV 16/18: 28.6 Controls: LSIL all HPV : 30.5 HPV 16/18: 2.3 HSIL all HPV :20.4 HPV 16/18: 3.7			
Temmerman et al., 1999	Nairobi, Kenya Family planning clinics	28 HSIL +5 cancers 28 LSIL + 583 normal cytology	PCR. GP 5/6 primers	Cases (HSIL/Ca) 69.7 Control (LSIL/normal) 16.9		14.9 (6.8–32.8) 10.9 (5.4–30.1)[1]	[1]Adjusted for HIV status
Mayaud et al., 2001	Mwanza, Tanzania Antenatal clinics	43 SIL (16 HSIL, 27 LSIL) 564 normal cytology	PCR (L1 primer) Reverse blot typing	Cases: Any HPV: 61.9 HR HPV: 42.0 Controls: Any HPV: 0.7 HR HPV: 18.9		3.7 (1.8–7.4) 3.3 (1.4–6.6)[1]	[1]Adjusted for HIV status

Infection has been shown to be linked to sexual behaviour (e.g., number of recent partners) or presence of other sexually transmitted diseases (Mayaud *et al.*, 2001; Temmerman *et al.*, 1999).

HIV

None of the case–control studies of HIV and cancer conducted in Africa have shown an excess risk of invasive cervix cancer and HIV. There is, however, evidence that the risk of pre-invasive disease (CIN) is increased in the presence of HIV infection, and that this is confined to women who are infected with HPV. The evidence is reviewed in Chapter 6.

Other infections

In a hospital-based study in Kampala, Uganda, Adam *et al.* (1972) investigated prevalence of antibodies to HSV-2 in cases of cervix cancer and in control subjects (matched for age and cervix cancer risk factors). Prevalence of infection in this population was high, with rather little difference between the cases and controls. Schmauz *et al.* (1989) investigated the prevalence of infection with HPV types 16 and 18, HSV-1 and -2, cytomegalovirus, Epstein–Barr virus and *C. trachomatis* in 34 cases of cervix cancer and 23 controls seen in Mulago hospital, Kampala. They found that the risk of cervix cancer increased with the number of concurrent infections, suggesting that chronic cervico-vaginal inflammation might increase the oncogenicity of HPV infection.

There is no evidence that the risk of cervix cancer is augmented by infection of the cervix with *Schistosoma* (Edington, 1970; Freedman *et al.*, 1974; Szela *et al.*, 1993).

Prevention

Control of cervix cancer has traditionally been through programmes of detection and treatment of precursor lesions (dysplasia/carcinoma *in situ*, CIN, SIL) by cytology. Organized screening programmes in many European countries have been successful in reducing incidence and mortality rates from levels which, before they were introduced, were not so different from those seen today in much of Africa. That the traditional Pap smear can give significant protection against development of invasive cancer has been demonstrated in many case–control studies (Parkin, 1997), including one in Morocco (Chaouki *et al.*, 1998). In this study, about one third of control women reported having had a Pap smear at some past time, and this was associated with a significantly reduced risk of invasive cancer (OR = 0.31, 95% CI 0.18–0.55).

However, screening programmes in Africa have been very limited in scope, and all have been 'opportunistic', centred on hospital or family planning clinics, rather than population-based. Reports on limited screening projects from various countries have been published: South Africa (Leiman,1987; Baile *et al.*, 1995; Heystek *et al.*, 1995; Lancaster *et al.*, 1999), Lesotho (Schneider & Meinhardt, 1984), Kenya (Mati *et al.*, 1984; Engels *et al.*, 1992), Nigeria (Ayangade & Akinyeme,1989) and Egypt (Mohga *et al.*, 1987). However, population coverage remains very low. In a survey of cytology laboratories in four countries (Côte d'Ivoire, Guinea, Mali, Senegal) in about 1995, Woto-Gaye *et al.* (1996) estimated that less than 1% of women aged at least 15 years had received a smear test that year. The results of these programmes, in terms of the yield of abnormal smears requiring follow-up or treatment, are difficult to compare, because of the selected nature of the clientèle in many 'screening' projects. However, in previously unscreened populations with a high incidence of cervix cancer, prevalence of lesions may be very high indeed. In the University of Zimbabwe/JHPIEGO Cervix Cancer Project (1999), among 10 934 women aged 25–55 years examined at 15 primary care clinics in Chitungwiza, Zimbabwe, 11% were found to have SIL, about equal numbers having LSIL and HSIL, and there were 20 prevalent cancers (1.8 per 1000).

The difficulties in implementing community programmes of screening in developing countries using the Pap smear have become increasingly obvious in recent years. The reasons lie in the logistics of organization, for all phases of the programme (screening, diagnosis and follow-up) and in the problems of maintaining good-quality cytology laboratories (Sankaranarayanan & Pisani, 1997). For this reason, there has been increasing interest in alternative screening strategies which may be easier to apply. In particular, much attention has focused on the value of screening with visual inspection following acetic acid impregnation of the cervix (VIA). One of the earliest studies to suggest that this technique might be as effective as cytology in detecting SIL was carried out in Cape Town, South Africa (Megevand *et al.*, 1996). The experience has been repeated in studies elsewhere, notably in the University of Zimbabwe/JHPIEGO Cervical Cancer Project (1999). In the second phase of this study, 2203 women underwent a Pap smear test, VIA and HPV testing, and all received diagnostic colposcopy, as well as biopsy when indicated. VIA was more sensitive (76.7%) than cytology (44.3%) in detecting HSIL or worse lesions, but specificity was lower (64.1% versus 90.6%). The relatively large number of false positives in this study may have been related to the high prevalence of sexually transmitted diseases in this particular population. Nevertheless, the high negative predictive value of VIA (96.3%) means that few significant lesions will be missed, and, if simple diagnostic triage and/or treatment can be immediately available to women who test positive, the technique holds considerable promise as a means of reducing the toll of cervix cancer in low-resource countries.

References

Adam, E., Sharma, S.D., Zeigler, O., Iwamoto, K., Melnick, J.L., Levy, A.H. & Rawls, W.E. (1972) Seroepidemiologic studies of herpesvirus type 2 and carcinoma of the cervix. II. Uganda. *J. Natl Cancer Inst.*, **48**, 65–72

Adelusi, B. (1977) Carcinoma of the cervix uteri in Ibadan: coital characteristics. *Int. J. Gynaecol. Obstet.*, **15**, 5–11

Ayangade, O. & Akinyeme, A. (1989) Cervical cytology in an urban Nigerian population. *E. Afr. Med. J.*, **66**, 50–56

Bailie, R.S., Barron, P. & Learmonth, G. (1995) Cervical cytology screening – a case study in a peri-urban settlement. *S. Afr. Med. J.*, **85**, 30–33

Bailie, R.S., Selvet, C.E., Bourne, D. & Bradshaw, D. (1996) Trends in cervical cancer mortality in South Africa. *Int. J. Epidemiol.*, **25**, 488–493

Bayo, S., Bosch, F.X., de Sanjose, S., Muñoz, N., Combita, A.L., Coursaget, P., Diaz, M., Dolo, A., van den Brule, A.J., Meijer, C.J. (2002) Risk factors of invasive cervical cancer in Mali. *Int. J. Epidemiol.*, **31**, 202–209

Bouchardy, C., Wanner, P. & Parkin, D.M. (1995) Cancer mortality among sub-Saharan African migrants in France. *Cancer Causes Control*, **6**, 539–544

Bouchardy, C., Parkin, D.M., Wanner, P. & Khlat, M. (1996) Cancer mortality among North African migrants in France. *Int. J. Epidemiol.*, **25**, 5–13

Bradshaw, E. & Harington, J.S. (1985) The changing pattern of cancer mortality in South Africa, 1949-1979. *S. Afr. Med. J.*, **68**, 455–465

Chaouki, N., Bosch, F.X., Munoz, N., Meijer, C.J.L.M., el Gueddari, B., el Ghazi, A., Deacon, J., Castellsague, X. & Walboomers, J.M.M. (1998) The viral origin of cervical cancer in Rabat, Morocco. *Int. J. Cancer*, **75**, 546–554

Cook-Mozaffari, P. (1982) Symposium on Tumours in the Tropics. Carcinomas of the oesophagus, bladder, cervix uteri and penis. *Trans. R. Soc. Trop. Med. Hyg.*, **76**, 157–163

Dodge, O.G., Owor, R. & Templeton, A.C. (1973) Tumours of the male genitalia. *Recent Results Cancer Res.*, **41**, 132–144

Edington, G.M. 1970, Cancer of the uterus in the Western State of Nigeria. *Afr. J. Med. Sci.*, **1**, 67–77

Engels, H., Nyongo, A., Temmerman, M., Quint, W.G.V., van Marck, E.V. & Eylenbosch, W.J. (1992) Cervical cancer screening and detection of genital HPV infection and chlamydial infection by PCR in different groups of Kenyan women. *Ann. Soc. Belg. Med. Trop.*, **72**, 53–62

Franceschi, S., Dal Maso, L., Arniani, S., Crosignani, P., Vercelli, M., Simonato, L., Falcini, F., Zanetti, R., Barchielli, A., Serraino, D. & Rezza, G. (1998) Risk of cancer other than Kaposi sarcoma and non-Hodgkin's lymphoma in persons with AIDS in Italy. *Br. J. Cancer*, **78**, 966–970

Frisch, M., Biggar, R.J. & Goedert, J.J. (2000) Human papillomavirus-associated cancers in patients with human immunodeficiency virus infection and acquired immunodeficiency syndrome. *J. Natl Cancer Inst.*, **92**, 1500–1510

Freedman, R.S., Joosting, A.C.C., Ryan, J.T. & Nkoni, S. (1974) A study of associated factors, including genital herpes, in black women with cervical carcinoma in Johannesburg. *S. Afr. Med. J.*, **48**, 1747–1752

Goedert, J.J., Cote, T.R., Virgo, P., Scoppa, S.M., Kingma, D.W., Gail, M.H., Jaffe, E.S. & Biggar, R.J. (1998) Spectrum of AIDS-associated malignant disorders. *Lancet*, **351**, 1833–1839

Grulich, A.E., Swerdlow, A.J., Head, J. & Marmot, M.G. (1992).Cancer mortality in African and Caribbean migrants to England and Wales. *Br. J. Cancer*, **66**, 905–911

Grulich, A.E., Wan, X., Law, M.G., Coates, M. & Kaldor, J.M. (1999) Risk of cancer in people with AIDS. *AIDS*, **13**, 839–843

Gustafsson, L., Ponten, J., Bergström, R. & Adami, H.O. (1997) International incidence rates of invasive cervical cancer before cytological screening. *Int. J. Cancer*, **71**, 159–165

Heystek, M.J., de Jonge, E.T., Meyer, H.P. & Lindeque, B.G. (1995) Screening for cervical neoplasia in Mamelodi – lessons from an unscreened population. *S. Afr. Med. J.*, **85**, 1180–1182

Kapiga, S.H., Msamanga, G.I., Spiegelman, D., Mwakyoma, H., Fawzi, W.W. & Hunter, D.J. (1999) Risk factors for squamous intraepithelial lesions among HIV seropositive women in Dar es Salaam, Tanzania. *Int. J. Gynaecol. Obstet.*, **67**, 87–94

Kitinya, J.N., Lauren, P.A. & Kajembe, A.H. (1988) Differential rates of carcinoma of cervix uteri among the Chagga and Pares of Kilimanjaro region, Tanzania. *Int. J. Gynecol. Obstet.*, **27**, 395–399

Kreiss, J.K., Kiviat, N.B., Plummer, F.A., Roberts, P.L., Waiyaki, P., Ngugi, E., & Holmes, K.K. (1992) Human immunodeficiency virus, human papillomavirus and cervical intraepithelial neoplasia in Nairobi prostitutes. *Sex. Trans. Dis.*, **19**, 54–59

Laga, M., Icenogle, J.P., Marsella, R., Manoka, A.T., Nzila, N., Ryder, R.W., Vermund, S.H., Heyward, W.L., Nelson, A. & Reeves, W.C. (1992) Genital papillomavirus infection and cervical dysplasia – opportunistic complications of HIV infection. *Int. J. Cancer*, **50**, 45–48

Lancaster, E.J., Banach, L., Lekalakala, T. & Mandiwana, I. (1999) Carcinoma of the uterine cervix: results of Ka-Ngwane screening programme and comparison btewen the results obtained from urban and other unscreened rural communities. *E. Afr. Med. J.*, **76**, 101–104

La Ruche, G., Ramon, R., Mensah-Ado, I., Bergeron, C., Diomande, M., Sylla-Koko, F., Ehouman, A., Toure-Coulibaly, K., Wellfens-Ekra, C. & Dabis, F. (1998a) Squamous intraepithelial lesions of the cervix, invasive cervical carcinoma and immunosuppression induced by human immunodeficiency virus in Africa. *Cancer*, **82**, 2410–2408

La Ruche, G., You, B., Mensah-Ado, I., Bergeron, C., Montcho, C., Ramon, R., Toure-Coulibaly, K., Wellfens-Ekra, C., Dabis, F. & Orth, G. (1998b) Human papillomavirus, and human immunodeficiency virus infections: relation with cervical dysplasia-neoplasia in African women. *Int. J. Cancer*, **76**, 480–486

Langley, C.L., Benga-De, E., Critchlow, C.W., Ndoye, I., Mbengue-Ly, M.D., Kuypers, J., Woto-Gaye, G., Mboup, S., Bergeron C.,

Holmes K.K. & Kiviat, N.B. (1996) HIV-1, HIV-2, human papillomavirus infection and cervical neoplasia in high-risk African women. *AIDS*, **10**, 413–417

Leiman, G. (1987) "Project screen Soweto" – a planned cervical cancer screening programme in a high risk population. *S. Afr. J. Epidemiol. Infect.*, **61**, 819–822

Leroy, V., Ladner, J., De Clercq, A., Meheus, A., Nyirazinje, M., Karita, E. & Dabis, F. (1999) Cervical dysplasia and HIV type 1 infection in African pregnant women: a cross sectional study, Kigali, Rwanda. The Pregnancy and HIV Study Group (EGE). *Sex. Trans. Infect.*, **75**, 103–106

Lomalisa, P., Smith, T. & Guidozzi, F. (2000) Human immunodeficiency virus infection and invasive cervical cancer in South Africa. *Gynecol. Oncol.*, **77**, 460–463

Maggwa, B.N., Hunter, D.J., Mbugua, S., Tukei, P. & Mati, J.K. (1993) The relationship between HIV infection and cervical intraepithelial neoplasia among women attending two family planning clinics in Nairobi, Kenya. *AIDS*, **7**, 733–738

Mandelblatt, J.S., Kanetsky, P., Eggert, L., & Gold, K. (1999) Is HIV infection a cofactor for cervical squamous cell neoplasia? *Cancer Epidemiol. Biomarkers Prev.*, **8**, 97–106

Martin, P.M.D., & Hill, G.B. (1984) Cervical cancer in relation to tobacco and alcohol consumption in Lesotho, southern Africa. *Cancer Detect. Prev.*, **7**, 109–115

Mati, J.K.G., Mbugaua, S. & Ndavi, M. (1984) Control of cancer of the cervix: feasibility of screening for premalignant lesions in an African environment. In: Williams, A.O., O'Conor, G.T., De Thé, G.T. & Johnson, C.A., eds, *Virus-Associated Cancers in Africa* (IARC Scientific Publications No. 63), Lyon, IARC, pp. 451–463

Mayaud, P., Gill, D.K., Weiss, H.A., Uledi, E., Kopwe, L., Todd, J., ka-Gina, G., Grosskurth, H., Hayes, R.J., Mabey, D.C. m& Lacey, C.J. (2001) The interrelation of HIV, cervical human papillomavirus, and neoplasia among antenatal clinic attenders in Tanzania. *Sex. Transm. Infect.*, **77**, 248–254

Megevand, E., Denny, L., Dehaeck, K., Soeters, R. & Bloch, B. (1996) Acetic acid visualisation of the cervix: an alternative to cytologic screening. *Obstet. Gynecol.*, **88**, 383–386

Miotti, P.G., Dallabetta, G.A., Daniel, R.W., Canner, J.K., Chiphangwi, J.D., Liomba, G., Yang, L.-P. & Shah, K.V. (1996) Cervical abnormalities, human papillomavirus, and human immunodeficiency virus infections in women in Malawi. *J. Inf. Dis.*, **173**, 714–717

Mohga, M.A., Hammad, M.D., Jones, H.W. & Zayed, M. (1987) Low prevalence of cervical intraepithelial neoplasia among Egyptian females. *Gynecol. Oncol.*, **28**, 300–304

Oettlé, A.G. (1961) Malignant neoplasms of the uterus in the white, "coloured", Indian and Bantu races of the Union of South Africa. *Acta Un. Int. Contra Cancrum*, **17**, 915–933

Parkin, D.M. (1997) The epidemiological basis for evaluating screening policies. In: Franco, E. & Monsonego, J., eds, *New Developments in Cervical Cancer Screening and Prevention*, Oxford, Blackwell, pp. 51–69

Parkin, D.M. & Iscovich, J.A. (1997) The risk of cancer in migrants and their descendants in Israel: II Carcinomas and germ cell tumours. *Int. J. Cancer*, **70**, 654–660

Parkin, D.M., Vizcaino, A.P., Skinner, M.E.G. & Ndhlovu, A (1994) Cancer patterns and risk factors in the African population of southwestern Zimbabwe, 1963–1977. *Cancer Epidemiol. Biomarkers Prev.*, **3**, 537–547

Rogo, K.O. & Kavoo-Linge (1990) Human immunodeficiency virus seroprevalence among cervical cancer patients. *Gynecol. Oncol.*, **37**, 87–92

Rogo, K.O., Omany, J., Onyango, J.N., Ojwang, S.B. & Stendahl, U. (1990) Carcinoma of the cervix in the African setting. *Int. J. Gynecol. Obstet.*, **33**, 249–255

Sankaranarayanan, R. & Pisani, P. (1997) Prevention measures in the third world; are they practicable? In: Franco, E. &

Monsonego, J., eds, *New Developments in Cervical Cancer Screening and Prevention*, Oxford, Blackwell Science, pp. 70–83

Schmauz, R. & Owor, R. (1984) Epidemiological aspects of cervical cancer in tropical Africa. In: Williams, A.O., O'Conor, G.T., De Thé, G.T. & Johnson, C.A., eds, *Virus-Associated Cancers in Africa* (IARC Scientific Publications No. 63), pp. 413–431

Schmauz, R., Okong, P., de Villiers, E.M., Dennin, R., Brade, L., Lwanga, S.K. & Owor, R. (1989) Multiple infections in cases of cervical cancer from a high incidence area in tropical Africa. *Int. J. Cancer*, **43**, 805–809

Schonland, M. & Bradshaw, E. (1969) Some observations on cancer of the uterine cervix in Africans and Indians of Natal. *S. Afr. J. Med. Sci.*, **34**, 61–71

Schneider, A. & Meinhardt, G. (1984) Screening for cervical cancer in Butha Buthe, Lesotho. A study of Papanicolaou (Pap) smears in a previously unsceened community over a one year period. *Trop. Doctor*, **14**, 170–174

Seck, A.C., Faye, M.A., Critchlow, C.W., Mbaye, A.D., Kuypers, J., Woto-Gaye, G., Langley, C., De, E.B., Holmes, K.K. & Kiviat, N.B. (1994) Cervical intraepithelial neoplasia and human papillomavirus infection among Senegalese women seropositive for HIV-1 or HIV-2 or seronegative for HIV. *Int. J. STD AIDS*, **5**, 189–193

Serraino, D., Carrieri, P., Pradier, C., Bidoli, E., Dorrucci, M., Ghetti, E., Schiesari, A., Zucconi, R., Pezzotti, P., Dellamonica, P., Franceschi, S. & Rezza, G.C. (1999) Risk of invasive cervical cancer among women with or at risk for HIV infection. *Int. J. Cancer*, **82**, 334–337

Serwadda, D., Wawer, M.J., Shah, K.V., Sewankambo, N.K., Daniel, R., Li, C., Lorincz, A., Meehan, M.P., Wabwire-Mangen, F. & Gray, R.H. (1999) Use of a hybrid capture assay of self-collected vaginal swabs in rural Uganda for detection of human papillomavirus. *J. Infect. Dis.*, **180**, 1316–1319

Sitas, F., Pacella-Norman, R., Carrara, H., Patel, M., Ruff, P., Sur, R., Jantsch, U., Hale, M., Rowji, P., Saffer, D., Connor, M., Bull, D., Newton, R. & Beral, V. (2000) The spectrum of HIV-1 related cancers in South Africa. *Int. J. Cancer*, **88**, 489–492

Skinner, M.E.G., Parkin, D.M., Vizcaino, A.P. & Ndhlovu, A. (1993) *Cancer in the African Population of Bulawayo, Zimbabwe, 1963–1977* (IARC Technical Report No. 15), Lyon, IARC

Szela, E., Bachiicha, J., Miller, D., Till, M. & Wilson, J.B. (1993) Schistosomiasis and cervical cancer in Ghana. *Int. J. Gynecol. Obstet.*, **42**, 127–130

Temmerman, M., Tyndall, M.W., Kidula, N., Claeys, P., Muchiri, L. & Quint, W. (1999) Risk factors for human papillomavirus and cervical precancerous lesions, and the role of concurrent HIV-1 infection. *Int. J. Gynaecol. .Obstet.*, **65**, 171–181

Ter Meulen, J., Eberhardt, H.C., Luande, J., Mgaya, H.N., Chang-Claude, J., Mtiro, H., Mhina, M., Kashaija, P., Ockert, S., Yu, X., Meinhardt, G., Gissman, L. & Pawlita, M. (1992) Human papillomavirus (HPV) infection, HIV infection and cervical cancer in Tanzania, East Africa. *Int. J. Cancer*, **52**, 515–521

University of Zimbabwe/JHPIEGO Cervical Cancer Project (1999) Visual inspection with acetic acid for cervical cancer screening: test qualities in a primary care setting. *Lancet*, **353**, 869–873

Vernon, S.D., Unger, E.R., Piper, M.A., Severin, S.T., Wiktor, S.Z., Ghys, P.D., Miller, D.L., Horowitz, I.R., Greenberg, A.E. & Reeves, W.C. (1999) HIV and human papillomavirus as independent risk factors for cervical neoplasia in women with high or low numbers of sex partners. *Sex. Transm. Infect.*, **75**, 258–260

Wabinga, H.R., Parkin, D.M., Wabwire-Mangen, F., & Nambooze, S. (2000) Trends in incidence in Kyadondo County, Uganda, 1960–1997. *Br. J. Cancer*, **82**, 1585–1592

Walboomers, J.M.M., Jacobs, M.V., Manos, M.M., Bosch, F.X., Kummer, J.A., Shah, K.V., Snijders, P.J., Peto, J., Meijer, C.J. & Muñoz, N. (1999) Human papillomavirus is a necessary cause of invasive cervical cancer worldwide. *J. Pathol.*, **189**, 12–19

Williams, M.A., Kenya, P.R., Mati, J.K.G. & Thomas, D.B. (1994) Risk factors for invasive cervical cancer in Kenyan women. *Int. J. Epidemiol.*, **32**, 906–912

Womack, S.D., Chirenje, Z.M., Blumenthal, P.D., Gaffikin, L., McGrath, J.A., Chipato, T., Ngwalle, E. & Shah, K.V. (2000a) Evaluation of a human papillomavirus assay in cervical screening in Zimbabwe. *Br. J. Obstet. Gynaecol.*, **107**, 33–38

Womack, S.D., Chirenje, Z.M., Gaffikin, L., Blumenthal, P.D., McGrath, J.A., Chipato, T., Ngwalle, E., Munjoma, M. & Shah, K.V. (2000b) HPV-based cervical cancer screening in a population at high risk for HIV infection. *Int. J. Cancer*, **85**, 206–210

Woto-Gaye, G., Critchlow, C., Kiviat, N., & Ndiaya, P.D. (1996) Le depistage cytologique des cancers du col uterin en Afrique noire; quelles perspectives? *Bull. Cancer*, **83**, 407–409

4.4 Colorectal cancer

Introduction

Large bowel cancer is predominant in affluent societies and most frequent in North America, western Europe, Australia/New Zealand and the southern part of South America. In 2000, colorectal cancer was estimated to be the fourth most common cancer in the world in both sexes, and the second in developed countries, with an estimated 943 000 new cases (9.4% of the total). In Africa, colorectal cancers account for just 2.5% of all cancers. Almost all colorectal cancers are adenocarcinomas.

Descriptive epidemiology in Africa

Incidence is very low in Africa, except in white populations. Rates are a little higher in North Africa than in sub-Saharan Africa. The higher rates seen in the French department of La Réunion may be due to the influence of European lifestyle factors and the ethnically diverse population. Table 1 presents age-standardized incidence from cancer registries reported in this volume, with comparison data from Europe and North America. Table 2 shows incidence data from registries for the 1950s to 1970s.

Figure 1 illustrates estimated incidence rates by country, based on the incidence data available. The high incidence in the south is due to the high rates in the white populations of South Africa.

Early data from Africa show that large bowel cancers were rare. A review of published data and four hospital series obtained from doctors in up-country hospitals in Africa summarized the frequency of cancer of the colon and rectum in the 1950s and 1960s (Burkitt, 1971) (Table 3).

Davies *et al.* (1965) compared the very low rate of intestinal cancer in Kyadondo County, Uganda for the period 1954–60 with US and Norwegian rates. In Uganda, the ASR per 100 000 for colon cancer was 0.2 in males and 0.6 in females, and for rectal cancer 0.6 and 1.8, compared with 12.4 and 14.0 (colon) and 10.6 and 7.8 (rectum) in US whites. It was suggested that the paucity of gastrointestinal cancer in Ugandan Africans, particularly in the older age groups, could be attributed to lack of death certification, as 22% of the US cases were based on death certificate diagnoses. This does not suffice to explain the difference, however, since the US rates remain much higher even if the cases based on a death certificate alone are excluded.

Cancer of the rectum is more common than cancer of the colon in Africa, as in other low-risk populations, such as those in India and China (Parkin *et al.*, 2001). This is the reverse of the pattern in high-incidence populations, notably the very high incidence of colon cancer in US blacks. This difference may be influenced by easier diagnosis of rectal cancer.

Time trends

The few long data series available for Africa show an increasing trend in incidence and mortality. Rates in the long series from Kampala, Uganda (Wabinga *et al.*, 2000) rose from ASR 3.0 (1960–66) to 6.8 (1995–97) in males and from 2.7 to 6.6 in females.

Colorectal cancer is one of the leading cancers in South African whites, but 10 times rarer in the black population than in the white (2.3 and 22 per 100 000 respectively). In South Africa, changes in exposure to environmental factors have resulted in the African population overtaking the whites in prevalence of obesity in women, hypertension and diabetes (Walker, 1996). However chronic bowel diseases, and occurrence of appendicitis, diverticular disease and colon cancer have risen only slightly (Walker & Segal, 1997).

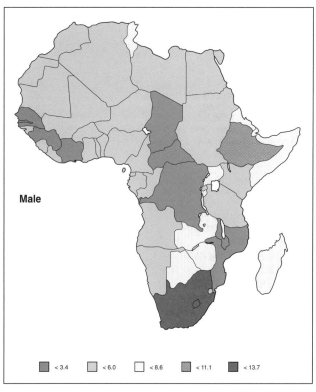

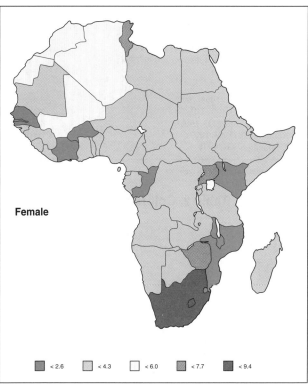

Figure 1. Age-standardized incidence of colorectal cancer in Africa

Migrant studies

Low mortality from colorectal cancer has been found among North African migrants in France (Bouchardy *et al.*, 1996) and Egyptian migrants to Australia (McCredie & Coates, 1989; Khlat *et al.*, 1993).

Table 1. Age-standardized (world) and cumulative (0-64) incidence
Colon, rectum and anus (C18-21)

	MALE				FEMALE			
	Cases	CRUDE (per 100,000)	ASR(W) (per 100,000)	Cumulative (%)	Cases	CRUDE (per 100,000)	ASR(W) (per 100,000)	Cumulative (%)
Africa, North								
Algeria, Algiers (1993-1997)	284	5.2	**7.1**	0.41	248	4.6	**6.1**	0.42
Algeria, Constantine (1994-1997)	42	2.7	**4.1**	0.28	43	2.8	**4.2**	0.24
Algeria, Oran (1996-1998)	87	4.9	**7.2**	0.51	83	4.7	**6.1**	0.39
Algeria, Setif (1993-1997)	82	2.7	**4.6**	0.36	89	3.0	**4.3**	0.32
Tunisia, Centre, Sousse (1993-1997)	65	5.6	**7.7**	0.45	77	6.8	**8.8**	0.58
Tunisia, North, Tunis (1994)	109	5.0	**6.2**	0.41	113	5.4	**7.0**	0.37
Tunisia, Sfax (1997)	28	7.1	**8.9**	0.38	31	8.2	**9.6**	0.54
Africa, West								
The Gambia (1997-1998)	8	0.8	**1.5**	0.10	14	1.4	**2.5**	0.16
Guinea, Conakry (1996-1999)	35	1.5	**3.2**	0.23	30	1.4	**3.2**	0.16
Mali, Bamako (1988-1997)	97	2.5	**5.0**	0.34	59	1.6	**3.5**	0.27
Niger, Niamey (1993-1999)	37	2.0	**4.8**	0.35	24	1.3	**3.6**	0.23
Nigeria, Ibadan (1998-1999)	29	2.0	**3.8**	0.35	24	1.6	**2.8**	0.22
Africa, Central								
Congo, Brazzaville (1996-1999)	34	2.8	**4.4**	0.25	25	2.1	**2.8**	0.23
Africa, East								
France, La Reunion (1988-1994)	199	9.5	**12.6**	0.65	199	9.2	**10.0**	0.58
Kenya, Eldoret (1998-2000)	24	2.6	**6.3**	0.45	10	1.1	**2.2**	0.09
Malawi, Blantyre (2000-2001)	11	1.2	**2.7**	0.12	13	1.5	**2.7**	0.12
Uganda, Kyadondo County (1993-1997)	68	2.4	**8.0**	0.39	61	2.1	**7.0**	0.47
Zimbabwe, Harare: African (1990-1993)	84	3.5	**8.5**	0.47	47	2.2	**7.1**	0.53
Zimbabwe, Harare: African (1994-1997)	82	2.9	**7.4**	0.34	52	2.0	**6.7**	0.42
Zimbabwe, Harare: European (1990-1997)	133	87.0	**49.8**	2.48	118	70.0	**35.5**	1.90
Africa, South								
Namibia (1995-1998)	85	2.7	**4.4**	0.30	67	2.1	**3.3**	0.21
South Africa: Black (1989-1992)	981	1.7	**3.0**	0.18	870	1.5	**2.3**	0.15
South Africa: Indian (1989-1992)	161	8.3	**14.2**	0.66	132	6.7	**9.4**	0.56
South Africa: Mixed race (1989-1992)	252	3.9	**7.5**	0.46	280	4.2	**6.4**	0.33
South Africa: White (1989-1992)	2414	24.0	**22.2**	1.06	2295	22.5	**17.1**	0.91
South Africa, Transkei, Umtata (1996-1998)	10	2.8	**4.9**	0.37	5	1.2	**1.5**	0.05
South Africa, Transkei, 4 districts (1996-1998)	6	0.8	**1.6**	0.14	6	0.7	**0.9**	0.03
Swaziland (1996-1999)	39	2.2	**4.2**	0.22	26	1.3	**2.4**	0.20
Europe/USA								
USA, SEER: White (1993-1997)	26300	54.0	**40.0**	1.79	26334	52.5	**30.3**	1.31
USA, SEER: Black (1993-1997)	2601	38.9	**45.0**	2.40	2844	38.3	**35.7**	1.84
France, 8 registries (1993-1997)	8500	61.8	**42.2**	1.91	7215	50.0	**27.0**	1.29
The Netherlands (1993-1997)	21001	55.0	**39.3**	1.76	20703	53.0	**29.9**	1.41
UK, England (1993-1997)	71079	59.2	**36.8**	1.62	65948	51.6	**25.0**	1.09

In italics: histopathology-based registries

Table 2. Colorectal cancer pre-1980. Age-standardized incidence (all ages)

Registry	Period	Colon Male	Colon Female	Rectum/anus Male	Rectum/anus Female	Source (see Chap. 1)
Senegal, Dakar	1969–74	*0.6*	0.7	1.5	1.0	4
Mozambique, Lourenço Marques	1956–60	*1.9*	*1.9*	*0.0*	*0.0*	1
Nigeria, Ibadan	1960–69	1.3	1.2	1.2	2.0	3
SA, Cape Province: Bantu	1956–59	*2.3*	*4.6*	*4.6*	*4.2*	2
SA, Cape Province: Coloured	1956–59	4.4	7.7	3.5	3.5	2
SA, Cape Province: White	1956–59	13.8	16.9	4.5	5.4	2
SA, Johannesburg, Bantu	1953–55	*1.8*	*4.1*	2.0	2.2	1
SA, Natal Province: African	1964–66	*2.0*	*2.1*	*1.1*	*3.9*	2
SA, Natal Province: Indian	1964–66	*2.7*	*7.6*	3.5	*10.3*	2
Uganda, Kyadondo	1954–60	*0.3*	*0.6*	*1.1*	*2.5*	1
Uganda, Kyadondo	1960–71	1.7	1.3	2.2	3.3	5
Zimbabwe, Bulawayo	1963–72	4.8	*4.1*	1.2	0.0	6

Italics: Rate based on less than 10 cases

Table 3. Proportion of cancer of the colon and rectum among total cancer in different parts of Africa

Place	Period	Total cases	Colorectal as % of total
Johannesburg (S. Africa)	1952-54	1076	2.6
Johannesburg (S. Africa)	1962-64	2407	2.4
Durban (S. Africa)	1964-66	1040	2.1
Lourenço Marques (Mozambique)	1956-60	603	1.3
Sudan	1954-61	2234	2.8
Accra (Ghana)	1942-55	1192	1.8
Kampala (Uganda)	1954-60	615	2.8
Nairobi (Kenya)	1957-63	4206	2.5
Dakar (Senegal)	1955-64	1838	2.5
Salisbury (Rhodesia)	1963-65	1415	1.6
Ilesha (Nigeria)	1954-67	465	5.8
Stanleyville (Congo Kinshasa)	1939-55	2536	1.1
Kenya (5 hospitals)	Questionnaire survey	934	1.5
Uganda (7 hospitals)	Questionnaire survey	613	2.1
Tanzania (23 hospitals)	Questionnaire survey	1743	2.3
Malawi (22 hospitals)	Questionnaire survey	827	1.7

Source: Burkitt (1971)

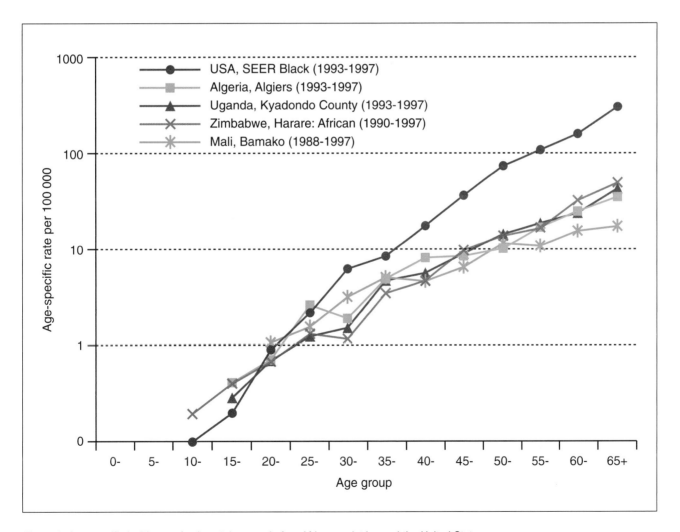

Figure 2. Age-specific incidence of colorectal cancer in four African registries and the United States

North African Arab immigrants have maintained their traditional diet, rich in cereals, legumes, green vegetables and fruit and poor in animal fats and grilled meat. The incidence in migrants from North Africa to Israel is half that of European migrants (Steinitz *et al.*, 1989).

Age-specific incidence
In many case series from Africa, e.g. in Uganda (Hutt *et al.*, 1967), Zaire (Kenda, 1976), Sudan (Elmasri & Boulos, 1975), Nigeria (Ojo *et al.*, 1991; Iliyasu *et al.*, 1996) and Egypt (Soliman *et al.*, 1999), the average age of patients with large bowel cancer was lower than in western countries. In the Egyptian study, 30.6% of cancers occurring in patients under the age of 40 years were mucin-producing tumours, compared with 13.7% in patients over the age of 40.

These differences may simply reflect the young age structure of African populations. However, age-specific incidence rates from this volume (Figure 2) do suggest that the increase of incidence wth age is much slower in African populations than in western countries (the data for the black population of the United States are shown). This may represent a cohort effect, due to increasing risk in successive generations of Africans. In South Africa, there is an eight-fold difference in incidence between the older black and white populations (e.g., males 55–64 years: 276.3 vs 33 per 100 000), but no difference in the younger age groups (e.g., 15–24 years: 1.6 vs 1.6 per 100 000), which suggests that the same lifestyle factors affecting the younger white generation may be affecting the younger black generation.

Location of lesions
The distribution of cancers within the large bowel shows marked differences according to geographical region. Evidence on the location of colorectal tumours in Africans is confusing. The distribution of carcinomas of the large intestine among the Bantu in the 1960s was reported to resemble that in westernized populations, over two thirds occurring on the left side, with the rectum as most common site followed by the caecum (Oettlé, 1964). Similarly, a report of 76 cases in Benin described 92% of malignancies occurring in the left side of the colon, 86.8% of which were in the sigmoid colon and rectum (Osime *et al.*, 1988) and in a ten-year pathology review of cases in Ile-Ife, Nigeria, the site distribution was 57.3% recto-sigmoid, 23.2% descending colon, 12.2% caecum and 3.7% for both ascending and transverse colon (Ojo *et al.*, 1991).

On the other hand, in a 20-year hospital series of 526 histologically confirmed colorectal cancers from Ibadan, Nigeria between 1971 and 1990, Iliyasu *et al.* (1996) found that neoplasms were predominantly right-sided (34.3% caecal). Colorectal cancer accounted for 3.7% of all neoplasms recorded during the period. An excess of cancer of caecum and ascending colon and a 'marked deficiency' in the sigmoid and rectosigmoid were observed by Davies (1959) in Ugandan Africans. Templeton (1973) observed that epithelial tumours were considerably more frequent in the right colon than in the left in Uganda. Muir Grieve (1967) reported a similar finding in the Cape Division of South Africa. A report on cases of colorectal cancer recorded in the Kampala Cancer Registry for the period 1964–76 described 36 (20%) of cancers of the colon as mucoid carcinomas, of which 19 were in the caecum, 7 in the ascending colon, 3 in the transverse, 2 in the descending and 5 in the sigmoid (Owor, 1983).

Risk factors
Diet
The increases in incidence in migrant populations point to an environmental causation, probably due to dietary factors, with a possible link to exercise. The roles of fat, fibre and protein and the protective effect of vegetables have been extensively examined. Protein and fat, notably from meat, are related consistently to risk of colon cancer, but inverse associations have been reported with physical activity and with intake of fish and shellfish (Potter, 1996; Hill, 1999; Kato *et al.*, 1997). There may be an association with alcohol consumption, and processed meat may confer more risk than red meat. The risk factors for cancers of both colon and rectum do not appear to be very different, but physical activity does not appear to play a role in rectal cancer.

The low incidence of cancer of the colon and rectum in Africans has frequently been related to the characteristics of the African diet, with high cereal and low animal protein consumption. Davies *et al.* (1965) described the population of Kyadondo, with its low rates, as 'peasant agriculturalists, minimally exposed to urbanization and industrialization, living on high-carbohydrate, low-protein, low-fat diets of largely unprocessed foodstuffs'. A variety of plantains remains the major source of carbohydrate in the area (Wabinga *et al.*, 2000).

Burkitt proposed a mechanism whereby fibre might protect against colorectal cancer, after measuring intestinal transit time in African villagers, boys on a semi-European diet and boys in an English boarding school and finding a clear correlation between transit time, stool bulk and the fibre content of food (Burkitt, 1971). A further factor suggested as capable of enhancing bowel motility was frequent use of emetics, laxatives and enemas (Oettlé, 1964). This was investigated in a survey among 584 residents in Lourenço Marques in the period 1956–61, which found that 9.7% of this population used emetics, 31.7% used laxatives and 3.8% enemas (Prates & Torres, 1965).

However, Walker and Segal (1997) noted that stool frequency in Africans in urban areas now averages about one motion daily, much the same as in the white population, and transit times are similar between the two populations. Mean levels of all components of faecal short-chain fatty acids (FSCH) with the exception of butyrate are significantly higher in Africans than in whites and FSCH are associated with a reduction in pH. Faecal pH values remain significantly lower in African adults and children than in the white population, which may be a protective factor (Segal, 1998).

It has been postulated that, although the dietary fibre content of the typical diet has fallen, the proportion of 'resistant' starch remains high and that this, allied with colonic microflora which seem to be more effective in fermenting fibre in Africans, may provide continuing protection (Segal *et al.*, 2000).

A dietary survey in South Africa compared nutrients in fishermen with a westernized white control group. While total fat intake in the two groups was similar, the fishermen (at low risk of colorectal cancer) had markedly higher polyunsaturated fat intake, notably of the omega-3 fatty acids docosahexaenoic acid and eicosapentaenoic acid, and it was postulated that these fatty acids might be protective (Schloss *et al.*, 1997).

Intestinal bacteria
Burkitt (1971) reported that the stools of developing country populations were bulky, soft and non-odorous compared to those of populations in western countries, perhaps indicating a lower rate of bacterial decomposition. Individuals seem to maintain their own distinctive flora compositions, so there may be a genetic element to this factor.

Faecal specimens were examined in an ecological study of individuals (non-randomized) from four populations at different risk of colon cancer. *Bacteroides vulgatus*, *Bacteroides stercoris*, *Bifidobacterium longum* and *Bifidobacterium angulatum* were found to be significantly associated with high risk of colon cancer, *Lactobacillus S06* and *Eubacterium aerofaciens* with low risk, and total lactobacilli were inversely related to risk (Moore & Moore, 1995). Diet and output of methane (from fermented complex carbohydrate) have been studied in adult white and black South Africans (O'Keefe *et al.*, 1999). Both fasting and food-induced breath methane production was two to three times higher in blacks, and it was concluded that differences in colonic bacterial fermentation might influence the cancer risk.

Adenomatous polyps

Adenomatous polyps and villous papillomas are strongly correlated with bowel cancer. It is probable that genetic and environmental factors interact in the formation and transformation of polyps. The hereditary cancer syndromes hereditary nonpolyposis colon cancer (HNPCC), involving a familial pattern of early onset, and the rare condition familial adenomatous polyposis coli (FAP), associated with multiple polyps in the large intestine which show a high frequency of malignant transformation, have been well characterized. It seems probable that most tumours occur in a section of the population with increased genetic susceptibility, a fact that complicates the interpretation of epidemiological studies of diet.

It has been repeatedly reported that premalignant diseases such as polyposis coli, ulcerative colitis, villous papilloma and adenoma are rare in Africans. No evidence of polyps was found in a series of 76 cases of colorectal cancer cases reported from a hospital series in Benin (Osime *et al.*, 1988). A search for polyps in the colon and rectum was made in a series of 343 post mortems of Africans over age 25 years in Uganda and no adenomatous polyps, villous papillomas or hyperplastic polyps were found (Hutt & Templeton, 1971). Owor (1983) found 18 cases of adenomatous polyps in biopsy material, and one at autopsy, in 180 cases of carcinoma of colon and 238 of rectum recorded in the Kampala Cancer Registry for the years 1964–76. In addition he noted six cases of carcinoma in the rectum and two in the colon which appeared to arise from pre-existing polyps.

In a comparison of colorectal polyps in surgical biopsies from American blacks and Nigerians in the 1960s, only 7.5% of the polyps in Nigerians were neoplastic, compared with 87% in the Americans. However, the average age of the two case series was very different, most of the Nigerian patients being under 20 years of age, and juvenile polyps accounted for about 60% of the total compared with only 9% in Americans (Williams *et al.*, 1975). In a Nigerian hospital series of 526 colorectal neoplasms, two isolated cases of familial polyposis were observed, at ages 22 and 36 years (Iliyasu *et al.*, 1996). Reports of this condition in Africans are very rare.

References

Bouchardy, C., Parkin, D.M., Wanner, P. & Khlat, M. (1996) Cancer mortality among North African migrants in France. *Int. J. Epidemiol.*, **25**, 5–13

Burkitt, D.P. (1971) Epidemiology of cancer of the colon and rectum. *Cancer*, **28**, 3–13

Davies, J.H.P. (1959) Cancer in Africans. In: Collins, D.H., ed., *Modern Trends in Pathology*, London, Butterworth, pp. 132–160

Davies, J.N.P., Knowelden, J. & Wilson, B.A. (1965) Incidence rates of cancer in Kyadondo County, Uganda 1954-1960. *J. Natl Cancer Inst.*, **35**, 789–821

Elmasri, S.H. & Boulos, P.B. (1975) Carcinoma of the large bowel in the Sudan. *Br. J. Surg.*, **62**, 284–286

Hill, M.J. (1999) Diet, physical activity and cancer risk. *Public Health Nutr.*, **2**, 397–401

Hutt, M.S.R. & Templeton, A.C. (1971) The geographical pathology of bowel cancer and some related diseases. *Proc. Roy. Soc. Med.*, **64**, 962–964

Hutt, M.S.R., Burkitt, D.P., Shepherd, J.J., Wright, B., Mati, J.K.G. & Auma, S. (1967) Malignant tumors of the gastrointestinal tract in Ugandans. *National Cancer Institute Monographs* No. 25, 41–67

Iliyasu, Y., Ladipo, J.K., Akang, E.E.U., Adebamowo, C.A., Ajao, O.G. & Aghadiuno, P.U. (1996) A twenty-year review of malignant colorectal neoplasms at University College Hospital, Ibadan, Nigeria. *Dis. Colon Rectum*, **39**, 536–540

Kato, I., Akhmedkhanov, A., Koenig, K., Toniolo, P.G., Shore, R.E. & Riboli, E. (1997) Prospective study of diet and female colorectal cancer: the New York University Women's Health Study. *Nutr. Cancer*, **28**, 276–281

Kenda, J.F. (1976) Cancer of the large bowel in the African: a 15-year survey at Kinshasa University Hospital, Zaire. *Br. J. Surg.*, **63**, 966–968

Khlat, M., Bouchardy, C. & Parkin, D.M. (1993) Mortalité par cancer chez les immigrés du Proche-Orient en Australia. *Rev. Epidemiol. Santé publ.*, **41**, 208–217

McCredie, M. & Coates, M.S. (1989) *Cancer Incidence in Migrants to New South Wales*. 1972-1984, Sydney, NSW Cancer Council

Moore, W.E.C. & Moore, L.H. (1995) Intestinal floras of populations that have a high risk of colon cancer. *Appl. Environ. Microbiol.*, **61**, 3202–3207

Muir Grieve, J. (1967) *Cancer in the Cape Division, South Africa*, London, Oxford University Press

O'Keefe, S.J.D., Kidd, M., Espitalier-Noel, G. & Owira, P. (1999) Rarity of colon cancer in Africans is associated with low animal product consumption, not fiber. *Am. J. Gastroenterol.*, **94**, 1373–1380

Oettlé, A.G. (1964) Cancer in Africa, especially in regions south of the Sahara. *J. Natl Cancer Inst.*, **33**, 383–439

Ojo, O.S., Odesanmi, W.O. & Akinola, O.O. (1991) The surgical pathology of colorectal carcinomas in Nigerians. *Trop. Gastroenterol.*, **12**, 180–184

Osime, U., Morgan, A. & Guirguis, M. (1988) Colorectal cancer in Africans (a report of 76 cases). *J. Indian Med. Assoc.*, **86**, 270–272

Owor, R. (1983) Carcinoma of colon and rectum in Uganda Africans. *E. Afr. Med. J.*, **60**, pp???

Parkin, D.M., Bray, F.I. & Devesa, S.S. (2001) Cancer burden in the year 2000. The global picture. *Eur. J. Cancer*, **37**, S4–S66

Potter, J.D. (1996) Nutrition and colorectal cancer. *Cancer Causes Control*, **7**, 127–146

Prates, M.D. & Torres, F.O. (1965) Malignant tumors of the alimentary canal in Africans of Mozambique. *National Cancer Institute Monographs* No. 25, pp. 73–82

Schloss, I., Kidd, M.S.G., Tichelaar, H.Y., Young, G.O. & O'Keefe, S.J.D. (1997) Dietary factors associated with a low risk of colon cancer in coloured West Coast fishermen. *S. Afr. Med. J.*, **87**, 152–158

Segal, I. (1998) Rarity of colorectal adenomas in the African black population. *Eur. J. Cancer Prev.*, **7**, 387–391

Segal, I., Edwards, C.A. & Walker, A.R. (2000) Continuing low colon cancer incidence in African populations. *Am. J. Gastroenterol.*, **95**, 859–860

Soliman, A.S., Bondy, M.L., Raouf, A.A., Makram, M.A., Johnston, D.A. & Levin, B. (1999) Cancer mortality in Menofeia, Egypt: comparison with US mortality rates. *Cancer Causes Control*, **10**, 349–354

Steinitz, R., Parkin, D.M., Young, J.L., Bieber, C.A. & Katz, L., eds (1989) *Cancer Incidence in Jewish Migrants to Israel 1961–1981* (IARC Scientific Publications No. 98), Lyon, IARC

Templeton, A.C. (1973) Tumours of the alimentary canal. In: Templeton, A.C., ed., *Tumours in a Tropical Country. A Survey of Uganda 1964-1968*, Heidelberg, Springer-Verlag, pp???

Wabinga, H.R., Parkin, D.M., Wabwire-Mangen, F. & Nambooze, S. (2000) Trends in cancer incidence in Kyadondo County, Uganda, 1960-1997. *Br. J. Cancer*, **82**, 1585–1592

Walker, A.R.P. (1996) The nutritional challenges in the New South Africa. *Nutr. Res. Rev.*, **9**, 33–65

Walker, A.R.P. & Segal, I. (1997) Effects of transition on bowel diseases in sub-Saharan Africans. *Eur. J. Gastroenterol. Hepatol.*, **9**, 207–210

Williams, A.O., Chung, E.B., Agbata, A. & Jackson, M.A. (1975) Intestinal polyps in American Negroes and Nigerian Africans. *Br. J. Cancer*, **31**, 485–491

4.5 Cancers of the eye and orbit

Introduction

The ICD-10 code C69 includes several anatomically distinct structures, (conjunctiva, cornea, retina, choroid, ciliary body, lacrimal gland, and orbit). The skin of the eyelid (C44.1) and the optic nerve (C72.3) are excluded, as well as lymphomas and leukaemias occurring in the orbit. Table 1 shows the incidence rates of tumours of the eye in the population-based series in this volume, and Table 2 the results from older series.

Particularly in the more recent data, the incidence rates for all eye cancers combined are rather higher in many of the sub-Saharan populations than in Europe or the United States. Table 3 shows the histological subtypes for the data-sets published in this volume, indicating that there is a relatively high percentage of squamous-cell carcinomas, which occur almost entirely on the conjunctiva. The predominance of retinoblastoma and squamous-cell conjunctival cancers in African case series has been noted many times before, as has the rarity of uveal melanomas in African populations. Case series are generally concerned with the percentages of different histological types of eye and orbital tumours, but comparison between them is complicated by lack of information on the age distribution of the series (those containing many children will include more retinoblastomas), the inclusion of tumours of surrounding structures, and lymphomas (particularly Burkitt lymphomas). Involvement of the orbit is frequently seen in Burkitt lymphoma, but involvement of the globe itself is very infrequent.

Templeton (1973) reported a series of 314 invasive tumours of the eye and adnexae in Uganda, comprising 59 cases of Burkitt lymphoma of the orbit, 53 squamous-cell carcinomas of the conjunctiva and 57 retinoblastomas. Three melanomas (one uveal) and four Kaposi sarcomas (one of eyelid) were noted in this series. No rhabdomyosarcomas were reported. Klauss and Chana (1983) reported on 470 cases of orbital disease, including 187 malignant tumours, in Kenya. The histological profile was similar to that in the Uganda series (39% retinoblastomas, 23% Burkitt lymphomas and 6.4% squamous cell carcinomas).

Retinoblastomas are found mainly in children (see Chapter 5), and are very rare after the age of 5 years.

Melanoma of the eye

As noted earlier, melanomas of the eye are rare in black African populations. For example, in the South African series, in whites, melanomas of the eye comprised 19% of all eye cancers, while only 1.9% of eye cancers in blacks were melanomas. Similar results were found in other series, reviewed by Klauss and Chana (1983): melanoma of the eye comprised 0.7% of 1487 eye cancer cases seen in Kenya (Awan & Shah, 1980), 0.3% of 312 cases in Uganda (Templeton, 1967), 1.6% of 191 cases in Nigeria (Olurin & Williams, 1972) and 0.7% of 279 cases seen in Sudan (Malik & Sheikh, 1979).

Northern European ancestry, presence of naevi and intense sun exposure and UV radiation appear to be risk factors for uveal melanoma (Seddon et al., 1990; Holly et al., 1990); this could explain the 10-fold higher relative frequency among white South Africans than among blacks. In the United States, the incidence of melanoma of the eye is at least ten times higher in whites (adults) than blacks (Parkin et al., 1997). Reasons for the variations among Africans are unclear, and are more likely to relate to the unsystematic nature of data collection than to any real trend. Nevertheless, in the Sudan all six cases of intra-ocular melanoma occurred in the Arab population, and none in Africans (Malik & Sheikh, 1979). No geographical association was found between ultraviolet radiation and melanoma incidence in cancer registries from the United States (Sun et al., 1997).

Squamous-cell carcinoma of the conjunctiva

This tumour appears to be common in many parts of Africa. Klauss and Chana (1983) reported relative frequencies of squamous-cell conjunctival cancers, which appeared to vary from place to place. Conjunctival cancers comprised 21.8% of eye cancers in Kenya (Awan & Shah, 1980), 16.0% in Uganda (Templeton, 1967), 6.2% in Nigeria (Olurin & Williams, 1972) and 50% in Sudan (Malik & Shah, 1979). The tumours occur close to the limbus, usually on the nasal aspect. They are preceded by a spectrum of lesions, showing progression from slight acanthosis and hyperkeratosis (pterygium), through progressive degrees of epithelial dysplasia and intra-epithelial carcinoma, to frank invasion (Clear et al., 1979). It has long been suspected that increased exposure to ultraviolet light is responsible, although roles for other factors, such as dust, dry air, wind, trachoma and vernal catarrh have been suggested (Klauss & Chana, 1983).

Human papillomavirus (HPV) has been measured in a variety of ways in a number of small studies and types 6, 16, 11 and 18 were found in lesions of dysplasia and conjunctival cancer (Newton, 1996; IARC, 1995), but the results are inconsistent. Bovine papillomaviruses infect the conjunctiva of cattle (Ford et al., 1982) and it is plausible that certain HPV types may infect the conjunctiva and cause cancer. However, in a case–control study in Uganda, comparing 60 conjunctival neoplasms (60% with histological confirmation) with 1214 controls (subjects with a variety of proved or suspected cancers, excluding those known to be associated with HIV, HPV or human herpes virus 8 (HHV-8)), Newton et al. (2002) found no association with presence of antibody to HPV-16 (OR 1.5, 95% CI 0.5–4.3). There was no association either with antibody to HPV 18 and 45, although seroprevalence to these two types was low, so that the confidence intervals were wide.

Ecological studies have shown that there is a significant association between cloud-adjusted UV-B ultraviolet B radiation and incidence of squamous-cell conjunctival cancers internationally (Newton et al., 1996) and in the United States (Sun et al., 1997). Newton et al. (1996) estimated that the incidence of squamous-cell conjunctival cancer declines by 49% for each 10° increase in latitude, falling from about 12 cases per million in Uganda (0.3°N) to less than 0.2 cases per million in the northern European countries. In the case–control study described above (Newton et al., 2002), risk was increased in individuals who spent a lot of time cultivating; this perhaps indicates higher exposures to UV radiation.

The incidence of squamous-cell carcinoma of the conjunctiva has been greatly increased by the epidemic of HIV/AIDS. This topic has been reviewed by Newton (1996) and IARC (1996), and is described in Chapter 6. Incidence rates of conjunctival carcinoma in the registry series in this volume are shown in Table 4.

References

Awan, A.M. & Shah, A.K. (1980) Orbito-ocular tumours in Kenya Africans. E. Afr. J. Ophthalmol., 65, 720–722

Clear, A.S., Chirambo, M.C. & Hutt, M.S.R. (1979) Solar keratosis, pterygium, and squamous cell carcinoma of the conjunctiva in Malawi. Br. J. Ophthalmol., 63, 102–109

Ford, J.N., Jennings, P.A. & Spradbrow, P.B. (1982) Evidence for papillomaviruses in ocular lesions in cattle. Res. Vet. Sci., 32, 257–259

Table 1. Age-standardized (world) and cumulative (0-64) incidence
Eye (C69)

	MALE				FEMALE			
	Cases	CRUDE	ASR(W) (per 100,000)	Cumulative (%)	Cases	CRUDE	ASR(W) (per 100,000)	Cumulative (%)
Africa, North								
Algeria, Algiers (1993-1997)	20	0.4	**0.5**	0.02	22	0.4	**0.5**	0.03
Algeria, Constantine (1994-1997)	2	0.1	**0.2**	0.01	2	0.1	**0.2**	0.03
Algeria, Oran (1996-1998)	18	1.0	**1.2**	0.04	8	0.5	**0.6**	0.02
Algeria, Setif (1993-1997)	4	0.1	**0.2**	0.02	5	0.2	**0.2**	0.00
Tunisia, Centre, Sousse (1993-1997)	5	0.4	**0.5**	0.04	5	0.4	**0.5**	0.02
Tunisia, North, Tunis (1994)	9	0.4	**0.5**	0.03	6	0.3	**0.4**	0.02
Tunisia, Sfax (1997)	2	0.5	**0.5**	0.03	1	0.3	**0.2**	0.02
Africa, West								
The Gambia (1997-1998)	6	0.6	**1.0**	0.06	5	0.5	**0.6**	0.05
Guinea, Conakry (1996-1999)	31	1.4	**1.7**	0.11	10	0.5	**0.4**	0.02
Mali, Bamako (1988-1997)	28	0.7	**0.9**	0.05	25	0.7	**1.1**	0.05
Niger, Niamey (1993-1999)	15	0.8	**1.1**	0.11	7	0.4	**0.6**	0.03
Nigeria, Ibadan (1998-1999)	15	1.0	**1.3**	0.03	7	0.5	**0.5**	0.03
Africa, Central								
Congo, Brazzaville (1996-1999)	6	0.5	**0.6**	0.02	9	0.7	**0.7**	0.04
Africa, East								
France, La Reunion (1988-1994)	7	0.3	**0.4**	0.01	7	0.3	**0.4**	0.03
Kenya, Eldoret (1998-2000)	9	1.0	**0.9**	0.07	5	0.5	**0.6**	0.04
Malawi, Blantyre (2000-2001)	18	2.0	**2.5**	0.10	25	2.9	**4.2**	0.34
Uganda, Kyadondo County (1993-1997)	76	2.7	**2.9**	0.22	64	2.2	**2.8**	0.23
Zimbabwe, Harare: African (1990-1993)	17	0.7	**1.0**	0.05	17	0.8	**0.9**	0.07
Zimbabwe, Harare: African (1994-1997)	67	2.4	**2.6**	0.16	73	2.8	**3.6**	0.27
Zimbabwe, Harare: European (1990-1997)	6	3.9	**2.7**	0.15	-	-	**-**	-
Africa, South								
Namibia (1995-1998)	45	1.4	**1.8**	0.14	42	1.3	**1.6**	0.13
South Africa: Black (1989-1992)	271	0.5	**0.6**	0.04	206	0.4	**0.4**	0.02
South Africa: Indian (1989-1992)	7	0.4	**0.5**	0.02	3	0.2	**0.2**	0.01
South Africa: Mixed race (1989-1992)	12	0.2	**0.2**	0.01	23	0.3	**0.4**	0.02
South Africa: White (1989-1992)	102	1.0	**1.0**	0.05	77	0.8	**0.7**	0.04
South Africa, Transkei, Umtata (1996-1998)	-	-	**-**	-	-	-	**-**	-
South Africa, Transkei, 4 districts (1996-1998)	1	0.1	**0.1**	0.00	4	0.4	**0.5**	0.02
Swaziland (1996-1999)	16	0.9	**1.4**	0.11	13	0.7	**0.9**	0.06
Europe/USA								
USA, SEER: White (1993-1997)	459	0.9	**0.8**	0.04	372	0.7	**0.6**	0.04
USA, SEER: Black (1993-1997)	13	0.2	**0.2**	0.01	15	0.2	**0.3**	0.01
France, 8 registries (1993-1997)	141	1.0	**0.9**	0.05	108	0.7	**0.5**	0.03
The Netherlands (1993-1997)	353	0.9	**0.8**	0.05	336	0.9	**0.7**	0.04
UK, England (1993-1997)	1025	0.9	**0.7**	0.04	969	0.8	**0.6**	0.03

In italics: histopathology-based registries

Table 2. Incidence of cancer of the eye in Africa, 1953–74

Registry	Period	ASR (per 100 000)		Source
		Male	Female	(see Chap. 1)
Senegal, Dakar	1969–74	1.5	0.9	4
Mozambique, Lourenço Marques	1956–60	*2.4*	*0.6*	1
Nigeria, Ibadan	1960–69	*0.3*	0.5	3
SA, Cape Province: Bantu	1956–59	0.0	*1.5*	2
SA, Cape Province: Coloured	1956–59	*0.2*	*0.6*	2
SA, Cape Province: White	1956–59	*1.5*	*0.6*	2
SA, Johannesburg, Bantu	1953–55	*0.7*	*0.3*	1
SA, Natal Province: African	1964–66	*0.6*	*1.0*	2
SA, Natal Province: Indian	1964–66	*1.3*	*0.0*	2
Uganda, Kyadondo	1954–60	1.0	1.6	1
Uganda, Kyadondo	1960–71	0.8	*0.3*	5
Zimbabwe, Bulawayo	1963–72	*0.7*	*0.4*	6

Italics: Rate based on less than 10 cases

Table 3. Percentage distribution of microscopically verified cases by histological type
Eye (C69) - Both sexes

	Retino-blastoma	Melanoma	Carcinoma Squamous	Carcinoma Other	Unspec.	Sarcoma	Other	Unspecified	Number of cases MV	Number of cases Total
Algeria, Algiers	59.5	5.4	13.5	2.7	13.5	5.4	-	-	37	42
Algeria, Batna	50.0	50.0	-	-	-	-	-	-	2	3
Algeria, Constantine	25.0	25.0	25.0	25.0	-	-	-	-	4	4
Algeria, Oran	65.4	3.8	19.2	-	7.7	-	-	3.8	26	26
Algeria, Setif	44.4	-	55.6	-	-	-	-	-	9	9
Burkina Faso, Ouagadougou	28.6	-	28.6	28.6	-	14.3	-	-	7	16
Congo, Brazzaville	50.0	-	16.7	16.7	-	-	-	16.7	6	15
France, La Reunion	30.8	23.1	30.8	-	7.7	7.7	-	-	13	14
The Gambia	16.7	-	50.0	-	-	33.3	-	-	6	11
Guinea, Conakry	-	-	75.0	-	25.0	-	-	-	4	41
Kenya, Eldoret	21.4	14.3	50.0	-	-	14.3	-	-	14	14
Malawi, Blantyre	8.3	2.8	80.6	-	2.8	2.8	-	2.8	36	43
Mali, Bamako	67.7	-	19.4	-	3.2	9.7	-	-	31	53
Namibia	12.9	1.2	80.0	-	-	3.5	-	2.4	85	87
Niger, Niamey	25.0	16.7	41.7	-	16.7	-	-	-	12	22
Nigeria, Ibadan	71.4	-	28.6	-	-	-	-	-	14	22
Rwanda, Butare	8.3	8.3	16.7	-	-	8.3	-	58.3	12	14
South Africa: Black	33.1	1.9	45.9	2.1	0.4	3.6	0.2	12.8	477	477
South Africa: White	20.7	19.0	52.5	1.1	2.8	2.2	0.6	1.1	179	179
South Africa: Indian	60.0	-	10.0	-	10.0	-	-	20.0	10	10
South Africa: Mixed race	48.6	14.3	31.4	2.9	-	2.9	-	-	35	35
South Africa, Elim	36.8	5.3	52.6	-	5.3	-	-	-	19	21
South Africa, Transkei, Umtata	-	-	-	-	-	-	-	-	-	-
South Africa, Transkei, 4 districts	40.0	-	40.0	-	-	-	-	20.0	5	5
Swaziland	7.7	3.8	84.6	3.8	-	-	-	-	26	29
Tanzania, Dar Es Salaam	23.5	-	58.8	5.9	2.9	4.4	2.9	1.5	68	68
Tanzania, Kilimanjaro	14.1	-	78.1	1.6	6.3	-	-	-	64	66
Tunisia, Centre, Sousse	40.0	10.0	50.0	-	-	-	-	-	10	10
Tunisia, North, Tunis	15.4	23.1	61.5	-	-	-	-	-	13	15
Tunisia, Sfax	-	-	-	66.7	-	-	33.3	-	3	3
Uganda, Mbarara	45.0	5.0	40.0	10.0	-	-	-	-	20	22
Uganda, Kyadondo County	14.0	2.2	78.5	1.1	2.2	-	-	2.2	93	140
Zimbabwe, Harare: African	20.9	-	73.4	1.3	1.9	1.9	0.6	-	158	174
Zimbabwe, Harare: European	-	16.7	66.7	-	-	-	16.7	-	6	6

Holly, E., Aston, D.A., Char, D.H., Kristiansen, J.J. & Ahn, D.K. (1990) Uveal melanoma in relation to ultraviolet light exposure and host factors. *Cancer Res.*, **50**, 5773–5777

IARC (1995) IARC *Monographs on the Evaluation of Carcinogenic Risks to Humans,* Vol. 64, *Human Papillomaviruses,* Lyon, IARC

IARC (1996) IARC *Monographs on the Evaluation of Carcinogenic Risks to Humans,* Vol. 67, *Human Immunodeficiency Viruses and Human T-cell Lymphotropic Viruses,* Lyon, IARC

Klauss, V. & Chana, H.S. (1983) Ocular tumors in Africa. *Soc. Sci. Med.*, **17**, 1743–1750

Malik, M.O.A. & Sheikh, E.H. (1979) Tumours of the eye and adnexa in Sudan. *Cancer*, **44**, 293–303

Newton, R. (1996) A review of the aetiology of squamous cell carcinoma of the conjunctiva. *Br. J. Cancer*, **74**, 1511–1513

Newton, R., Ferlay, J., Reeves, G., Beral, V. & Parkin, D.M. (1996) Effect of ambient ultraviolet radiation on incidence of squamous cell carcinoma of the eye. *Lancet*, **347**, 1450–1451

Newton, R., Ziegler, J., Ateenyi-Agaba, C., Bousarghin, L., Casabonne, D., Beral, V., Mbidde, E., Carpenter, L., Reeves, G., Parkin, D.M., Wabinga, H., Mbulaiteye, S., Jaffe, H., Bourboulia, D., Boshoff, C., Touze, A. & Coursaget, P. (2002) The epidemiology of conjunctival squamous cell carcinoma in Uganda. *Br. J. Cancer*, **87**, 301–308

Olurin, O. & Williams, A.O. (1972) Orbito-ocular tumors in Nigeria. *Cancer*, **30**, 580–587

Parkin, D.M., Whelan, S.L., Ferlay, J., Raymond, L. & Young, J., eds (1997) *Cancer Incidence in Five Continents,* Vol. VII (IARC Scientific Publications No. 143) Lyon, IARC

Seddon, J.M., Gragoudas, E.S., Glynn, R.J., Egan, K.M., Albert, D.M. & Blitzer, P.H. (1990) Host factors, UV radiation, and risk of uveal melanoma. A case control study. *Arch. Ophthalmol.*, **108**, 1274–1280

Sun, E.C., Fears, T.R. & Goedert, J.J. (1997) Epidemiology of squamous cell conjunctival cancer. *Cancer Epidemiol. Biomarkers Prev.*, **6**, 73–77

Templeton, A.C. (1967) Tumours of the eye and adnexa in Africans of Uganda. *Cancer*, **20**, 1689-1698.

Templeton, A.C. (1973) Tumours of the eye and adnexa. In: Templeton, A.C., ed. Tumours of a Tropical Country: a Survey of Uganda 1964–1968. *Recent Results in Cancer Research*, pp. 203–214

Wabinga, H.R., Parkin, D.M., Wabwire-Mangen, F. & Nambooze, S. (2000) Trends in incidence in Kyadondo County, Uganda, 1960–1997. *Br. J. Cancer*, **82**, 1585–1592

Table 4. Age-standardized (world) and cumulative (0-64) incidence
Conjunctiva: squamous cell carcinoma*

	MALE				FEMALE			
	Cases	CRUDE	ASR(W)	Cumulative	Cases	CRUDE	ASR(W)	Cumulative
		(per 100,000)		(%)		(per 100,000)		(%)
Africa, North								
Algeria, Algiers (1993-1997)	1	0.0	**0.0**	-	2	0.0	**0.0**	0.00
Algeria, Constantine (1994-1997)	-	-	**-**	-	-	-	**-**	-
Algeria, Oran (1996-1998)	2	0.1	**0.2**	-	2	0.1	**0.1**	0.00
Algeria, Setif (1993-1997)	1	0.0	**0.0**	0.00	2	0.1	**0.1**	0.00
Tunisia, Centre, Sousse (1993-1997)	1	0.1	**0.1**	0.02	-	-	**-**	-
Tunisia, North, Tunis (1994)	1	0.0	**0.1**	0.01	-	-	**-**	-
Tunisia, Sfax (1997)	-	-	**-**	-	-	-	**-**	-
Africa, West								
The Gambia (1997-1998)	2	0.2	**0.4**	0.03	2	0.2	**0.2**	0.01
Guinea, Conakry (1996-1999)	13	0.6	**0.9**	0.08	3	0.1	**0.1**	0.01
Mali, Bamako (1988-1997)	5	0.1	**0.2**	0.01	1	0.0	**0.1**	-
Niger, Niamey (1993-1999)	1	0.1	**0.2**	0.02	1	0.1	**0.3**	-
Nigeria, Ibadan (1998-1999)	3	0.2	**0.4**	0.00	-	-	**-**	-
Africa, Central								
Congo, Brazzaville (1996-1999)	1	0.1	**0.1**	0.01	-	-	**-**	-
Africa, East								
France, La Reunion (1988-1994)	2	0.1	**0.1**	0.00	-	-	**-**	-
Kenya, Eldoret (1998-2000)	4	0.4	**0.5**	0.04	3	0.3	**0.4**	0.03
Malawi, Blantyre (2000-2001)	13	1.4	**2.0**	0.07	17	2.0	**2.6**	0.23
Uganda, Kyadondo County (1993-1997)	57	2.0	**2.3**	0.20	47	1.6	**2.0**	0.16
Zimbabwe, Harare: African (1990-1993)	5	0.2	**0.3**	0.02	5	0.2	**0.2**	0.02
Zimbabwe, Harare: African (1994-1997)	43	1.5	**1.5**	0.12	56	2.1	**2.5**	0.17
Zimbabwe, Harare: European (1990-1997)	2	1.3	**0.7**	0.05	-	-	**-**	-
Africa, South								
Namibia (1995-1998)	35	1.1	**1.5**	0.12	33	1.0	**1.3**	0.11
South Africa: Black (1989-1992)	84	0.1	**0.2**	0.01	63	0.1	**0.1**	0.01
South Africa: Indian (1989-1992)	1	0.1	**0.1**	-	-	-	**-**	-
South Africa: Mixed race (1989-1992)	2	0.0	**0.1**	-	8	0.1	**0.1**	0.01
South Africa: White (1989-1992)	57	0.6	**0.5**	0.03	20	0.2	**0.2**	0.01
South Africa, Transkei, Umtata (1996-1998)	-	-	**-**	-	-	-	**-**	-
South Africa, Transkei, 4 districts (1996-1998)	-	-	**-**	-	2	0.2	**0.3**	0.01
Swaziland (1996-1999)	14	0.8	**1.2**	0.11	9	0.5	**0.6**	0.06
Europe/USA								
USA, SEER: White (1993-1997)	40	0.1	**0.1**	0.00	9	0.0	**0.0**	0.00
USA, SEER: Black (1993-1997)	-	-	**-**	-	-	-	**-**	-
France, 8 registries (1993-1997)	9	0.1	**0.0**	0.00	4	0.0	**0.0**	-
The Netherlands (1993-1997)	6	0.0	**0.0**	0.00	1	0.0	**0.0**	0.00
UK, England (1993-1997)	23	0.0	**0.0**	0.00	10	0.0	**0.0**	0.00

* Includes conjunctival neoplasm (C69.0) with unspecified histology or carcinoma NOS (M8000-8034), and
squamous cell carcinoma (M8070) of eye, NOS (C69.9)
In italics: histopathology-based registries

4.6 Kaposi sarcoma

Introduction

Kaposi sarcoma is a tumour arising from a pluripotential angioformative cell, or angioblast. The cells of the tumour show features of venous endothelial, fibroblastic, smooth muscle and peripheral cell differentiation. The early patch-stage macular lesions contain abnormally shaped, dilated vessels surrounded by a mononuclear-cell infiltrate containing plasma cells; nuclear atypia and mitoses are rarely seen. In the plaque-stage lesions, there is proliferation of spindle-shaped cells in the superficial-to-deep dermis, with rare proliferation of spindle-shaped cells, nuclear atypia and mitoses. Spindle cells, which often surround slit-like vascular spaces, are characteristic of more advanced nodular lesions.

Epidemiologically, Kaposi sarcoma has been classified into sporadic (classic), endemic (African), epidemic (AIDS-related) and immunosuppression-associated (usually in transplant recipients) types; however, the histopathology of all of these types is identical (Templeton, 1981).

The earliest reports from Africa describe the presence of Kaposi sarcoma (KS) histopathology slides in South Africa as early as 1912 (Oettlé, 1962) and in the Cameroon in 1914 (Gigase, 1984). Since about 1950, it was noted that this tumour had an unusual worldwide distribution, with the highest incidence in central Africa. Although rarer, KS was also found in southern and northern Africa and countries around the Mediterranean littoral and the Middle East. It was almost non-existent elsewhere, except in immigrants from these endemic countries (Biggar et al., 1984, Grulich et al., 1992, Hjalgrim et al., 1996) and a few isolated clusters elsewhere.

In developed countries, KS was one of the most common cancers occurring among recipients of organ transplants (Penn, 1995; Margolius, 1995), especially if the recipients were of Mediterranean or Middle Eastern origin. Immune suppression caused by cancer chemotherapeutic drugs was found to be a risk factor for KS, and these observations led to suspicion that KS was caused by an infection (e.g., Kinlen, 1982). The appearance of an aggressive form of KS in 1981 in the United States among homosexual men heralded the onset of the HIV/AIDS epidemic (Centers for Disease Control, 1981) and it was suggested that KS was caused by a combination of a sexually transmitted agent and immune suppression (Peterman et al., 1993). In the meanwhile, as the HIV epidemic spread in East and then Southern Africa, KS became increasingly common. For example, in Kampala in 1989–92, KS was the most common cancer in males and the second most common cancer in females (Wabinga et al., 1993) and it is now the commonest cancer in males in Harare, Malawi, Rwanda, Zambia and possibly other central, eastern and southern African countries where cancer registration is non-existent. In 1996, a new virus of the herpes virus family (human herpesvirus 8 (HHV-8)) was found to be present in almost all tissues of KS (Chang et al., 1994) and this virus is now thought to be the cause of KS (Chang et al., 1994; Whitby et al., 1995). The close association between KS and immune suppression (post-transplant, cancer chemotherapy or HIV-induced) suggests that KS is under tight immunological control (Boshoff & Moore, 1998).

Distribution in Africa before the advent of HIV: endemic KS

'Classic' or endemic Kaposi sarcoma affects predominantly the skin of the lower limbs; internal organs are rarely involved, Figure 1. The disease typically follows an indolent course, patients surviving for an average of 10–15 years (Templeton & Bhana, 1975). Young children tend to have more severe disease than adults, with a corresponding poorer prognosis. The sex distribution is more equal than in adults and the lesions often affect the lymphatic system and

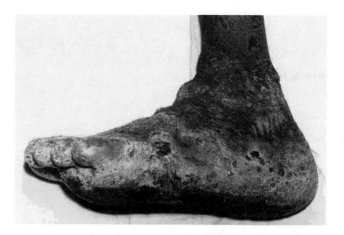

Figure 1. Kaposi sarcoma.

internal organs rather than the skin (Oettlé, 1962; Slavin et al., 1970; Olweny et al., 1976; Ziegler & Katongole-Mbidde, 1996).

A number of reviews described the striking distribution of KS in Africa before the advent of HIV, defined here for practical reasons as before 1980 (Oettlé, 1962; Templeton, 1981; Hutt, 1981, 1984; Gigase, 1984; Cook-Mozzaffari et al., 1998). Figure 2 draws together results of these early studies, in terms of relative frequency of KS in clinical series from different regions.

KS appeared to have an 'epicentre' around the West Nile district in Uganda and the north-west of the Democratic Republic of the Congo (former Zaire), with relative frequencies ranging between 5% and 18% of all cancers (Oettlé, 1962; Templeton, 1981; Hutt & Burkitt, 1965; Hutt 1981; Oates et al., 1984) stretching to the west

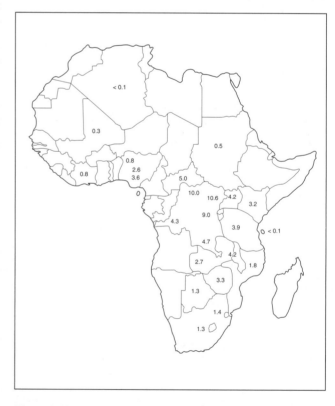

Figure 2. Map showing percentage frequency of Kaposi sarcoma (both sexes combined) (from Hutt, 1984)

286

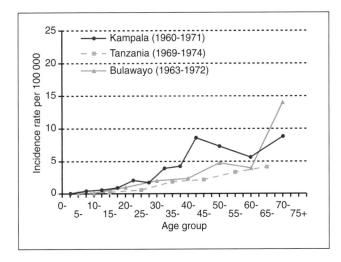

Figure 3. Kaposi sarcoma: estimated incidence in males
Sources: Wabinga *et al.*, 2000; Bland *et al.*, 1977; Skinner *et al.*, 1993

coast of the Cameroon (Jensen *et al.*, 1978) and to the south along the rift valley to southern Africa (Oettlé, 1962). The cumulative incidence rate of KS around the West Nile district was estimated to be about 6–15 per 1000, i.e. similar to the incidence of colon cancer in certain developed countries (Cook-Mozzaffari *et al.*, 1998). Cook-Mozzaffari *et al.* (1998) speculate that the distribution of KS shows an original focus in the high altitudes of north-eastern Zaire spreading via trade or migration routes to North Africa, Mecca and the Mediterranean littoral, and to the mines of southern Africa.

KS was rare (comprising about 1% of all cancers or less) in western, northern and southern Africa, although even in these places the estimated cumulative incidence of about 1 per 1000 was much greater than that seen in countries such as the United Kingdom, United States, Norway and Sweden, where the cumulative incidence of KS was typically around 0.005 per thousand or less, comprising about 0.3% of male and 0.1% or less of female cancers (Hjalgrim *et al.*, 1996; Grulich *et al.*, 1992; Gigase, 1984).

Age and sex
Endemic KS in Africa was primarily a disease of the elderly, with incidence rates rising progressively after the age of 30–35 years. In older age groups, KS was about 10 times more common in men than women (Oettlé, 1962; Hutt, 1981). Figure 3 shows estimated incidence in men in Kampala Uganda in 1960–71 (Wabinga *et al.*, 2000), in Tanzania in 1972–74 (Bland *et al.*, 1977) and in Bulawayo, Zimbabwe in 1963–72 (Skinner *et al.*, 1993).

The sex ratio (M:F) of sporadic KS in developed countries varies from about 3:1 in the United States and Sweden to 1:1 in the United Kingdom (Grulich *et al.*, 1992). Hormonal factors have been postulated as the reason for the male:female differences but possible mechanisms underlying these findings remain unclear.

Within-country contrasts
Striking within-country distributions of KS were documented within Uganda and the Democratic Republic of the Congo, with populations around the West Nile district and the areas bordering Lake Kivu showing the greatest relative frequencies in Africa and worldwide. In Kenya and Tanzania, KS comprised about 3–5% of all cancers, whereas on the island of Zanzibar, 0.1% of all cancers (Hutt, 1984; Oettlé, 1962). In the early reviews, KS was reported to be common in southern Sudan, but absent in the north (Malik *et al.*, 1974).

Geographical and/or ethnic differences in frequency of KS have been described in Uganda (Hutt & Burkitt, 1965; Cook & Burkitt, 1971; Taylor *et al.*, 1972; Owor & Hutt, 1977), Tanzania (Bland *et al.*, 1977) and Kenya (Rogoff, 1968). Hutt (1981), however, suggested that geographical rather than ethnic or sociocultural factors appeared more important. It is unclear whether these and the within-country differences suggest some lifestyle, genetic or geographical difference in environmental exposure. In South Africa, pre-AIDS KS was rarer in whites, coloureds and Indians than in blacks, suggesting that some sociodemographic factors may play an important role in certain places.

Migrant studies
Pre-AIDS reports from developed countries suggested that KS was a disease of men of Italian or Jewish origin (Rothman, 1962). Nevertheless, in the United Kingdom, immigrants from central and west Africa, the Middle East and the Caribbean had greater relative risks of developing KS (about 8- to 50-fold) compared with, e.g., Irish immigrants (RR = 1.1; Grulich *et al.*, 1992). No cases of KS were found in the American negro population of Washington, DC in 1965–69 (Kovi & Heshmat, 1972). Similarly in Haiti, inhabited by black populations originating from the West African coast, no cases of KS were recorded before 1979; however, between 1979 and 1984, KS comprised 4.3% of all male and 1.3% of all female cancers (Mitacek *et al.*, 1986). Reasons for the absence of KS among migrants of African origin in France, Haiti and the United States before the advent of AIDS are unclear, but it is possible that these populations originated from places where the pre-AIDS incidence of KS was low.

Environmental and genetic determinants of risk
On the basis of the geographical distribution of KS, high rainfall (Gigase, 1984), humidity or proximity to water (Ziegler *et al.*, 1997), high rural density and altitudes over 600 m (Cook-Mozzaffari *et al.*, 1998) and residence on volcanic soils (Ziegler, 1993) have been suggested as risk factors for development of KS, but confounding by other factors associated with these exposures cannot be ruled out. In rural Africa, many of these features are closely correlated (Cook-Mozzaffari *et al.*, 1998), as they are found in the most fertile and therefore the most populated places.

There have been disappointingly few individual-based studies of potential risk factors for endemic KS. Early studies in Europe and the United States suggested that markers of infection by cytomegalovirus (CMV) were more frequent in cases of KS than in control subjects (Giraldo *et al.*, 1984). However, in Africa, although subjects with KS also had high titres of antibody to CMV, they were not significantly different from those in the age–sex-matched control subjects (Giraldo *et al.*, 1981). The tiny case–control study of McHardy *et al.* (1984) in the West Nile district of Uganda (19 cases, 19 controls) had insufficient power to detect all but the grossest risks. Cases were more prone to drink water from rivers or to have received bites from various types of insect, though neither was close to statistical significance. Kestens *et al.* (1985) studied 27 cases of clinically endemic KS (histologically confirmed) and 41 age-, sex- and tribe-matched controls from Katana in eastern Zaire (Congo). All were HIV (HTLV III)-negative and the authors found no association with immune status (as judged by immunoglobulin levels, counts of different lymphocyte subsets, skin test reactivity, etc.) and antibody titres to various viruses (Epstein–Barr, CMV, hepatitis B) were similar in cases and controls. In a later report on 23 of these KS cases and 23 matched controls, Melbye *et al.* (1987) found no difference with respect to HLA antigens, notably DR5 and DR3. These had been suspected as being linked to KS (sporadic and AIDS-related) susceptibility in earlier studies in the United States and Europe.

KS after HIV: epidemic KS
In the 'epidemic' form of KS, the lesions are usually multiple, progress rapidly and may affect any area of the skin as well as internal organs. The tumours frequently begin as dusky red or violet macules, progressing over weeks or months to plaques and raised, usually painless, firm nodules and plaques. Although the tumour may affect

the legs, as seen with 'classic' KS, lesions of the trunk, arms, genitalia and face are also common. Lymph nodes and the oral cavity, most notably the palate, may be extensively involved. Oral KS is often associated with involvement elsewhere in the gastrointestinal tract (Levine, 1993). Pulmonary KS generally presents with shortness of breath and cough and is clinically difficult to distinguish from other pulmonary complications of AIDS (Levine, 1993).

Although the incidence of KS has increased a thousand-fold or more in populations at high risk of HIV in, for example, the United States (Biggar et al., 1984; Rabkin et al., 1991), in the rest of the population the tumour still remains relatively rare (Rabkin et al., 1991; Grulich et al., 1992). In Africa, an increase in the frequency of KS cases, with the clinical features described above, was noted first in Zambia in the early 1980s (Bayley, 1984). In the following 10–15 years, in areas with a high prevalence of HIV infection and where KS was relatively common before the era of AIDS, the incidence of KS has increased about 20-fold, for example in Malawi, Swaziland, Uganda and Zimbabwe, and it is now the most common cancer in men and the second most common in women (Wabinga et al., 1993; Bassett et al., 1995; Banda et al., 2001; Wabinga et al., 2000).

The incidence of KS (age-standardized incidence per 100 000 person years) from the series presented in this volume is shown in Table 1. Age-standardized incidence of KS is highest in Kyadondo county in Uganda (M = 37.7, F = 20.5), Blantyre, Malawi (M = 49.9, F = 31.7), Harare, Zimbabwe (African) (M = 50.9, F = 21.6) and Swaziland (M = 17.2, F = 9.5). In the black population in South Africa, the incidence of KS (until 1992) was low (males = 0.7, females = 0.2, Sitas et al., 1997), but about a three-fold increase occurred between 1993 and 1995 (Sitas et al., 1998), in keeping with the increases seen in Uganda and other central African countries at the beginning of the HIV epidemic. In West Africa the incidence of KS is low—less than 2/100 000 in males and 1 per 100 000 in females. In both South and West Africa, however, HIV was introduced later than in the countries of East and Central Africa. Overall, there does appear to be a geographical association between the median prevalence of HIV in different countries (see Chapter 6, Table 1) and the incidence of KS.

Age-specific incidence

Since the early 1990s, the age-specific incidence rates in countries of East and Central Africa have been markedly influenced by the prevalence of infection with HIV. Thus, incidence shows a pattern reminiscent of the prevalence of HIV infection, with a modest peak for children aged zero to four years, a decline until age 15 years and then a progressive increase to a peak at age 35–39 years in men and 25–29 years in women (Figure 4).

KS in children

A few reports have described the incidence of KS in children in Africa. Bland et al. (1977) reported an incidence of KS in children (0–9 years) in Tanzania between 1969 and 1974 of 1.1 per million in boys and 0.6 per million in girls, whereas in Nigeria it appeared to be rare (< 0.1% of childhood cancers; see Chapter 3.2.13, Table 6). The incidence of KS in children In Zambia has increased since the HIV epidemic (Chintu et al., 1995) and in the rest of Africa, KS in childhood comprises about 10% of all childhood cancers and has increased to about 10 per million (see tables).

Risk factors

HIV

Four case–control studies in Africa have assessed the relationship between HIV and KS. All found elevated relative risks between HIV and KS: 35 in Rwanda (Newton et al., 1995), 62 in Johannesburg (Sitas et al., 1997), 95 in children from Uganda (Newton et al., 2001) and 22 in a later study in Johannesburg (Sitas et al., 2000). The relative risks found in the African studies are much lower than those found among HIV-infected people in developed countries, which are

usually 300 or more (Goedert et al., 1998). Complex pathology and rapid mortality may hide some of the cancers that occur in association with HIV in Africa. However, as the pre-AIDS incidence of KS in Africa was much greater than elsewhere, it is not surprising that the relative risks in Africa in association with HIV and the magnitude of the increase over time are much lower in Africa. In the Gambia, Ariyoshi et al. (1998) observed 15 cases of KS among 609 HIV-1-positive subjects diagnosed in 1986–96 in two hospitals, compared with one case among 636 persons found to be positive for HIV-2. This corresponds to an OR (adjusted for sex and CD4%) of 12.4 (95% CI 1.5–100.6) for KS in HIV-1 infection, relative to HIV-2.

Human herpes virus 8 (HHV-8)/Kaposi sarcoma herpes virus

Occurrence: Human herpesvirus-8 (HHV-8), a recently discovered human herpesvirus (Chang et al., 1994), has been consistently associated with KS and is now considered to be the principal cause of the disease (Whitby et al., 1995; Boshoff, 1999). Hayward (1999) suggests that HHV-8 is an ancient human virus and its distribution using nucleotide sequence analysis of the ORF K1 subtype reflects the migration of human populations 35 000–60 000 years ago.

A number of assays have been developed to measure the presence of antibodies to HHV-8 in human sera for diagnostic and epidemiological purposes. There is variation in both the sensitivity and the specificity of these assays (Engels et al., 2000a), but in general, HHV-8 seroprevalence in 'normal' populations (i.e., blood donors, patients without KS and population samples) appears to be highest in Africa (prevalence varying from 10 to 100%, depending on the assay), intermediate in the Middle East and Mediterranean littoral and lowest in northern Europe (Chatlynne & Ablashi, 1999). In Uganda, for example, the prevalences of HHV-8 infection were between 53% and 77% (Gao et al., 1996b; Lennette et al., 1996; Simpson et al., 1996). Testing sera obtained from a variety of different patient groups in the West Nile district of Uganda in 1972–75, de The et al. (1999) found a seroprevalence of 84% in adults. In the high-incidence areas of eastern Congo (Zaire), prevalence of HHV-8 was 82% in 1984 (Engels et al., 2000b).

In all reported series, there has been no difference in seroprevalence between men and women.

Epidemiology: HHV-8 appears to be transmitted by sexual contact in developed countries (Martin et al., 1998). Men who develop KS tend to be more sexually active and to have more sexual partners from epicentres of the AIDS epidemic. In conjunction with the much higher risk for KS among homosexual men than among other HIV transmission groups, these data indicate that an infectious sexually transmitted agent (independent of HIV) is associated with KS. Transmission of such an agent via the blood is apparently less common, since KS occurs in only 3% of people who acquire HIV through a blood transfusion (IARC, 1996). Several serological studies have suggested that, irrespective of the type of antigen used, HHV-8 infection is more common among people attending sexually transmitted disease clinics than among blood donors (Kedes et al., 1996; Lennette et al., 1996; Simpson et al., 1996). Among Danish homosexual men, variables such as promiscuity and receptive anal intercourse increased the risk for HHV-8 infection, while, in the United States in the early 1980s, contact with homosexual men markedly enhanced the likelihood of having or acquiring antibodies to HHV8 (Melbye et al., 1998).

In Africa, sexual transmission is probably important in adolescents and young adults. In Uganda, increased risk for KS was seen in HIV-seropositive adults of each sex who had a history of sexually transmitted diseases, and especially those who were relatively affluent, well educated, and had travelled (Ziegler et al., 1997). In Cameroon, Rezza et al. (2000) found that a history of sexually transmitted diseases was an independent determinant of HHV-8 infection (adjusted odds ratio 2.47; 95% CI 1.09–4.91) and seroprevalence was higher in prostitutes than in pregnant women at

Table 1. Age-standardized (world) and cumulative (0-64) incidence
Kaposi sarcoma (C46)

	MALE				FEMALE			
	Cases	CRUDE	ASR(W) (per 100,000)	Cumulative (%)	Cases	CRUDE	ASR(W) (per 100,000)	Cumulative (%)
Africa, North								
Algeria, Algiers (1993-1997)	16	0.3	**0.4**	0.02	3	0.1	**0.1**	0.01
Algeria, Constantine (1994-1997)	2	0.1	**0.3**	-	2	0.1	**0.3**	0.02
Algeria, Oran (1996-1998)	3	0.2	**0.2**	0.02	1	0.1	**0.1**	0.01
Algeria, Setif (1993-1997)	-	-	**-**	-	1	0.0	**0.1**	-
Tunisia, Centre, Sousse (1993-1997)	11	1.0	**1.2**	0.05	3	0.3	**0.3**	0.00
Tunisia, North, Tunis (1994)	2	0.1	**0.1**	-	2	0.1	**0.1**	0.01
Tunisia, Sfax (1997)	1	0.3	**0.3**	-	1	0.3	**0.3**	0.04
Africa, West								
The Gambia (1997-1998)	4	0.4	**0.6**	0.04	4	0.4	**0.4**	0.03
Guinea, Conakry (1996-1999)	2	0.1	**0.2**	0.02	1	0.0	**0.0**	0.00
Mali, Bamako (1988-1997)	46	1.2	**1.8**	0.10	16	0.4	**0.7**	0.06
Niger, Niamey (1993-1999)	5	0.3	**0.3**	0.03	4	0.2	**0.2**	0.02
Nigeria, Ibadan (1998-1999)	3	0.2	**0.2**	0.02	1	0.1	**0.1**	0.00
Africa, Central								
Congo, Brazzaville (1996-1999)	37	3.1	**4.3**	0.34	14	1.2	**1.4**	0.11
Africa, East								
France, La Reunion (1988-1994)	9	0.4	**0.4**	0.03	-	-	**-**	-
Kenya, Eldoret (1998-2000)	35	3.7	**5.8**	0.51	15	1.6	**2.4**	0.21
Malawi, Blantyre (2000-2001)	385	42.8	**49.9**	4.15	234	27.0	**31.7**	2.58
Uganda, Kyadondo County (1993-1997)	843	30.0	**37.7**	2.94	533	18.4	**20.5**	1.49
Zimbabwe, Harare: African (1990-1993)	679	28.6	**31.3**	2.45	185	8.7	**9.4**	0.75
Zimbabwe, Harare: African (1994-1997)	1278	45.8	**50.9**	4.15	482	18.3	**21.6**	1.70
Zimbabwe, Harare: European (1990-1997)	2	1.3	**1.3**	0.09	-	-	**-**	-
Africa, South								
Namibia (1995-1998)	158	5.0	**6.8**	0.53	54	1.7	**1.9**	0.13
South Africa: Black (1989-1992)	232	0.4	**0.7**	0.04	69	0.1	**0.2**	0.01
South Africa: Indian (1989-1992)	2	0.1	**0.2**	0.00	2	0.1	**0.1**	0.00
South Africa: Mixed race (1989-1992)	23	0.4	**0.6**	0.03	5	0.1	**0.1**	0.00
South Africa: White (1989-1992)	68	0.7	**0.6**	0.03	17	0.2	**0.1**	0.01
South Africa, Transkei, Umtata (1996-1998)	1	0.3	**0.3**	0.02	-	-	**-**	-
South Africa, Transkei, 4 districts (1996-1998)	2	0.3	**0.7**	0.07	1	0.1	**0.1**	0.01
Swaziland (1996-1999)	209	11.9	**17.2**	1.37	164	8.4	**9.5**	0.70
Europe/USA								
USA, SEER: White (1993-1997)	2788	5.7	**4.4**	0.36	70	0.1	**0.1**	0.00
USA, SEER: Black (1993-1997)	560	8.4	**6.8**	0.55	32	0.4	**0.3**	0.02
France, 8 registries (1993-1997)	204	1.5	**1.2**	0.09	26	0.2	**0.1**	0.01
The Netherlands (1993-1997)	425	1.1	**0.8**	0.07	25	0.1	**0.0**	0.00
UK, England (1993-1997)	672	0.6	**0.5**	0.04	68	0.1	**0.0**	0.00

In italics: histopathology-based registries

an antenatal clinic (Bestetti *et al.*, 1998). In South Africa, Sitas *et al.* (1999a) found an association with number of lifetime sexual partners. Ariyoshi *et al.* (1998) did not, however, find any association between infection with HHV-8 and serological evidence (treponema pallidum antibody; TPA) of syphilis in Gambia.

Other risk factors for HHV-8 include lower standard of education (Olsen *et al.*, 1998; Sitas *et al.*, 1999a), birth in a rural area (Sitas *et al.*, 1999a) and having an HHV-8-positive mother (Bourboulia *et al.*, 1998), especially if the mother has high antibody titres against HHV-8 (Sitas *et al.*, 1999b).

Antibody to HHV-8 is transmitted transplacentally, so that most children born to seropositive mothers have antibody present at birth, although titres fall rapidly thereafter (Gessain *et al.*, 1999; Mantina *et al.*, 2001). However, prevalence of antibody to HHV-8 is higher in older children whose mothers are HHV-8-positive, suggesting that transmission of HHV-8 from mother to child is possible. A study of South African mothers and their children revealed that about 30% of the children (under 10 years) of HHV-8-seropositive mothers were themselves HHV-8-seropositive, whereas none of the children of HHV-8-seronegative mothers were HHV-8-seropositive

(Bourboulia *et al.*, 1998) Furthermore, the proportion of children who were seropositive for HHV-8 increased in relation to their mothers' HHV-8 antibody titre; the data suggested that HHV-8 seropositive mothers with high titer may be about twice as likely to have HHV-8-seropositive children as mothers with a low titre (Sitas *et al.*, 1999b). In a study of 89 HHV-8-seropositive mothers and their children in Lusaka, Zambia, Mantina *et al.* (2001) observed 13 mothers (14.6%) with HHV-8 DNA detectable in peripheral blood mononuclear cells. 83% of the neonates (< 24 hours old) were seropositive and two also had HHV-8 DNA detectable in peripheral blood mononuclear cells. This suggests that vertical mother-to-child transmission does occur, but that it is rather rare.

On the other hand, the steady increase in the prevalence of HHV-8 infection throughout childhood suggests that transmission of the virus from person to person, via non-sexual routes, may be more important (Wilkinson *et al.*, 1999; Mayama *et al.*, 1998; Olsen *et al.*, 1998; de Thé *et al.*, 1999; Sitas *et al.*, 1999a). The presence of HHV-8 DNA sequences in mucosal secretions (oral, vaginal) of women with KS lesions in Zimbabwe suggests possible routes of transmission (Lampinen *et al.*, 2000).

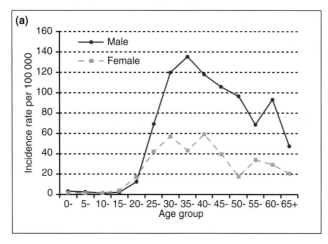

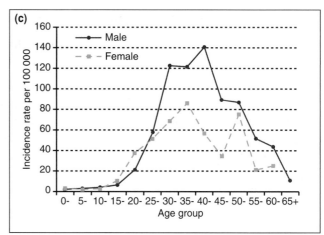

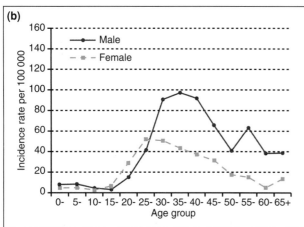

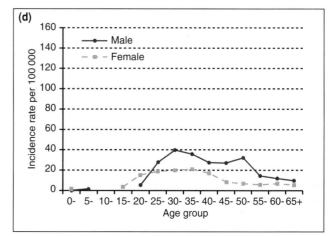

Figure 4. Incidence of Kaposi sarcoma in (a) Zimbabwe, (b) Uganda, (c) Malawi and (d) Swaziland

A recent study in Uganda showed that HHV-8-seropositivity in children was strongly correlated with the presence of antibodies to hepatitis B core antigen (Mayama *et al.*, 1998) Hepatitis B virus is known to be transmitted from person to person and this finding may suggest a similar route for HHV-8 (Abdool Karim *et al.*, 1988). The linear increase of HHV-8 infection with age of child suggests a causal horizontal pattern of infection, similar to that of other herpes viruses, between mothers and possibly other family members before puberty (Gessain *et al.*, 1999; Lyall *et al.*, 1999; Mayama *et al.*, 1998). In Egypt, young children (1–3 years) had higher titres of anti-lytic antibodies, suggesting the time of greatest risk of HHV-8 acquisition and/or viral activity in this group (Andreoni *et al.*, 1999)

In South Africa, the lower seroprevalence of HHV-8 in whites compared with blacks, and the decrease in seroprevalence with increasing education (Sitas *et al.*, 1999a) suggests that factors associated with poverty contribute to transmission of the virus. In contrast to this association between poverty and acquisition of HHV-8, in Uganda the development of KS, irrespective of HIV status, appears to be associated with markers of higher social class, such as better education and wealth (Ziegler *et al.*, 1997, 1998).

If high social status protects an individual from early infection with HHV-8, it could imply that the age at which infection occurs (or even the route of infection) could affect the subsequent risk of KS. This hypothesis is reminiscent of the effect of late infection with Epstein-Barr virus (a closely related gamma herpesvirus) in relation to the risk of infectious mononucleosis (Sitas *et al.*, 1999a).

Pathology: Kaposi sarcoma: DNA analysis has consistently demonstrated the presence of HHV-8 at high (>90%) rates in KS lesions (whether or not the patients are HIV-infected) and at a generally low rate in neoplastic and non-neoplastic tissues from

control patients (Boshoff & Weiss, 2001). The load of viral DNA is higher in tissue from KS than in unaffected tissues from the same patients. When mononuclear cells from KS patients and controls are examined using a polymerase chain reaction (PCR) method, HHV-8 is detected in significantly more cases (up to 50%) than controls (IARC, 1997). Detection of HHV-8 in peripheral blood correlates with, and in asymptomatic HIV-infected individuals predicts the development of, KS (Whitby *et al.*, 1995; Moore *et al.*, 1996), and sero-conversion (acquisition of anti-HHV-8 antibody) during HIV infection is predictive of development of KS (Renwick *et al.*, 1998).

Despite the differences in the antigens examined by the different serological tests for HHV-8, and in the sensitivity and specificity of these tests, all studies are consistent in showing high rates of antibody-positivity in KS patients and lower rates of seropositivity among various controls. A case–control study of black cancer patients in South Africa found that the presence of antibodies against HHV-8 was strongly associated with KS, but not with any other major cancer site or type, including prostate cancer and multiple myeloma (Sitas *et al.*, 1999a). In addition, the risk of KS increased with increasing antibody titre (as measured by the intensity of the fluorescent signal) to HHV-8, but, for a given titre, the risk was much greater in HIV-seropositive than in HIV-seronegative subjects. The highest fluorescent signal intensity for HHV-8, corresponding to an antibody titre of 1:204 800, was associated with a 12-fold increase in risk of KS among HIV-seronegative subjects, but with a more than 1600-fold increase in risk among HIV-seropositive subjects

No data on the relationship between HHV-8 antibody titre and viral load are available, but it can be presumed that a high anti-HHV-8 antibody titre reflects a high viral load and that it is this, rather than antibody titre, that primarily determines the risk of KS. Nevertheless, the relationship between high antibody titre and disease is reminiscent of the association between the related Epstein–Barr virus and African Burkitt lymphoma (de Thé *et al.*, 1978a) and nasopharyngeal cancer (de Thé *et al.*, 1978b), where individuals with high titres appear to be at highest risk of developing these cancers.

Nevertheless, it is clear that HHV-8 is not the only determinant of KS. Prevalence of infection is much the same in both sexes, despite the male excess of KS, especially the endemic form, in most of sub-Saharan Africa, but KS was rare in women before the AIDS epidemic (Serraino *et al.*, 2001). Furthermore, as far as one can tell from the data available, there does not seem to have been a close geographical correlation between prevalence of antibody to HHV-8 and the incidence of KS in the pre-AIDS era. Serraino *et al.* (2001) compared prevalence of lytic and latent antigens to HHV-8 in sera from subjects in northern Cameroon, northern Uganda, and Alexandia, Egypt. Prevalence of lytic antibody in adolescents (aged 13–19 years) was highest in Egypt (56.2% positive), an area where KS is rare, but prevalence of latent antibody was lower (8.3%) than in Cameroon and Uganda (19–26%). In adults, sero-prevalence was higher in Cameroon than in northern Uganda, although endemic KS is almost certainly more common in the latter. Ablashi *et al.* (1999) found no difference in prevalence of IgG antibody to HHV-8 (38–42%) between healthy adult subjects from Uganda, Zambia (areas of moderate to high risk of endemic KS) and Ghana (a low-risk area). A high prevalence of HHV-8 has been found in Gambia (Ariyoshi *et al.*, 1998) and Botswana (Engels *et al.*, 2000b), countries where KS was not a common cancer (see Chapters 3.2.5 and 3.5.1 and Figure 1).

Mechanisms: HHV-8 has numerous genes capable of deregulating mitosis, interrupting apoptosis (programmed cell death), increasing angiogenesis and blocking presentation of antigenic epitopes. It is conjectured that the virus may establish a persistent infection which (as with EBV) is normally controlled by the immune system. When immune control declines (e.g., due to AIDS), the number of HHV-8-infected cells increases, with subsequent unchecked proliferation and tumour development (Boshoff & Weiss, 2001).

Joint effects of HIV and HHV-8
It seems clear from the studies cited above that the risk of KS is increased both by infection with HIV and with HHV-8. However, most studies in Africa suggest that the association between infection with the two viruses is either weakly positive or inconsistent (Gao *et al.*, 1996a, b; Simpson *et al.*, 1996; Bestetti *et al.*, 1998; He *et al.*, 1998). In Gambia, Ariyoshi *et al.* (1998) found very little difference in prevalence of HHV-8 infection (by serology, or PCR to detect HHV-8 genome in peripheral blood mononuclear cells) between pregnant women who were HIV-1-positive (73% seropositive for HHV-8), HIV-2-positive (83% seropositive) or HIV-negative (79% seropositive). In South Africa, prevalence of antibody to HHV-8 was 30% in HIV-seropositive subjects and 33% in seronegative (Sitas *et al.*, 1999a). The latter study suggests that the effect of the two viruses on risk is independent (and more or less multiplicative). The effect of HIV is probably through immunosuppression, for example by allowing HHV-8 to escape control and increase viral load. In cohort studies in the United States and Europe, the risk of developing KS in HIV-positive subjects is related to the degree of immunosuppression, as measured by CD4+ lymphocyte counts (Goedert *et al.*, 1987; Hermans *et al.*, 1996; Rezza *et al.*, 1999).

The possible role of immunodeficiency in the etiology of endemic KS is clearly of interest, given the supposed role of immune surveillance in the control of latent infection with HHV-8. Early studies in Uganda (Master *et al.*, 1970; Taylor & Ziegler,

1974) suggested some impairment in skin reactivity to dinitrochlorobenzene. However, in their study in East Kivu (Congo) in 1984, Kestens *et al.* (1985), comparing 27 cases of endemic KS with 41 age–sex–tribe-matched control subjects (all HIV-negative), did not find any significant difference in terms of skin reactivity to a variety of recall antigens, and serum levels of immunoglobulin and complement factors. White blood cell counts and lymphocyte counts, as well as the absolute counts of CD4+ cells and CD8+ cells were slightly higher in cases than in controls, but there was no difference in the CD4/CD8 ratios. Conversely, a study of sporadic KS in Greece (Touloumi *et al.*, 1999) showed slightly lower white cell and lymphocyte counts in the KS cases, with a significantly low CD4+ lymphocyte count (mean 812 cells per µl compared with 1009 per µl in controls) that was not explained by overall lymphopenia. There were also significantly increased levels of neopterin and ß2-microglobulin, which are interferon-induced products suggesting immune activation.

A study in Tanzania (Urassa *et al.*, 1998) reported on lymphocyte counts in 39 endemic KS patients, 93 AIDS–KS patients and 82 unmatched controls. The HIV status of the cases was not reported. The main finding was a low CD4-T lymphocyte count in endemic KS, who also had a CD8-T lymphocyte count higher than the controls. However, the results are sometimes inconsistent and the very low CD4 count (mean 104 cells/µl) in endemic KS—significantly lower than in the AIDS–KS cases (mean 340 per µl)—suggests that some of the former group may have been HIV-positive.

The effect of HIV may also occur through different mechanisms. In vitro studies suggest that HIV-1 Tat may have angiogenic properties (Ensoli *et al.*, 1994), and that it may be responsible for activating HHV-8 (Harrington *et al.*, 1997). Nevertheless, the reasons for the dramatic increase in risk of developing KS among HHV-8-infected individuals who are HIV-seropositive remain unclear.

References

Abdool-Karim, S.S., Coovadia, H.C., Windsor, I.M., Thejpal, R., van der Ende, J. & Fouche, A. (1988) The prevalence and transmission of hepatitis B virus infection in urban, rural and institutional black children of Natal/KwaZulu, South Africa. *Int. J. Epidemiol.*, **17**, 168–173

Ablashi, D., Chatlynne, L., Cooper, H., Thomas, D., Yadav, M., Norhanom, A.W., Chandana, A.K., Churdboonchart, V., Kulpradist, S.A., Patnaik, M., Liegmann, K., Masood, R., Reitz, M., Cleghorn, F., Manns, A., Levine, P.H., Rabkin, C., Biggar, R., Jensen, F., Gill, P., Jack, N., Edwards, J., Whitman, J. & Boshoff, C. (1999) Seroprevalence of human herpesvirus-8 (HHV-8) in countries of Southeast Asia compared to the USA, the Caribbean and Africa. *Br. J. Cancer*, **81**, 893–897

Andreoni, M., El-Sawaf, G., Rezza, G., Ensoli, B., Nicastri, E., Ventura, L., Ercoli, L., Sarmati, L. & Rocchi, G. (1999) High seroprevalence of antibodies to human herpesvirus-8 in Egyptian children: evidence of nonsexual transmission. *J. Natl Cancer Inst.*, **91**, 465–469

Ariyoshi, K., Schim van der Loeff, M., Cook, P., Whitby, D., Corrah, T., Jaffar, S., Cham, F., Sabally, S., O'Donovan, D., Weiss, R.A., Schulz, T.F. & Whittle H. (1998) Kaposi's sarcoma in the Gambia, West Africa, is less frequent in human immunodeficiency virus type 2 than in human immunodeficiency virus type I infection despite a high prevalence of human herpesvirus 8. *J. Hum. Virol.*, **1**, 193–199

Banda, L.T., Parkin, D.M., Dzamalala, C.P. & Liomba, N.G. (2001) Cancer incidence in Blantyre, Malawi 1994-1998. *Trop. Med. Int. Health*, **6**, 296–304

Bassett, M.T., Chokunonga, E., Mauchaza, B., Levy, L., Ferlay, J. & Parkin, D.M. (1995) Cancer in the African population of Harare, Zimbabwe in 1990-92. *Int. J. Cancer*, **63**, 29–36

Bayley, A.C. (1984) Aggressive Kaposi's sarcoma in Zambia, 1983. *Lancet*, **i**, 1318–1320

Bestetti, G., Renon, G., Mauclere, P., Ruffie, A., Mbopi Keou, F.X., Eme, D., Parravicini, C., Corbellino, M., de Thé, G., Gessain, A. (1998) High seroprevalence of human herpesvirus-8 in pregnant women and prostitutes from Cameroon. *AIDS*, **12**, 541–543

Biggar, R.J., Horm, J., Fraumeni, J.F., Greene, M.H. & Goedert, J.J. (1984) Incidence of Kaposi's sarcoma and mycosis fungoides in the United States including Puerto Rico, 1973-1981. *J. Natl Cancer Inst.*, **73**, 89-94

Bland, J.M., Mutoka, C. & Hutt, M.S.R. (1977) Kaposi's sarcoma in Tanzania. *E. Afr J. Med. Sci.*, **4**, 47–53

Boshoff, C. (1999) Kaposi's sarcoma associated herpesvirus. In: Newton, R., Beral, V. & Weiss, R., eds, *Cancer Surveys, volume 33, Infections and Human Cancer*, Cold Spring Harbor Laboratory Press

Boshoff, C. & Moore, P.S. (1998) Kaposi_s sarcoma-associated herpesvirus: a newly recognized pathogen. In: Volberding, P. & Jacobson, M.A., eds, *AIDS Clinical Review 1997/1998*, New York, Marcel Dekker, pp. 323–347

Boshoff, C. & Weiss, R.A. (2001) Epidemiology and pathogenesis of Kaposi sarcoma-associated herpesvirus. *Phil. Trans. R. Soc. Lond. B. Biol. Sci.*, **356**, 517–534

Bourboulia, D., Whitby, D., Boshoff, C., Newton, R., Beral, V., Carrara, H., Lane, A. & Sitas, F. (1998) Serologic evidence for mother to child transmission of Kaposi sarcoma associated herpesvirus infection. *J. Am. Med. Assoc.*, **280**, 31–32

Centers for Disease Control (1981) Kaposi's sarcoma and Pneumocystis pneumonia among homosexual men—New York City and California. *MMWR*, **30**, 305–308

Chang, Y., Cesarman, E., Pessin, M.S., Lee, F., Culpepper, J., Knowles, D.M. & Moore, P.S. (1994) Identification of Herpesvirus-like DNA sequences in AIDS-associated Kaposi's sarcoma. *Science*, **266**, 1865–1869

Chatlynne, L.G. & Ablashi, D.V. (1999) Seroepidemiology of Kaposi's sarcoma-associated herpesvirus (KSHV). *Semin. Cancer Biol.*, **9**, 175–185

Chintu, C. Atale, U.H. & Patil, P.S. (1995) Childhood cancers in Zambia before and after the HIV epidemic. *Arch. Dis. Child.*, **73**, 100–104

Cook-Mozaffari, P.J. & Burkitt, D.P. (1971) Cancer in Africa. *Br. Med. Bull.*, **27**, 14–20

Cook-Mozaffari, P., Newton, R., Beral, V. & Burkitt, D.P. (1998) The geographical distribution of Kaposi's sarcoma and of lymphomas in Africa before the AIDS epidemic. *Br. J. Cancer*, **78**, 1521–1528

de Thé, G., Geser, A., Day, N.E., Tukei, P.M., Williams, E.H., Beri, D.P., Smith, P.G., Dean, A.G., Bronkamm, G.W., Feorino, P. & Henle, W. (1978a) Epidemiological evidence for causal relationship between Epstein Barr virus and Burkitt's lymphoma from Ugandan prospective study. *Nature*, **274**, 751–761

de Thé, G., Lavoue, M.F. & Muenz, L. (1978b) Differences in EBV antibody titres of patients with nasopharyngeal carcinoma originating from areas of high, intermediate and low incidence areas. In: de Thé, G. & Ito, Y., eds, *Nasopharyngeal Carcinoma: Etiology and Control* (IARC Scientific Publications no. 20), Lyon, IARC, pp. 471–481

de Thé, G., Bestetti, G., van Beveren, M. & Gessain, M. (1999) Prevalence of human herpes virus 8 infection before the acquired immunodeficiency disease syndrome-related epidemic of Kaposi's sarcoma in East Africa. *J. Natl Cancer Inst.*, **91**, 1888–1889

Engels, E.A., Whitby, D., Goebel, P.B., Stossel, A., Waters, D., Pintus, A., Conti, L., Biggar, R.J. & Goedert, J.J. (2000a) Identifying human herpesvirus 8 infection: performance characteristics of serological assays. *J. Acquir. Immune Defic. Syndr.*, **23**, 346–354

Engels, E.A., Sinclair, M.D., Biggar, R.H., Whitby, D., Ebbesen, P., Goedert, J.J. & Gastwirth, J.L. (2000b) Latent class analysis of human herpesvirus 8 assay performance and infection prevalence in sub-Saharan African and Malta. *Int. J. Cancer*, **88**, 1003–1008

Ensoli, B., Gendelmen, R., Markhem, P., Fiorelli, V., Colombini., S., Raffeld, M., Cafaro, A., Chang, H.K., Brady, J.N. & Gallo, R.C. (1994) Synergy between basic fibroblast growth factor as HIV-1 Tat protein in induction of Kaposi's sarcoma. *Nature*, **371**, 674–680

Fife, K. & Bower, M. (1996) Recent insights into the pathogenesis of Kaposi's sarcoma. *Br. J. Cancer*, **73**, 1317–1322

Gao, S.J., Kingsley, L., Hoover, D.R., Spira, T.J., Rinaldo, C.R., Saah, A., Phair, J., Detels, R., Parry, P., Chang, Y. & Moore, P.S. (1996a) Seroconversion of antibodies to Kaposi's sarcoma-associated herpesvirus-related latent nuclear antigens prior to onset of Kaposi's sarcoma. *New Engl. J. Med.*, **335**, 233–241

Gao, S.-J., Kingsley, L., Li, M., Zheng, W., Parravicini, C., Ziegler, J.L., Newton, R., Rinaldo, C.R., Saah, A., Phair, J., Detels, R., Chang, Y. & Moore, P.S. (1996b) Seroprevalence of Kaposi's sarcoma-associated herpesvirus antibodies among Americans, Italians and Ugandans with and without Kaposi's sarcoma. *Nature Med.*, **2**, 925–928

Gessain, A., Mauclere, P., van Beveren, M., Plancoulaine, S., Ayouba, A., Essame-Oyono, J.L., Martin, P.M. & de The, G. (1999) Human herpesvirus 8 primary infection occurs during childhood in Cameroon, Central Africa. *Int. J. Cancer*, **81**, 189–192

Gigase, P.L. (1984) Epidemiologie du sarcome de Kaposi en Afrique. *Bull. Soc. Pathol. Ex.*, **77**, 546–559

Giraldo, G., Beth, E. & Kyalwazi, S.K. (1981) Etiological implications on Kaposi's sarcoma. In: Olweny, C.L.M., Hutt, M.S.R. & Owor R., eds, *Kaposi's Sarcoma. 2nd KS Symposium, Kampala, 1980. Antibiot. Chemother.*, **29**, 12–29

Giraldo, G., Beth, E. & Kyalwazi, S.K. (1984) Role of cytomegalovirus in Kaposi's sarcoma. In: Williams, A.O., O'Conor, G.T., De Thé, G.T. & Johnson, C.A., eds, *Virus-Associated Cancers in Africa* (IARC Scientific Publications No. 63), Lyon, IARC, pp. 583–606

Goedert, J.J., Biggar, R.J., Melbye, M.Mann, D.L., Wilson, S., Gail, M.H., Grossman, R.J., DiGioia, R.A., Sanchez, W.C., Weiss, S.H. & Blattner, W.A. (1987) Effect of T4 count and cofactors on the incidence of AIDS in homosexual men infected with human immunodeficiency virus. *J. Am. Med. Assoc.*, **257**, 331–334

Goedert, J.J., Coté, T.R., Virgo, P., Scoppa, S.M., Kingma, D.W., Gail, M.H., Jaffe, E.S. & Biggar, R.J. (1998) Spectrum of AIDS-associated malignant disorders. *Lancet*, **351**, 1833–1839

Grulich, A.E., Beral, V., Swerdlow, A.J. (1992) Kaposi's sarcoma in England and Wales before the AIDS epidemic. *Br. J. Cancer*, **66**, 1135–1137

Harrington, W., Sieczkowski, L., Sosa, C., Chan-a-Sue, S., Cai, J.P., Cabral, L., Wood, C. (1997) Activation of HHV-8 by HIV-1 tat. *Lancet*, **349**, 774–778

Hayward, G.S. (1999) KSHV strains: the origins and global spread of the virus. In: Weiss, R.A. & Boshoff, C., eds, *Seminars in Cancer Biology: Kaposi's Sarcoma-Associated Herpesvirus*, vol. 9, London, Academic Press, pp. 187-199

He, J., Bhat, G., Kanasa, C., Chistu, C., Mitchell, C., Dvan, W. & Wood, C. (1998) Seroprevalence of human herpesvirus 8 among Zambian women of childbearing age without Kaposi's sarcoma (KS) and mother-child pairs with KS. *J. Infect. Dis.*, **178**, 1787–1790

Hermans, P., Lundgren, J., Somnereijns, B., Pedersen, C., Vella, S., Katlama, C., Luthy, R., Pinching, A.J., Gerstoft, J., Pehrson, P. & Clumeck, N. (1996) Epidemiology of AIDS-related Kaposi's sarcoma in Europe over 10 years. AIDS in Europe study group. *AIDS*, **10**, 911–917

Hjalgrim, H., Melbye, M., Pukkala, E., Langmark, F., Frisch, M., Dictor, M. & Ekbom, A. (1996) Epidemiology of Kaposi's sarcoma in the Nordic countries prior to the AIDS epidemic. Br. J. Cancer, 74, 1499–1502

Hutt, M.S. (1981) The epidemiology of Kaposi's sarcoma. Antibiot. Chemother., 29, 3–11

Hutt, M.S.R. (1984) Kaposi's sarcoma. Br. Med. Bull., 40, 355–358

Hutt, M.S.R. & Burkitt, D.P. (1965) Geographical distribution of cancer in East Africa. Br. Med. J., ii, 719–722

IARC (1996) IARC Monographs on the Evaluation of Carcinogenic Risks to Humans. Volume 67, Human Immunodeficiency Viruses and Human T-cell Lymphotropic Viruses, Lyon, IARC

IARC (1997) IARC Monographs on the Evaluation of Carcinogenic Risks to Humans. Volume 70. Epstein–Barr Virus and Kaposi Sarcoma Herpes Virus/Human Herpes Virus 8, Lyon, IARC

Jensen, O.M., Tuyns, A.J. & Ravisse, P. (1978) Cancer in Cameroon: a relative frequency study. Rev. Epid. Santé Publ., 26, 147–159

Kedes, D.H., Operskalski, E., Busch, M., Kohn, R., Flood, J. & Ganem, D. (1996) The seroepidemiology of human herpesvirus 8 (Kaposi's sarcoma- associated herpesvirus): distribution of infection in KS risk groups and evidence for sexual transmission. Nature Med., 2, 918–924

Kestens, L., Melbye, M., Biggar, R.J., Stevens, W.J., Piot, P., De Muynck, A., Taelman, H., De Feyter, M., Paluku, L. & Gigase, P.L. (1985) Endemic African Kaposi's sarcoma is not associated with immunodeficiency. Int. J. Cancer, 36, 49–54

Kinlen, L. (1992) Immunosuppressive therapy and acquired immunological disorders. Cancer Res., 52 (Suppl.) 5474s–5476s

Kovi, J. & Heshmat, M.Y. (1972) Incidence of cancer in negroes in Washington, D.C. and selected African cities. Am. J. Epidemiol., 96, 401–413

Lampinen, T.M., Kulasingam, S., Min, J., Borok, M., Gwanzura, L., Lamb, J., Mahomed, K., Woelk, G.B., Strand, K.B., Bosch, M.L., Edelman, D.C., Constantine, N.T., Katzenstein, D. & Williams, M.A. (2000) Detection of Kaposi's sarcoma-associated herpesvirus in oral and genital secretions of Zimbabwean women. J. Infect. Dis., 181, 1785–1790

Lennette, E.T., Blackbourn, D.J. & Levy, J.A. (1996) Antibodies to human herpesvirus type 8 in the general population and in Kaposi's sarcoma patients. Lancet, 348, 858–861

Levine, A.M. (1993) AIDS-related malignancies: the emerging epidemic. J. Natl Cancer Inst., 85, 1382–1397

Lyall, E.G., Patton, G.S., Sheldon, J., Stainsby, C., Mullen, J., O'Shea, S., Smith, N.A., De Ruiter, A., McClure, M.O. & Schulz, T.F. (1999) Evidence for horizontal and not vertical transmission of human herpesvirus 8 in children born to human immunodeficiency virus-infected mothers. Pediatr. Infect. Dis. J., 18, 795–799

Malik, M.O., Hidaytalla, A., Daoud, E.H. & el-Hassan, A.M. (1974) Superficial cancer in the Sudan. A study of 1225 primary malignant superficial tumours. Br. J. Cancer, 30, 355–364

Mantina, H., Kankasa, C., Klaskala, W., Brayfield, B., Campbell, J., Du, Q., Bhat, G., Kasolo, F., Mitchell, C. & Wood, C. (2001) Vertical transmission of Kaposi's sarcoma-associated herpesvirus. Int. J. Cancer, 94, 749–752

Margolius, L.P. (1995) Kaposi's sarcoma in renal transplant recipients. J. Nephrol., 8, 300–304

Martin, J.N., Ganem, D.E., Osmond, D.H., Page-Shafer, K.A., Macrae, D. & Kedes, D.H. (1998) Sexual transmission and the natural history of human herpesvirus-8 infection. New Engl. J. Med., 338, 948–954

Master, S.P., Taylor, J.F., Kyalwazi, S.K. & Ziegler, J.L. (1970) Immunological studies in Kaposi's sarcoma in Uganda. Br. Med. J., 1, 600–602

Mayama, S., Cuevas, L., Sheldon, J., Omar, O.H., Smith, D.H., Okong, P., Silvel, B., Hart, C.A. & Schulz, T.F. (1998) Prevalence and transmission of Kaposi's sarcoma-associated herpesvirus (human herpesvirus 8) in Ugandan children and adolescents. Int. J. Cancer, 77, 817–820

McHardy, J., Williams, E.H., Geser, A., de-The, G., Beth, E. & Giraldo, G. (1984) Endemic Kaposi's sarcoma: incidence and risk factors in the West Nile District of Uganda. Int. J. Cancer, 33, 203–212

Melbye, M., Kestens, L., Biggar, R.J., Schreuder, G.M.T. & Gigase, P.L. (1987) HLA studies of endemic African Kaposi's sarcoma patients and matched controls: no association with HLA-DR5. Int. J. Cancer, 39, 182–184

Melbye, M., Cook, P.M., Hjalgrim, H., Begtrup, K., Simpson, G.R., Biggar, R.J., Ebbesen, P. & Schulz, T.F. (1998) Risk factors for Kaposi's-sarcoma-associated herpesvirus (KSHV/HHV-8) seropositivity in a cohort of homosexual men, 1981-1996. Int. J. Cancer, 77, 543–548

Mitacek, E.J., St Vallieres, D. & Polednak, A.P. (1986) Cancer in Haiti 1979-84: distribution of various forms of cancer according to geographical area and sex. Int. J. Cancer, 38, 9–16

Moore, P.S., Kingsley, L.A., Holmberg, S.D., Spira, T., Gupta, P., Hoover, D.R., Parry, J.P., Conley, L.J., Jaffe, H.W. & Chang, Y. (1996) Kaposi's sarcoma-associated herpesvirus infection prior to onset of Kaposi's sarcoma. AIDS, 10, 175–180

Newton, R., Grulich, A., Beral, V., Sindikubwabo, B., Ngilimana, P.-J., Nganyira, A. & Parkin, D.M. (1995) Cancer and HIV infection in Rwanda. Lancet, 345, 1378–1379

Newton, R., Ziegler, J., Beral, V., Mbidde, E., Carpenter, L., Wabinga, H., Mbuletieye, Appleby, P., Reeves, G., Jaffe, H. & Uganda Kaposi's sarcoma Study Group (2001) A case-control study of HIV infection and cancer in adults and children in Kampala Uganda. Int. J. Cancer, 91, 622–627

Oates, K., Dealler, S., Dickey, R. & Wood, P. (1984) Malignant neoplasms in 1971-1983 in northeastern Zaire with particular reference to Kaposi's sarcoma and malignant melanoma. Ann. Soc. Belge Trop. Med., 64, 373–378

Oettlé, A.G. (1962) Geographical and racial differences in the frequency of Kaposi's sarcoma as evidence of environmental or genetic causes. Acta unio. int. contra cancrum, 18, 330–363

Olsen, S.J., Chang, Y., Moore, P.S., Biggar, R.J. & Melbye, M. (1998) Increasing Kaposi's sarcoma-associated herpesvirus seroprevalence with age in a highly Kaposi's sarcoma endemic region, Zambia 1985. AIDS, 12, 1921–1925

Olweny, C.L.M., Kaddumukasa, A., Atine, O., Owor, R., Magrath, I.T. & Ziegler, J. (1976) Childhood Kaposi's sarcoma in Uganda: clinical features and treatment. Br. J. Cancer, 33, 555–560

Owor, R. & Hutt, M.S.R. (1977) Kaposi's sarcoma in Uganda. Further epidemiological observations. E. Afr. J. Med. Sci., 4, 55–57

Penn, I. (1995) Sarcomas in organ allograft recipients. Transplantation, 60, 1485–1491

Peterman, T.A., Jaffe, H.W. & Beral, V. (1993) Epidemiologic clues to the etiology of Kaposi's sarcoma. AIDS, 7, 605–611

Rabkin, C.S., Biggar, R.J. & Horm, J.W. (1991) Increasing incidence of cancers associated with the human immunodeficiency virus epidemic. Int. J. Cancer, 47, 692–696

Renwick, N., Halaby, T., Weverling, G.J., Dukers, N.H., Simpson, G.R., Coutinho, R.A., Lange, J.M., Schulz, T.F. & Goudsmit, J. (1998) Seroconversion for human herpesvirus 8 during HIV infection is highly predictive of Kaposi's sarcoma. AIDS, 12, 2481–2488

Rezza, G., Andreoni, M., Dorrucci, M., Pezzoti, P., Monini, P., Zerboni, R., Salassa, B., Colangeli, V., Sarmati, L., Nicastri, E., Barbanera, M., Pristera, R., Aiuti, F., Ortona, L. & Encoli, B. (1999) Human herpesvirus 8 seropositivity and risk of Kaposi's sarcoma and other acquired immunodeficiency syndrome-related diseases. J. Natl Cancer Inst., 91, 1468–1474

Rezza, G., Tchangmena, O.B., Andreoni, M., Bugarini, R., Toma, L., Bakary, D.K., Glikoutou, M., Sarmati, L., Monini, P., Pezzotti, P. & Ensoli, B. (2000) Prevalence and risk factors for human herpesvirus 8 infection in northern Cameroon. *Sex. Transm. Dis.*, **27**, 159–164

Rogoff, M.G. (1968) Kaposi's sarcoma. Age, sex, and tribal incidence in Kenya. In: Clifford, P., Linsell, C.A. & Timms, G.L., eds, *Cancer in Africa*, Nairobi, East African Publishing House, pp. 445–448

Rothman, S. (1962) Some clinical aspects of Kaposi's sarcoma in the European and American population. In: Ackerman, L.V. & Murray, J.F., eds. Symposium on Kaposi's sarcoma. *Acta unio. int. contra cancrum*, **18**, 51–58

Serraino, D., Toma, L., Andreoni, M., Butto, S., Tchangmena, O., Sarmati, L., Monini, P., Franceschi, S., Ensoli, B. & Rezza, G. (2001) A seroprevalence study of human herpesvirus type 8 (HHV8) in eastern and Central Africa and in the Mediterranean area. *Eur. J. Epidemiol.*, **17**, 871–876

Simpson, G.R., Schulz, T.F., Whitby, D., Cook, P.M., Boshoff, C., Rainbow, L., Howard, M.R., Gao, S.J., Bohenzky, R.A., Simmonds, P., Lee, C., De Ruiter, A., Hatzakis, A., Tedder, R.S., Weller, L.V.D., Weiss, R.A. & Moore, P.S. (1996) Prevalence of Kaposi's sarcoma associated herpesvirus infection measured by antibodies to recombinant capsid protein and latent immunofluorescence antigen. *Lancet*, **348**, 1133–1138

Sitas, F., Bezwoda, W.R., Levin, V., Ruff, P., Kew, M.C., Hale, M.J., Carrara, H., Beral, V., Fleming, G., Odes, R. & Weaving, A. (1997) Association between human immunodeficiency virus type 1 infection and cancer in the black population of Johannesburg and Soweto, South Africa. *Br. J. Cancer;* **75**, 1704–1707

Sitas, F., Madhoo, J. & Wessie, J. (1998) *Incidence of Histologically Diagnosed Cancer in South Africa, 1993-1995. National Cancer Registry of South Africa*, Johannesburg, South African Institute of Medical Research

Sitas, F., Carrara, H., Beral, V., Newton, R., Reeves, G., Bull, D., Jentsch, U., Pacella-Norman, R., Bourboulia, D., Whitby, D., Boshoff, C. & Weiss, R. (1999a) The seroepidemiology of HHV-8/KSHV in a large population of black cancer patients in South Africa. *New Engl. J. Med.*, **340**, 1863–1871

Sitas, F., Newton, R. & Boshoff, C. (1999b) Probability of mother-to-child transmission of HHV-8 increases with increasing maternal antibody titre for HHV-8. *New Engl. J. Med.*, **340**, 1923

Sitas, F., Pacella-Norman, R., Carrara, H., Patel, M., Ruff, P., Sur, R., Jentsch, U., Hale, M., Rowji, P., Saffer, D., Connor, M., Bull, D., Newton, R. & Beral, V. (2000) The spectrum of HIV-1 related cancers in South Africa. *Int. J. Cancer*, **88**, 489–492

Skinner, M.E.G., Parkin, D.M., Vizcaino, A.P. & Ndhlovu, A. (1993) *Cancer in the African Population of Bulawayo, Zimbabwe, 1963-1977* (IARC Technical Report No. 15), Lyon, IARC

Slavin, G., Cameron, H.M., Forbes, C. & Mitchell, R.M. (1970) Kaposi's sarcoma in East African children. A report of 51 cases. *J. Pathol.*, **100**, 187–199

Taylor, J.F., Smith, P.G., Bull, D. & Pike, M.C. (1972) Kaposi's sarcoma in Uganda: geographic and ethnic distribution. *Br. J. Cancer*, **26**, 483–497

Taylor, J.F. & Ziegler, J.L. (1974) Delayed cutaneous hypersensitivity reactions in patients with Kaposi's sarcoma. *Br. J. Cancer*, **30**, 312–318

Templeton, A.C. & Bhana, D. (1975) Prognosis in Kaposi's sarcoma. *J. Natl Cancer Inst.*, **55**, 1301–1304

Templeton, A.C. (1981) Kaposi's sarcoma. In: Sommers, S.C. & Rosen, P.P., eds, *Pathology Annual*, New York, Appleton: Century-Crofts, pp. 315–336

Touloumi, G., Hatzakis, A., Potouridou, I., Milona, I., Strarigos, J., Katsambas, A., Giraldo, G., Beth-Giraldo, E., Biggar, E.J., Mueller, N. & Trichopoulos, D. (1999) The role of immunosuppression and immune-activation in classic Kaposi's sarcoma. *Int. J. Cancer*, **82**, 817–821

Urassa, W.K., Kaaya, E.E., Kitinya, J.N., Lema, L.L., Amir, H., Luande, J., Biberfeld, G., Mhalu, F.S. & Biberfeld, P. (1998) Immunological profile of endemic and epidemic Kaposi's sarcoma patients in Dar-es-Salaam, Tanzania. *Int. J. Mol. Med.*, **1**, 979–982

Wabinga, H.R., Parkin, D.M., Wabwire-Mangen, F., Mugerwa, J.W. (1993) Cancer in Kampala, Uganda, in 1989-91: Changes in incidence in the era of AIDS. *Int. J. Cancer*, **54**, 26–36

Wabinga, H.R., Parkin, D.M., Wabwire-Mangen, F. & Nambooze, S. (2000) Trends in cancer incidence in Kyadondo County, Uganda, 1960-1997. *Br. J. Cancer*, **82**, 1585–1592

Whitby, D., Howard, M.R., Tenant-Flowers, M., Brinks, N.S., Copas, A., Boshoff, C., Hatzioannou, T., Suggett, F.E., Aldam, D.M., Denton, A.S., *et al.*, (1995) Detection of Kaposi's sarcoma-associated herpesvirus in peripheral blood of HIV-infected individuals and progression to Kaposi's sarcoma. *Lancet*, **346**, 799–802

Wilkinson, D., Sheldon, J., Gilks, C. & Schulz, T.F. (1999) Prevalence of infection with human herpesvirus 8 (HHV8)/Kaposi's sarcoma herpesvirus (KSHV) in rural South Africa. *S. Afr. Med. J.*, **89**, 554–557

Ziegler, J.L. (1993) Endemic Kaposi's sarcoma in Africa and local volcanic soils. *Lancet*, **342**, 1348–1351

Ziegler, J.L. & Katongole-Mbidde, E. (1996) Kaposi's sarcoma in childhood: an analysis of 100 cases from Uganda, and relationship to HIV infection. *Int. J. Cancer*, **65**, 200–203

Ziegler, J.L., Newton, R., Katongole-Mbidde, E., Mbulataiye, S., De Cock, K., Wabinga, H., Mugerwa, J., Katabira, E., Jaffe, H., Parkin, D.M., Reeves, G., Weiss, R. & Beral, V. (1997) Risk factors for Kaposi's sarcoma in HIV-positive subjects in Uganda. *AIDS*, **11**, 1619–1626

Ziegler, J. and the Uganda Kaposi's Sarcoma Study Group (1998) Wealth and soil exposure are risk factors for endemic Kaposi's sarcoma in Uganda. *J. Acquir. Immune Defic. Synd. Hum. Retrovirol.*, **17**, A12

4.7 Leukaemia

The features of childhood leukaemia in Africa have been discussed in the chapter on childhood cancer.

In adults, there seem to be few features of note in the epidemiology of these cancers in Africa. Overall incidence rates are lower than those recorded in western countries (Tables 1a–c). Most descriptions of leukaemia in Africa are based upon clinical series. It is difficult to know how much the age structure of the population, selective factors influencing access to hospital and diagnostic facilities influence the pattern by age, sex and cell type. The literature up to 1985 was summarized by Fleming (1986).Older data on incidence in Africa are presented in Table 2.

In many series, chronic leukaemias apparently outnumber acute leukaemias; this possibly reflects the deficit of childhood acute lymphocytic leukaemia (ALL) and possibly the poor prognosis or misdiagnosis of acute leukaemias, especially in earlier data.

In some African series (mainly from east Africa), chronic myeloid leukaemia (CML) appears to be more frequent than chronic lymphocytic leukaemia (CLL) (Edington & Hendrickse, 1973; Williams, 1984). CML occurs with peak frequency in the third and fourth decades of life in most case series, although this presumably relates to the age structures of the populations, rather than to any special feature of age-specific incidence rates. These seem to be similar to the rates in the United States (Figure 1).

It is difficult to be certain of the reality of the descriptive features of CLL reported from Africa, because of the arbitrary distinction from the common B-cell lymphomas. Fleming (1985) considered that there are two forms of CLL in tropical Africa. About half the patients described are aged less than 45 years, and in this age group, the male to female ratio is 1:2, and CLL is reported more commonly in

west than in east Africa. Over the age of 45 years, most cases are in men (ratio 2:1), as in European populations. Williams (1985) found that CLL cases in Ibadan, Nigeria, were of lower social status than subjects with other forms of leukaemia or than the general population.

In north Africa, the pattern seems to be much the same as in European populations (Bellabes *et al.*, 1983; El Bolkainy *et al.*, 1984)

The epidemiology of acute T-cell leukaemia-lymphoma (ATLL) in Africa is described in the chapter on lymphomas.

References

Bellabes, S., Hamman, P., Desablens, B., Collonna, P. & Messerschmitt, J. (1983) Chronic lymphatic leukaemia in Maghreb and Europe. *Acta Haematol.*, **46**, 89–94

Edington, G.M. & Hendrickse, M. (1973) Incidence and frequency of lymphoreticular tumors in Ibadan and the Western State of Nigeria. *J. Natl Cancer Inst.*, **50**, 1623–1631

El Bolkainy, M., Gad-El-Mawla, N., Tawfik, H.N., & Aboul-Enein, M.I. (1984) Epidemiology of lymphoma and leukaemia in Egypt. In: Magrath, I., O'Conor, G.T. & Ramot, B., eds, *Pathogenesis of Leukemias and Lymphomas: Environmental Influences* (Progress in Cancer Research and Therapy, Vol. 27), pp. 9–16, New York, Raven Press, pp. 9–16

Fleming, A.F. (1985) The epidemiology of lymphomas and leukaemias in Africa—an overview. *Leuk. Res.*, **9**, 735–740

Fleming, A.F. (1986) A bibliography of the leukaemias in Africa, 1904-1985. *Leuk. Res.*, **10**, 1353–1365

Williams, C.K.O. (1985) Influence of life-style on the pattern of leukaemia and lymphoma subtypes among Nigerians. *Leuk. Res.*, **9,** 741–745

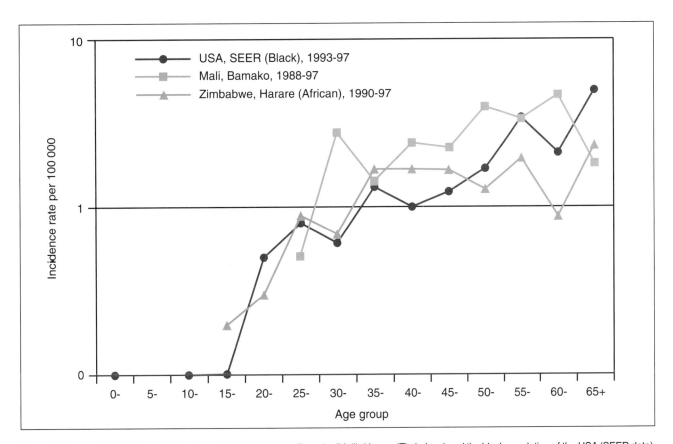

Figure 1. Age-specific incidence of chronic myeloid leukaemia in Bamako (Mali), Harare (Zimbabwe) and the black population of the USA (SEER data)

Williams, C.K.O. (1984) Some biological and epidemiological characteristics of human leukaemia in Africans. In: Williams, A.O., O'Conor, G.T., De Thé, G.T. & Johnson, C.A., eds, *Virus-* *Associated Cancers in Africa* (IARC Scientific Publications No. 63), Lyon, IARC, pp. 687–711

Table 1a. Age-standardized (world) and cumulative (0-64) incidence
Lymphoid leukaemia (C91)

	MALE				FEMALE			
	Cases	CRUDE (per 100,000)	ASR(W)	Cumulative (%)	Cases	CRUDE (per 100,000)	ASR(W)	Cumulative (%)
Africa, North								
Algeria, Algiers (1993-1997)	56	1.0	1.2	0.07	29	0.5	0.7	0.03
Algeria, Constantine (1994-1997)	29	1.9	2.7	0.15	13	0.9	1.1	0.05
Algeria, Oran (1996-1998)	25	1.4	1.5	0.09	12	0.7	0.8	0.03
Algeria, Setif (1993-1997)	43	1.4	1.5	0.08	22	0.7	0.7	0.03
Tunisia, Centre, Sousse (1993-1997)	25	2.2	2.5	0.14	13	1.2	1.3	0.07
Tunisia, North, Tunis (1994)	42	1.9	2.2	0.12	32	1.5	1.7	0.13
Tunisia, Sfax (1997)	19	4.8	5.3	0.19	11	2.9	3.2	0.15
Africa, West								
The Gambia (1997-1998)	1	0.1	0.1	0.01	-	-	-	-
Guinea, Conakry (1996-1999)	12	0.5	0.6	0.05	10	0.5	1.0	0.03
Mali, Bamako (1988-1997)	1	0.0	0.0	0.00	2	0.1	0.1	0.00
Niger, Niamey (1993-1999)	18	1.0	1.6	0.11	16	0.9	2.1	0.15
Nigeria, Ibadan (1998-1999)	2	0.1	0.1	0.01	2	0.1	0.2	0.03
Africa, Central								
Congo, Brazzaville (1996-1999)	18	1.5	1.8	0.13	19	1.6	2.2	0.17
Africa, East								
France, La Reunion (1988-1994)	32	1.5	1.8	0.11	29	1.3	1.5	0.08
Kenya, Eldoret (1998-2000)	21	2.2	4.1	0.24	5	0.5	1.2	0.12
Malawi, Blantyre (2000-2001)	-	-	-	-	2	0.2	0.4	0.04
Uganda, Kyadondo County (1993-1997)	6	0.2	0.2	0.01	7	0.2	0.5	0.05
Zimbabwe, Harare: African (1990-1993)	26	1.1	2.2	0.08	16	0.7	1.7	0.14
Zimbabwe, Harare: African (1994-1997)	25	0.9	1.2	0.06	15	0.6	1.3	0.06
Zimbabwe, Harare: European (1990-1997)	11	7.2	5.4	0.27	5	3.0	2.2	0.05
Africa, South								
Namibia (1995-1998)	20	0.6	1.0	0.06	9	0.3	0.4	0.03
South Africa: Black (1989-1992)	449	0.8	1.2	0.07	302	0.5	0.7	0.04
South Africa: Indian (1989-1992)	37	1.9	2.2	0.13	21	1.1	1.1	0.06
South Africa: Mixed race (1989-1992)	70	1.1	1.3	0.07	39	0.6	0.7	0.04
South Africa: White (1989-1992)	347	3.4	3.6	0.19	225	2.2	2.2	0.12
South Africa, Transkei, Umtata (1996-1998)	1	0.3	0.2	0.01	-	-	-	-
South Africa, Transkei, 4 districts (1996-1998)	-	-	-	-	-	-	-	-
Swaziland (1996-1999)	5	0.3	0.2	0.02	2	0.1	0.1	0.00
Europe/USA								
USA, SEER: White (1993-1997)	3361	6.9	5.9	0.29	2326	4.6	3.5	0.16
USA, SEER: Black (1993-1997)	252	3.8	4.3	0.21	162	2.2	2.1	0.09
France, 8 registries (1993-1997)	890	6.5	5.3	0.29	633	4.4	3.2	0.17
The Netherlands (1993-1997)	2100	5.5	4.8	0.24	1287	3.3	2.6	0.12
UK, England (1993-1997)	7370	6.1	4.7	0.22	5259	4.1	2.8	0.12

In italics: histopathology-based registries

Table 1b. Age-standardized (world) and cumulative (0-64) incidence
Myeloid leukaemia (C92-94)

	MALE				FEMALE			
	Cases	CRUDE	ASR(W) (per 100,000)	Cumulative (%)	Cases	CRUDE	ASR(W) (per 100,000)	Cumulative (%)
Africa, North								
Algeria, Algiers (1993-1997)	37	0.7	**0.8**	0.05	26	0.5	**0.5**	0.04
Algeria, Constantine (1994-1997)	25	1.6	**2.4**	0.13	24	1.6	**2.0**	0.16
Algeria, Oran (1996-1998)	13	0.7	**0.9**	0.05	10	0.6	**0.6**	0.06
Algeria, Setif (1993-1997)	22	0.7	**1.0**	0.06	34	1.1	**1.6**	0.12
Tunisia, Centre, Sousse (1993-1997)	21	1.8	**2.1**	0.11	12	1.1	**1.3**	0.08
Tunisia, North, Tunis (1994)	37	1.7	**1.9**	0.10	47	2.2	**2.6**	0.21
Tunisia, Sfax (1997)	13	3.3	**3.8**	0.17	4	1.1	**1.2**	0.06
Africa, West								
The Gambia (1997-1998)	-	-	**-**	-	-	-	**-**	-
Guinea, Conakry (1996-1999)	14	0.6	**0.9**	0.06	11	0.5	**0.6**	0.05
Mali, Bamako (1988-1997)	30	0.8	**1.0**	0.08	24	0.7	**1.5**	0.14
Niger, Niamey (1993-1999)	10	0.5	**0.8**	0.07	15	0.8	**1.4**	0.09
Nigeria, Ibadan (1998-1999)	9	0.6	**0.7**	0.04	3	0.2	**0.3**	0.01
Africa, Central								
Congo, Brazzaville (1996-1999)	9	0.7	**0.9**	0.06	6	0.5	**0.7**	0.07
Africa, East								
France, La Reunion (1988-1994)	59	2.8	**3.4**	0.18	51	2.4	**2.5**	0.14
Kenya, Eldoret (1998-2000)	16	1.7	**2.2**	0.19	19	2.1	**3.9**	0.35
Malawi, Blantyre (2000-2001)	2	0.2	**0.2**	0.01	-	-	**-**	-
Uganda, Kyadondo County (1993-1997)	8	0.3	**0.2**	0.02	7	0.2	**0.6**	0.06
Zimbabwe, Harare: African (1990-1993)	38	1.6	**1.9**	0.13	26	1.2	**2.4**	0.12
Zimbabwe, Harare: African (1994-1997)	35	1.3	**1.4**	0.09	35	1.3	**1.6**	0.10
Zimbabwe, Harare: European (1990-1997)	14	9.2	**5.3**	0.31	7	4.1	**2.3**	0.13
Africa, South								
Namibia (1995-1998)	21	0.7	**0.9**	0.06	19	0.6	**0.8**	0.07
South Africa: Black (1989-1992)	504	0.9	**1.1**	0.07	388	0.7	**0.8**	0.06
South Africa: Indian (1989-1992)	28	1.4	**1.4**	0.09	21	1.1	**1.2**	0.07
South Africa: Mixed race (1989-1992)	86	1.3	**1.8**	0.11	71	1.1	**1.3**	0.09
South Africa: White (1989-1992)	329	3.3	**3.1**	0.18	275	2.7	**2.3**	0.16
South Africa, Transkei, Umtata (1996-1998)	1	0.3	**0.3**	-	1	0.2	**0.3**	-
South Africa, Transkei, 4 districts (1996-1998)	-	-	**-**	-	2	0.2	**0.3**	0.03
Swaziland (1996-1999)	-	-	**-**	-	4	0.2	**0.3**	0.02
Europe/USA								
USA, SEER: White (1993-1997)	3095	6.4	**4.9**	0.24	2550	5.1	**3.4**	0.19
USA, SEER: Black (1993-1997)	258	3.9	**4.1**	0.21	249	3.4	**3.1**	0.17
France, 8 registries (1993-1997)	735	5.3	**4.0**	0.21	610	4.2	**2.8**	0.16
The Netherlands (1993-1997)	1935	5.1	**3.9**	0.20	1494	3.8	**2.5**	0.14
UK, England (1993-1997)	6616	5.5	**3.8**	0.19	5877	4.6	**2.7**	0.15

In italics: histopathology-based registries

Table 1c. Age-standardized (world) and cumulative (0-64) incidence
Leukaemia, unspecified

	MALE				FEMALE			
	Cases	CRUDE	ASR(W)	Cumulative	Cases	CRUDE	ASR(W)	Cumulative
		(per 100,000)		(%)		(per 100,000)		(%)
Africa, North								
Algeria, Algiers (1993-1997)	18	0.3	**0.4**	0.02	14	0.3	**0.3**	0.02
Algeria, Constantine (1994-1997)	2	0.1	**0.2**	0.01	-	-	**-**	-
Algeria, Oran (1996-1998)	5	0.3	**0.3**	0.01	-	-	**-**	-
Algeria, Setif (1993-1997)	9	0.3	**0.4**	0.03	11	0.4	**0.5**	0.03
Tunisia, Centre, Sousse (1993-1997)	1	0.1	**0.1**	0.01	1	0.1	**0.1**	-
Tunisia, North, Tunis (1994)	3	0.1	**0.2**	0.00	3	0.1	**0.1**	0.01
Tunisia, Sfax (1997)	1	0.3	**0.3**	-	2	0.5	**0.5**	0.01
Africa, West								
The Gambia (1997-1998)	3	0.3	**0.2**	0.01	3	0.3	**0.4**	0.04
Guinea, Conakry (1996-1999)	2	0.1	**0.1**	0.01	3	0.1	**0.3**	0.04
Mali, Bamako (1988-1997)	9	0.2	**0.3**	0.02	11	0.3	**0.4**	0.03
Niger, Niamey (1993-1999)	-	-	**-**	-	3	0.2	**0.1**	0.01
Nigeria, Ibadan (1998-1999)	3	0.2	**0.3**	0.03	2	0.1	**0.1**	0.01
Africa, Central								
Congo, Brazzaville (1996-1999)	9	0.7	**0.9**	0.06	7	0.6	**0.6**	0.05
Africa, East								
France, La Reunion (1988-1994)	7	0.3	**0.4**	0.01	3	0.1	**0.1**	0.00
Kenya, Eldoret (1998-2000)	4	0.4	**0.5**	0.03	2	0.2	**0.2**	0.01
Malawi, Blantyre (2000-2001)	3	0.3	**0.8**	0.08	3	0.3	**0.2**	0.01
Uganda, Kyadondo County (1993-1997)	9	0.3	**0.4**	0.04	10	0.3	**0.5**	0.02
Zimbabwe, Harare: African (1990-1993)	2	0.1	**0.4**	0.01	-	-	**-**	-
Zimbabwe, Harare: African (1994-1997)	6	0.2	**0.5**	0.01	5	0.2	**0.4**	0.03
Zimbabwe, Harare: European (1990-1997)	5	3.3	**1.7**	0.10	-	-	**-**	-
Africa, South								
Namibia (1995-1998)	1	0.0	**0.0**	0.00	1	0.0	**0.1**	-
South Africa: Black (1989-1992)	319	0.6	**0.8**	0.05	263	0.5	**0.6**	0.04
South Africa: Indian (1989-1992)	30	1.5	**1.6**	0.11	23	1.2	**1.2**	0.08
South Africa: Mixed race (1989-1992)	12	0.2	**0.2**	0.01	10	0.1	**0.2**	0.01
South Africa: White (1989-1992)	126	1.3	**1.2**	0.07	124	1.2	**1.2**	0.08
South Africa, Transkei, Umtata (1996-1998)	1	0.3	**0.3**	-	1	0.2	**0.3**	-
South Africa, Transkei, 4 districts (1996-1998)	1	0.1	**0.4**	0.04	-	-	**-**	-
Swaziland (1996-1999)	19	1.1	**1.6**	0.05	15	0.8	**1.1**	0.07
Europe/USA								
USA, SEER: White (1993-1997)	451	0.9	**0.7**	0.02	431	0.9	**0.5**	0.01
USA, SEER: Black (1993-1997)	31	0.5	**0.5**	0.02	23	0.3	**0.3**	0.01
France, 8 registries (1993-1997)	47	0.3	**0.2**	0.01	35	0.2	**0.2**	0.01
The Netherlands (1993-1997)	103	0.3	**0.2**	0.01	94	0.2	**0.1**	0.00
UK, England (1993-1997)	572	0.5	**0.3**	0.01	545	0.4	**0.2**	0.01

In italics: histopathology-based registries

Table 2. Incidence of leukaemia in Africa, 1953–74

Registry	Period	ASR (per 100 000)		Source
		Male	Female	(see Chap. 1)
Senegal, Dakar	1969–74	*0.7*	*0.2*	4
Mozambique, Lourenço Marques	1956–60	*3.8*	2.3	1
Nigeria, Ibadan	1960–69	4.0	3.9	3
SA, Cape Province: Bantu	1956–59	*7.9*	*0.7*	2
SA, Cape Province: Coloured	1956–59	5.4	3.4	2
SA, Cape Province: White	1956–59	6.5	5.2	2
SA, Johannesburg, Bantu	1953–55	2.7	3.8	1
SA, Natal Province: African	1964–66	2.4	9.2	2
SA, Natal Province: Indian	1964–66	4.7	*3.6*	2
Uganda, Kyadondo	1954–60	2.4	3.2	1
Uganda, Kyadondo	1960–71	2.7	2.4	5
Zimbabwe, Bulawayo	1963–72	5.5	8.2	6

Italics: Rate based on less than 10 cases

4.8 Liver cancer

Introduction

Liver cancer is estimated to be the fifth most common cancer worldwide, responsible for around 564 000 new cases (398 000 in men and 166 000 in women) in the year 2000 (Ferlay *et al.*, 2001). Because it has a very poor prognosis, the number of deaths (549 000) is not far short of the number of new cases, and it represents the third most common cause of death from cancer. The geographical distribution of liver cancer is very uneven; 81% of cases occur in the developing countries. The highest incidence rates are in West and central Africa (where it accounts for almost one fifth of cancer in men), eastern and south-eastern Asia, and Melanesia. China alone accounts for 54% of the total cases in the world. With the exception of Japan, the incidence rates are low in developed countries, with the highest incidence found in southern Europe, especially in Greece.

Liver cancer comprises a variety of different cancers, which show different epidemiological features (see Table 3). The most frequent subtype in most areas is hepatocellular carcinoma, and much of the geographical variation worldwide is linked to this cancer. Cholangiocarcinoma, a tumour of the epithelium of the intrahepatic bile ducts, is generally less frequent, comprising around 10–25% of liver cancers in men in Europe and North America, but a rather higher proportion in women, because although the incidence rates of cholangiocarcinoma are rather similar in males and females, the rates of hepatocellular carcinoma are some 2–3 times higher in males in low-incidence areas (Europe, North America) and up to fivefold higher in the high-risk populations of Asia and sub-Saharan Africa. The incidence of cholangiocarcinoma shows rather little variation worldwide, with rates in males between 0.5 and 2.0 per 100 000 and somewhat lower in females (Parkin *et al.*, 1993), although incidence in some local areas of Asia (e.g., north-east Thailand) is high.

Other types of liver cancer are much less common. Hepatoblastoma is a tumour of young children, with overall 82% of cases occurring in the first five years of life. There is very little geographical variation in incidence. Malignant vascular tumours (haemangiosarcomas) are even rarer and affect principally adults.

Descriptive epidemiology in Africa

The high frequency of liver cancer in sub-Saharan Africa has been clear for as long as records have been kept (Oettlé, 1964; Cook & Burkitt, 1971). Reports from cancer registries in the 1980s and 1990s have helped to establish the contemporary pattern (Figure 1).

In West Africa, the data from the Gambia, Mali and Guinea, and previous publications from these registries (Bah *et al.*, 1990; Bayo *et al.*, 1990; Koulibaly *et al.*, 1997) have shown liver cancer to be the most common tumour in males. Incidence rates, standardized to the world standard population (ASR), range from 38 to 49 in males and 12 to 18 per 100 000 in females (Table 1). In Abidjan (Côte d'Ivoire) and Niamey (Niger), the recorded rates are lower, probably due to some under-registration, but liver cancer comprises 15% and 24% of cancers in men. These observations confirm early reports from the region, indicating a high incidence of the disease in men (Edington, 1978; Fakunle *et al.*, 1977).

Data from East Africa suggest that incidence rates are not as high as in West Africa. The long time series from Kampala, Uganda, from 1960 to 1997 (Wabinga *et al.*, 2000), suggests a rather fluctuating incidence, with the rates in men between 6 and 12 per 100 000, and in women between 2 and 6 per 100 000. This is consistent with the low incidence reported from Malawi: 4.6 in men and 2.2 in women per 100 000 in 1994–98 (Banda *et al.*, 2001).

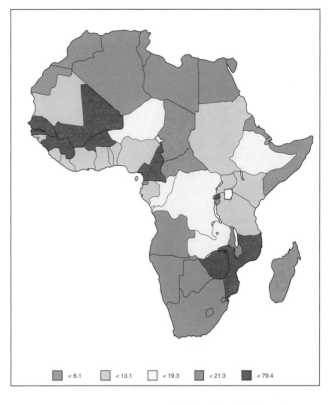

< 6.1	< 13.1	< 19.3	< 21.3	< 79.4

Figure 1. Incidence of liver cancer: ASR (world)-male (all ages)

In central Africa, the actual incidence is uncertain, but liver cancer is the commonest tumour of men in Butare (Rwanda) and in Brazzaville (Congo), where the recorded incidence was 17.2 per 100 000 in men and 8.4 in women. Kocheleff *et al.* (1984) estimated the crude incidence rate of liver cancer in Burundi to be 8.8 per 100 000.

In southern Africa, there are marked differences in the incidence of liver cancer between the different races. Populations of European origin living in Zimbabwe for the past 30 years show lower incidence rates than the native African populations (albeit with a much higher rate than their European counterparts living in Europe or North America (Bassett *et al.*, 1995a, b)). A similar phenomenon has been observed for the Asian population, largely of Indian origin, living in Natal, South Africa (Akoojee *et al.*, 1990). The native black African population in Zimbabwe exhibits high rates of 30.7 and 17.1 per 100 000 for males and females, respectively, in 1993–97.

Older data confirm the high rates in the region (Table 2). The highest recorded rate was 100.8 per 100 000 in males in Maputo (then Lourenço Marques), Mozambique, in 1956–60. In Bulawayo, Zimbabwe, the incidence was 52.1 in men and 20.6 in women per 100 000 in 1963–72 (Parkin *et al.*, 1994).

In North Africa, the incidence of liver cancer is low. Age-standardized rates in Algeria are around 1 per 100 000 and range from 1 to 3 in males in Tunisia (Table 1).

Notwithstanding the tendency for deep-seated tumours to be under-diagnosed, and some methodological differences that exist between cancer registries (Burkitt, 1969; Parkin, 1986), the picture of high incidence and a 3–5-fold male excess in most of sub-Saharan Africa is clear.

In addition to the variation by region, age group, sex and race, some reports have suggested differences in occurrence between specific tribal groups. A study of Mozambican

Table 1. Age-standardized (world) and cumulative (0-64) incidence
Liver (C22)

	MALE				FEMALE			
	Cases	CRUDE	ASR(W)	Cumulative	Cases	CRUDE	ASR(W)	Cumulative
		(per 100,000)		(%)		(per 100,000)		(%)
Africa, North								
Algeria, Algiers (1993-1997)	34	0.6	**0.9**	0.04	34	0.6	**0.9**	0.03
Algeria, Constantine (1994-1997)	6	0.4	**0.6**	0.05	6	0.4	**0.6**	0.04
Algeria, Oran (1996-1998)	2	0.1	**0.2**	0.01	10	0.6	**0.9**	0.08
Algeria, Setif (1993-1997)	23	0.8	**1.4**	0.09	32	1.1	**1.9**	0.15
Tunisia, Centre, Sousse (1993-1997)	11	1.0	**1.3**	0.10	6	0.5	**0.7**	0.04
Tunisia, North, Tunis (1994)	49	2.3	**2.9**	0.13	29	1.4	**1.8**	0.10
Tunisia, Sfax (1997)	5	1.3	**1.4**	0.02	1	0.3	**0.3**	0.01
Africa, West								
The Gambia (1997-1998)	257	26.0	**48.9**	3.92	91	8.9	**17.6**	1.45
Guinea, Conakry (1996-1999)	453	19.8	**37.6**	3.02	144	6.5	**12.1**	1.02
Mali, Bamako (1988-1997)	752	19.4	**38.2**	2.85	283	7.8	**17.8**	1.26
Niger, Niamey (1993-1999)	135	7.3	**16.9**	1.30	65	3.6	**9.3**	0.67
Nigeria, Ibadan (1998-1999)	56	3.8	**7.7**	0.43	19	1.3	**2.1**	0.13
Africa, Central								
Congo, Brazzaville (1996-1999)	150	12.4	**17.2**	1.23	76	6.3	**8.4**	0.61
Africa, East								
France, La Reunion (1988-1994)	47	2.2	**2.9**	0.19	32	1.5	**1.6**	0.11
Kenya, Eldoret (1998-2000)	44	4.7	**10.0**	0.75	29	3.2	**7.3**	0.60
Malawi, Blantyre (2000-2001)	28	3.1	**5.1**	0.35	2	0.2	**0.6**	-
Uganda, Kyadondo County (1993-1997)	74	2.6	**6.5**	0.48	59	2.0	**5.5**	0.46
Zimbabwe, Harare: African (1990-1993)	289	12.2	**30.7**	1.51	93	4.4	**17.1**	1.39
Zimbabwe, Harare: African (1994-1997)	281	10.1	**26.0**	1.22	84	3.2	**10.6**	0.51
Zimbabwe, Harare: European (1990-1997)	23	15.1	**8.4**	0.48	15	8.9	**4.1**	0.18
Africa, South								
Namibia (1995-1998)	59	1.9	**3.2**	0.21	37	1.2	**1.8**	0.11
South Africa: Black (1989-1992)	1863	3.3	**5.6**	0.38	736	1.3	**1.9**	0.13
South Africa: Indian (1989-1992)	47	2.4	**3.8**	0.20	16	0.8	**1.2**	0.07
South Africa: Mixed race (1989-1992)	124	1.9	**3.5**	0.24	52	0.8	**1.1**	0.07
South Africa: White (1989-1992)	353	3.5	**3.2**	0.22	210	2.1	**1.6**	0.10
South Africa, Transkei, Umtata (1996-1998)	35	9.8	**16.0**	1.16	15	3.5	**4.5**	0.35
South Africa, Transkei, 4 districts (1996-1998)	19	2.6	**5.5**	0.42	7	0.8	**1.2**	0.09
Swaziland (1996-1999)	193	11.0	**22.0**	1.65	63	3.2	**5.2**	0.37
Europe/USA								
USA, SEER: White (1993-1997)	2505	5.1	**3.9**	0.19	1301	2.6	**1.5**	0.07
USA, SEER: Black (1993-1997)	412	6.2	**7.1**	0.49	177	2.4	**2.2**	0.10
France, 8 registries (1993-1997)	1810	13.2	**9.1**	0.46	425	2.9	**1.6**	0.08
The Netherlands (1993-1997)	853	2.2	**1.6**	0.08	476	1.2	**0.7**	0.04
UK, England (1993-1997)	4676	3.9	**2.5**	0.12	3176	2.5	**1.3**	0.05

In italics: histopathology-based registries

Shangaans has shown primary hepatocellular carcinoma to occur at a significantly younger age (mean 33.4 years) than among non-Shangaans (mean 40.0 years) (Kew *et al.*, 1977). In Uganda, a significantly higher frequency of liver cancer has long been noted among the largely immigrant Bantu tribes from Rwanda and Burundi and the Nilohamitic tribes of the northwest of the country than in neighbouring and racially related tribes (Alpert *et al.*, 1968; Templeton & Hutt, 1973). Kew *et al.* (1983) drew attention to the markedly younger age at incidence among rural versus urban populations in southern African blacks (and inferred a higher incidence in the former, too). There was no apparent difference, however, with respect to age-specific prevalence of markers of infection with hepatitis B virus (see below).

Age-specific incidence
Although one must be careful in interpreting age-specific cancer incidence rates, because of differential diagnosis and reporting of liver cancer with age, as well as the uncertainty of many older persons concerning their actual age, it is clear that, in countries with a high incidence, the risk of liver cancer begins to rise quite early in life. Figure 2 shows data from the Gambia (where special attention has been paid to identification of cases), which suggest an increase in incidence in young adults, reaching a peak about age 50 years. A similar pattern of a sharp rise in young males is observed in Conakry and Bamako (although in Bamako the peak is at a much later age, 60–74 years). In contrast, in Kampala, Uganda, an area of low risk for PHC, there is a less dramatic rise in age-specific incidence, with a plateau at ages above 55 years (see chapter on Uganda).

Migrants
Studies of cancer mortality in migrants to France have shown a high death rate from liver cancer among migrants from West and Central Africa (Bouchardy *et al.*, 1995). A similar observation was made for migrants to England and Wales from West Africa, but not for East Africans, who were largely of Asian ethnicity (Grulich *et al.*, 1992).

Table 2. Incidence of liver cancer in Africa, 1953–74

| Registry | Period | ASR (per 100 000) | | Source |
		Male	Female	(see Chap. 1)
Senegal, Dakar	1969–74	25.6	9.0	4
Mozambique, Lourenço Marques	1956–60	100.8	30.8	1
Nigeria, Ibadan	1960–69	10.4	3.9	3
SA, Cape Province: Bantu	1956–59	26.3	8.4	2
SA, Cape Province: Coloured	1956–59	1.5	0.7	2
SA, Cape Province: White	1956–59	1.2	0.6	2
SA, Johannesburg, Bantu	1953–55	19.2	9.9	1
SA, Natal Province: African	1964–66	28.4	6.9	2
SA, Natal Province: Indian	1964–66	9.5	3.8	2
Uganda, Kyadondo	1954–60	-	-	1
Uganda, Kyadondo	1960–71	8.9	3.1	5
Zimbabwe, Bulawayo	1963–72	52.1	20.6	6

Italics: Rate based on less than 10 cases

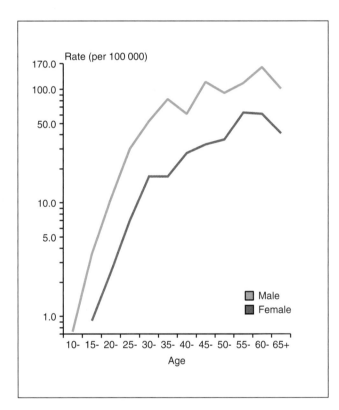

Figure 2.. Age-specific incidence rates per 100 000 of liver cancer, by sex (Gambia, 1988–97) (Bah *et al.*, 2001)

Time trends

There are very few long time series of data from Africa. Comparing the incidence rates in Ibadan, Nigeria, in 1960–69 (Table 2) with those reported for 1998–99 (Table 1) suggests almost no change in the intervening 30 years, although the rates are very low. The long series from Kampala, Uganda (Wabinga *et al.*, 2000) suggests that, in the most recent period (1995–97), there has been a small decline in recorded incidence in men, but not in women. In the 15-year observation period in Bulawayo from 1963 to 1977 (Skinner *et al.*, 1993), there was little to suggest any marked change in incidence.

In the studies of incidence rates of cancer among black gold miners in South Africa (Bradshaw *et al.*, 1982; Harington *et al.*, 1983),

quite marked declines in incidence of liver cancer were observed, especially among miners from Mozambique. The crude incidence fell from 80.4 per 100 000 in 1964–71 to 40.8 per 100 000 in 1972–79 and 29.9 per 100 000 in 1981.

Risk factors

The major risk factors implicated in the very high incidence of liver cancer in sub-Saharan Africa are infection with the hepatitis viruses, especially hepatitis B, and exposure to aflatoxins. Other known risk factors probably play more minor roles.

Hepatitis B virus infection

Chronic carriage of the hepatitis B virus (HBV), as shown by seropositivity for HBV surface antigen (HBsAg), is associated with a large increase in risk of liver cancer, specifically of hepatocellular carcinoma. The earliest reports were case series that noted the rather higher prevalence of HBsAg in liver cancer cases than in the general population (Szmuness, 1978). Since then, many case–control studies have confirmed the relationship; the IARC (1994a) review summarized more than 20 studies in Africa alone, between the study of Prince *et al.* (1970) in Uganda and 1992 (Table 4). In most, the odds ratio associated with the carrier state was between 6 and 20. Since then, at least three more case–control studies have been published from South Africa (Kew *et al.*, 1997), from Nigeria (Olubuyide *et al.*, 1997), and from Egypt (Badawi and Michael 1999), with similar findings (Table 4).

In general, cohort studies yield rather greater relative risks than case–control studies. This is partly because the cases occurring during follow-up of apparently healthy individuals tend to be those detected at young ages, and hence are more likely to be related to HBV carrier status. It is also the result of misclassification of HBV infection status – there is a tendency for HBsAg titre to decline with age, becoming undetectable in some subjects, so that there will be misclassification in case–control studies, where HBsAg status is assessed only at the time of diagnosis.

Only one cohort study has been reported from Africa (London *et al.*, 1995; Evans *et al.*, 1998). The paucity of studies reflects the difficulties in identifying suitable population cohorts, and in conducting prospective follow-up, in the African situation. In Senegal, 13 036 soldiers aged 20–55 years were screened for HBsAg. The only published results are the age-standardized incidence rate of liver cancer in the 2611 men who were HBsAg-positive (68.3 per 100 000 person years). The rate in non-carriers was not reported, but, if we assume that these men (mean

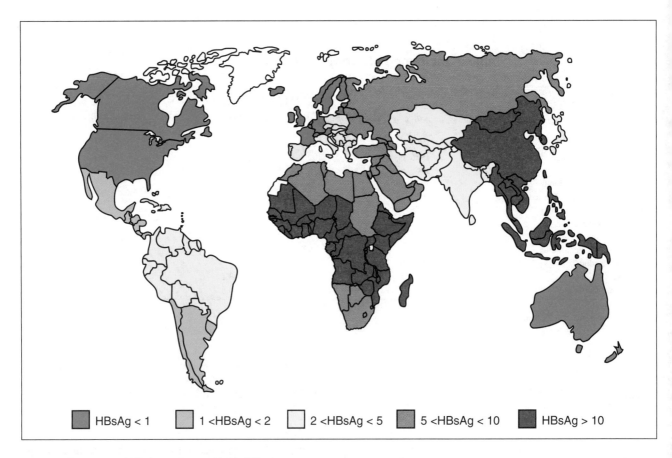

HBsAg < 1   1 <HBsAg < 2   2 <HBsAg < 5   5 <HBsAg < 10   HBsAg > 10

Figure 3. Prevalence of HBsAg carriers worldwide (%)

age 30 years) had the same incidence of liver cancer as men aged 25–34 in Dakar in 1969–74 (Waterhouse *et al.*, 1982)—26.0 per 100 000—then, with an HBsAg prevalence of 0.20, we may estimate the rate in non-carriers as [26.0 – (0.2 x 68.3)]/0.8 or 12.3, and the relative risk about 5–6. Evans *et al.* (1998) drew attention to the very much lower risk (one tenth) of liver cancer in the Senegal cohort than in carriers in China (or in Asian Americans). The Senegalese carriers have a much lower prevalence of serum HBV DNA than Chinese (mainly due to a more rapid decline with age); serum HBV DNA is associated with serum glutathione *S*-transferase titres, a marker of liver damage.

Figure 3 shows prevalence of HBsAg carriers among adults in different countries around 1993 (data supplied by WHO). Prevalence of chronic infection with hepatitis B virus is high in sub-Saharan Africa (average for all countries in the region is 11.6%), but lower in the north (average 5.4%). Because of this, the proportion of liver cancer cases attributable to hepatitis B infection can be estimated to vary from 50% in North Africa to 70% in West Africa, with a continent-wide average of 66% (28 000 cases per year).

Chronic carriage of HBV implies the persistence of replication of the virus, as reflected by the continued presence of HBsAg in the blood, although the titres of serum HBsAg in infected individuals decline with age (Evans *et al.*, 1998). The most important factor influencing this persistence is age at infection, with the likelihood of becoming a chronic carrier decreasing with age (Edmunds *et al.*, 1993). The high prevalence of HBV chronic carriage in Africa is a reflection of the high rates of infection in the first decade of life (Kew *et al.*, 1982). Perinatal infection seems to be rather uncommon, accounting for only 5–10% of carriers. It is possible that age at infection also determines the intensity of viraemia in chronic carriers—as noted above, Chinese subjects, infected perinatally, have higher and more persistent levels of serum HBV DNA than Senegalese. However, unlike in adults, in whom parenteral and sexual transmission are the most common, the modes of

transmission in children are not clear (IARC, 1994a). In rural Africa, risk of infection in childhood is associated with the number of siblings in a household (Whittle *et al.*, 1990). Late birth order has also been shown to influence the risk of becoming a carrier of

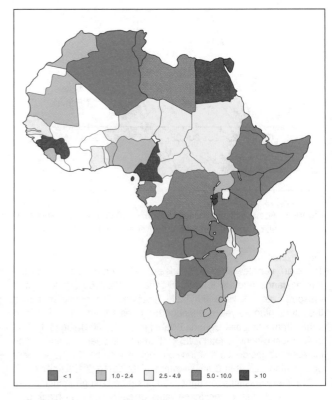

< 1   1.0 - 2.4   2.5 - 4.9   5.0 - 10.0   > 10

Figure 4. Prevalence of hepatitis C (source: WHO, 1999)

Table 3. Percentage distribution of microscopically verified cases by histological type
Liver (C22) - Both sexes

	Carcinoma				Hepato-blastoma	Sarcoma		Other	Unspec.	Number of cases	
	Hepato	Cholangio	Other	Unspec.		Haemangio	Other			MV	Total
Algeria, Algiers	57.1	20.4	-	12.2	8.2	-	2.0	-	-	**49**	68
Algeria, Batna	33.3	50.0	-	-	-	-	-	-	16.7	**6**	33
Algeria, Constantine	11.1	22.2	-	44.4	11.1	-	-	-	11.1	**9**	12
Algeria, Oran	40.0	30.0	10.0	10.0	-	-	-	-	10.0	**10**	12
Algeria, Setif	5.0	60.0	-	5.0	-	-	5.0	-	25.0	**20**	55
Burkina Faso, Ouagadougou	100.0	-	-	-	-	-	-	-	-	**9**	66
Congo, Brazzaville	75.9	16.5	1.3	6.3	-	-	-	-	-	**79**	226
France, La Reunion	54.8	19.4	3.2	12.9	-	-	-	-	9.7	**62**	79
The Gambia	100.0	-	-	-	-	-	-	-	-	**11**	348
Guinea, Conakry	94.4	2.2	1.1	-	2.2	-	-	-	-	**89**	597
Kenya, Eldoret	92.6	7.4	-	-	-	-	-	-	-	**27**	73
Malawi, Blantyre	63.2	10.5	10.5	5.3	-	-	-	-	10.5	**19**	29
Mali, Bamako	90.9	-	-	6.1	-	-	-	-	3.0	**33**	1035
Namibia	65.1	22.9	1.2	4.8	-	-	4.8	-	1.2	**83**	96
Niger, Niamey	85.7	7.1	-	7.1	-	-	-	-	-	**14**	200
Nigeria, Ibadan	87.5	4.2	-	8.3	-	-	-	-	-	**24**	75
Rwanda, Butare	43.8	3.1	-	-	-	-	-	-	53.1	**32**	53
South Africa: Black	65.0	13.6	3.6	5.7	0.5	0.0	0.9	0.3	10.3	**2599**	2599
South Africa: White	32.0	43.7	7.3	11.5	0.7	0.5	1.2	0.9	2.1	**563**	563
South Africa: Indian	54.0	20.6	3.2	11.1	-	-	-	1.6	9.5	**63**	63
South Africa: Mixed race	60.2	21.6	4.5	7.4	2.3	-	0.6	1.1	2.3	**176**	176
South Africa, Elim	93.6	2.1	-	4.3	-	-	-	-	-	**47**	48
South Africa, Transkei, Umtata	84.6	7.7	-	-	-	-	-	-	7.7	**13**	50
South Africa, Transkei, 4 districts	93.8	-	-	-	-	-	6.3	-	-	**16**	26
Swaziland	70.6	23.5	-	-	5.9	-	-	-	-	**17**	256
Tanzania, Dar Es Salaam	87.5	6.3	-	6.3	-	-	-	-	-	**16**	16
Tanzania, Kilimanjaro	90.0	6.7	-	3.3	-	-	-	-	-	**30**	77
Tunisia, Centre, Sousse	76.5	5.9	-	5.9	5.9	5.9	-	-	-	**17**	17
Tunisia, North, Tunis	78.0	10.0	2.0	2.0	4.0	-	2.0	-	2.0	**50**	78
Tunisia, Sfax	83.3	-	-	-	-	-	-	16.7	-	**6**	6
Uganda, Mbarara	50.0	-	-	50.0	-	-	-	-	-	**2**	41
Uganda, Kyadondo County	78.0	14.0	4.0	2.0	-	-	-	-	2.0	**50**	133
Zimbabwe, Harare: African	96.0	1.3	-	-	1.3	-	1.3	-	-	**150**	747
Zimbabwe, Harare: European	100.0	-	-	-	-	-	-	-	-	**11**	38

HBsAg (Ryder et al., 1992). This presumably reflects the fact that children with many older siblings are likely to be exposed to infection at a very young age. The possibility that biting insects (specifically bed bugs) play a role was tested in a randomized study in the Gambia, but the result was negative (Vall-Mayans et al., 1994). Moreover, low socioeconomic status plays a major role in the perpetuation of HBV endemicity in Africa. This factor was shown to be important elsewhere in both developed (Szmuness, 1978) and developing countries (Toukan, 1987).

HBV sub-type ad is associated with long-term carriage of HBsAg while ay is associated with short-term carriage (Rioche, 1986) and a significant relationship exists between sub-types and ethnic group in Africa. Reports from West Africa, where incidence of PHC is highest, show a high preponderance of ayw, which is also known to be common among non-Bantu West Africans in Uganda (Lwanga et al., 1977). To what extent these sub-types determine the incidence of PHC in Africa is worth further investigation (Wild & Hall, 1997).

The mechanism of carcinogenesis of HBV remains uncertain. The virus is not integrated into any specific part of the genome of the host, and some hepatocellular carcinomas in HBV carriers do not contain integrated HBV DNA (Matsubara & Tokino, 1990). One possibility is that cell proliferation associated with chronic hepatitis and cirrhosis is the important factor, the increased rate of cell turnover favouring accumulation of genetic alterations in liver cells.

In Africa, liver cancer is practically always preceded by cirrhosis, and it seems likely that the main role of HBV (as for HCV; see below) is in inducing cirrhosis, although there is evidence for an effect independent of this (Wild & Hall, 2000).

Hepatitis C virus infection

The recognition of the hepatitis C virus (HCV) and its role in hepatocarcinogenesis is much more recent than for HBV (IARC, 1994a). Presence of infection can be recognized by detecting antibody to the virus, or, more sensitively, by testing for viral RNA. The early tests for antibody (first-generation tests) were rather non-specific, so there is some doubt about the true prevalence of infection in studies that used them. Now, a large number of case–control studies (using second-generation tests) have been carried out in many countries. Overall, they suggest that the presence of antibody to HCV is associated with a relative risk of about 25. The results of seven studies in Africa are shown in Table 5. In a further study in Somalia (Bile et al., 1993), the cases were subjects with chronic liver disease and, although most were liver cancers, results were not reported separately. Several cohort studies have also been reported, but none from Africa. The prevalence of antibody-positive subjects in the population is rather lower than for HBsAg (see below); worldwide, prevalence seems to be highest in Japan, Egypt and parts of sub-Saharan Africa. Thus, although the relative risk associated with HCV infection is high, the proportion of cases of

Table 4. Summary of results of case–control studies of hepatocellular carcinoma and presence versus absence of hepatitis B surface antigen (HBsAg)

Reference and location	Subjects	Seroprevalence of HBsAg				OR	95% CI	Comments*
		Cases		Controls				
		No.	%	No.	%			
Prince et al. (1970); Uganda	Sex unspecified	4	12	6	2	[6.8]	[1.8–25]	Blood donor controls
Vogel et al. (1972); Uganda	Women and men	90	40	224	3	[19]	17.6–451	Adjusted for age and sex; testing by CF, CEP and PHA
Kew et al. (1974); South Africa	Men	75	40	18377	7	[8.7]	[5.3–14]	Mineworkers; testing by CEP and CF
Michon et al. (1975); Prince et al. (1975); Senegal	Women and men Controls with other cancer	165	61	154	12	[11]	[5.8–19]	Adjusted for age
	Controls without cancer	165	61	328	11	[14]	[8.7–24]	
Larouzé et al. (1976); Senegal	Women and men	28	79	28	57	[2.8]	[0.74–10]	
Tsega et al. (1976); Tsega (1977); Ethiopia	Women and men	46	50	90	7	[14]	[4.6–44]	
Tabor et al. (1977)	Women and men							
Uganda		47	47	50	6	[14]	[3.8–51]	
Zambia		19	63	40	8	[21]	[4.7–96]	
USA		27	30	6726	0.02	[134]	[53–337]	
Reys et al. (1977); Mozambique	Women and men	32	60	231	9	[15]	[5.9–37]	Male controls; solid-phase RIA + CEP
Van Den Heever et al. (1978); South Africa	Women and men	92	34	92	9	[5.3]	12.2–14]	Blacks
Kew et al. (1979); South Africa	Women and men	289	62	213	11	[13]	[7.6–21]	Blacks; solid-phase RIA
Bowry and Shah (1980); Kenya	Women	76	51	33	6	[16]	[3.4–106]	Testing by PHA
Coursaget et al. (1981); Senegal	Women and men Blood donor controls	134	63	100	12	[12]	[5.9–26]	
	Rural controls	134	63	833	14	[11]	[6.9–16]	
	Leprosy patient controls	134	63	560	25	[5.0]	[3.3–7.5]	
Gombe (1984); Congo	Women and men Blood donor controls	65	74	120	9	[32]	[11–87]	Adjusted for sex; testing by RIA or PHA
	Other cancer controls	65	74	71	3	[55]	[12–256]	
Sebti (1984); Morocco		46	17	379	5	[4.2]	[1.6–11]	Adjusted for sex
Kew et al. (1986a); South Africa	Women and men	62	40	62	3	[20]	[4.3–132]	Blacks
Otu (1987); Nigeria	Women and men	200	49	400	7.5	[12]	[7.3–19]	
Gashau & Mohammed (1991); Nigeria	Women and men	65	65	69	36	[3.2]	[1.5–7.0]	Testing by ELISA and reverse PHA
Mohamed et al. (1992); South Africa	Men	77	35	77	5	7.5	2.2–25	Adjusted for alcohol intake and smoking; blacks
	Women	24	25	24	4	12	1.0–154	
Tswana & Moyo (1992); Zimbabwe	Women and men	182	56	100	11	[10]	[5.0–22]	Testing by ELISA
Ryder et al. (1992); Gambia	Women and men	70	63	70	21	6.9		Adjusted for age; p < 0.01; 64 cases, 67 controls tested
Kashala et al. (1992); Zaire	Women and men	40	57.6	68	7.4	[17]	[5.7–51]	Testing by immunoperoxidase
Kew et al. (1997); South Africa	Women and men	231	53.3	231	8.2	21.8	8.9–53.4	Matched for age ± 2 years
Olubuyide et al. (1997); Nigeria	Men and women	64	59	64	50	1.0	0.5–8.0	Adjusted for age
Badawi & Michael, (1999); Egypt	Women and men	102	91	96	7	12.5	6.1–25.6	Adjusted for "confounders". Testing by ELISA

OR, odds ratio
CI, confidence interval
HCV, hepatitis C virus
NR, not reported
NS not significant
[ ], calculated values, unadjusted unless otherwise indicated in the comments
*, serological testing for HBV markers by radioimmunoassay unless otherwise specified:
ID, immunodiffusion,; CF complement fixation; CEP countercurrent immunoelectrophoresis; PHA passive haemagglutination; ELISA enzyme-linked immunoabsorbent assay

Table 5. Summary of results of case-control studies of hepatocellular carcinoma and the prevalence of antibody to HCV

Reference and location	Subjects	Seroprevalence of antibodies to HCV				OR[a]	95% CI	Comments*
		Cases		Controls				
		No.	%	No.	%			
Coursaget et al. (1990); Senegal	NR	80	37.5	136	3	[20]	[6.9–57]*	1982–86; stringent cut-off used for assay*
Kew et al. (1990); South Africa	Men and women	380	29	152	0.7	[62]	[11–353]*	Unmatched hospital controls
Dazza et al. (1993); Mozambique	NR	178	6	194	2	1.1	0.4–3.1	Blood donor controls; adjusted for age; mean age of cases, 40.8 years; controls, 31.3 years
Coursaget et al. (1992); Senegal	NR	49	4	134	1	[5.7]	[0.5–69]	General population controls
Kew et al. (1997); South Africa	Men and women	231	20.7	231	5.2	6.1	2.8–13.7	Age-matched hospital controls
Olubuyide et al. (1997); Nigeria	Men and women	64	19	64	11	1.1	0.4–7.8	Adjusted for age
Yates et al. (1999); Egypt	Men and women	31	67	26	30	[4.7]	[1.4–17.2]	Hospital cases, healthy controls. Confined to ages 42–52 for age-matching

[a]Cornfield limits
* As measured by first-generation assays

Table 6. Separate effects of HBV and HCV on risk for hepatocellular carcinoma

Reference and location	HBsAg seronegative HCV Ab seronegative		HBsAg seronegative HCV Ab seropositive			HBsAg seropositive HCV Ab seronegative			HBsAg seropositive HCV Ab seropositive		
	Cases	Controls	Cases	Controls	OR	Cases	Controls	OR	Cases	Controls	OR
Coursaget et al. (1992); Senegal	23	82	4	0	[•]	20	50	[1.4]	2	2	[3.6]
Dazza et al. (1993); Mozambique	52	163	8	4	1.4	115	27	[13]	3	0	[•]
Kew et al. (1997); South Africa	69	197	39	15	6.6	103	18	23.3	20	1	82.5
Olubuyide et al. (1997) Nigeria	21	29	5	3	[2.3]	31	28	[1.5]	7	4	[2.4]

liver cancer due to the virus is rather less than for HBV—perhaps 20–25% worldwide. Hepatitis C virus is transmitted mainly by blood and blood products, and most infection worldwide seems to be a consequence of blood transfusion or injections with unsterilized equipment. HCV is an RNA virus, and is not, therefore, integrated into the host cell DNA. Several different genotypes exist, which differ in their geographic distribution and, reportedly, in the severity of the hepatitis they cause. It seems that HCV causes liver cancer by causing chronic hepatitis and cirrhosis, both known to act as precursors of liver cancer through the intense hepatocyte regeneration occurring in these conditions.

The epidemiology of HCV infection on the African continent is not clearly described, and must be deduced from rather non-systematic small-scale studies of seroprevalence and surveys of blood donors and pregnant women. The available data (from WHO, 1999) are summarized in Figure 4.

One striking finding is the extraordinarily high prevalence of infection in Egypt. The average seroprevalence is about 15%, but there is considerable regional variation within the country, with the highest seroprevalence in the governorates (provinces) in the Nile delta (20–40%) and along the Nile valley (Arthur, 1996; Arthur et al., 1997). This is now recognized to be a result of campaigns of eradication of schistosomiasis, with inadequate sterilization of the

syringes and needles used for injection of antimonal compounds (Tartar emetic) between 1950 and 1982, when oral praziquantel became available (Attia, 1998). Seroprevalence increases with age, reaching a plateau around age 40 years (Hibbs et al., 1993; Yates et al., 1999). Frank et al. (2000) have shown that the birth-cohort-specific prevalence of HCV can be well explained by exposure to parenteral anti-schistosomal therapy in the 1960s and 1970s. For individuals in two large surveys of HCV prevalence, a regression model adjusting for region and age showed that there is a significant association between seroprevalence, and an index of exposure to such therapy. The high prevalence of infection in the general population—(35–55% at age 40–50 years in the non-metropolitan areas of the Nile valley) implies that continuing transmission may be maintained through blood transfusion and other, ill-defined, parenteral means.

The effects of combined infection with HBV and HCV are not very clear. Although joint infection occurs more often than would be expected by chance, it is still relatively rare in the general population, so that stable estimates of associated odds ratios are difficult to obtain. Four studies from Africa are summarized in Table 6. A further case–control study in Khartoum, Sudan (Omer et al., 2001) compared 115 hospital cases of liver cancer (probably mainly histologically confirmed) with 199 unmatched community controls with respect to positivity for HBsAg and/or anti-HCV. The crude OR was 12.9 (95% CI 6.9–24.2), although results for the two viruses separately, or together, were not given. A meta-analysis of case–control studies suggests that the combined effect lies somewhere between additive and multiplicative effects (Donato et al., 1998), and the results of a cohort study (Wang et al., 1996) are also compatible with this conclusion.

Aflatoxin B_1

Aflatoxins are produced by moulds of the Aspergillus species, which infect stored grains and nuts, and one of these, aflatoxin B_1, long known to cause liver tumours in animals, has been classified by IARC as a human carcinogen (IARC, 1993, 2002).

In Africa, high levels of contamination have been found particularly in groundnuts and maize. Human exposure to aflatoxin B1 in tropical Africa is in the range 3–200 ng/kg bw per day (Hall & Wild, 1994). Aflatoxins and their metabolites can be detected in various human tissues and body fluids. Thus, their presence in urine samples from Zimbabwe (Nyathi et al., 1987), Gambia (Wild et al., 1988), Kenya (Autrup et al., 1987) has been described. In the Gambia, urinary excretion was shown to correlate with dietary intake over the previous 24–48 hours (Groopman et al., 1992). Aflatoxins have been detected in blood samples in Nigeria (Denning et al., 1988), Sudan (Hendrickse et al., 1982) and Nigeria and Ghana (Lamplugh et al., 1988). The levels of covalently bound aflatoxin–albumin adducts in serum from subjects in the Gambia, Senegal and Kenya were much higher than those found in Europe or south-east Asia (Wild et al., 1990). Exposure levels did not vary with age and sex in the Gambia, but there were strong seasonal effects and higher levels in rural than urban dwellers (Allen et al., 1992; Wild et al., 2000). Aflatoxins can also be detected in human milk, as observed in Sudan (Coulter et al., 1984), Zimbabwe (Wild et al., 1987) and the Gambia (Zarba et al., 1992).

The first evidence for a carcinogenic effect in humans came from ecological studies that compared aflatoxin levels in foodstuffs with liver cancer incidence rates in different geographical locations. There are inherent problems in deducing probable effects in individuals from observations at the ecological level. In addition, the studies in Africa suffer from problems of estimating exposure (usually from some measures in foodstuffs) and outcome (data on liver cancer incidence are often very imprecise) and in taking into account such other important factors as exposure to HBV. Table 7 summarizes eight ecological studies carried out in Africa. They include studies comparing different population groups within Uganda (Alpert et al., 1971), Kenya (Peers & Linsell, 1973; Autrup et al., 1987), Swaziland (Peers et al., 1976, 1987), Mozambique (van Rensburg et al., 1985), South Africa (van Rensburg et al., 1990) and Sudan (Omer et al., 1998). For example, in Swaziland, aflatoxin intake was estimated from dietary samples and crop surveys; it varied more than five-fold between the four topographic regions of the country. Liver cancer incidence in 10 sub-regions was more closely related to mean estimated aflatoxin intake than to mean HBsAg prevalence (Peers et al., 1987).

Measurement of aflatoxins in body fluids and tissues has provided a more accurate measure of dietary exposure. In the Gambia, the levels of aflatoxin–albumin adducts in blood correlated well with dietary intake in the preceding seven days (Wild et al., 1992). In Kenya, Autrup et al. (1987) observed a significant correlation between liver cancer "incidence" (as estimated from attendance at a liver clinic in Kenyatta Hospital, Nairobi) and aflatoxin levels in the urine of patients attending outpatient departments in nine different district hospitals.

The ability to measure aflatoxin bound to cellular macromolecules, including DNA and proteins in urine and serum, has sharpened the measure of exposure, providing a biomarker that does reflect individual intake of aflatoxin (Hall & Wild, 1994). These measures have been used in cohort studies to study the

association between aflatoxin exposure and liver cancer risk. Thus, using urinary aflatoxin N7-guanine as a marker in a cohort study carried out in Shanghai, China, an increased risk of liver cancer was observed in individuals positive for the marker at enrolment compared with those who were negative (Qian et al., 1994). Furthermore, there appeared to be a multiplicative interaction with chronic HBV infection (also a clear risk factor in this study), suggesting a different mechanism of action from the virus. The effect of aflatoxin alone, in the absence of HBV, was rather weak. One mechanism for the interaction may be the diminished activity of aflatoxin-metabolizing enzymes in the presence of chronic infection by HBV. Thus, some studies in West Africa have suggest that there are higher levels of aflatoxin–albumin adducts in serum of HBsAg-positive subjects than in HBsAg-negative subjects, especially in children (Wild & Hall, 1997).

Recent work has focused on the role of polymorphisms of the genes responsible for aflatoxin metabolism in modifying risk due to aflatoxin exposure. Chen et al. (1996) observed that, among HBsAg carriers, the risk of liver cancer was related to serum aflatoxin B–albumin levels, but only in individuals with the null genotype for the enzymes glutathione S-transferase (GST) M1 and GST T1, possibly responsible for conjugation and detoxification of aflatoxin. Wild et al. (2000) found that blood levels of aflatoxin–albumin adducts in Gambian subjects were higher in those with GSTM1 null genotype in the absence of HBV infection. In a case–control study in China (McGlynn et al., 1995), a mutation in one or both alleles of the gene coding for epoxide hydrolase—another detoxifying enzyme—had a stronger association with hepatocellular carcinoma (OR = 3.3) than did the null genotype of GSTM1 (OR = 1.9).

Three case–control studies have been conducted in Africa to compare intake of aflatoxin in liver cancer patients with that in control subjects (Table 7). Case–control studies are much less satisfactory that the cohort studies mentioned earlier, since it is highly probable that dietary habits are profoundly altered in patients suffering from liver cancer. Even when serum or urine levels of aflatoxin adducts are used to measure exposure, only relatively recent intake (days or weeks) of aflatoxin is being evaluated. This may not reflect exposures during the etiologically relevant period (years earlier). Moreover, the presence of liver disease may modify the levels of aflatoxin found in serum or urine, biasing comparisons between cases and controls.

In small studies in Nigeria (Olubuyide et al., 1993a,b), cases were 22 patients at a university hospital in Ibadan in 1988 and controls were 22 patients from the gastroenterology ward of the same hospital with acid peptic disease, matched to cases on sex and age. Blood samples were collected and analysed for HBsAg and a variety of aflatoxins (B_1, B_2, M_1, M_2, G_1, G_2 and aflatoxicol). HBsAg was detected in 16 cases and 8 controls. Elevated levels of aflatoxins were detected in five (23%) cases and one (5%) control, the difference being significantly different (p < 0.05).

Mandishona et al. (1998) carried out a small case–control study in South Africa aiming primarily to determine the role of dietary iron overload in the etiology of hepatocellular carcinoma (see below), which included information on exposure to aflatoxin B_1. Cases were 24 consecutive patients with HCC in two hospitals of one province of South Africa. There were two sets of controls: a matched (sex, age, race) series of 48 (two controls per case) selected from patients hospitalized with trauma or infection, and 75 relatives of the cases. Analyses of blood samples yielded measures of serum aflatoxin B_1–albumin adducts, iron overload, HBsAg, HCV and other biochemical parameters. The median level of aflatoxin B_1–albumin adducts was lower among cases (7.3; range 2.4–91.2) than among hospital controls (21.7; range 0–45.6) and family controls (8.7; range 0.7–82.1). The use of median values to compare the groups may have obscured differences in the distribution of values between them.

Table 7. Summary of principal ecological and cross-sectional studies on liver cancer and aflatoxins in Africa

Reference	Area	Units of observation/ number of units	Exposure measure(s)	Outcome measure(s)	Covariate	Results	Comments
Alpert et al. (1971)	Uganda	Main tribes and districts of Uganda; 7	Aflatoxin contamination of nearly 500 food samples taken from randomly selected native homes and markets; 1966–67	Hepatoma incidence identified from hospital records; 1963–66	Nil	The highest incidence of hepatoma occured in areas with highest levels of aflatoxin contamination.	
Peers & Linsell (1973)	Kenya	Areas of Murang'a district; 3	Aflatoxin extracted from food samples, repeated sampling over 21 months	Incident hepatocellular cancers ascertained from local hospital; 1967–70	Nil	Using 6 data points (3 areas, both sexes), correlation ($r = 0.87$) between aflatoxin intake and liver cancer	Questionable completeness of liver cancer registration. Small number of units of observation
Peers et al. (1976)	Swaziland	Altitude areas; 4	Aflatoxin from food and beer samples: every 2 months for period 1 year, over 1000 samples analysed; 1972–73	Primary liver cancer (PLC) incidence rates, from national cancer registry, 1964–68	Nil	Correlation ($r = 0.99$) between aflatoxin and PLC rates	Exposure post-dated cancer data
Van Rensberg et al. (1985)	Southern Africa	7 regions in Mozambique and 1 in South Africa	Mean aflatoxin contamination of food samples, over 2500 samples analysed; 1969–74	Incidence rates of hepatocellular carcinoma (HCC); 1968–75. A variety of sources including local hospitals and South African mines	Nil	Rank correlations between HCC and mean total aflatoxin 0.64 ($p < 0.05$) in men and 0.71 ($p < 0.01$) in women	
Autrup et al. (1987)	Kenya	Districts of Kenya; 9	Prevalence of urinary AFB-Gual adducts as ascertained in surveys of local clinic patients in the various districts (total sample, 983); 1981–84	Primary hepatocellular carcinoma (PHC) incidence diagnosed at one large hospital in Nairobi; 1978–82	HBV measured by HBsAg in same sample as used for AFB	Spearman rank correlation showed moderate association ($r = 0.75$) between rate of AFB exposure and incidence of PHC. Using the same type of analysis, no correlation between HBV and PHC ($r = 0.19$). No interaction detected between AFB and HBV	Possible confounding by ethnic characteristics
Peers et al. (1987)	Swaziland	Administrative regions; 10	Aflatoxin measured in food samples from households and crop samples from the fields over 1200 samples analysed; 1982–83.	Incidence rates of PLC; 1979–83	Serum samples from the Swaziland blood bank HBsAg	Significant correlation between mean aflatoxin contamination and PLC; little effect of HBsAg on PLC.	
Van Rensberg et al. (1990)	South Africa	Natives of districts of the Transkei, working as goldminers; 4	Aflatoxin contamination of local food samples, based on over 600 samples; 1976–77	PLC incidence	Nil	Rank order correlations between aflatoxin intake and PLC incidence in goldminers from the Transkei were significant at $p < 0.05$.	
Omer et al. (1998)	Sudan	Two areas, one high risk, one low risk	Peanut butter samples collected in markets and analysed for AFB1. Type of storage assessed	Clinical experience and Khartoum hospital records	Nil	Aflatoxin consumption levels were much higher in the presumed high risk area than in the presumed low risk area	Only two areas compared. Unreliable measures of liver cancer incidence

Table 8. Summary of case-control studies on liver cancer and aflatoxins in Africa

Reference	Area	Study base	Cases	Controls	Exposure measures	Covariate	Results				Comments
Olubidye et al. (1993)	Nigeria	Hospital in Ibadan	Primary hepatocellular cancer diagnosed in 1988; $n = 22$	Matched patients from gastro-enterology ward; $n = 22$	Serum levels of aflatoxin	HBsAg was measured but not included in analysis of aflatoxins	High aflatoxin levels were detected in 5 cases and 1 control ($p < 0.05$)				
Mandishona et al. (1998)	South Africa	Two hospitals in one province of South Africa	Suspected cases of HCC; $n = 24$	Two control series: one hospital-based (trauma or infection patients), $n = 48$; family-based (including related and unrelated family members), $n = 75$	Measured AFB_1–albumin adducts	Several measured, but not used in analysis of aflatoxin	Levels of AFB_1–albumin adducts were lower among cases than among both sets of controls				High risks of HCC found for subjects with HBV, alcohol, and iron overload. Questionable comparability of hospital control series, and possible overmatching with family control series
Omer et al. (2001)	Sudan	Residents of two regions of Sudan	Cases of hepatocellular cancer diagnosed in 5 hospitals in Khartoum; $n = 150$	Community-based, selected from lists in 'sugar shops' in same localities as cases; $n = 205$	Questionnaire on peanut butter consumption and on storage of peanuts	HBsAg, HCV, smoking alcohol, $GSTM_1$ genotype	High peanut butter intake High peanut butter intake $+GSTM_1$ null genotype	OR 3.0 16.7	95% CI 1.6–5.5 2.7–104	No. 63 –	Questionable comparability of cases and controls

Omer *et al.* (2001) conducted a case–control study in Sudan to assess the association between peanut butter intake as a source of aflatoxin and the GSTM$_1$ genotype in the etiology of HCC. Cases were 150 patients with HCC who were diagnosed in one of the six major hospitals of Khartoum and whose place of residence was in one of two regions: West Sudan which is about 650 km from Khartoum and Central Sudan which is about 500 km from Khartoum. Controls were 205 residents of the two study areas, selected by a two-stage process, the second stage of which involved random selection from local village 'sugar shops'. Consumption of peanut butter (and some other factors) was obtained by interview by the principal investigator and transformed into a quantitative cumulative index. Usable blood samples were collected from 110 cases and 189 controls, and were analysed for HBsAg and genotyped for GSTM. In West Sudan, the cases consumed more peanut butter than controls, and there was a dose–response relationship between cumulative consumption and risk for HCC. In the highest quartile of consumption, the odds ratio was 8.7. However, peanut butter consumption conferred no increased risk in Central Sudan. GSTM$_1$ was not a risk factor for HCC, but it was a strong effect modifier; the excess risk due to peanut butter consumption was restricted to subjects with the GSTM$_1$ null genotype; the odds ratio in the high peanut butter exposure group among GSTM1 null genotype subjects was 16.7 (95% CI 2.7–105). There was no interaction between "hepatitis infection" (positivity for HBsAg or anti-HCV) and estimated consumption of peanut butter.

Some liver tumours have a highly specific point mutation involving a GC to TA transversion in codon 249 of the *TP53* tumour-suppressor gene (Greenblatt *et al.*, 1994; Montesano *et al.*, 1997). This mutation appears to be more frequent in populations where aflatoxin intake is thought to be high, for example, in Senegal (Coursaget *et al.*, 1993) and Mozambique and South Africa (Bressac *et al.*, 1991). In addition, the same base pair has been shown to be a hot-spot for mutation by aflatoxin in hepatocytes in vitro (Aguilar *et al.*, 1993) and to be more frequently mutated in non-tumorous liver tissue of patients originating from regions of supposed high aflatoxin exposure than those from low-exposure regions (Aguilar *et al.*, 1994). Kirk *et al.* (2000) observed the same mutation in DNA extracted from plasma of 36% patients with hepatocellular carcinoma in Gambia (but not in European patients), as well as in patients with cirrhosis (15%) and apparently normal subjects (6%). To date, no positive correlation has been made at the individual level between aflatoxin exposure and *TP53* mutation.

Iron overload

The role of iron overload as a cause of hepatocellular carcinoma has been of particular interest on the African continent. The observation that cases of liver cancer are often associated with elevated levels of serum ferritin, the principal iron storage protein (Kew *et al.*, 1978; Ola *et al.*, 1995), does not clarify whether this is a cause or an effect of the liver damage. However, prospective observation of subjects with haemochromatosis, a common inherited disorder of increased intestinal iron absorption and progressive parenchymal iron overload, shows that they have a high risk of developing cirrhosis and hepatocellular carcinoma (Niederau *et al.*, 1985).

Iron overload appears to be relatively frequent in some populations of sub-Saharan Africa, especially in South Africa (Bothwell *et al.*, 1964; Friedman *et al.*, 1990) and Zimbabwe (Gordeuk *et al.*, 1986), but has been reported also from Uganda (Owor, 1974) and Tanzania (Haddock, 1965) in East Africa, and Ghana (Dodu *et al.*, 1958) and Nigeria (Isak *et al.*, 1985) in West Africa. It is ascribed to excessive intake of iron derived from preparation of food and drink in iron vessels. Traditional beer has been particularly implicated (Walker & Segal, 1999). However, it has been suggested that, in addition to the quantity of iron consumed, there is also a familial predisposition, presumably implicating a genetic mechanism, though the responsible gene does not appear to be linked to HLA (as is the haemochromatosis gene) (Gordeuk *et al.*, 1992; Moyo *et al.*, 1998a).

Most of the evidence relating hepatocellular carcinoma to iron overload derives from autopsy studies in southern Africa. The initial observation by Strachan (1929) that hepatic iron concentrations were higher in subjects dying with hepatocellular carcinoma than in those with other causes of death has been confirmed in later studies (Friedman *et al.*, 1990; Jaskiewicz *et al.*, 1991; Gordeuk *et al.*, 1996). Moyo *et al.* (1998b) measured hepatocellular iron in a series of 215 liver biopsies in Harare, Zimbabwe; the odds of hepatocellular carcinoma (36 cases) were 3.1 times (95% CI 1.05–9.4) higher in the presence of iron overload. Mandishona *et al.* (1998), in a case–control study in Mpumulanga Province of South Africa, compared 24 biopsy-proved liver cancer cases with 48 hospital controls and 75 family members of the cases. Iron overload (defined as markedly raised serum transferrin saturation combined with an elevated serum ferritin concentration) was present in five cases and three controls, corresponding to an odds ratio of 10.6 (95% CI 1.5–76.8) after adjustment for alcohol consumption, infection with HBV and HCV, and exposure to aflatoxin B. Compared with the 75 family members, the risk conferred by iron overload was 4.1 (95% CI 0.5–32.2).

There have been no prospective studies in Africa. In a nested case–control study within a cohort of male government employees in Taiwan, the risk of developing liver cancer was increased 1.4-fold (95% CI 1.0–2.0) in subjects with elevated serum ferritin at entry (Stevens *et al.*, 1986). However, HBV carriers have higher mean iron levels than the general population (Israel *et al.*, 1989) and no adjustment was made for HBV infection status, possibly because almost all of the liver cancer cases were HBsAg carriers. In a prospective study of subjects with chronic liver disease in Korea, Hann *et al.* (1989) observed an odds ratio of 4.4 (95% CI 1.3–14.5) of developing liver cancer eight months or more after entry among 93 chronic carriers of HBsAg with the highest tertile of serum ferritin at entry, compared with those having lower levels.

Mechanisms by which a high level of serum or tissue iron may predispose to liver cancer are not yet clear; it may act by promoting tissue damage and cirrhosis, by enhancing chronic carriage of HBV and/or HCV, or by a direct mutagenic effect of iron (Gangaidzo & Gordeuk, 1995).

Other risk factors

Excessive alcohol consumption is an important cause of hepatocellular carcinoma in western countries; in an evaluation in 1988, IARC (1988) considered four cohort studies and six case–control studies, and concluded that the evidence was sufficient to indicate a causative association. Since that time, other work has suggested that the effects of alcohol on HBsAg-positivity are independent and have a multiplicative effect (Chen *et al.*, 1991), and that the same may be true for alcohol and infection with HCV (Yu *et al.*, 1991). In South Africa, habitual drinking of more than 80g of ethanol daily in the presence of HBV infection was associated with increased risk in urban men aged over 40 years (Mohammed *et al.*, 1992). Alcohol is believed to operate through its action as a hepatotoxin, promoting liver cirrhosis and regeneration with rapid cell division, favouring oncogenic mutations.

Because of the close association between alcohol consumption and tobacco smoking, it has been difficult to establish whether tobacco smoking plays an independent role in the etiology of liver cancer. In general, the evidence suggests a weak association, independent of alcohol and hepatitis B infection (Doll, 1996), with only a two- to three-fold increase in risk. In South Africa, Kew *et al.* (1985) did not find any association between smoking and risk of hepatocellular carcinoma, and no significant association was observed for cigarette smoking or alcohol consumption in a study in Nigeria (Olubuyide & Bamgboye, 1990).

Use of oral contraceptives is well known to increase the risk of hepatic adenomas. The evidence is less convincing for hepatocellular carcinoma, although several studies suggest that there is an increased risk (Kew *et al.*, 1990) that is higher with more prolonged use (Schlesselman, 1995). A WHO multicentre study, which included countries in which hepatitis B is endemic, found no association, although adjustment for HBV status was not done or was inadequate (WHO, 1989).

Evidence linking schistosomal infection with liver cancer has come mainly from observations in China and Japan, where *S. japonicum* is involved. The studies are not convincing (IARC, 1994b). In a hospital-based case–control study in Cairo, Egypt, Badawi and Michael (1999) found infection with *S. mansoni* to be more common in liver cancer cases (59%) than in control subjects (11%), corresponding to an odds ratio of 5.2. The estimate may have been adjusted for HBV infection, but there was no adjustment for HCV infection, common in this population and known to be associated with schistosomal infection (Darwish *et al.*, 1993).

Several studies have suggested that ingestion of inorganic arsenic is a risk factor for hepatocellular carcinoma.

There is also evidence that membranous obstruction of inferior vena cava (MOIVC) has a minor causal association with primary hepatocellular carcinoma in Africa, in a manner similar to that thought to occur with cirrhosis elsewhere (Kew *et al.*, 1989).

Prevention

Prevention of chronic carriage of HBV became a reality with the development of vaccines in the early 1970s (Krugman *et al.*, 1970, 1971). Early trials suggested that vaccination could prevent approximately 70–75% transmission of hepatitis B virus infection from carrier mother to infant. If hepatitis B immune globin (HBIG) was given with vaccine in the neonatal period, 90–95% of transmission was prevented (Beasley *et al.*, 1983; Wong *et al.*, 1984).

Two randomized studies were set up in Qidong county, China (Sun *et al.*, 1991) and in the Gambia, West Africa (GHIS, 1987), to formally establish the effectiveness of vaccination against hepatitis B in preventing liver cancer later in life. It will be many years before results are available. However, follow-up of the vaccinated children does demonstrate that there is a much lower rate of natural infection and a greatly reduced prevalence of chronic HBsAg carriers (Viviani *et al.*, 1999). In Taiwan, mass vaccination against hepatitis B was introduced in the 1980s, first to neonates born of HBsAg-positive mothers, then, in 1984, for all new-borns. By 1994, it was possible to compare liver cancer incidence in children aged 6–9 years born before vaccination was introduced with those born after. There was a fourfold difference in incidence (Chang *et al.*, 1997). These results suggest that vaccination will, indeed, be as successful as hoped.

Wild and Hall (2000) have reviewed measures to prevent aflatoxin-induced liver disease. They distinguish individual-level and community-level preventive measures, with the latter category subdivided into pre- and post-harvest actions. Pre-harvest measures include reducing crop vulnerability to fungal infection (using irrigation, insecticides and fungicides), introduction of non-aflatoxigenic strains of *A. flavus* to compete with aflatoxin-producing strains (biocontrol) and use of genetically modified crops (*Aspergillus*-resistant).

Post-harvest, the objective is to minimize aflatoxin accumulation due to food storage in hot and humid conditions, with rodent or insect damage. Improved drying and storage are key elements, along with use of pesticides and biological pest control.

At the individual level, consumers can be educated to avoid obviously mouldy grains, and to consume a more varied diet, with less reliance on staple crops (especially maize and peanuts) that are heavily contaminated with aflatoxin. Chemoprevention is a different approach to prevention of aflatoxin toxicity; the aim is to enhance detoxification of ingested aflatoxin by modulating expression of enzymes such as glutathione S-transferases. Oltipraz is a drug which induces these enzymes in animals (rats) and results in enhanced excretion of aflatoxin–glutathione conjugates in bile, lowered formation of aflatoxin–DNA adducts in liver and inhibition of aflatoxin B_1-mediated hepatocarcinogenesis. In a small-scale trial in China (Wang *et al.*, 1999), a relatively large dose of oltipraz was observed to reduce the level of albumin–aflatoxin adducts in humans and to increase excretion of glutathione conjugates. However, it is doubtful whether this type of chemoprevention will have a practical application in the control of liver cancer.

Screening for liver cancer among high-risk subjects (HBsAg carriers, patients with chronic liver disease) using serum alpha-fetoprotein (AFP) and/or abdominal ultrasound has been tried in a number of settings, but there is no evidence of benefit from a properly conducted randomized trial (Brown & Scharschmitt, 1999). A small study in Cameroon (Biwole-Sida *et al.*, 1992) using both ultrasound and AFP (cut-off > 1000 ng/ml) found a high prevalence of liver cancer in subjects with clinical cirrhosis (20/48) and chronic hepatitis (9/45), but no cases in 70 otherwise healthy carriers of HBsAg.

References

Aguilar, F., Harris, C.C., Sun, T., Hollstein, M. & Cerutti, P. (1994) Geographic variation of p53 mutational profile in nonmalignant human liver. *Science*, **264**, 1317–1319

Aguilar, F., Hussain, S.P. & Cerutti, P. (1993) Aflatoxin B1 induces the transversion of G_T in codon 249 of the p53 tumor suppressor gene in human hepatocytes. *Proc. Natl. Acad. Sci. USA*, 90, 8586–8590

Akoojee S.S., Seebaran A.R., Akerman B.S., Rajput M.C., Kandar M.C. (1990) Hepatocellular carcinoma in South African Indians resident in Natal. *Trop. Geogr. Med.*, **42**, 265–268

Allen, S.J., Wild, C.P., Wheeler, J.G., Riley, E.M., Montesano, R., Bennett, S., Whittle, H.J., Hall, A.J. & Greenwood, B.M. (1992) *Trans. Roy. Soc. Trop. Med. Hyg.*, **86**, 426–430

Alpert, M.E., Hutt, M.S.R. & Davidson, C.S. (1968) Hepatoma in Uganda. A study in geographic pathology. *Lancet*, i, 1265–1267

Alpert, M.E., Hutt, M.S., Wogan, G.N. & Davidson, C.S. (1971) Association between aflatoxin content of food and hepatoma frequency in Uganda. *Cancer*, **28**, 253–260

Arthur, R.R. Epidemiology of HCV infections in Egypt. *Medicine and the Community*, **6**, 4–7 (1996)

Arthur, R.R., Hassan, N.F., Abdallah, M.Y., el-Sharkawy, M.S., Saad, M.D., Hackbart, B.G., Imam, I.Z. (1997) Hepatitis C antibody prevalence in blood donors in different governorates in Egypt. *Trans. R. Soc. Trop. Med. Hyg.*, **91**, 271–274

Attia, M.A. (1998) Prevalence of hepatitis B and C in Egypt and Africa. *Antiviral Therapy*, **3** (suppl. 2), 1–9

Autrup, H., Seremet, T., Wakhisi, J. & Wasunna, A. (1987) Aflatoxin exposure measured by urinary excretion of aflatoxin B1-guanine adduct and hepatitis B virus infection in areas with different liver cancer incidence in Kenya. *Cancer Res.*, **47**, 3430–3433

Badawi, A.F. & Michael, M.S. (1999) Risk factors for hepatocellular carcinoma in Egypt: the role of hepatitis-B viral infection and schistosomiasis. *Anticancer Res.*, **19**, 4563–4568

Bah, E., Hall, A.J. & Inskip, H.M. (1990) The first 2 years of the Gambian National Cancer Registry. *Br. J. Cancer*, **62**, 647–650

Bah, E., Parkin, D.M., Hall, A.J., Jack, A.D. & Whittle, H. (2001) Cancer in The Gambia: 1988-97. *Br. J. Cancer*, **84**, 1207–1214

Banda, L.T., Parkin, D.M., Dzamalala, C.P. & Liomba, N.G. (2001) Cancer incidence in Blantyre, Malawi 1994–1998. *Trop. Med. Int. Health*, **6**, 296–304

Bassett, M.T., Chokunonga, E., Mauchaza, B., Levy, L., Ferlay, J. & Parkin, D.M. (1995a) Cancer in the African population of Harare, Zimbabwe, 1990–1992. *Int. J. Cancer*, **63**, 29–36

Bassett, M.T., Levy, L., Chokunonga, E., Mauchaza, B., Ferlay, J. & Parkin, D.M. (1995b) Cancer in the European population of Harare, Zimbabwe, 1990–1992. *Int. J. Cancer*, **63**, 24–28

Bayo, S., Parkin, D.M. & Koumare, A.K. (1990) Cancer in Mali, 1987–1988. *Int. J. Cancer*, **45**, 679–684

Beasley, R.P., Hwang, L.Y., Lee, G.C., Lan, C.C., Roan, C.H., Huang, F.Y., Chen, C.L. (1983) Prevention of perinatally transmitted hepatitis B virus infections with hepatitis B virus infections with hepatitis B immune globulin and hepatitis B vaccine. *Lancet*, **2**, 1099–1102

Bile, K., Aden, C., Norder, H., Magnius, L., Lindberg, G. & Nilsson, L. (1993) Important role of hepatitis C virus infection as a cause of chronic liver disease in Somalia. *Scand. J. Infect. Dis.*, **25**, 559–564

Biwole-Sida, M., Amvene, M., Oyono, E., Mbakop, A., Manfo, C., Tapko, J.B., Edzoa, T. & Ngu, K.B. (1992) Dépistage de carcinome hépatocellulaire au sein d'une population de sujets à haut risque au Cameroun. *Ann. Gastroentérol. Hépatol.*, **28**, 213–216

Bothwell, T.H., Seftel, H. & Jacobs, P. (1964) Iron overload in Bantu subjects: studies on the availability of iron in bantu beer. *Am. J. Clin. Nutr.*, **14**, 47–51

Bouchardy, C., Wanner, P. & Parkin, D.M. (1995) Cancer mortality among sub-Saharan African migrants in France. *Cancer Causes Control*, **6**, 539–544

Bowry, T.R. & Shah, M.V. (1980) A study of hepatitis Bs antigen titres and alpha foetoprotein levels in primary hepatocellular carcinoma in Kenya. *E. Afr. Med. J.*, **57**, 382–389

Bradshaw, E., McGlashan, N.D., Fitzgerald, D. & Harington, J.S. (1982) Analyses of cancer incidence in black gold miners from Southern Africa (1964–79). *Br. J. Cancer*, **46**, 737–748

Bressac, B., Kew, M., Wands, J. & Ozturk, M. (1991) Selective G to T mutations of p53 gene in hepatocellular carcinoma from southern Africa. *Nature*, **350**, 429–431

Brown, R.S. & Scharschmitt, B.F. (1999) Liver cancer. In Kramer, B.S., Gohagan, J.K. & Prorok, P.C., eds, *Cancer Screening: Theory and Practice*, New York, Basel, Marcel Dekker, pp. 299–326

Burkitt, D.P. (1969) A study of cancer patterns in Africa. *Sci. Basis Med. Annu. Rev.*, 82–94

Chang, M.H., Chen, C.J., Lai, M.S., Hsu, H.M., Wu, T.C., Kong, M.S., Liang, D.C., Shau, W.Y. & Chen, D.S. (1997) Universal hepatitis B vaccination in Taiwan and the incidence of hepatocellular carcinoma in children. Taiwan Childhood Hepatoma Study Group. *New Engl. J. Med.*, **336**, 1855–1859

Chen, J.G., Zhang, B.C., Jiang, Y.H., Chen, Q.C., Yun, Z.X. & Shen, Q.J. (1991) Study on screening for primary liver cancer in high-risk populations of an endemic area. *Chin. J. Prev. Med.*, **25**, 326–328

Chen, C.-J., Yu, M.W., Liaw, Y.F., Wang, L.W., Chiamprasert, S., Matin, F., Hirvonen, A., Bell, D.A. & Santella, R.M. (1996) Chronic hepatitis B carriers with null genotypes of glutathione S-transferase M1 and T1 polymorphisms who are exposed to aflatoxin are at increased risk of hepatocellular carcinoma. *Am. J. Hum. Genet.*, **59**, 128–134

Cook, P.J. & Burkitt, D.P. (1971) Cancer in Africa. *Br. Med. Bull.*, **27**, 14–20

Coulter, J.B., Lamplugh, S.M., Suliman, G.I., Omer, M.I. & Hendrickse, R.G. (1984) Aflatoxins in human breast milk. *Ann. Trop. Paediatr.*, **4**, 61–66

Coursaget, P., Maupas, P., Goudeau, A., Chiron, J.P., Raynaud, B., Drucker, J., Barin, F., Denis, F., Diop Mar, I. & Diop, B. (1981) A case/control study of hepatitis B virus serologic markers in Senegalese patients suffering from primary hepatocellular carcinoma. *Prog. Med. Virol.*, **27**, 49–59

Coursaget, P., Bourdil, C., Kastally, R., Yvonnet, B., Rampanarivo, Z., Chiron, J.P., Bao, O., Diop-Mar, I., Perrin, J. & Ntareme, F. (1990) Prevalence of hepatitis C virus infection in Africa: anti-HCV antibodies in the general population and in patients suffering from cirrhosis or primary liver cancer. *Res. Virol.*, **141**, 449–454

Coursaget, P., Leboulleux, D., Le Cann, P., Bao, O. & Coll-Seck, A.M. (1992) Hepatitis C virus infection in cirrhosis and primary hepatocellular carcinoma in Senegal. *Trans. R. Soc. Trop. Med. Hyg.*, **86**, 552–553

Coursaget, P., Depril, N., Chabaud, M., Nandi, R., Mayelo, V., LeCann, P., Yvonnet, B. (1993) High prevalence of mutations at codon 249 of the p53 gene in hepatocellular carcinomas from Senegal. *Br. J. Cancer*, **67**, 1395–1397

Darwish, M.A., Raouf, T.A., Rushdy, P., Constantine, N.T., Rao, M.R. & Edelman, R. (1993) Risk factors associated with a high seroprevalence of hepatitis C virus infection in Egyptian blood donors. *Am. J. Trop. Med. Hyg.*, **49**, 440–447

Dazza, M.C., Meneses, L.V., Girard, P.M., Astagneau, P., Villaroel, C., Delaporte, E., Larouze, B. (1993) Absence of a relationship between antibodies to hepatitis C virus and hepatocellular carcinoma in Mozambique. *Am. J. Trop. Med. Hyg.*, **48**, 237–242

Denning, D.W., Onwubalili, J.K., Wilkinson, A.P. & Morgan, M.R. (1988) Measurement of aflatoxin in Nigerian sera by enzyme-linked immunosorbent assay. *Trans. R. Soc. Trop. Med. Hyg.*, **82**, 169–171

Dodu, S.R.A. (1958) Diabetes and haeosiderosis – haemochromatosis in Ghana. *Trans. R. Soc. Trop. Med. Hyg.*, **52**, 425–431

Doll, R. C(1996) ancers weakly related to smoking. *Br. Med. Bull.*, **52**, 35–49

Donato, F., Boffetta, P. & Puoti, M. (1998) A meta-analysis of epidemiological studies on the combined effect of hepatitis B and C virus infections in causing hepatocellular carcinoma. *Int. J. Cancer*, **75**, 347–354

Edington, G.M. (1978) The pattern of cancer in the Northern Savannah of Nigeria with special reference to primary liver cell carcinoma and the Burkitt lymphoma. *Niger. Med. J.*, **8**, 281–289

Edmunds, W.J., Medley, G.F., Nokes, D.J., Hall, A.J. & Whittle, H.C. (1993) The influence of age on the development of the hepatitis B carrier state. *Proc. R. Soc. Lond. B*, **253**, 197–201

Evans, A.A., O'Connell, A.P., Pugh, J.C., Mason, W.S., Shen, F.M., Chne, G.C., Lin, W.Y., Dia, W.Y., M'Boup, S., Drame, B. & London, W.T. (1998) Geographic variation in viral load among hepatitis B carriers with differing risks of hepatocellular carcinoma. *Cancer Epidemiol. Biomarkers Prev.*, **7**, 559–565

Fakunle, Y.M., Ajdukiewicz, A.B. & Greenwood, B.M. (1977) Primary liver cell carcinoma (PLCC) in the northern Guinea savanna of Nigeria. *Trans. R. Soc. Trop. Med. Hyg.*, **71**, 335–337

Ferlay, J., Bray, F., Pisani, P. & Parkin, D.M. (eds) (2001) *Globocan2000: Cancer Incidence, Mortality and Prevalence Worldwide* (CD-ROM) (IARC Cancer Base No.5), Lyon, International Agency for Research on Cancer

Frank, C., Mohamed, M.K., Strickland, G.T., Lavanchy, D., Arthur, R.R., Magder, L.S., El Khoby, T., Abdel-Wahab, Y., Aly Ohn, E.S., Anwar, W. & Sallam, I. (2000) The role of parenteral antischistosomal therapy in the spread of hepatitis C virus in Egypt. *Lancet*, **355**, 887–891

Friedman, B.M., Baynes, R.D., Bothwell, T.H., Gordeuk, V.R., Macfarlane, B.J., Lamparelli, R.D., Robinson, E.J., Sher, R. & Hamberg, S. (1990) Dietary iron overload in southern African rural blacks. *S. Afr. Med. J.*, **78**, 301–305

Gambia Hepatitis Study Group (1987) The Gambia Hepatitis Intervention Study. *Cancer Res.*, **47**, 5782–5787

Gangaidzo, I.T. & Gordeuk, V.R. (1995) Hepatocellular carcinoma and African iron overload. *Gut*, **37**, 727–730

Gashau, W. & Mohammed, I. (1991) Hepatitis B viral markers in Nigerian patients with primary liver carcinoma. *Trop. Geogr. Med.*, **43**, 64–67

Gombe, C.M. (1984) L'antigène HBs: marqueude la relation entre le virus de l'hépatitis B et le cancer primitif du foie: situation à Brazzaville en 1984. In: Williams, A.O., O'Conor, G.T., De Thé, G.T. & Johnson, C.A., eds, *Virus-Associated Cancers in Africa* (IARC Scientific Publications No. 63), Lyon, IARC, pp. 221–226

Gordeuk, V., Mukiibi, J., Hasstedt, S.J., Samowitz, W., Edwards, C.Q., West, G., Ndambire, S., Emmanual, J., Nkanza, N., Chapanduka, Z., Randall, M., Boone, P., Romano, P., Martell, R.W., Yamashita, T., Effler, P. & Brittenham, G. (1992) Iron overload in Africa. Interaction between a gene and dietary iron content. *New Engl. J. Med.*, **326**, 95–100

Gordeuk, V.R., Boyd, R.D. & Brittenham, G.M. (1986) Dietary iron overload persists in rural sub-Saharan Africa. *Lancet*, **i**, 1310–1313

Gordeuk, V.R., McLaren, C.E., MacPhail, A.P., Deichsel, G. & Bothwell, T.H. Associations of iron overload in Africa with hepatocellular carcinoma and tuberculosis; Strachan's 1929 thesis revisited. *Blood* 87, 3470–3476 (1996)

Greenblatt, M.S., Bennett, W.P., Hollstein, M. & Harris, C.C. (1994) Mutations in the p53 tumor suppressor gene: clues to cancer etiology and molecular pathogenesis. *Cancer Res.*, **54**, 4855–4878

Groopman, J.D., Roebuck, B.D. & Kensler, T.W. (1992) Molecular dosimetry of aflatoxin DNA adducts in humans and experimental rat models. *Prog. Clin. Biol. Res.*, **374**, 139–155

Grulich, A.E., Swerdlow, A.J., Head, J. & Marmot, M.G. (1992) Cancer mortality in African and Caribbean migrants to England and Wales. *Br. J. Cancer*, **66**, 905–911

Haddock, D.R.W. (1965) Bantu siderosis in Tanzania. *E. Afr. Med. J.*, **42**, 67–71

Hall, A.J. & Wild, C.P. (1994) Epidemiology of aflatoxin related disease. In: Eaton D.L. & Groopman J.D., eds, *The Toxicology of Alfatoxins: Human Health, Veterinary and Agricultural Significance*, San Diego, CA, Academic Press, pp. 233–258

Hann, H.-W., Kim, C.Y., London, T. & Blumberg, B.S. (1989) Increased serum ferritin in chronic liver disease: a risk factor for primary hepatocellular carcinoma. *Int. J. Cancer*, **43**, 376–379

Harington, J.S., Bradshaw, E.M. & McGlashan, N.D. (1983) Changes in primary liver and oesophageal cancer rates among black goldminers, 1964–1981. *S. Afr. Med. J.*, **64**, 650

Hendrickse, R.G., Coulter, J.B., Lamplugh, S.M., Macfarlane, S.B., Williams, T.E., Omer, M.I., Suliman, G.I. (1982) Aflatoxins and kwashiorkor: a study in Sudanese children. *Br. Med. J.*, **285**, 843–846

Hibbs, R.G., Corwin, A.L., Hassan, N.F., Kamel, M., Darwish, M., Edelman, R., Constantine, N.T., Rao, M.R., Khalifa, A.S., Mokhtar, S., Fam, N.S., Ekladious, E.M. & Bassily, S.B. (1993) The epidemiology of antibody to hepatitis C in Egypt. *J. Infect. Dis.*, **168**, 789–790

IARC (1988) *IARC Monographs on the Evaluation of the Carcinogenic Risks to Humans*, Vol. 44, *Alcohol Drinking*, Lyon, IARC

IARC (1993) *IARC Monographs on the Evaluation of the Carcinogenic Risks to Humans*, Vol. 56, *Some Naturally Occurring Substances: Food Items and Constituents, Heterocyclic Aromatic Amines and Mycotoxins*, Lyon, IARC

IARC (1994a) *IARC Monographs on the Evaluation of the Carcinogenic Risks to Humans*, Vol. 59, *Hepatitis Viruses*, Lyon, IARC

IARC (1994b) *IARC Monographs on the Evaluation of the Carcinogenic Risks to Humans*, Vol. 61, *Schistosomes, liver flukes and Helicobacter pylori*, IARC, Lyon

IARC (2002) *IARC Monographs on the Evaluation of the Carcinogenic Risks to Humans*, Vol. 82, *Some Traditional Herbal Medicines, Some Mycotoxins, Naphthalene and Styrene*, Lyon, IARCPress

Isak, H.S. & Fleming, A.F. (1985) Anaemia and iron status of symptom-free adult males in northern Nigeria. *Ann. Trop. Med. Parasitol.*, **79**, 479–484

Israel, J., McGlynn, K., Hann, H.-W.L. & Blumberg, B.S. (1989) Iron-related markers in liver cancer. In: de Sousa, M. & Brock, J.H., eds, *Iron in Immunity, Cancer and Inflammation*, New York, John Wiley, pp. 301–316

Jaskiewicz, K., Stepien, A. & Banach, L. (1991) Hepatocellular carcinoma in a rural population at risk. *Anticancer Res.*, **11**, 2187–2189

Kashala, L.O., Conne, B., Kapanci, Y., Frei, P.C., Lambert, P.H., Kalengayi, M.R. & Essex, M. (1992) Hepatitis B virus, alpha-fetoprotein synthesis, and hepatocellular carcinoma in Zaire. *Liver*, **12**, 330–340

Kew, M.C., Geddes, E.W., Macnab, G.M., Bersohn, I. (1974) Hepatitis-B antigen and cirrhosis in Bantu patients with primary liver cancer. *Cancer*, **34**, 538–541

Kew, M.C., Marcus, R. & Geddes, E.W. (1977) Some characteristics of Mozambican Shangaans with primary hepatocellular cancer. *S. Afr. Med. J.*, **51**, 306–309

Kew, M.C., Torrance, J.D., Derman, D., Simon, M., Macnab, G.M., Charlton, R.W. & Bothwell, T.H. (1978) Serum and tumour ferritins in primary liver cancer. *Gut*, **19**, 294–299

Kew, M.C., Desmyter, J., Bradburne, A.F. & Macnab, G.M. (1979) Hepatitis B virus infection in southern African blacks with hepatocellular cancer. *J. Natl Cancer Inst.*, **62**, 517–520

Kew, M.C., Hodkinson, J. & Paterson, A.C. (1982) Hepatitis-B virus infection in black children with hepatocellular carcinoma. *J. Med. Virol.*, **9**, 201–207

Kew, M.C., Rossouw, E. & Hodkinson, J. (1983) Hepatitis B virus status of Southern African blacks with hepatocellular carcinoma: comparison between rural and urban patients. *Hepatology*, **3**, 65–68

Kew, M.C., DiBisceglie, A.M. & Paterson, A.C. (1985) Smoking as a risk factor in hepatocellular carcinoma. A case-control study in Southern African blacks. *Cancer*, **56**, 2315–2317

Kew, M.C., Kassianides, C., Hodkinson, J., Coppin, A. & Paterson, A.C. (1986) Hepatocellular carcinoma in urban born blacks: frequency and relation to hepatitis B virus infection. *Br. Med. J. (Clin. Res. Ed.)*, **293**, 1339–1341

Kew, M.C., McKnight, A., Hodkinson, J., Bukofzer, S. & Esser, J.D. (1989) The role of membranous obstruction of the inferior vena cava in the etiology of hepatocellular carcinoma in Southern African blacks. *Hepatology*, **9**, 121–125

Kew, M.C., Song, E., Mohammed, A. & Hodkinson, J. (1990) Contraceptive steroids as a risk factor for hepatocellular carcinoma: case/control study in South African black women. *Hepatology*, **11**, 298–302

Kew, M.C., Yu, M.C., Kedda, M.A., Coppin, A., Sarkin, A. & Hodkinson, J. (1997) The relative roles of hepatitis B and C viruses in the etiology of hepatocellular carcinoma in southern African blacks. *Gastroenterology*, **112**, 184–187

Kirk, G.D., Camus-Randon, A.M., Mendy, M., Goedert, J., Merle, P., Trepo, C., Brechot, C., Hainaut, P. & Montesano, R. (2000) Ser-249 mutations in plasma DNA of patients with hepatocellular carcinoma from The Gambia. *J. Natl. Cancer Inst.*, **92**, 148–153

Kocheleff, P., Carteron, B., Constant, J.L. & Bedere, C. (1984) Incidence rate and geographic distribution of hepatoma in Burundi. *Ann. Soc. Belge Med. Trop.*, **64**, 299–307

Koulibaly, M., Kabba, I.S., Cisse, A., Diallo, S.B., Diallo, M.B., Keita, N., Camara, N.D., Diallo, M.S., Sylla, B.S. & Parkin, D.M. (1997) Cancer incidence in Conakry, Guinea: first results from the cancer registry 1992–1995. *Int. J. Cancer*, **70**, 39–45

Krugman, S., Gilles, G.P. & Hammond, J. (1970) Hepatitis virus: effect of heat on the infectivity and antigenicity of the MS-1 and MS-2 strains. *J. Infect. Dis.*, **122**, 432–436

Krugman, S., Gilles, G.P. & Hammond, J. (1971) Viral hepatitis type B (MS-2 strain): studies on effective immunization. *J. Am. Med. Assoc.*, **217**, 41–45

Lamplugh, S.M., Hendrickse, R.G., Apeagyei, F. & Mwanmut, D.D. (1988) Aflatoxins in breast milk, neonatal cord blood, and serum of pregnant women. *Br. Med. J.*, **296**, 968

Larouzé, B., Saimot, G., Lustbader, E.D., London, W.T., Werner, B.G. & Payet, M. (1976) Host responses to hepatitis-B infection in patients with primary hepatic carcinoma and their families. A case/control study in Senegal, West Africa. *Lancet*, **2**, 534–538

London, W.T., Evans, A.A., Buetow, K., Litwin, S., McGlynn, K., Zhou, T., Clapper, M., Ross, E., Wild, C., Shen, F.M., et al. (1995) Molecular and genetic epidemiology of hepatocellular carcinoma: studies in China and Senegal. Princess Takamatsu Symp., 25, 51–60

Lwanga, S.K., Olweny, C.L. & Tukei, P.M. (1977) Hepatitis B surface antifen (HBsAg) subtypes in Uganda. A preliminary report. Trop. Geogr. Med., 29, 381–385

Mandishona, E., MacPhail, A.P., Gordeuk, V.R., Kedda, M.A., Paterson, A.C., Rouault, T.A., Kew, M.C. (1998) Dietary iron overload as a risk factor for hepatocellular carcinoma in black Africans. Hepatology, 27, 1563–1566

Matsubara, K. & Tokino, T. (1990) Integration of hepatitis B DNA and its implications to (sic) hepatocarcinogenesis Mol. Biol. Med., 7, 243–260

Michon, J., Prince, A.M., Szmuness, W., Demaille, J., Diebolt, G., Linhard, J., Quenum, C. & Sankale, M. (1975) Primary liver cancer and hepatitis B infection in Senegal. Comparison of cancer patients with 2 control groups. Biomedicine, 23, 263–266

McGlynn, K.A., Rosvold, E.A., Lustbader, E.D., Hu, Y., Clapper, M.L., Zhou, T., Wild, C.P., Xia, X.L., Baffoe Bonnie, A., Ofori Adjei, D., Chen, G.C., London, W.T., Shen, F.M. & Buetow, K.H. (1995) Susceptibility to hepatocellular carcinoma is associated with genetic variation in the enzymatic detoxification of aflatoxin B1. Proc. Natl Acad. Sci. USA, 92, 2384–2387

Mohammed, A.E., Kew, M.C. & Groeneveld, H.T. (1992) Alcohol consumption as a risk factor for hepatocellular carcinoma in urban southern African blacks. Int. J. Cancer, 51, 537–541

Montesano, R., Hainaut, P. & Wild, C.P. (1997) Hepatocellular carcinoma: from gene to public health. J. Natl Cancer Inst., 89, 1844–1851

Moyo, V.M., Mandishona, E., Hasstedt, S.J., Gangaidzo, I.T., Gomo, Z.A., Khumalo, H., Saungweme, T., Kiire, C.F., Paterson, A.C., Bloom, P., MacPhail, A.P., Rouault, T. & Gordeuk, V.R. (1998a) Evidence of genetic transmission in African iron overload. Blood, 91, 1076–1082

Moyo, V.M., Makunike, R., Gangaidzo, I.T., Gordeuk, V.R., McLaren, C.E., Khumalo, H., Saungweme, T., Rouault, T. & Kiire, C.F. (1998b) African iron overload and hepatocellular carcinoma . Eur. J. Haematol., 60, 28–34

Niederau, C., Fischer, R., Sonnenberg, A., Stremmel, W., Trampisch, H.J., Strohmeyer, G. (1985) Survival and causes of death in cirrhotic and in noncirrhotic patients with primary hemochromatosis. New Engl. J. Med., 313, 1256–1262

Nyathi, C.B., Mutiro, C.F., Hasler, J.A. & Chetsanga, C.J. (1987) A survey of urinary aflatoxin in Zimbabwe. Int. J. Epidemiol., 16, 516–519

Oettlé, A.G. (1964) Cancer in Africa, especially in regions south of the Sahara. J. Natl Cancer Inst., 33, 383–439

Ola, S.O., Akanji, A.O., Ayoola, E.A. (1995) The diagnostic utility of serum ferritin estimation in Nigerian patients with primary hepatocellular carcinoma. Nutrition, 11 (5 Suppl.), 532–534

Olubuyide, I.O. & Bamgboye, E.A. (1990) A case-controlled study of the current role of cigarette smoking and alcohol consumption in primary liver cell carcinoma in Nigerians. Afr. J. Med. Med. Sci., 19, 191–194

Olubuyide, I.O., Maxwell, S.M., Akinyinka, O.O., Hart, C.A., Neal, G.E. & Hendrickse, R.G. (1993a) HbsAgs and aflatoxins in sera of rural (Ibgo-Ora) and urgan (Ibadan) populations in Nigeria. Afr. J. Med. Med. Sci., 22, 77–80

Olubuyide, I.O., Maxwell, S.M., Hood, H., Neal, G.E. & Hendrickse, R.G. (1993b) HbsAg, aflatoxins and primary hepatocellular carcinoma. Afr. J. Med. Med. Sci., 22, 89–91

Omer, R.E., Bakker, M.I., van't-Veer, P., Hoogenboom, R.L., Polman, T.H., Alink, G.M., Idris, M.O., Kadaru, A.M. & Kok, F.J. (1998) Aflatoxin and liver cancer in Sudan. Nutr. Cancer, 32, 174–180

Omer, R.E., Verhoef, L., Van't Veer, P., Idris, M.O., Kadaru, A.M.Y., Kampman, E., Bunschoten, A. & Kok, F.J. (2001) Peanut butter intake, GSTM1 genotype and hepatocellular carcinoma: a case-control study in Sudan. Cancer Causes Control, 12, 23–32

Otu, A.A. (1987) Hepatocellular carcinoma, hepatic cirrhosis, and hepatitis B virus infection in Nigeria. Cancer, 60, 2581–2585

Owor, R. (1974) Haemosiderosis in Uganda: autopsy study. E. Afr. Med. J., 51, 388–391

Parkin, D.M., ed. (1986) Cancer Occurrence in Developing Countries (IARC Scientific Publications No. 75), Lyon, IARC

Parkin, D.M., Ohshima, H., Srivatanakul, P. & Vatanasapt, V. (1993) Cholangiocarcinoma: epidemiology, mechanisms of carcinogenesis and prevention. Cancer Epidemiol. Biomarkers Prev., 2, 537–544

Parkin, D.M., Vizcaino, P., Skinner, M.E.G. & Ndhlovu, A. (1994) Cancer patterns and risk factors. Cancer Epidemiol. Biomarkers Prev., 3, 537–547

Peers, F.G. & Linsell, C.A. (1973) Dietary aflatoxins and liver cancer – a population based study in Kenya. Br. J. Cancer, 27, 473–484

Peers, F., Bosch, X., Kaldor, J., Linsell, A. & Pluijmen, M. (1987) Aflatoxin exposure, hepatitis B virus infections and liver cancer in Swaziland. Int. J. Cancer, 39, 545–553

Prince, A.M., Leblanc, L., Krohn, K., Masseyeff, R., Alpert, M.E. (1970) S.H. antigen and chronic liver disease. Lancet, 2, 717–718

Prince, A.M., Szmuness, W. & Michon, J. (1975) A case/control study of the association between primary liver cancer and hepatitits B infection in Senegal. Int. J. Cancer, 16, 376–383

Qian, G.S., Ross, R.K., Yu, M.C., Yuan, J.M., Gao, Y.T., Henderson, B.E., Wogan, G.N. & Groopman, J.D. (1994) A follow-up study of urinary markers of aflatoxin exposure and liver cancer risk in Shanghai, People's Republic of China. Cancer Epidemiol. Biomarkers Prev., 3, 3–10

Reys, L.L., Purcell, R.H. & Holland, P.V. (1977) The relationship between hepatitis B virus infection and infections and hepatic cell carcinoma in Mozambique. Trop. Geogr. Med., 29, 251–256

Rioche, M. (1986) Subtypes of HBsAG in Morocco: general distribution in HBsAg carries in Casablanca in terms of their clinical state. Relations with the markers of the Hbe system. Bull. Soc. Pathol. Filiales, 79, 191–198

Ryder, R.W., Whittle, H.C. & Sanneh, A.B. (1992) Persistent hepatitis B virus infections and hepatoma in The Gambia, west Africa. A case–control study of 140 adults and their 603 family contacts. Am. J. Epidemiol., 136, 1122–1131

Schlesselman, J.J. (1995) Net effect of oral contraceptive use on the risk of cancer in women in the United States. Obstet. Gynecol., 85, 793–801

Sebti, M.F. (1984) Hépatites virales aigües et marqueurs du virus HB dans les maladies chroniques du foie et dans les cancers primitifs du foie. In: Williams, A.O., O'Conor, G.T., De Thé, G.T. & Johnson, C.A., eds, Virus-Associated Cancers in Africa (IARC Scientific Publications No. 63), Lyon, IARC, pp. 227–236

Skinner, M.E.G., Parkin, D.M., Vizcaino, P. & Ndhlovu, A. (1993) Cancer in the African ppulation of Bulawayo, Zimbabwe, 1963–1977 (IARC Technical Report No. 15), Lyon, IARC

Stevens, R.G., Beasley, R.P., & Blumberg, B.S. (1986) Iron-binding proteins and risk of cancer in Taiwan. J. Natl Cancer Inst., 76, 605–610

Strachan, A.S. (1929) Haemosichtosis and Haemochromatosis in South African Natives with a Comment on the Aetiology of Haemochromatosis, M.D. Thesis, University of Glasgow

Sun, Z., Zhu, Y. Stjernsward, J., Hilleman, M., Zhen, Y., Hsia, C.C., Lu, J., Huang, F., Ni, Z., Ni, T., Chen, J.G., Yu, Z., Liu, Y., Liu, G., Chen, J.M. & Peto, R. (1991) Design and compliance of HBV vaccination trial on newborns to prevent hepatocellular carcinoma and five-year results of its pilot study. Cancer Detection Prev., 15, 313–318

Szmuness, W. (1978) Hepatocellular carcinoma and the hepatitis B virus: evidence for a causal association. *Prog. Med. Virol.*, **24**, 40–69

Tabor, E., Gerety, R.J., Vogel, C.L., Bayley, A.C., Anthony, P.P., Chan, C.H., Barker, L.F. (1977) Hepatitis B virus infection and primary hepatocellular carcinoma. *J. Natl Cancer Inst.*, **58**, 1197–1200

Templeton, A.C. & Hutt, M.S.R. (1973) Introduction: Distribution of tumours in Uganda. In: Templeton, A.C., ed., *Tumours in a Tropical Country. Recent Results in Cancer Research* No. 41. Berlin, Springer Verlag, pp. 1–22

Toukan, A.U. (1987) Hepatitis B virus infection in urban residents of Jordan with particular reference to socioeconomic factors. *Trop. Gastroenterol.*, **8**, 161–166

Tsega, E., Gold, P., Shuster, J., Whittemore, B. & Lester, F.T. (1976) Hepatitis B antigen, alpha-fetoglobulins and primary hepatocellular carcinoma in Ethiopia. *J. Trop. Med. Hyg.*, **79**, 230–234

Tsega, E. (1977) Hepatocellular carcinoma in Ethiopia. A prospective clinical study of 100 patients. *E. Afr. Med. J.*, **54**, 281–292

Tswana, S.A. & Moyo, S.R. (1992) The interrelationship between HBV-markers and HIV antibodies in patients with hepatocellular carcinoma. *J. Med. Virol.*, **37**, 161–164

Vall Mayans, M., Hall, A.J. & Inskip, H.M. (1994) Do bedbugs transmit hepatitis B? *Lancet*, **344**, 962

Van Den Heever, A., Pretorius, F.J., Falkson, G. & Simson, I.W. (1978) Hepatitis B surface antigen and primary liver cancer. *S. Afr. Med. J.*, **54**, 359–361

Van Rensburg, S.J., Cook-Mozaffari, P., Van Schalkwyk, D.J., Van der Watt, J.J., Vincent, T.J. & Purchase, I.F. (1985) Hepatocellular carcinoma and dietary aflatoxin in Mozambique and Transkei. *Br. J. Cancer*, **51**, 713–726

Van Rensburg, S.J., Van Schalkwyk, G.C. & Van Schalkwyk, D.J. (1990) Primary liver cancer and aflatoxin intake in Transkei. *J. Envir. Pathol. Toxicol. Oncol.*, **10**, 11–16

Viviani, S., Jack, A., Hall, A.J., Maine, N., Mendy, M., Montesano, R. & Whittle, H.C. (1999) Hepatitis B vaccination in infancy in the Gambia: protection against carriage at 9 years of age. *Vaccine*, **17**, 2946–295

Vogel, C.L., Anthony, P.P., Sadikali, F., Barker, L.F. & Peterson, M.R. (1972) Hepatitis-associated antigen and antibody in hepatocellular carcinoma: results of a continuing study. *J. Natl Cancer Inst.*, **48**, 1583–1588

Wabinga, H.R., Parkin, D.M., Wabwire-Mangen, F. & Nambooze, S. (2000) Trends in cancer incidence in Kyadondo County, Uganda, 1960–1997. *Br. J. Cancer*, **82**, 1585–1592

Walker, A.R. & Segal, I. (1999) Iron overload in Sub-Saharan Africa: to what extent is it a public health problem? *Br. J. Nutr.*, **81**, 427–434.

Wang, L.Y., Hatch, M., Chen, C.J., Levin, B., You, S.L., Lu, S.N., Wu, M.H., Wu, W.P., Wang, L.W., Wang, Q., Huang, G.T., Yang, P.M., Lee, H.S. & Santella, R.M. (1996) Aflatoxin exposure and risk of hepatocellular carcinoma in Taiwan. *Int. J. Cancer*, **67**, 620–625

Wang, J.S., Shen, X., He, X., Zhu, Y.R., Zhang, B.C., Wang, J.B., Qian, G.S., Kuang, S.Y., Zarba, A., Egner, P.A., Jacobson, L.P., Muñoz, A., Helzlsouer, K.J., Groopman, J.D. & Kensler, T.W. (1999) Protective alterations in phase 1 and 2 metabolism of aflatoxin B1 by oltipraz in residents of Qidong, People's Republic of China. *J. Natl Cancer Inst.*, **91**, 347–354

Whittle, H., Inskip, H. & Bradley, A.K. (1990) The pattern of childhood hepatitis B infection in two Gambian villages. *J. Infect. Dis.*, **161**, 1112–1115

WHO (1989) Combined oral contraceptives and liver cancer. The WHO Collaborative Study of Neoplasia and Steroid Contraceptives. *Int. J. Cancer*, **43**, 254–259

WHO (1999) Hepatitis-C global prevalence (update). *Weekly Epidemiological Record*, **49**, 425–427 (10 Dec.1999)

Wild, C.P. & Hall, A.J. (1997) Hepatitis B virus and liver cancer: unanswered questions. *Cancer Surveys,* Vol. 33, Infections and Human Cancer, 1–29

Wild, C.P. & Hall, A.J. (2000) Primary prevention of hepatocellular carcinoma in developing countries. *Mutat Res.*, **462**, 381–393

Wild, C.P., Pionneau, F.A., Montesano, R., Mutiro, C.F. & Chetsanga, C.J. (1987) Aflatoxin detected in human breast milk by immunoassay. *Int. J. Cancer*, **40**, 328–333

Wild, C.P., Chapot, B., Scherer, E., Den Engelse, L. & Montesano, R. (1988) Application of antibody methods to the detection of aflatoxin in human bodyfluids. In: Bartsch, H., Hemminki, K. & O'Neill, I.K., eds, *Methods for Detecting DNA Damaging Agents in Humans: Applications in Cancer Epidemiology and Prevention* (IARC Scientific Publications No. 89), Lyon, IARC, pp. 67–74

Wild, C.P., Jiang, Y.Z., Allen, S.J., Jansen, L.A., Hall, A.J. & Montesano, R. (1990) Aflatoxin–albumin adducts in human sera from different regions of the world. *Carcinogenesis*, **11**, 2271–2274

Wild, C.P., Hudson, G.J., Sabbioni, G., Chapot, B., Hall, A.J., Wogan, G.N., Whittle, H., Montesano, R. & Groopman, J.D. (1992) Dietary intake of aflatoxins and the level of albumin-bound aflatoxin in peripheral blood in The Gambia, West Africa. *Cancer Epidemiol. Biomarkers Prev.*, **1**, 229–234

Wild, C.P., Yin, F., Turner, P.C., Chemin, I., Chapot, B., Mendy, M., Whittle, H., Kirk, G.D. & Hall, A.J. (2000) Environmental and genetic determinants of aflatoxin–albumin adducts in the Gambia. *Int. J. Cancer*, **86**, 1–7

Wong, V.C., Ip, H.M., Reesink, H.W., Lelie, P.N., Reerink-Brongers, E.E., Yeung, C.Y. & Ma, H.K. (1984) Prevention of the HBsAg carrier state in newborn infants of mothers who are chronic carriers of HBsAg and HBeAg by administration of hepatitis-B vaccine and hepatitis-B immunoglobulin. Double-blind randomised placebo-controlled study. *Lancet*, **1**, 921–926

Yates, S.C., Hafez, M., Beld, M., Lukashov, V.V., Hassan, Z., Carboni, G., Khaled, H., McMorrow, M., Attia, M. & Goudsmit, J. (1999) Hepatocellular carcinoma in Egyptians with and without a history of hepatitis B virus infection: association with hepatitis C virus (HCV) infection but not with (HCV) RNA level. *Am. J. Trop. Med. Hyg.*, **60**, 714–720

Yu, M.W., You, S.L., Chang, A.S., Lu, S.N., Liaw, Y.F. & Chen, C.J. (1991) Association between hepatitis C virus antibodies and hepatocellular carcinoma in Taiwan. *Cancer Res.*, **51**, 5621–5625

Zarba, A., Wild, C.P., Hall, A.J., Montesano, R., Hudson, G.J. & Groopman, J.D. (1992) Aflatoxin M1 in human breast milk from The Gambia, west Africa, quantified by combined monoclonal antibody immunoaffinity chromatography and HPLC. *Carcinogenesis*, **13**, 891–894

4.9 Lung cancer

Introduction

Lung cancer is now the leading cancer worldwide, with an estimated 1.24 million new cases (12.3% of all cancers) occurring in the year 2000 (Ferlay *et al.*, 2001). However, only a small proportion of this burden (19 500 cases; 1.9% of the world total) is estimated to occur in Africa.

Descriptive epidemiology in Africa

A summary of the age-standardized incidence rates from the registries reporting results in this volume is presented in Table 1 and old data from the 1950s and 60s are given in Table 2.

Incidence rates in women are very low (except among the populations of European origin in Zimbabwe and South Africa) and are indeed considerably lower than the rates among non-smoking women in the United States (4.8 per 100 000; Parkin *et al.*, 1994). In men, the rates are, in general, rather higher in North Africa (Algeria and Tunisia) than in sub-Saharan Africa. In West Africa, incidence rates are low, ranging from 0.7 per 100 000 in Ibadan, Nigeria to 8.2 in Conakry, Guinea. In southern Africa, the rates are higher. In Zimbabwe, the incidence rates recorded in Bulawayo in the 1960s were very high, but in Harare, the incidence among the African population in 1993–97 is very much lower (12.1 per 100 000) and only about half that reported in the first results from this cancer registry (24.6 per 100 000) (Bassett *et al.*, 1995). In an early study of 'Bantu' gold miners in Gwanda (Zimbabwe), Osburn (1957) noted that lung cancers comprised more than 40% of malignancies found at autopsy, and estimated incidence as 18 per 100 000. In South Africa, the incidence rates recorded in Cape Province and Natal in the 1950s and 1960s (Table 2) were very high by African standards. In the recent data (1989–92) from the histopathology-based National Cancer Register (Table 1), the incidence is higher in the white, mixed-race and Indian populations than in the black population. In a study by Bradshaw *et al.* (1983), age-standardized mortality rates (per 100 000) from lung cancer were 42.8 in whites, 45.3 in mixed race and 13.2 in populations of 'Asian/Indian' origin. Among females, rates were 9.5 in whites, 6.3 in mixed-race populations and 6.8 in populations of Asian/Indian origin.

The island populations of Reunion, Mauritius and the Seychelles all have high lung cancer incidence and mortality rates. For example, in the Seychelles, age-standardized mortality rates of 45.7 in males and 14.0 per 100 000 in females have been reported for the period 1985–87 (WHO, 1988).

Based on these incidence/mortality data, and frequencies in various clinical series, estimated incidence and mortality by country have been prepared (Figure 1).

Within-country/regional variation

Oettlé (1964) described increased mortality ratios from lung cancer in the South African asbestos districts of the Northern Cape in white and mixed-race populations. McGlashan & Harington (1985) used death certification data from South Africa, excluding the 'homeland' areas, to describe the geographical distribution of lung cancer. While the representativity of these findings is unclear (only blacks resident on white farms or in townships and urban areas were included), a higher standardized mortality ratio (SMR) compared with the national rate was observed in urban areas (SMR = 1.80) and in the predominantly rural northwestern Cape (SMR = 1.84), an area rich in asbestos. McGlashan and Harington (1985) also found inter-ethnic differences, with the Xhosa having higher SMR (1.48) than the Zulu (0.79), Tswana (0.77), South Sotho (0.57) North Sotho (0.16) and the Swazi (0.88) groups.

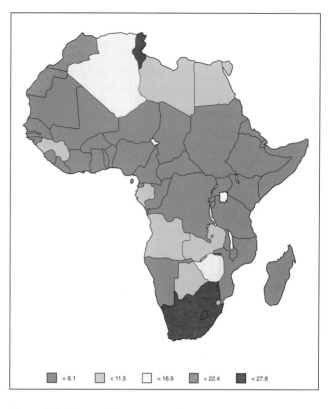

Figure 1. Incidence of lung cancer: ASR (world)- male (all ages)

Bradshaw *et al.* (1982) described cancer patterns among African gold miners from southern Africa. In this group, 'respiratory' cancer (including primary and secondary cancer of the larynx, bronchus, trachea and antrum) comprised 11.2% of all cancers (up from 5.4% of all cancers in an earlier survey; Harington *et al.*, 1975). The crude incidence was higher among miners recruited from the former Natal, Transvaal and the Cape, and lower in those from Botswana, Lesotho, Malawi, 'Northern Territories' (mainly Namibia, Angola, Zimbabwe and Zambia) and Mozambique. Using the same data, McGlashan *et al.* (1982) found a close geographic correlation between the occurrence of respiratory and oesophageal cancers (r = 0.66), suggesting that the two cancers share some etiological factors. Bradshaw *et al.* (1982) examined the geographical variation of lung (and stomach) cancers in white and mixed-race (coloured) populations in South Africa. No reliable mortality data were available for Africans. No striking geographical differences were found except for urban/rural contrasts. However, in a study by Botha *et al.* (1986), elevated standardized mortality ratios were again observed in districts in the Northern Cape where crocidolite asbestos was mined. (SMR white males = 1.75, coloured males =1.28, and in white and coloured females 1.87 and 2.47, respectively).

Trends over time

In South Africa, there have been marked increases in lung cancer mortality rates among males of all ethnic groups, with the rates among whites increasing almost three-fold between 1949 and 1979, and the increase in coloured males is even more dramatic (see Figure 1 in South Africa chapter). Some much smaller increases are also seen among females.

Data from Kampala, Uganda show an increase in age-standardized lung cancer rates over time, from 0.8 in 1960–66 to

Table 1. Age-standardized (world) and cumulative (0-64) incidence
Trachea, bronchus and lung (C33-34)

	MALE				FEMALE			
	Cases	CRUDE	ASR(W) (per 100,000)	Cumulative (%)	Cases	CRUDE	ASR(W) (per 100,000)	Cumulative (%)
Africa, North								
Algeria, Algiers (1993-1997)	635	11.5	**17.2**	1.08	73	1.3	**1.9**	0.12
Algeria, Constantine (1994-1997)	108	7.0	**13.1**	0.96	20	1.3	**2.2**	0.12
Algeria, Oran (1996-1998)	263	14.8	**23.7**	1.48	30	1.7	**2.4**	0.18
Algeria, Setif (1993-1997)	246	8.2	**15.5**	1.04	31	1.0	**1.7**	0.07
Tunisia, Centre, Sousse (1993-1997)	255	22.1	**30.6**	1.70	16	1.4	**1.8**	0.08
Tunisia, North, Tunis (1994)	437	20.2	**26.6**	1.78	37	1.8	**2.3**	0.16
Tunisia, Sfax (1997)	76	19.3	**24.2**	1.32	7	1.9	**2.2**	0.15
Africa, West								
The Gambia (1997-1998)	22	2.2	**5.1**	0.25	3	0.3	**0.5**	0.04
Guinea, Conakry (1996-1999)	101	4.4	**8.2**	0.61	20	0.9	**1.7**	0.14
Mali, Bamako (1988-1997)	60	1.5	**3.7**	0.27	14	0.4	**0.9**	0.09
Niger, Niamey (1993-1999)	23	1.2	**4.9**	0.22	2	0.1	**0.4**	0.05
Nigeria, Ibadan (1998-1999)	5	0.3	**0.7**	0.05	2	0.1	**0.3**	0.04
Africa, Central								
Congo, Brazzaville (1996-1999)	28	2.3	**3.9**	0.29	4	0.3	**0.5**	0.03
Africa, East								
France, La Reunion (1988-1994)	522	24.9	**34.4**	1.80	64	3.0	**3.3**	0.17
Kenya, Eldoret (1998-2000)	15	1.6	**4.0**	0.28	10	1.1	**3.0**	0.24
Malawi, Blantyre (2000-2001)	9	1.0	**2.5**	0.13	1	0.1	**0.5**	0.06
Uganda, Kyadondo County (1993-1997)	33	1.2	**3.6**	0.28	23	0.8	**2.3**	0.20
Zimbabwe, Harare: African (1990-1993)	156	6.6	**20.9**	1.03	32	1.5	**7.2**	0.29
Zimbabwe, Harare: African (1994-1997)	120	4.3	**12.1**	0.66	40	1.5	**5.9**	0.25
Zimbabwe, Harare: European (1990-1997)	112	73.3	**38.4**	1.70	86	51.0	**24.5**	1.24
Africa, South								
Namibia (1995-1998)	104	3.3	**6.1**	0.40	45	1.4	**2.3**	0.19
South Africa: Black (1989-1992)	3347	5.9	**11.2**	0.79	841	1.5	**2.3**	0.16
South Africa: Indian (1989-1992)	288	14.8	**22.5**	1.69	50	2.5	**3.3**	0.24
South Africa: Mixed race (1989-1992)	627	9.8	**19.2**	1.43	220	3.3	**5.1**	0.40
South Africa: White (1989-1992)	2187	21.7	**20.3**	1.23	1120	11.0	**8.8**	0.60
South Africa, Transkei, Umtata (1996-1998)	33	9.2	**15.7**	1.03	10	2.4	**3.6**	0.30
South Africa, Transkei, 4 districts (1996-1998)	15	2.1	**4.9**	0.46	4	0.4	**0.7**	0.06
Swaziland (1996-1999)	81	4.6	**10.1**	0.68	15	0.8	**1.4**	0.10
Europe/USA								
USA, SEER: White (1993-1997)	36165	74.3	**55.6**	2.58	28036	55.9	**34.5**	1.89
USA, SEER: Black (1993-1997)	4879	72.9	**86.5**	4.95	2789	37.6	**36.4**	2.26
France, 8 registries (1993-1997)	10080	73.3	**52.8**	3.21	1681	11.6	**7.2**	0.46
The Netherlands (1993-1997)	35244	92.2	**66.0**	3.01	9501	24.3	**15.8**	1.13
UK, England (1993-1997)	104901	87.4	**53.1**	2.08	57382	44.9	**22.1**	1.04

In italics: histopathology-based registries

Table 2. Incidence of lung cancer in Africa, 1953–74

Registry	Period	ASR (per 100 000)		Source
		Male	Female	(see Chap. 1)
Senegal, Dakar	1969–74	1.1	*0.1*	4
Mozambique, Lourenço Marques	1956–60	*4.1*	*1.6*	1
Nigeria, Ibadan	1960–69	0.8	0.8	3
SA, Cape Province: Bantu	1956–59	26.9	*0.0*	2
SA, Cape Province: Coloured	1956–59	42.8	0.7	2
SA, Cape Province: White	1956–59	44.7	0.5	2
SA, Johannesburg, Bantu	1953–55	7.4	*3.1*	1
SA, Natal Province: African	1964–66	41.2	10.2	2
SA, Natal Province: Indian	1964–66	20.0	*3.3*	2
Uganda, Kyadondo	1954–60	*0.9*	*0.0*	1
Uganda, Kyadondo	1960–71	1.5	*1.0*	5
Zimbabwe, Bulawayo	1963–72	48.4	*3.0*	6

Italics: Rate based on less than 10 cases

3.2 per 100 000 in 1995–97 among males and from 0.6 in 1960–66 to 3.2 in 1995–1997 among females.

Migrant studies

Dean (1959) found that the mortality rate due to lung cancer among whites in South Africa was higher among British immigrants than in persons of local descent, and was higher in populations of urban rather than rural origin. Given that the current tobacco consumption of these groups was similar, Dean concluded that air pollution in urban centres was responsible, at least in part, for the excess lung cancers. (At the time, the effect of duration of smoking had not been investigated). However, noting that white females in highly polluted urban areas did not have excess lung cancer mortality rates and that British-born whites had rates intermediate between those in the United Kingdom and South Africa, Oettlé (1964) argued that pollution was not an important cause of lung cancer in these populations.

Risk factors

Tobacco smoking

Tobacco smoking is by far the most important cause of lung cancer (IARC, 1986; US DHHS, 1989). It has been estimated that in 1985 about 76% of all lung cancer worldwide (84% of cases in men and 46% in women) could be attributed to tobacco smoking (Parkin et al., 1994). However in Africa, because smoking is a relatively recently acquired habit in most areas, the proportion of tobacco-attributed lung cancers is still low. Only where the habit has been established in a significant percentage of the population for a long time is there a high proportion of tobacco-attributable cancers – 85% of cases in males in southern Africa and 68% in North Africa, for example.

Because of the small proportion of lung cancers estimated to occur in Africa (and the low prevalence of tobacco consumption in most places in Africa), there is a widespread misconception that the hazards of tobacco are relevant only in developed countries. The increase in consumption of tobacco, and particularly of manufactured cigarettes, has occurred relatively recently in most of Africa. In a WHO survey, over two decades from 1970–72 to 1990–92, consumption of cigarettes increased in 15 African countries, decreased in six, and remained unchanged in five (data were unavailable for the rest of Africa). In comparison, among 'more developed' countries, 12 increased their consumption, 18 decreased and one remained the same, and the bulk of the increase in developed countries occurred decades earlier (WHO, 1997). Adult smoking rates also varied significantly, prevalence among men ranging from 10 to 50% and among women from 1 to 10% (WHO, 1997). An exception is the mixed-race population of South Africa, where there has been a high prevalence (currently 40–50%) of smoking among women.

In a continuation of his previous work, Dean (1961) interviewed the next-of-kin of (white) individuals who died from lung cancer, and a group of controls who died from other causes, about their smoking habits. Among South African-born men, compared with those who

Table 3. Percentage distribution of microscopically verified cases by histological type
Bronchus and lung (C34) - Both sexes

	Squamous	Adeno	Carcinoma Small cell	Large cell	Other	Unspec.	Sarcoma	Other	Unspec.	Number of cases MV	Total
Algeria, Algiers	32.7	20.9	4.9	4.3	2.6	34.4	-	0.2	-	575	707
Algeria, Batna	70.0	6.7	3.3	8.3	-	8.3	-	-	3.3	60	75
Algeria, Constantine	43.3	12.4	1.0	5.2	1.0	22.7	-	-	14.4	97	128
Algeria, Oran	49.6	5.9	2.9	18.5	0.4	18.1	0.4	-	4.2	238	265
Algeria, Setif	70.2	6.3	-	2.7	-	11.0	-	-	9.8	255	277
Burkina Faso, Ouagadougou	50.0	25.0	-	-	-	25.0	-	-	-	12	12
Congo, Brazzaville	-	50.0	20.0	-	-	20.0	-	-	10.0	10	32
France, La Reunion	46.7	21.5	6.4	11.6	2.7	9.1	0.5	-	1.5	550	579
The Gambia	50.0	-	50.0	-	-	-	-	-	-	2	24
Guinea, Conakry	16.1	12.9	-	-	-	71.0	-	-	-	31	121
Kenya, Eldoret	7.1	35.7	14.3	14.3	7.1	14.3	-	-	7.1	14	25
Malawi, Blantyre	75.0	25.0	-	-	-	-	-	-	-	4	10
Mali, Bamako	56.3	6.3	-	6.3	-	31.3	-	-	-	16	73
Namibia	36.2	33.1	11.5	12.3	0.8	3.1	0.8	-	2.3	130	146
Niger, Niamey	50.0	-	-	50.0	-	-	-	-	-	4	25
Nigeria, Ibadan	50.0	25.0	-	-	-	-	25.0	-	-	4	6
Rwanda, Butare	-	-	-	-	-	-	-	-	-	-	1
South Africa: Black	38.9	18.6	8.1	6.5	4.9	7.0	0.3	0.3	15.5	4122	4122
South Africa: White	32.5	28.8	14.5	8.8	4.1	8.5	0.5	0.6	1.6	3275	3275
South Africa: Indian	33.8	19.3	12.1	10.0	5.7	7.3	0.6	0.3	10.9	331	331
South Africa: Mixed race	37.9	27.3	11.5	8.5	3.6	9.1	0.2	-	1.9	836	836
South Africa, Elim	21.4	14.3	21.4	28.6	-	7.1	-	-	7.1	14	17
South Africa, Transkei, Umtata	66.7	5.6	-	-	-	5.6	-	-	22.2	18	43
South Africa, Transkei, 4 districts	55.6	22.2	11.1	-	-	11.1	-	-	-	9	19
Swaziland	54.5	9.1	18.2	-	-	9.1	-	9.1	-	11	94
Tanzania, Dar Es Salaam	25.0	25.0	12.5	25.0	-	12.5	-	-	-	8	8
Tanzania, Kilimanjaro	50.0	50.0	-	-	-	-	-	-	-	2	6
Tunisia, Centre, Sousse	41.9	24.7	18.0	6.4	1.5	7.1	0.4	-	-	267	269
Tunisia, North, Tunis	51.2	15.8	13.3	2.4	1.2	12.1	-	-	3.9	412	474
Tunisia, Sfax	44.2	35.1	10.4	2.6	-	6.5	1.3	-	-	77	83
Uganda, Mbarara	-	-	-	-	-	-	-	-	-	-	1
Uganda, Kyadondo County	17.1	17.1	11.4	-	-	40.0	-	-	14.3	35	56
Zimbabwe, Harare: African	44.2	27.5	10.1	5.1	-	10.9	2.2	-	-	138	348
Zimbabwe, Harare: European	40.6	28.1	20.8	6.3	-	3.1	1.0	-	-	96	197

Table 4. Summary of case–control studies on lung cancer in Africa
Odds ratio vs. non exposed (with 95% CI)

Exposure		Parkin *et al.*, 1994	Mzileni *et al.*, 1999	Pacella-Norman *et al.*, 2002
Ex-smoker	M	3.4 (1.9–5.8)	2.6 (1.0–4.6)	6.8 (2.9–16.0)
	F		5.8 (1.3–25.8)	7.1 (2.6–19.4)
Current smoker	M		10.7 (6.6–17.3)	9.7 (4.3–22.2)
	F		5.5 (2.6–11.3)	13.7 (5.7–32.8)
Current smoker,	M	3.9 (3.0–5.0)	9.4 (5.9–16.4)	6.2 (2.6–14.9)
0–14 g/day	F		–	10.7 (4.2–27.6)
Current smoker,	M	5.2 (3.5–7.7)	12.0 (6.5–22.3)	24.2 (9.6–61.0)
15+ g/day	F		–	50.8 (12.7–203.4)
Wood, coal	M		1.9 (0.9–3.3)	1.6 (0.7–3.8)
	F		1.4 (0.6–3.2)	0.7 (0.2–1.8)
Dusty occupation	M	1.2 (0.9–1.4)*	3.2 (1.8–5.8)	2.8 (1.1–7.6)
	F		0.5 (0.3–1.1)	5.8 (0.7–45.6)
Asbestos residence	M		2.1 to 2.8	–
	F		1.1 to 5.4	
Asbestos birth	M		2.9 (1.2–6.7)	–
	F		3.1 (0.4–21.4)	–
Asbestos mine	M	0.7 (0.5–1.0)		–
Gold mine	M	1.5 (0.9–2.3)		–
Other mines	M	Nickel (2.6; 1.6–4.2), Copper (1.5; 1.0–2.2)		–

*Mining

had never smoked, the odds ratio of lung cancer associated with smoking was 1.8 in those whose family reported consumption of 1–20 cigarettes per day, 6.6 in those who smoked 25–45 per day and 11.8 in those who smoked 50 cigarettes or more. The corresponding odds ratios for British-born immigrants of 2.1, 6.3 and 9.0 were similar. Individuals dying from lung cancer were not employed in occupations with likely air pollution more frequently than the controls. However, the differences in lung cancer rates between British- and South African-born males was still poorly understood at that time and it was still thought that aside from tobacco consumption, environmental pollution played an important role.

In a cancer registration survey in Lourenço Marques (now Maputo) in Mozambique covering 1956–61, Prates and Torres (1964) found that three out of four male lung cancer cases were smokers compared with 206 out of 757 non-cancerous subjects (OR = 8); in females the single case of lung cancer was reported to be a smoker, compared with 7 out of 328 non-cancer controls (O/E = 46).

In studies among Rhodesian (Zimbabwean) Africans, Gelfand *et al.* (1968) found that 28/32 males with lung cancer admitted to Harare Hospital were regular smokers, compared with 7/32 age- and sex-matched controls (OR with respect to non-smokers = 32.6, 95% CI 5.3–324). Osburn (1968) noted that the majority of lung cancer patients in Gwanda, near Bulawayo were also miners (although no comparison group was used).

Three case–control studies of lung cancer in relation to smoking in Africa have been conducted (Table 4). In a study based on interview of cancer cases (or their relatives) recorded in the Bulawayo cancer registry between 1963 and 1977, Parkin *et al.* (1994) compared 877 lung cancers with 4434 other cancers (excluding those cancers related to smoking). After adjustment for confounding factors, the odds ratios for lung cancer in relation to smoking were 3.4 in ex-smokers, 3.9 in those smoking less than 15 g tobacco per day, and 5.2 in those smoking 15 g per day or more. Prevalence of smoking in men in the control group was 41%, but consumption was not high: 86% of smokers were smoking less than 15 cigarettes daily.

In a case–control study of 288 males and 60 females with lung cancer and 183 male and 197 female controls in the Northern Province of South Africa, Mzileni *et al.* (1999) found that although

tobacco smoking is the most important risk factor for the development of lung cancer, environmental exposure to asbestos, a 'dusty' occupation in men, and indoor pollution may also contribute to the development of lung cancer in this province. In males, compared with non-smokers, the risks associated with lung cancer were 9.4 in smokers of 0–14 g cigarettes daily and 12.0 in men who smoked 15 g or more. In females, the risk in current smokers was 5.5.

In a South African case–control study of 105 cases of lung cancer in males and 816 controls, and 41 females and 1383 controls, Pacella-Norman *et al.* (2002) found that in males, the risks for lung cancer relative to non-smokers were 6.8 in ex-smokers, 6.2 in current light smokers and 24.2 in current heavy smokers, while among females, the corresponding figures were 7.1, 10.7 and 50.8. The mean daily cigarette consumption by current smokers in this study was 9.7 ± 7.2 in the male control group and 8.1 ± 7.6 in the female control group. This is rather higher than was previously reported among the control groups in a study of oesophagus cancer in Soweto in 1988: 4.73 ± 0.4 in males and 1.1 ± 0.3 in females (Segal *et al.*, 1988).

Occupational exposures

Other factors known to increase risk of lung cancer are occupational exposures to asbestos, some metals (e.g., nickel, arsenic and cadmium), radon (particularly among miners) and ionizing radiation. Some of these have been addressed in African studies.

In one of the South African case–control studies, lung cancer was associated with birth or residence in areas where asbestos was mined (Mzileni *et al.*, 1999). In the study by Parkin *et al.* (1994), however, no association between lung cancer and occupation in asbestos mines was found, perhaps because in Zimbabwe mainly chrysotile is mined, whereas in South Africa, the asbestos is crocidolite and amosite (which pose a much higher risk of lung cancer) as well as chrysotile. Indeed, South African incidence rates of mesothelioma are high and similar to rates in other asbestos-rich countries (Zwi *et al.*, 1989) and excess lung cancer risks related to asbestos exposure have been found in white miners (SMR 1.4 for amosite and 2.0 for crocidolite) (Sluis-Cremer *et al.*, 1992).

Gold miners in South Africa have been observed to be at increased risk of lung cancer. In a cohort of 3971 white middle-aged miners, followed up over nine years, a standardized mortality ratio of 1.61 (95% CI 1.15–2.20) was reported (Wyndham et al., 1986). When follow-up was extended to 20 years, the SMR was 1.39 (95% CI 1.18–1.65) and the relative risk of exposure to dust was estimated as 1.08 (95% CI 0.94–1.20) per 10 000 particle-years (Reid & Sluis-Cremer, 1996). A second study, in which a cohort of 2209 white miners aged 45–54 years was followed up for 16 years, found a statistically significant association with cumulative dust exposure (RR 1.02, 95% CI 1.00–1.04) per 1000 particle-years (Hnizdo et al., 1991). Two case–control studies of deceased white gold miners did not show any association between lung cancer and exposure to dust, radiological silicosis or silicosis identified at necropsy; most of the excess risk in the miners was due to smoking (Hessel et al., 1986, 1990). Hnizdo et al. (1997) compared 78 lung cancer cases identified in their cohort of 45–54-year-old miners, with 386 matched controls. An increased risk of lung cancer was found in patients with prior silicosis (RR = 2.45, 95% CI 1.2–5.2, after adjustment for smoking) (Hnidzo et al., 1997), but not with uranium production.

In the study based on records from the Bulawayo cancer registry in 1963–77, Parkin et al. (1994) found an increased risk of lung cancer (after adjustment for smoking) in subjects who reported having worked in mines extracting nickel (OR = 2.6; 95% CI 1.6–4.2) or copper (OR = 1.5; 95% CI 1.0–2.2), but not gold (OR 1.5; 95% CI 0.9–2.3), chrome (OR 1.1) or coal (OR 1.1). The copper/nickel ores mined in Matabeleland (served by the hospital in Bulawayo) contain varying amounts of arsenic; the ores are converted locally to matte form in furnaces before transport elsewhere for refining and this process has been associated with an increased incidence of lung cancer in studies elsewhere (IARC, 1990). In a mortality study among South African white iron moulders, a significantly increased proportional mortality ratio (1.71) was found for lung cancer in those dying after the age of 65 (Sitas et al., 1989).

Exposure to smoke from wood or coal appears to be important in certain settings. In the Northern Province of South Africa, where 80% of the population use it as a primary source of energy for heating and cooking, Mzileni et al. (1999) found a significant association between lung cancer and indoor pollution (RR 2.0, 95% c.i., 1.1-3.6) for both sexes combined. The study of Pacella Norman et al. (2002) in Soweto found no association, which may be due to low-levels of exposure, in an area where heating is rarely required in winter.

References

Bassett, M.T., Chokunonga, E., Mauchaza, B., Levy, L., Ferlay, J. & Parkin, D.M. (1995) Cancer in the African population of Harare, Zimbabwe, 1990-1992. Int. J. Cancer, 63, 29–36

Botha, J.L., Irwig, L. & Strebel, P. (1986) Excess mortality from stomach cancer lung cancer and asbestosis and/or mesothelioma in crocidolite mining districts in South Africa. Am. J. Epidemiol., 123, 30–40

Bradshaw, E., McGlashan, N.D., Fitzgerald, D. & Harington, J.S. (1982) Analyses of cancer incidence in black gold miners from Southern Africa 1964-79. Br. J. Cancer, 46, 737–748

Bradshaw, E., Harington, J.S. & McGlashan, N.D. (1983) Geographical distribution of lung and stomach cancers in South Africa, 1968-1972. S. Afr. Med. J., 64, 655–663

Dean, G. (1959) Lung cancer among white south Africans. Br. Med. J., 852–857

Dean G 1961 Lung cancer among white South Africans. Report on a further study. Br. Med. J., 1599–1605

Ferlay, J., Bray, F., Pisani, P. & Parkin, D.M. (2001) GLOBOCAN 2000: Cancer Incidence, Mortality and Prevalence Worldwide, Version 1.0 (CD-ROM) (IARC CancerBase No. 5), Lyon, IARCPress

Gelfand, M., Graham, A.J.P. & Lightman, E. (1968) Carcinoma of the bronchus and the smoking habit in Rhodesian Africans. Br. Med. J., 3, 468–469

Harington, J.S., McGlashan, N.D., Bradshaw, E., Geddes, E.W. & Purves, L.R. (1975) A spatial and temporal analysis in African gold miners from Southern Afirca. Br. J. Cancer, 31, 665–678

Hessel, P.A., Sluis-Cremer, G.K. & Hnidzo, E. (1986) Case–control study of silicosis, silica exposure and lung cancer in white South African gold miners. Am. J. Ind. Med., 10, 57–62

Hessel, P.A., Sluis-Cremer, G.K. & Hnidzo, E. (1990) Silica exposure, silicosis and lung cancer: a necropsy study. Br. J. Ind. Med., 47, 4–9

Hnidzo, E. & Sluis-Cremer, G.K. (1991) Silica exposure, silicosis, and lung cancer: a mortality study of South African gold miners. Br. J. Ind. Med., 48, 53–60

Hnidzo, E., Murray, J. & Klempman, S. (1997) Lung cancer in relation to exposure to silica dust, silicosis, and uranium production in South African gold miners. Thorax, 52, 271–275

IARC (1986) IARC Monographs on the Evaluation of the Carcinogenic Risk of Chemicals to Humans, Vol. 38, Tobacco Smoking, Lyon, IARC

IARC (1990) IARC Monographs on the Evaluation of the Carcinogenic Risks to Humans, Vol. 49, Chromium, Nickel and Welding, Lyon, IARC

McGlashan, N. & Harington, J. (1985) Lung cancer 1978-1981 in the black peoples of South Africa. Br. J. Cancer, 52, 339–346

McGlashan, N.D., Harington, J.S. & Bradshaw, E. (1982) Eleven sites of cancer in black gold miners from Southern Africa. A geographic enquiry. Br. J. Cancer, 46, 947–954

Mzileni, O., Sitas, F., Steyn, K., Carrara, H. & Bekker, P. (1999) Lung cancer, tobacco, and environmental factors in the African population of the Northern Province, South Africa. Tobacco Control, 8, 398–401

Oettlé, A.G. (1964) Cancer in Africa, especially in regions south of the Sahara. J. Natl Cancer Inst., 33, 383-439

Osburn, H.S. (1957) Cancer of the lung in Gwanda. Cent. Afr. J. Med., 3, 215–223

Osburn, H.S. (1968) Carcinoma, smoking and Rhodesian Africans. Br. Med. J., 702

Pacella-Norman, R., Urban, M.I., Sitas, F., Carrara, H., Sur, R., Hale, M., Ruff, P., Patel, M., Newton, R., Bull, D. & Beral, V. (2002) Risk factors for oesophageal, lung, oral and laryngeal cancers in black South Africans. Br. J. Cancer, 86, 1751–1756

Parkin, D.M., ed. (1986) Cancer Occurrence in Developing Countries (IARC Scientific Publications No. 75), Lyon, IARC

Parkin, D.M., Pisani, P., Lopez, A.D. & Masuyer, E. (1994) At least one in seven cases of cancer is caused by smoking. Global estimates for 1985. Int. J. Cancer, 59, 494–504

Parkin, D.M., Vizcaino, A.P., Skinner, M.E.G. & Ndhlovu, A. (1994) Cancer patterns and risk factors in the African population of South Western Zimbabwe, 1963-1977. Cancer Epidemiol. Biomarkers Prev., 3, 537–547

Prates, M.D. & Torres, F.O. (1965) A cancer survey in Laurenco Marques. J. Natl Cancer Inst., 35, 729–757

Reid, P.J. & Sluis-Cremer, G.K. (1996) Mortality of South African gold miners. Occup. Environ Med., 53, 11–16

Segal, I., Reinach, S.G. & de Beer, M. (1988) Factors associated with oesophageal cancer in Soweto, South Africa. Br. J. Cancer, 58, 681–686

Sitas, F., Douglas, A.J. & Webster, E.C. (1989) Respiratory disease mortality patterns among South African Iron moulders. Br. J. Ind. Med., 46, 310–315

Sluis-Cremer, G.K., Liddell, F.D.K., Logan, W.P.D. & Bezuidenhout, B.N. (1992) The mortality of amphibole miners in South Africa, 1946–1980. Br. J. Ind. Med., 49, 566–575

US DHHS (1989) *Reducing the Health Consequences of Smoking. 25 Years of Progress. A Report of the Surgeon General* (USDHSS publication 89-8411), Washington DC, Government Printing Office

WHO (1988) *World Health Statistics Annual 1988*, Geneva

Wyndham, C.H., Bezuidenhuit, B.N., Greenacre, M.J. & Sluis-Cremer, G.K. (1986) Mortality of middle-aged white South African gold miners. *Br. J. Indust. Med.*, 43, 677–684

Zwi, A.B., Reid, G., Landau, S.P., Kielkowski, D., Sitas, F. & Becklake, M.R. (1989) Mesothelioma in South Africa 1976-1984. Incidence and case characteristics. *Int. J. Epidemiol.*, **18**, 320–329

4.10 Lymphomas

Introduction

Advances in molecular biology, genetics and immunology have led to profound changes in the classification of neoplasms of lymphoid cells over the last 20 years. Previously, a sharp distinction was made between lymphomas (solid tumours) and leukaemias (involving bone marrow and peripheral blood), although it was recognized that some lymphomas developed into a 'leukaemic phase'. Now, in the Revised European-American Lymphoma (REAL) classification system (Harris et al., 1994) and its successor, the WHO classification (Jaffe et al., 2001), the unity of lymphoid neoplasms is stressed, and three broad categories are recognized: Hodgkin disease (in which the malignant cell is the Reed–Sternberg cells of lymph nodes) and T-cell and B-cell non-Hodgkin lymphomas. The lymphocytic leukaemias fall within the B-cell non-Hodgkin lymphoma group.

Hodgkin disease comprises about 18% of malignant lymphomas worldwide (about 62 000 annual cases). There is a strong male predominance (sex ratio 1.6:1). Two disease entities are recognized: nodular lymphocyte-predominant Hodgkin lymphoma and classical Hodgkin lymphoma. Within the latter, four subtypes have been distinguished: nodular sclerosis, mixed cellularity, lymphocyte-rich and lymphocyte-depleted (Jaffe et al., 2001). In developing countries, Hodgkin disease occurs mainly in children (most cases are the mixed cellularity subtype) and in the elderly, while in developed countries there is a peak in young adults, of the nodular sclerosing subtype. In Africa, there were an estimated 7200 new cases in the year 2000, representing 1.2% of all new cancer cases, compared with the frequency worldwide of 0.6%.

Non-Hodgkin lymphomas are a very heterogeneous group of neoplasms. The types which generally manifest as leukaemias (precursor lymphoblastic leukaemia/lymphoma, and B-cell chronic lymphocytic leukaemia/small lymphocytic lymphoma) are considered in the chapter on leukaemias. The remaining non-Hodgkin lymphomas comprise around 290 000 cases worldwide per year (2.9% of all cancers), rather more in males than females. Geographically, non-Hodgkin lymphomas are most common in developed countries (51% of the world total of cases), although in Africa, the frequency is above the world average: 5400 new cases in North Africa (3.9% of cancers) and 24 800 in sub-Saharan Africa (5.1% of new cancers). In part, this arises from the high incidence rates of Burkitt lymphoma (BL) in the tropical zone of Africa, where the incidence rates of this tumour in childhood may be very high.

In this chapter we describe the epidemiology of the lymphomas in Africa, and review also what is known about multiple myeloma on the continent. Myeloma is a multifocal neoplasm of plasma cells, responsible for about 74 000 new cases worldwide (0.75% of new cancers).

Hodgkin disease

Geographical distribution

In general, incidence rates in Africa appear to be rather low in comparison with those in developed countries. The rates in North Africa appear to be higher than in sub-Saharan African populations (Table 1(a)). Males are predominantly affected.

Table 2(a) shows rates from older series.

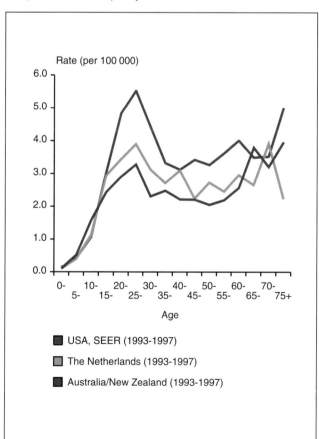

Figure 1. Hodgkin disease in male Caucasian populations

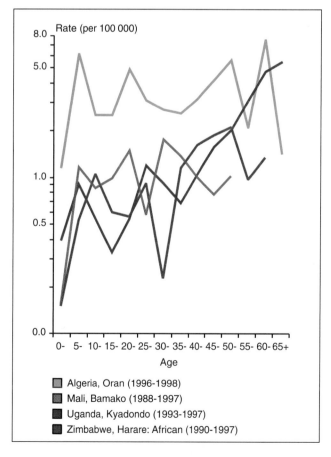

Figure 2.. Hodgkin disease in male African populations

Table 1a. Age-standardized (world) and cumulative (0-64) incidence
Hodgkin disease (C81)

	MALE				FEMALE			
	Cases	CRUDE	ASR(W) (per 100,000)	Cumulative (%)	Cases	CRUDE	ASR(W) (per 100,000)	Cumulative (%)
Africa, North								
Algeria, Algiers (1993-1997)	33	0.6	**0.5**	0.04	27	0.5	**0.5**	0.03
Algeria, Constantine (1994-1997)	19	1.2	**1.5**	0.10	16	1.1	**1.1**	0.08
Algeria, Oran (1996-1998)	56	3.2	**3.1**	0.22	20	1.1	**1.3**	0.08
Algeria, Setif (1993-1997)	55	1.8	**2.3**	0.16	29	1.0	**1.1**	0.09
Tunisia, Centre, Sousse (1993-1997)	20	1.7	**2.2**	0.16	15	1.3	**1.2**	0.07
Tunisia, North, Tunis (1994)	33	1.5	**1.6**	0.13	18	0.9	**0.9**	0.06
Tunisia, Sfax (1997)	10	2.5	**2.8**	0.23	4	1.1	**1.0**	0.03
Africa, West								
The Gambia (1997-1998)	6	0.6	**0.5**	0.03	3	0.3	**0.4**	0.00
Guinea, Conakry (1996-1999)	27	1.2	**1.6**	0.09	10	0.5	**0.4**	0.03
Mali, Bamako (1988-1997)	33	0.9	**0.8**	0.05	16	0.4	**0.7**	0.05
Niger, Niamey (1993-1999)	10	0.5	**0.6**	0.04	1	0.1	**0.1**	0.01
Nigeria, Ibadan (1998-1999)	7	0.5	**0.6**	0.06	1	0.1	**0.1**	0.01
Africa, Central								
Congo, Brazzaville (1996-1999)	2	0.2	**0.3**	0.02	2	0.2	**0.2**	0.02
Africa, East								
France, La Reunion (1988-1994)	21	1.0	**1.0**	0.07	12	0.6	**0.5**	0.03
Kenya, Eldoret (1998-2000)	15	1.6	**2.4**	0.17	8	0.9	**1.4**	0.12
Malawi, Blantyre (2000-2001)	5	0.6	**0.6**	0.06	3	0.3	**0.2**	0.01
Uganda, Kyadondo County (1993-1997)	18	0.6	**1.1**	0.06	20	0.7	**0.7**	0.05
Zimbabwe, Harare: African (1990-1993)	18	0.8	**0.9**	0.08	6	0.3	**0.4**	0.04
Zimbabwe, Harare: African (1994-1997)	18	0.6	**0.6**	0.04	15	0.6	**0.6**	0.04
Zimbabwe, Harare: European (1990-1997)	2	1.3	**2.0**	0.11	5	3.0	**2.8**	0.18
Africa, South								
Namibia (1995-1998)	15	0.5	**0.6**	0.04	9	0.3	**0.4**	0.03
South Africa: Black (1989-1992)	390	0.7	**0.8**	0.05	213	0.4	**0.4**	0.03
South Africa: Indian (1989-1992)	22	1.1	**1.1**	0.08	9	0.5	**0.4**	0.04
South Africa: Mixed race (1989-1992)	74	1.2	**1.2**	0.09	38	0.6	**0.7**	0.05
South Africa: White (1989-1992)	215	2.1	**2.0**	0.14	181	1.8	**1.6**	0.10
South Africa, Transkei, Umtata (1996-1998)	1	0.3	**0.2**	0.01	1	0.2	**0.2**	0.01
South Africa, Transkei, 4 districts (1996-1998)	-	-	**-**	-	-	-	**-**	-
Swaziland (1996-1999)	8	0.5	**0.4**	0.03	8	0.4	**0.5**	0.03
Europe/USA								
USA, SEER: White (1993-1997)	1661	3.4	**3.1**	0.22	1408	2.8	**2.6**	0.17
USA, SEER: Black (1993-1997)	187	2.8	**2.7**	0.20	162	2.2	**2.0**	0.14
France, 8 registries (1993-1997)	412	3.0	**2.7**	0.18	293	2.0	**1.8**	0.12
The Netherlands (1993-1997)	955	2.5	**2.2**	0.16	730	1.9	**1.7**	0.12
UK, England (1993-1997)	3084	2.6	**2.3**	0.16	2323	1.8	**1.7**	0.11

In italics: histopathology-based registries

Table 2(a). Incidence of Hodgkin disease in Africa, 1953–74

Registry	Period	ASR (per 100 000)		Source
		Male	Female	(see Chap. 1)
Senegal, Dakar	1969–74	2.2	1.5	4
Mozambique, Lourenço Marques	1956–60	*0.0*	*0.0*	1
Nigeria, Ibadan	1960–69	3.8	2.0	3
SA, Cape Province: Bantu	1956–59	2.6	*1.2*	2
SA, Cape Province: Coloured	1956–59	2.8	*0.8*	2
SA, Cape Province: White	1956–59	*0.9*	*0.0*	2
SA, Johannesburg, Bantu	1953–55	1.1	*1.4*	1
SA, Natal Province: African	1964–66	3.0	*0.4*	2
SA, Natal Province: Indian	1964–66	*0.7*	*0.5*	2
Uganda, Kyadondo	1954–60	1.7	*0.7*	1
Uganda, Kyadondo	1960–71	1.7	*0.7*	5
Zimbabwe, Bulawayo	1963–72	2.0	*0.1*	6

Italics: Rate based on less than 10 cases

Table 3. Percentage distribution of microscopically verified cases by histological type
Hodgkin disease (C81) - Both sexes

	Lymphocytic predominance	Nodular sclerosis	Mixed cellularity	Lymphocytic depletion	Unspecified	Number of cases MV	Total
Algeria, Algiers	3.3	10.0	10.0	-	76.7	60	60
Algeria, Batna	5.6	5.6	50.0	-	38.9	18	21
Algeria, Constantine	-	-	2.9	-	97.1	35	35
Algeria, Oran	1.3	3.9	1.3	1.3	92.1	76	76
Algeria, Setif	13.1	7.1	20.2	10.7	48.8	84	84
Burkina Faso, Ouagadougou	-	-	-	-	100.0	3	3
Congo, Brazzaville	-	25.0	-	-	75.0	4	4
France, La Reunion	12.1	48.5	21.2	-	18.2	33	33
The Gambia	14.3	-	57.1	-	28.6	7	9
Guinea, Conakry	2.7	2.7	5.4	-	89.2	37	37
Kenya, Eldoret	-	-	27.3	-	72.7	22	23
Malawi, Blantyre	-	20.0	-	-	80.0	5	8
Mali, Bamako	17.4	4.3	26.1	17.4	34.8	46	49
Namibia	-	16.7	37.5	29.2	16.7	24	24
Niger, Niamey	37.5	37.5	-	12.5	12.5	8	11
Nigeria, Ibadan	-	-	20.0	-	80.0	5	8
Rwanda, Butare	20.0	20.0	40.0	20.0	-	5	5
South Africa: Black	3.5	19.7	18.6	5.1	53.1	603	603
South Africa: White	3.8	21.0	12.4	3.0	59.8	396	396
South Africa: Indian	3.2	9.7	19.4	3.2	64.5	31	31
South Africa: Mixed race	1.8	20.5	14.3	6.3	57.1	112	112
South Africa, Elim	-	-	40.0	20.0	40.0	5	5
South Africa, Transkei, Umtata	-	50.0	-	-	50.0	2	2
South Africa, Transkei, 4 districts	-	-	-	-	-	-	-
Swaziland	-	8.3	-	-	91.7	12	16
Tanzania, Dar Es Salaam	-	-	-	-	100.0	13	13
Tanzania, Kilimanjaro	-	-	-	14.3	85.7	7	7
Tunisia, Centre, Sousse	2.9	85.7	11.4	-	-	35	35
Tunisia, North, Tunis	-	45.1	37.3	3.9	13.7	51	51
Tunisia, Sfax	-	7.1	-	-	92.9	14	14
Uganda, Mbarara	-	-	-	50.0	50.0	2	2
Uganda, Kyadondo County	-	11.4	-	5.7	82.9	35	38
Zimbabwe, Harare: African	-	14.8	22.2	7.4	55.6	54	57
Zimbabwe, Harare: European	-	42.9	14.3	-	42.9	7	7

In Caucasian populations, there is a clear bimodal pattern of incidence, with very few cases in childhood, a rising incidence to a 'young adult' peak at about age 25 years, a subsequent decrease, and then a further increase in old age. This pattern is observed in Europe, North America and Australia/New Zealand (Figure 1). Correa and O'Conor (1971) first observed that the pattern in developing countries is rather different, with an initial peak in childhood (especially in boys), no young adult peak, and then a rise in incidence to old age. They also described an 'intermediate' pattern, and a shift from the 'developing' to 'intermediate' patterns with economic development has been noted by others (Hartge et al., 1994).

Current patterns in African populations mainly conform to the 'developing' pattern (Figure 2), so that, in case series, a relatively high percentage of cases occur in children. Cohen and Hamilton (1980) noted that the age–incidence pattern among blacks in Johannesburg, South Africa was 'developing-intermediate' while that among whites was 'intermediate-developed'.

In Europe and North America, there is an association between risk of Hodgkin disease and socioeconomic status, but this is confined to cases in young adults, and to the nodular sclerosis subtype (Cozen et al., 1992). This is consistent with Mueller's (1996) observations that cases of Hodgkin disease in developing countries are predominantly of mixed cellularity and lymphocytic depletion subtypes, while the young adult peak of developed countries involves mainly the nodular sclerosing type (Figure 3).

The early data from Africa have been reviewed by Glaser (1990). Wright (1973), reviewing cases recorded by the Uganda Cancer Registry in 1964–68, noted the deficit of lymphocyte predominance (and nodular sclerosis) subtypes and an excess of mixed cellularity and lymphocyte-depleted groups, compared with series from the United States and the United Kingdom. Similar profiles have been observed in Ibadan, Nigeria (Edington et al., 1973; Okpala et al., 1991), Zimbabwe (Levy, 1988), Sudan (Abu El Hassan et al., 1993) and Egypt (El Bolkainy et al., 1984) and in black and 'coloured' children in South Africa (Vianna et al., 1977; Cohen & Hamilton, 1980; Hesseling et al., 1997).

Table 3 shows the distribution by cell type in the series presented in this volume. A large proportion of the cases in most centres are without specification of subtype. However, among the remainder, mixed cellularity is the predominant type of Hodgkin disease in most series.

Etiology

The epidemiological features of Hodgkin disease have given rise to hypotheses concerning an infectious etiology. Thus it has been suggested that early infection (associated with crowding and lower socioeconomic status) is associated with childhood Hodgkin disease, while delayed infection would explain the association of young adult Hodgkin disease (age 15–40 years) with higher socioeconomic status, small families, less crowding and low birth order.

Table 1b. Age-standardized (world) and cumulative incidence
Burkitt lymphoma (age 0-14)

	MALE				FEMALE			
	Cases	CRUDE (per 100,000)	ASR(W) (per 100,000)	Cumulative (%)	Cases	CRUDE (per 100,000)	ASR(W) (per 100,000)	Cumulative (%)
Africa, North								
Algeria, Algiers (1993-1997)	-	-	-	-	-	-	-	-
Algeria, Constantine (1994-1997)	-	-	-	-	-	-	-	-
Algeria, Oran (1996-1998)	-	-	-	-	-	-	-	-
Algeria, Setif (1993-1997)	2	0.1	**0.1**	0.00	1	0.0	**0.1**	0.00
Tunisia, Centre, Sousse (1993-1997)	1	0.1	**0.2**	0.00	-	-	-	-
Tunisia, North, Tunis (1994)	2	0.1	**0.3**	0.00	3	0.1	**0.5**	0.01
Tunisia, Sfax (1997)	-	-	-	-	-	-	-	-
Africa, West								
The Gambia (1997-1998)	4	0.4	**0.8**	0.01	6	0.6	**1.2**	0.02
Guinea, Conakry (1996-1999)	12	0.5	**1.3**	0.02	12	0.5	**1.3**	0.02
Mali, Bamako (1988-1997)	2	0.1	**0.1**	0.00	1	0.0	**0.1**	0.00
Niger, Niamey (1993-1999)	6	0.3	**0.7**	0.01	5	0.3	**0.6**	0.01
Nigeria, Ibadan (1998-1999)	12	0.8	**1.8**	0.03	2	0.1	**0.3**	0.00
Africa, Central								
Congo, Brazzaville (1996-1999)	5	0.4	**1.0**	0.01	6	0.5	**1.2**	0.02
Africa, East								
France, La Reunion (1988-1994)	6	0.3	**1.0**	0.01	-	-	-	-
Kenya, Eldoret (1998-2000)	3	0.3	**0.7**	0.01	5	0.5	**1.3**	0.02
Malawi, Blantyre (2000-2001)	10	1.1	**2.8**	0.05	2	0.2	**0.6**	0.01
Uganda, Kyadondo County (1993-1997)	53	1.9	**4.7**	0.07	37	1.3	**3.0**	0.05
Zimbabwe, Harare: African (1990-1993)	3	0.1	**0.4**	0.01	1	0.0	**0.1**	0.00
Zimbabwe, Harare: African (1994-1997)	-	-	-	-	2	0.1	**0.2**	0.00
Zimbabwe, Harare: European (1990-1997)	-	-	-	-	-	-	-	-
Africa, South								
Namibia (1995-1998)	2	0.1	**0.1**	0.00	1	0.0	**0.1**	0.00
South Africa: Black (1989-1992)	18	0.0	**0.1**	0.00	11	0.0	**0.1**	0.00
South Africa: Indian (1989-1992)	-	-	-	-	-	-	-	-
South Africa: Mixed race (1989-1992)	5	0.1	**0.3**	0.00	1	0.0	**0.1**	0.00
South Africa: White (1989-1992)	8	0.1	**0.3**	0.01	2	0.0	**0.1**	0.00
South Africa, Transkei, Umtata (1996-1998)	-	-	-	-	-	-	-	-
South Africa, Transkei, 4 districts (1996-1998)	-	-	-	-	-	-	-	-
Swaziland (1996-1999)	6	0.3	**0.8**	0.01	6	0.3	**0.7**	0.01
Europe/USA								
USA, SEER: White (1993-1997)	35	0.1	**0.3**	0.01	9	0.0	**0.1**	0.00
USA, SEER: Black (1993-1997)	7	0.1	**0.4**	0.01	1	0.0	**0.1**	0.00
France, 8 registries (1993-1997)	24	0.2	**0.8**	0.01	5	0.0	**0.2**	0.00
The Netherlands (1993-1997)	51	0.1	**0.7**	0.01	10	0.0	**0.1**	0.00
UK, England (1993-1997)	41	0.0	**0.2**	0.00	4	0.0	**0.0**	0.00

In italics: histopathology-based registries

Table 2(b). Incidence of BL in children aged 0–14 years (rates per million)

			Rate	Source
Uganda: Kampala		1960–71	9.5* (12 boys, 7 girls)	
		1992–95	36.0* (49 boys, 29 girls)	Wabinga *et al.*, 2000
	Lango District	1963–68	42.9* (65 boys, 26 girls)	
	Acholi District	1963–68	31.8* (36 boys, 28 girls)	Morrow *et al.*, 1977
Nigeria: Ibadan	1960–66		83.6* (113.9 boys, 58.5 girls)	Edington & Hendrikse 1973
		1985–92	18.0* (24 boys, 12 girls)	Parkin *et al.*, 1998
North Mara, Tanzania		1964–70	57 (62 boys, 51 girls)	Brubaker *et al.*, 1973
Harare, Zimbabwe		1991–95	2.4*	Parkin *et al.*, 1998
Algeria, Setif		1986–95	1.3*	Parkin *et al.*, 1998
Mali, Bamako		1987–95	1.7*	Parkin *et al.*, 1998
Namibia		1983–92	1.9*	Parkin *et al.*, 1998
USA (SEER)		1983–92		Parkin *et al.*, 1998
	White		2.5 (4.1 boys, 0.7 girls)*	
	Black		0.6*	

* Age-standardized rate

Much evidence points to an association between Hodgkin disease and Epstein–Barr virus (EBV) (IARC, 1997). A history of infectious mononucleosis (indicating adolescent infection with EBV) is associated with increased risk of Hodgkin disease. Many case–control studies have shown that Hodgkin disease subjects have higher prevalence and a higher titre of antibody to EBV than control subjects. In a large cohort study, Mueller et al. (1989) showed that elevated titres of antibodies to EBV were predictive of later development of Hodgkin disease.

Markers of EBV infection or EBV DNA can be detected in tumour tissue from a proportion of subjects. The virus appears to be located within the Reed–Sternberg cells or their variants, in up to 50% of patients. It has been difficult to distinguish patterns of EBV infection in relation to other features (geography, age, etc.), since most clinical series have been rather small. However, in a large multi-centre study including more than 1500 cases of Hodgkin disease, Glaser et al. (1997) concluded that the important determinants of presence of EBV, independently associated, were:

- Mixed cellularity versus nodular sclerosing or lymphocyte-predominant subtypes
- Age (lowest in young adults, higher in childhood and the elderly)
- Sex (higher in male than in female and in young adults)
- Socioeconomic development (higher in populations of lower socioeconomic status).

Data from clinical series in Africa are largely consistent with these observations. There is a higher prevalence of EBV in Hodgkin disease cases from Kenya than in European countries (Leoncini et al., 1996; Weinreb et al., 1996; Lazzi et al., 1998) and Japan (Kusuda et al., 1998), with almost all of the paediatric cases from Kenya being EBV-positive.

Burkitt lymphoma

Burkitt lymphoma (BL) was first described by Sir Albert Cook, who established the first mission hospital in Uganda in 1897. In the 1950s, various clinicians and pathologists working in Africa described facial 'sarcomas' and lymphomas occurring at high frequency in African children. Comprehensive clinical and pathological descriptions of "African lymphoma" were made by Denis Burkitt and his colleagues (Burkitt, 1958; O'Conor & Davies, 1960, Burkitt & O'Conor, 1961; O'Conor, 1961).

Soon after these reports, it was observed that the pathological features of 'African lymphoma' were present in certain childhood lymphomas in North America and Europe (O'Conor et al., 1965; Wright & Roberts, 1966). Comparative studies of the incidence or frequency of BL have been difficult because of the lack of a clear and consistent definition. For example, BL can be regarded as a clinical syndrome or as a pathological entity (the two will not exactly coincide) and the presence or absence of evidence of EBV infection has sometimes been taken into account in making the 'diagnosis'. In fact, comparative studies must still rely upon the entity as defined by histology.

Clinical features
The jaw is the most frequently involved site and the commonest presenting feature in patients with BL in sub-Saharan Africa (Burkitt, 1958, 1970) (Figure 3). Jaw involvement is age-dependent, occurring much more frequently in young children, and the tumour arises in close proximity to the developing molar tooth buds. In series of cases of Burkitt lymphoma in Uganda, 70% of children under five years of age and 25% of patients over 14 had jaw involvement (Burkitt, 1970). Very young children who do not have overt jaw tumours often have orbital involvement (Olurin & Williams, 1972). Jaw involvement appears to be more frequent in regions of higher incidence, and a decline in the incidence of BL may result in proportionately fewer jaw tumours in clinical series

(Biggar et al., 1981). Patients from highland regions, where incidence rates are relatively low (see below), are also of higher median age, and this probably accounts for the lower frequency of jaw tumours (Burkitt & Wright, 1966; Kitinya & Lauren, 1982). It has been suggested that the frequency of jaw tumours is decreasing in some regions of equatorial Africa, with a corresponding increase in the fraction of abdominal tumours but with no clear change in the age-related incidence (Nkrumah, 1984).

Abdominal involvement, often with ascites, is found in a little over half of equatorial African patients at presentation (Magrath, 1991; Williams, 1975). Bone-marrow involvement is seen in some 7–8% of cases in Uganda (Magrath & Ziegler, 1980). Central nervous system involvement, with cranial nerve palsy and paraplegia due to paraspinal disease, is relatively common in Africa, being found in about one third of patients at presentation (Ziegler et al., 1970).

Pathology
BL is characterized by a monomorphic cytoarchitecture composed of medium-sized cells with a high nucleus to cytoplasm ratio, a round or oval nucleus with a coarse or 'open' chromatin pattern and usually two to five readily discernible nucleoli. Histological sections often show the presence of tingible body macrophages scattered among the tumour cells, giving rise to a 'starry sky' appearance. This appearance is not pathognomonic of BL and may be seen in other lymphomas (O'Conor, 1961). BL is invariably of B-cell origin, the presence of surface immunoglobulin having first been shown by Klein et al. (1967). The surface immunoglobulin is usually IgM, but IgG and IgA are occasionally present and kappa or lambda immunoglobulin light chains are nearly always detected.

Cytogenetic studies have permitted the characterization of BL in terms of chromosomal translocation. These invariably involve the part of chromosome 8 (the q24 region) in which is located c-myc, an oncogene important in controlling cell proliferation. However, the breakpoint does not always concern the c-myc gene itself, although c-myc is moved adjacent to a region on a different chromosome concerned with production of part of the immunoglobulin molecules. These chromosomal breakpoint locations are quite different in BL cases in Africa and in America (Magrath, 1990); in the United States, for example, only 9% of tumours have a breakpoint outside c-myc, compared with 75% in Africa. This suggests that there are different subtypes of BL within the histopathological entity, in different parts of the world.

Incidence and geographical occurrence
Burkitt and O'Conor (1961) noted the age distribution (maximum occurrence in children age 5–9 years), predominance of boys over girls, and limited geographical extent. Table 1(b) shows incidence rates of BL in children reported from population-based cancer registries in this volume, and Table 2(b) data from other series published in the last 30–40 years. BL cases do occur in Africa after the childhood age range, but the rates are very much lower.

BL accounts for between one quarter and one half of all paediatric cancers in tropical East, Central and West Africa, but appears much less frequently in northern and southern Africa and in series from Europe and North America. Nevertheless, even in the latter areas, it may comprise 20–30% of non-Hodgkin lymphoma (NHL) in the childhood age range.

The geography of BL in Africa has been the subject of many reviews. The early work of Burkitt relied upon collecting information on the relative frequency of cancers in clinical series from hospitals in Africa. Crude and simple though this method may appear, it allowed detection of the striking geographical patterns seen for BL, for which incidence rates vary at least 100-fold. Thus, Burkitt delimited a zone 15° north and south of the equator (with a prolongation southward into Mozambique to the east) as the high-incidence area (Wright, 1967). Even within this area, however, BL

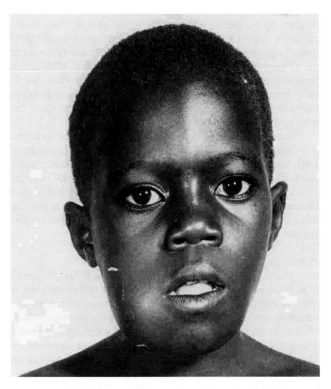

Figure 3. Typical presentation of Burkitt lymphoma

is infrequent in high-altitude regions, such as Rwanda and Burundi, the Kenya Highlands and the plateaux of Zambia and Zimbabwe. These limits are related to climate; areas of high BL incidence have been associated with an annual rainfall above 50 cm and an average temperature in the coolest month above 15.6°C (Haddow, 1963). It was initially thought that this might indicate the importance of an arthropod-borne virus (and the specific vector), but Burkitt (1969) and O'Conor (1970) drew attention to the close relationship to endemicity of malaria and malaria parasitaemia.

The interesting distribution in relation to climatic factors persists when the focus is on smaller geographical areas in Africa. The most detailed studies have been undertaken in Uganda (Wright, 1973), where there are marked differences in the incidence of BL between different districts. The highest rates are seen in the lowland areas around the Nile in the north-west (West Nile, Madi, Acholi and Lango), while mountainous districts in the south-west show low rates. This pattern closely reflects the endemicity of malaria (Kafuko & Burkitt, 1970); it cannot be explained by quality of communications and medical facilities, since the distribution of other lymphomas approximates to that expected on the basis of population density (Wright & Roberts, 1966). Within the West Nile district itself, the same phenomenon is seen, with an almost total absence of cases from the highlands in the south of the district (Williams, 1968).

In Kenya, the lowest incidence of BL was in the Kalenjin tribe, living in highland areas above 1500 m altitude, with higher incidence in tribes from lower-lying lakeshore or coastal areas (Dalldorf et al., 1964). This pattern coincided with prevalence of malaria (and associated splenomegaly).

In northern Tanzania, Kitinya and Lauren (1982) found a low frequency (2.2% of tumours) of BL around Mount Kilimanjaro, and most of the cases occurred at lower altitudes (under 1000 m). In this low-incidence area, the average age of patients was higher (16.4% over 20 years of age) and the frequency of jaw tumours lower (22%) than in the high-incidence areas of Uganda.

The link between BL and climate is supported by studies of migrant populations. Populations migrating from low- to high-incidence areas have a higher average age of onset of BL than those born in endemic areas (Burkitt & Wright, 1966; Morrow et al.,

1976, 1977). This, together with the lower rates observed in urban than rural populations in Ghana (Biggar & Nkrumah, 1979), has lent support to the concept of the etiological role of malaria (see below).

Space–time clustering
Pike et al. (1967) drew attention to space–time clustering of BL cases (pairs of cases occurring closer in space/time than would be expected by chance) in the West Nile District of Uganda in the period 1961–65. Morrow et al. (1971) also reported a remarkable outbreak of seven cases of BL in Bwamba County of Toro District in western Uganda. These observations provoked great interest, since clustering was thought to imply that infectious agents, spread from person to person, were somehow involved in etiology. Seasonal variation in presentation of BL cases, consistent from year to year (Williams et al., 1974; Morrow et al., 1976), also favours such a hypothesis, although seasonality was not seen in other studies (Morrow et al., 1977). The putative infectious agent was not supposed to be the ubiquitous EBV (see below), but it was thought that maybe the waxing and waning in intensity of malaria infection might be responsible. In fact, the latent period for an effect would have to be very short to generate clustering, if it were not to be masked by variation in latent period.

Williams et al. (1978) reviewed the observations in West Nile District from a 15-year period (1961–75), during which time an attempt was made to identify all new diagnosed cases in local hospitals and from the referral centres and pathology laboratory in Kampala. 202 cases were found (81% with histology) and there was no trend in incidence over time. As had been reported by Pike et al. (1967), marked clustering was evident in the first quinquennium, but not in the next 10 years (except for the two-year period 1972–73). The incidence of BL varied within the different subdivisions (counties of West Nile) between the three quinquennia, suggesting that the intensity of the precipitating factor varied over relatively wide areas with time.

Elsewhere in Uganda there has been no evidence of space–time clustering, either in the relatively low-incidence Mengo District in the south (Morrow et al., 1976) or in the high-risk districts of Acholi and Lango in the centre north (Morrow et al., 1977). Nor was any clustering observed in the high-incidence area of North Mara District, Tanzania (Siemiatycki et al., 1980). Biggar and Nkrumah (1979) did not observe any space–time clustering among 236 cases seen in the main teaching hospital of Ghana in 1970–75.

On the other hand, van den Bosch et al. (1993a) found limited evidence, based on interviews of 146 cases referred to Kamuzu Central Hospital in Lilongwe, Malawi, of space–time clustering (more pairs of cases <2.5 km distant and <60 days apart than expected by chance). The clustering was more marked when the analysis was confined to cases aged 8 years or more.

The significance and any biological explanation of the clustering found in West Nile and Malawi remain speculative; the possibility of biased case ascertainment and pure chance cannot be excluded.

Etiology
Role of EBV
EBV was first identified in an attempt to confirm the hypothesis that African BL is caused by a vectored virus. Evidence that EBV was associated with BL was based initially on serological evidence of the presence of viral antibodies (Henle & Henle, 1966). This test was later shown to reflect the level of viral capsid antigen (VCA) in the cells; cells that gave positive results in immunofluorescence assays were shown to contain viral particles by electron microscopy (Henle & Henle, 1967; Epstein & Achong, 1968). Later, EBV DNA was detected in tumour cells using a nucleic acid hybridization technique (zur Hausen & Schulte-Holthausen, 1970). Viral DNA is present in cells in which late viral antigens or viral particles cannot be detected, indicating that the virus can latently infect cells, i.e. remain within the cell without replicating viral particles.

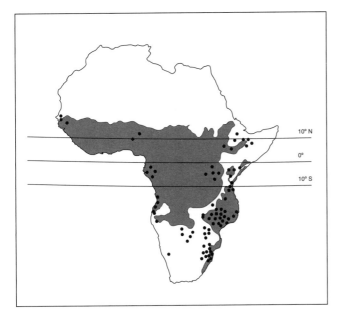

Figure 4. Distribution of Burkitt lymphoma in Africa (from Haddow, 1963) The shaded area represents the area in which, on climatological grounds, Burkitt lymphoma might be expected to occur. The black points show the distribution of the series of cases compiled by D. Burkitt. The method used was to fill in any degree-square in which the condition had been recorded, irrespective of the number of cases

Differences in the frequency of the association of BL with EBV, as determined by the presence of EBV DNA (or RNA) or EBV antigens, are found in different regions of the world. Case series from Africa have been reviewed by IARC (1997). In Africa, some 95% of BL are associated with EBV, as demonstrated by the presence of either EBV nuclear antigen (EBNA) or EBV DNA in the tumour cells, and such patients have higher geometric mean titres (GMT) of antibodies against EBV-associated antigens. In North Africa, around three quarters of BL is associated with EBV, compared with 15–20% in Europe and North America (Ladjadj et al., 1984, Anwar et al., 1995).

A number of case–control studies compared the prevalence of antibodies to EBV in cases of BL and in control subjects, but adjustment for the age of subjects being compared, necessary because the prevalence of antibodies to EBV changes with age, appears to have rarely been made (IARC, 1997). In all of these studies, the antibody was more often detected in cases than in controls, and antibody titres of cases were higher (Henle & Henle, 1967; Henle et al., 1969; Klein et al., 1970; Henle et al., 1971; Hirshaut et al., 1973; Nkrumah et al., 1976). Case–control studies cannot resolve whether the antibodies to EBV in BL cases represent a response to infection or re-activation of latent EBV following tumour onset (an effect rather than cause of disease).

In a large cohort study in West Nile District of Uganda, sera were obtained from 42 000 children aged 4–8 years, who were then followed up for up to seven years. In the initial analysis (de The et al., 1978), each of the the 14 cases of BL detected in the cohort was matched for age, sex and locality with five control subjects. The cases had significantly higher prediagnostic anti-VCA titres than control subjects (GMT, 425.5 versus 125.8), but no difference was observed between cases and controls in the titres of anti-early antigen (EA) and anti-EBNA. Two additional EBV-associated, histologically confirmed cases of BL were detected up to 1979, both of which had high anti-VCA titres before the onset of BL (Geser et al., 1982). This study showed that anti-VCA titres can be elevated as long as six years before the onset of BL and as early as three months after birth. The relative risk for developing BL increased multiplicatively by a factor of 5.1 for each two-fold

dilution in anti-VCA titre for all cases of BL and by a factor of 9.2 when the analysis was confined to cases in which EBV DNA was present in the tumour.

Role of malaria
The evidence linking risk of BL to malaria infection, derived from ecological comparisons, has been reviewed by Morrow (1985):

- The incidence of BL correlates within and between countries with the incidence of malaria and with parasitaemia rates.
- The age at which peak levels of antimalarial antibodies are acquired (5–8 years) corresponds to the age of peak incidence of BL.
- Individuals who live in urban areas where malarial transmission rates are lower also have a lower incidence of BL.
- In regions where death rates due to malaria have declined, BL incidence has also declined.
- The age at onset of BL in immigrants from malaria-free areas to malarious areas is higher than that of the original inhabitants.
- There is an inverse relationship between the age at onset of BL and the intensity of infection with Plasmodium falciparum.
- There is an apparently reduced incidence (though not statistically significant) of BL in individuals with sickle-cell trait, which also protects against malaria.
- There is some evidence for seasonal variation in the onset of BL and for time-space clustering.

Dalldorf (1962) appears to have been the first to suggest that malaria is relevant to the development of BL. In his ecological study in Kenya (Dalldorf et al., 1964), the highest incidence of BL occurred in areas where malaria was holoendemic, namely in the coastal and lakeside regions. Kafuko and Burkitt (1970) summarized the early geographical studies linking malaria infection to risk of BL, noting that the disease was not common in any area where malaria transmission occurs for less than six months in the year. In Ghana, a significant difference in malaria parasitaemia (*P. falciparum*) rates between urban (1.4%) and rural populations (22%) was accompanied by similar differences in antimalarial antibody titres (Biggar et al., 1981). Persons who had taken chloroquine for treatment of suspected malaria had a lower antibody frequency and lower titres than those who did not use chloroquine. This difference correlated with the distribution of BL in Ghana (Biggar & Nkrumah, 1979). Morrow (1985) reported a significant correlation between malaria parasitaemia (*P. falciparum*) rates and the incidence of BL in various districts in Uganda. Parasitaemia rates ranged from 7.9% (in Ankole) to 75.2% (in Madi), and the incidence of BL in children aged 0–14 years from 0.1 (in Ankole) to 6.0 (in Lango) per 100 000. In holoendemic areas, the peak age of prevalence and of the density of falciparum parasitaemia is two to three years, whereas the maximal level of antimalarial and non-antimalarial immunoglobulin occurs two to five years later, coinciding with the peak age of incidence of BL in these regions. Also in Uganda, immigrants into Mengo District (around Kampala) from highland regions with low malarial prevalence who developed BL were significantly older (median, 12 years) at the onset of BL than patients from meso-endemic Mengo (median, 8 years; p < 0.008), while patients from Mengo were significantly older than patients from hyper- or holoendemic regions at lower altitude (median, 6 years; p < 0.04) (Morrow et al., 1976; Morrow, 1985).

Despite these ecological observations, an association between risk of BL and malaria infection, or its intensity, has never been demonstrated at the individual level. No differences have been reported in the levels of malarial antibodies between BL patients and controls (Morrow, 1985).

Conclusive evidence exists regarding the role of haemoglobin S (HbS; beta6Glu → Val) heterozygosity in protecting against severe malaria. Furthermore, in a large case–control study in Burkina

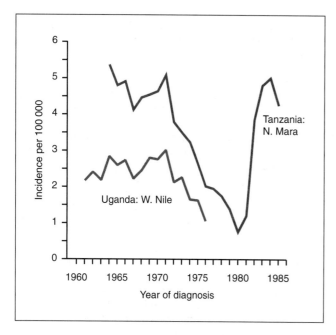

Figure 5. Trends in the incidence rate (three-year moving average) of Burkitt lymphoma in East Africa (data from Geser *et al.*, 1989)

Faso, Modiano *et al.* (2001) showed that HbC is associated with a 29% reduction in risk of clinical malaria in HbAC heterozygotes, and of 93% in HbCC homozygotes. If BL is associated with malaria, these haemoglobinopathies should, therefore, be associated with a decreased risk of BL. Williams (1966) compared the haemoglobin electrophoretic patterns of 100 Yoruba children (Nigeria) with BL with those of 331 children of the same ages from the same hospital. There was an significant excess of AA haemoglobin in BL cases (78%) compared with control children, 32% of whom were homo- or heterozygous for HbS or HbC. An earlier study (Gilles, 1963) had found no difference. The study has been criticized for using hospital controls, which could have introduced a selective bias in favour of children with AS haemoglobin. In Uganda, a case–control study by Pike *et al.* (1970), matching 36 cases of BL and controls by age, sex, tribe and place of residence, found that in children with AA haemoglobin, the risk of BL was about twice that of those with AS, but (due to the small study size), this increase was not significant (*p* = 0.16, one-sided). In Ghana, Nkrumah and Perkins (1976) compared 112 patients with BL with nearest neighbour controls of the same age, sex, and tribe, and with sibling controls. There was no significant protective advantage for sickle cell trait (HbAS) against BL. Haemoglobin C trait appeared to offer a slight protective advantage (*p* < 0.1).

The observational data are supported by the results of an intervention study in North Mara District, Tanzania (Geser *et al.*, 1989), during which, for a period of five years, chloroquine tablets were regularly distributed to a cohort of children below the age of 10 years. In the pre-trial period (1964–76), malarial parasitaemia was high in the lowlands (near Lake Victoria) where BL cases were occurring, and low in the high plateau (over 1500 m) bordering Kenya, where BL was rare. The prevalence of malarial parasitaemia, titres of antimalarial fluorescent antibody, and incidence of BL fell during the period of chloroquine administration (1977–82), the latter to the lowest level ever recorded in the region: 0.5 per 100 000 in 1980 and 1981 in comparison with 2.6–6.9 per 100 000 before the trial (Figure 5). When chloroquine distribution ceased, prevalence of malaria rapidly rose again to pre-trial levels, followed some two years later by an increase in incidence of BL, to reach a high of 7.1 in 1984 (Figure 5). There was no decline in the prevalence of malarial parasitaemia or incidence of BL in the neighbouring South Mara District during the period of the trial.

A possible mechanism for the link between BL and malaria is loss of cytotoxic T cell control of EBV in B cells following infection with *P. falciparum*, possibly due to the destruction or dysfunction of a subset of CD4 cells responsible for the induction of suppressor/cytotoxic CD8 cells. This could result in activation and proliferation of foci of B cells containing EBV. The expanded pool of B cells and their rapid turnover would increase the chance of genetic alterations involving the c-*myc* gene leading to malignant transformation (Whittle *et al.*, 1990; Pagano, 1992).

Other factors
Socioeconomic factors have been claimed to be important in BL. Williams (1988) noted an association with low socioeconomic status in Nigeria and suggested a reduced incidence following the economic boom in the country. Morrow *et al.* (1974) compared 56 BL cases with neighbourhood controls in Uganda. The BL cases lived in poorer houses, had more siblings (and sibling deaths) and shared their rooms with more people than the control children. However, Wood *et al.* (1988) found no association in southern Africa.

Family aggregation in siblings was described by Brubaker *et al.* (1980) in the North Mara District of Tanzania. The possibility of a genetic basis for familial cases is raised by the association with certain HLA phenotypes (Jones *et al.*, 1985).

Environmental exposure to the plant *Euphorbia tirucalli*, and other medicinal plants containing phorbol esters, has been suggested as a risk factor for BL. Osato *et al.* (1987, 1990) found *E. tirucalli* around almost all houses, fields and reservoirs in villages near Lake Victoria and in other high-incidence regions in Kenya and Tanzania. The plant was reported to be uncommon in areas of these countries where BL is rare. In Malawi, van den Bosch *et al.* (1993b) reported that *E. tirucalli* was found significantly more often near to the homes of cases of BL than to those of control subjects. Phorbol esters present in this plant have been reported to increase the ability of EBV to transform B lymphocytes and to increase the likelihood that a chromosomal translocation will develop in transformed cells.

The observation that the pattern of space–time clustering of BL cases in Malawi (see above) coincided with an epidemic of Chikungunya fever prompted van den Bosch and Lloyd (2000) to carry out a sero-epidemiological study of the association of the responsible arbovirus with BL. 108 BL cases (12 clinically diagnosed) were compared with two age-sex matched hospital controls and two neighbourhood (same village) controls per case. Comparing the BL cases with hospital controls, there was no difference in the presence of antibody at time of admission, but when antibody at the time of discharge was considered, the odds ratio was 2.36 (95% CI 1.28–4.56). For neighbourhood controls, recruited some 8–16 weeks after the case was first admitted, antibody presence was compared with BL cases at their third admission to hospital; the odds ratio was similar (2.28, 95% CI 1.14–5.07).

Burkitt lymphoma in relation to AIDS
In the United States and Europe, NHLs are the most common malignancy in children with AIDS and about one-third are BL (Mueller, 1998). AIDS-related BL resembles the form of the disease (sporadic; sBL) that comprised up to a third of NHL cases in childhood before the advent of the AIDS epidemic (Parkin *et al.*, 1985). It occurs with a peak at 10–19 years of age (Beral *et al.*, 1991) and frequently involves lymph nodes and the bone marrow (Knowles, 1996). The EBV genome is present in around 30% of cases, which is similar to the proportion in sBL cases (Hamilton-Dutoit *et al.*, 1993a; IARC, 1996). Molecular analyses of translocation breakpoints in the chromosomes of tumour cells suggest that the pattern in most cases of AIDS-related BL resembles that observed in sBL in Europe and America, and is quite different from that in endemic, EBV-related, African BL (Roithmann & Andrieu, 1992).

The effect of the AIDS epidemic on lymphoma in childhood is described in the chapter on AIDS and cancer in sub-Saharan Africa.

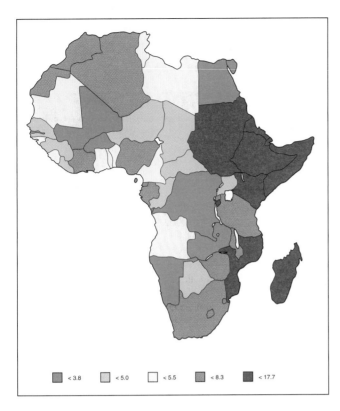

■ < 3.8	■ < 5.0	□ < 5.5	■ < 8.3	■ < 17.7

Figure 6. Incidence of non-Hodgkin lymphoma: ASR (world) - males, age 15–65+

Non-Hodgkin lymphomas

Pathology

The greatest problem in the study of NHLs has always been that these do not by any means constitute a single diagnostic entity. The very title indicates that it is a diagnosis of exclusion. Many attempts at classification of this group of neoplasms have been made, but the most usual criteria chosen, such as morphological pattern, immunological origin, histological grade and prognosis may have little or no relevance to etiology, the usual concern of epidemiologists. The most recent WHO classification attempts to incorporate morphological, immunophenotypic and molecular information to produce groupings with more relevance to cause (Jaffe et al., 2001).

Unfortunately, most studies, descriptive and analytic, use older terminologies that are impossible to translate into equivalents in more modern schemas. It is generally necessary, therefore, to group together all 'non-Hodgkin lymphomas', accepting that this will be grossly unsatisfactory for elucidating meaningful patterns.

Geography

Overall rates of NHL seem to be highest in the more developed areas of the world. Nevertheless, estimated rates of incidence (Ferlay et al., 2001) suggest that West and East Africa have relatively high incidence. Most studies of the relationship of NHL to socioeconomic status have been non-conclusive (Faggiano et al., 1997). Studies in the United States (e.g., Cantor & Fraumeni, 1980) have suggested that geographical distribution is associated with relative affluence of the population, but this has not been clearly shown in individual-based studies (La Vecchia et al., 1992).

Adult NHL in Africa

It is not clear whether or not there is significant variation in the incidence of NHL as an entity in Africa as a whole.

Figure 6 shows estimated incidence rates for adult NHL (excluding children) for males, by country. These estimates are derived largely from a knowledge of the contemporary incidence rates shown in Table 1(c).

Comparison of these rates with those observed in Europe and North America suggests that, in general, the incidence of NHL is relatively low in adults in African populations. Wright (1973) suggested, on the basis of data from Kyadondo county and Ibadan, that incidence in African populations was similar to that in Europe (at least up to age 50 years). In fact, this observation was only partly correct, as incidence in Ibadan at that time (1960–62), based on just 52 adult cases, was unusually high, and incidence rates in European populations were lower than in more recent years.

There seems to have been rather little change in incidence of NHL in African adults over time, as judged from a comparison of older (Table 2(c)) and the more recent series.

Therefore, it seems that, although lymphomas appear to be frequent in clinical or histopathology series, the actual incidence rates are not particularly high.

Clinical series show an excess of high-grade lymphomas in series from Africa, and a deficit of nodular lymphomas (El Bolkainy et al., 1984; Fleming, 1985; Okpala et al., 1991; Ngendahayo & Schmauz, 1992; Cool & Bitter, 1997). Few systematic studies have classified African lymphomas using modern techniques. In general, B-cell lymphomas predominate in both East Africa (Cool & Bitter, 1997), South Africa (Jacobs, 1985), North Africa (El Bolkainy et al., 1984) and Nigeria (Thomas et al., 1991).

The so-called Mediterranean lymphoma reported from countries of the Middle East (Rappaport et al., 1972) appears to be uncommon in North Africa, although the small intestine was noted to be the most common location for gastrointestinal lymphomas in Eqypt (El Bolkainy et al., 1984).

A relatively high prevalence of antibodies to HTLV-I has been reported from various parts of Africa (Saxinger et al., 1984; Delaporte et al., 1989), with particularly high prevalence in Gabon. It is estimated that sub-Saharan Africa constitutes the largest reservoir of the virus in the world—possibly as many as 10 million carriers (Hunsmann et al., 1984). Despite this, T-cell lymphomas in general, and acute T-cell leukaemia-lymphoma (ATLL) in particular, are not commonly observed. Williams et al. (1993) described four cases of ATLL from Nigeria, all positive for HTLV-I, and Fouchard et al. (1998) three HTLV-I positive cases (among 14 cutaneous T-cell lymphomas) from Bamako, Mali.

Etiology

Wright and Roberts (1966) and Schmauz et al. (1990) investigated whether BL and other NHLs had similar geographical distributions in Uganda (implying etiological similarities). Their conclusions were different (negative and positive, respectively). However, regional incidence rates were based upon dispatch of biopsy material to a central pathology laboratory, and must be subject to a number of unknown biases, as well as being considerable underestimates of the true incidence.

The role of EBV in NHL (other than BL) in immunocompetent subjects is unclear. Although viral DNA is found in a proportion of tumours, the evidence that reactivation of the virus precedes tumour development is sparse and the evaluation by IARC (1997) found no clear evidence for an etiological role.

Certain chemical exposures—particularly to pesticides/herbicides and petrol products have been implicated in several studies (reviewed by Cartwright & McNally, 1994). There have been reports of various drugs increasing risk (Bernstein & Ross, 1992).

Since 1992, there has been interest in a possible association between NHL and hepatitis C virus (HCV), mainly based upon observations from case–control studies (Silvestri et al., 2000). We are not aware of any such studies in Africa.

Table 1c. Age-standardized (world) and cumulative (15-64) incidence
Adult non-Hodgkin lymphoma (age 15+)

	MALE				FEMALE			
	Cases	CRUDE	ASR(W)	Cumulative	Cases	CRUDE	ASR(W)	Cumulative
		(per 100,000)		(%)		(per 100,000)		(%)
Africa, North								
Algeria, Algiers (1993-1997)	138	3.6	**4.7**	0.26	102	2.7	**3.3**	0.15
Algeria, Constantine (1994-1997)	50	5.4	**7.3**	0.30	33	3.5	**4.3**	0.23
Algeria, Oran (1996-1998)	91	7.6	**9.2**	0.45	72	6.0	**7.6**	0.40
Algeria, Setif (1993-1997)	58	3.4	**4.4**	0.23	38	2.1	**2.6**	0.14
Tunisia, Centre, Sousse (1993-1997)	73	9.6	**11.5**	0.56	46	6.1	**7.3**	0.35
Tunisia, North, Tunis (1994)	88	6.0	**7.3**	0.32	53	3.7	**4.5**	0.15
Tunisia, Sfax (1997)	15	5.7	**6.4**	0.24	11	4.3	**5.3**	0.26
Africa, West								
The Gambia (1997-1998)	9	1.9	**2.6**	0.13	5	0.9	**1.2**	0.02
Guinea, Conakry (1996-1999)	44	3.4	**4.9**	0.26	27	2.2	**2.6**	0.14
Mali, Bamako (1988-1997)	40	1.8	**2.4**	0.10	32	1.7	**2.1**	0.12
Niger, Niamey (1993-1999)	29	2.9	**4.4**	0.23	26	2.8	**4.2**	0.22
Nigeria, Ibadan (1998-1999)	35	4.1	**6.1**	0.32	23	2.5	**3.7**	0.21
Africa, Central								
Congo, Brazzaville (1996-1999)	31	4.5	**5.2**	0.30	16	2.2	**2.3**	0.13
Africa, East								
France, La Reunion (1988-1994)	83	5.7	**7.2**	0.32	69	4.5	**4.7**	0.12
Kenya, Eldoret (1998-2000)	39	7.4	**10.1**	0.40	20	3.9	**6.1**	0.35
Malawi, Blantyre (2000-2001)	30	5.4	**7.2**	0.41	23	4.6	**6.8**	0.40
Uganda, Kyadondo County (1993-1997)	57	3.4	**4.9**	0.22	49	3.0	**3.7**	0.17
Zimbabwe, Harare: African (1990-1993)	58	3.6	**5.3**	0.28	35	2.6	**6.1**	0.22
Zimbabwe, Harare: African (1994-1997)	111	5.9	**8.5**	0.44	69	4.2	**7.1**	0.33
Zimbabwe, Harare: European (1990-1997)	15	11.8	**8.9**	0.46	19	13.3	**8.3**	0.32
Africa, South								
Namibia (1995-1998)	47	2.6	**3.2**	0.16	35	1.9	**2.4**	0.09
South Africa: Black (1989-1992)	865	2.5	**3.5**	0.16	569	1.6	**2.1**	0.10
South Africa: Indian (1989-1992)	99	7.4	**10.3**	0.43	61	4.4	**6.0**	0.30
South Africa: Mixed race (1989-1992)	168	4.0	**5.5**	0.26	150	3.3	**4.7**	0.22
South Africa: White (1989-1992)	1094	14.1	**14.4**	0.61	995	12.5	**11.3**	0.52
South Africa, Transkei, Umtata (1996-1998)	5	2.5	**2.6**	0.08	4	1.5	**1.6**	0.08
South Africa, Transkei, 4 districts (1996-1998)	1	0.3	**0.4**	0.03	2	0.4	**0.5**	0.02
Swaziland (1996-1999)	32	3.4	**4.4**	0.24	21	1.9	**2.0**	0.09
Europe/USA								
USA, SEER: White (1993-1997)	10643	27.9	**24.4**	0.99	8639	21.5	**15.7**	0.59
USA, SEER: Black (1993-1997)	1002	20.7	**21.9**	1.08	590	10.5	**10.6**	0.47
France, 8 registries (1993-1997)	2107	19.3	**16.4**	0.67	1784	15.2	**10.8**	0.44
The Netherlands (1993-1997)	5407	17.5	**15.3**	0.62	4562	14.2	**10.3**	0.40
UK, England (1993-1997)	17200	17.9	**14.2**	0.59	15120	14.5	**9.6**	0.39

In italics: histopathology-based registries

Table 2(c). Incidence of non-Hodgkin lymphoma in Africa (adults), 1953–74

Registry	Period	ASR (per 100 000)		Source
		Male	Female	(see Chap. 1)
Senegal, Dakar	1969–74	4.4	1.3	4
Mozambique, Lourenço Marques	1956–60	5.7	*2.9*	1
Nigeria, Ibadan	1960–69	9.0	8.8	3
SA, Cape Province: Bantu	1956–59	3.8	*0.0*	2
SA, Cape Province: Coloured	1956–59	2.4	2.3	2
SA, Cape Province: White	1956–59	6.4	4.0	2
SA, Johannesburg, Bantu	1953–55	*1.7*	*2.4*	1
SA, Natal Province: African	1964–66	4.0	*2.7*	2
SA, Natal Province: Indian	1964–66	*2.4*	*1.0*	2
Uganda, Kyadondo	1954–60	3.5	2.8	1
Uganda, Kyadondo	1960–71	3.8	2.6	5
Zimbabwe, Bulawayo	1963–72	2.9	*0.6*	6

Italics: Rate based on less than 10 cases

Table 1d. Age-standardized (world) and cumulative (0-64) incidence
Multiple myeloma (C90)

	MALE				FEMALE			
	Cases	CRUDE	ASR(W) (per 100,000)	Cumulative (%)	Cases	CRUDE	ASR(W) (per 100,000)	Cumulative (%)
Africa, North								
Algeria, Algiers (1993-1997)	24	0.4	**0.7**	0.04	23	0.4	**0.6**	0.03
Algeria, Constantine (1994-1997)	13	0.8	**1.2**	0.08	7	0.5	**0.8**	0.01
Algeria, Oran (1996-1998)	13	0.7	**1.2**	0.11	16	0.9	**1.2**	0.08
Algeria, Setif (1993-1997)	6	0.2	**0.3**	0.01	3	0.1	**0.2**	0.02
Tunisia, Centre, Sousse (1993-1997)	4	0.3	**0.6**	0.04	10	0.9	**1.2**	0.09
Tunisia, North, Tunis (1994)	30	1.4	**1.8**	0.13	25	1.2	**1.6**	0.11
Tunisia, Sfax (1997)	3	0.8	**0.8**	0.01	3	0.8	**1.0**	0.07
Africa, West								
The Gambia (1997-1998)	-	-	**-**	-	-	-	**-**	-
Guinea, Conakry (1996-1999)	-	-	**-**	-	-	-	**-**	-
Mali, Bamako (1988-1997)	-	-	**-**	-	-	-	**-**	-
Niger, Niamey (1993-1999)	3	0.2	**0.2**	0.02	1	0.1	**0.1**	0.01
Nigeria, Ibadan (1998-1999)	1	0.1	**0.2**	-	5	0.3	**0.6**	0.05
Africa, Central								
Congo, Brazzaville (1996-1999)	9	0.7	**1.2**	0.08	12	1.0	**1.4**	0.12
Africa, East								
France, La Reunion (1988-1994)	52	2.5	**3.4**	0.18	64	3.0	**3.1**	0.12
Kenya, Eldoret (1998-2000)	8	0.9	**2.2**	0.17	3	0.3	**0.6**	0.00
Malawi, Blantyre (2000-2001)	2	0.2	**0.4**	0.05	1	0.1	**0.5**	0.06
Uganda, Kyadondo County (1993-1997)	2	0.1	**0.1**	0.01	9	0.3	**1.2**	0.08
Zimbabwe, Harare: African (1990-1993)	27	1.1	**2.6**	0.18	18	0.8	**4.1**	0.29
Zimbabwe, Harare: African (1994-1997)	27	1.0	**2.9**	0.15	25	0.9	**3.7**	0.25
Zimbabwe, Harare: European (1990-1997)	12	7.9	**3.9**	0.10	8	4.7	**2.0**	0.05
Africa, South								
Namibia (1995-1998)	12	0.4	**0.7**	0.03	16	0.5	**0.8**	0.05
South Africa: Black (1989-1992)	450	0.8	**1.5**	0.10	418	0.7	**1.2**	0.09
South Africa: Indian (1989-1992)	22	1.1	**1.9**	0.09	19	1.0	**1.2**	0.11
South Africa: Mixed race (1989-1992)	53	0.8	**1.7**	0.10	44	0.7	**1.1**	0.07
South Africa: White (1989-1992)	146	1.5	**1.3**	0.08	103	1.0	**0.8**	0.04
South Africa, Transkei, Umtata (1996-1998)	5	1.4	**3.1**	0.28	3	0.7	**0.9**	0.02
South Africa, Transkei, 4 districts (1996-1998)	1	0.1	**0.4**	0.03	1	0.1	**0.1**	-
Swaziland (1996-1999)	3	0.2	**0.4**	0.05	-	-	**-**	-
Europe/USA								
USA, SEER: White (1993-1997)	2648	5.4	**4.0**	0.19	2329	4.6	**2.7**	0.12
USA, SEER: Black (1993-1997)	517	7.7	**9.0**	0.46	552	7.4	**7.0**	0.37
France, 8 registries (1993-1997)	627	4.6	**3.2**	0.16	591	4.1	**2.2**	0.11
The Netherlands (1993-1997)	1978	5.2	**3.7**	0.17	1824	4.7	**2.6**	0.12
UK, England (1993-1997)	6832	5.7	**3.5**	0.16	6523	5.1	**2.5**	0.11

In italics: histopathology-based registries

Table 2(d). Incidence of myeloma in Africa, 1953–74

Registry	Period	ASR (per 100 000)		Source (see Chap. 1)
		Male	Female	
Senegal, Dakar	1969–74	0.2	0.2	4
Mozambique, Lourenço Marques	1956–60	*0.0*	*0.0*	1
Nigeria, Ibadan	1960–69	0.9	*0.8*	3
SA, Cape Province: Bantu	1956–59	*3.1*	*2.2*	2
SA, Cape Province: Coloured	1956–59	*1.7*	*0.4*	2
SA, Cape Province: White	1956–59	2.2	*0.3*	2
SA, Johannesburg, Bantu	1953–55	7.4	*3.1*	1
SA, Natal Province: African	1964–66	2.3	*4.3*	2
SA, Natal Province: Indian	1964–66	*1.2*	*1.4*	2
Uganda, Kyadondo	1954–60	*0.5*	*0.0*	1
Uganda, Kyadondo	1960–71	1.4	*0.6*	5
Zimbabwe, Bulawayo	1963–72	*2.5*	*2.8*	6

Italics: Rate based on less than 10 cases

Non-Hodgkin lymphoma and AIDS

In 1985, the United States Centers for Disease Control (CDC) revised the case definition for AIDS surveillance to include NHL of B-cell or indeterminate phenotype (Centers for Disease Control, 1985). In the USA and Europe, approximately 5–10% of HIV-infected persons will develop a lymphoma, and NHL is the AIDS-defining illness in about 3% of HIV-infected patients (Remick, 1995).

The epidemiology of AIDS-related lymphomas is summarized in the chapter on AIDS-related cancers in Africa, together with a review of the current status of research in this field in Africa.

Myeloma

Myeloma is more common in the black population of the United States than in whites. Incidence in the SEER registries in 1988–92 was 8.6 (males) and 6.1 (females) per 100 000 in blacks and 3.9 (males) and 2.3 (females) per 100 000 in whites. It used to be considered that the disease was rare in Africa, but Blattner *et al.* (1979) reported rates of 7.5 (males) and 5.1 (females) in the black population of South Africa.

Table 1(d) shows the rates from the population-based series in this volume and Table 2(d) presents data from the older series.

References

Abu El Hassan, M.S., Ahmed, M.E., A/Fatah, A/Gadir, Hidaytalla, A. & Ahmed, H.M. (1993) Differences in presentation of Hodgkin's disease in Sudan and Western countries. *Trop. Geogr. Med.*, **45**, 28–29

Anwar, N., Kingma, D.W., Bloch, A.R., Mourad, M., Raffeld, M., Franklin, J., Magrath, I., El Bolkainy, N. & Jaffe, E.S. (1995) The investigation of Epstein-Barr viral sequences in 41 cases of Burkitt's lymphoma from Egypt. Epidemiologic correlations. *Cancer*, **76**, 1245–1252

Beral, V., Peterman, T., Berkelman, R. & Jaffe, H. (1991) AIDS-associated non-Hodgkin lymphoma. *Lancet*, **337**, 805–809

Bernstein, L. & Ross, R.K. (1992) Prior medication use and health history as risk factors for non hodgkin's lymphomas: preliminary results from a case-control study in Los Angeles county. *Cancer Res.*, **52**, 5510s–5515s.

Biggar, R.J. & Nkrumah, F.K. (1979) Burkitt's lymphoma in Ghana: urban-rural distribution, time-space clustering and seasonality. *Int. J. Cancer*, **23**, 330–336

Biggar, R.J., Nkrumah, F.K., Neequaye, J. & Levine, P.H. (1981) Changes in presenting tumour site of Burkitt's lymphoma in Ghana, West Africa, 1965-1978. *Br. J. Cancer*, **43**, 632–636

Blattner, W.A., Jacobson, R.J. & Schulman, G. (1979) Multiple myeloma in South African Blacks. *Lancet*, **i**, 928

van den Bosch, C., Hills, M., Kazembe, P., Dziweni, C. & Kadzamira, L. (1993a) Time-space clusters of Burkitt's lymphoma in Malawi. *Leukaemia*, **7**, 1875–1878

van den Bosch, C., Griffin, B.E., Kazembe, P., Dziweni, C. & Kadzamira, L. (1993b) Are plant factors a missing link in the evolution of endemic Burkitt's lymphoma? *Br. J. Cancer*, **68**, 1232–1235

van den Bosch, C. & Lloyd G. (2000) Chikungunya fever as a risk factor for endemic Burkitt's lymphoma in Malawi. *Trans. R. Soc. Trop. Med. Hyg.*, **94**, 704–705

Brubaker, G., Geser, A. & Pike, M.C. (1973) Burkitt's lymphoma in the North Mara district of Tanzania 1964-70: Failure to find evidence of time–space clustering in a high risk isolated rural area. *Br. J. Cancer*, **28**, 469–472

Brubaker, G., Levin, A.G., Steel, C.M., Creasey, G., Cameron, H.M., Linsell, C.A. & Smith, P.G. (1980) Multiple cases of Burkitt's lymphoma and other neoplasms in families in the North Mara District of Tanzania. *Int. J. Cancer*, **26**, 165–170

Burkitt, D.P. (1958) A sarcoma involving the jaws in African children. *Br. J. Surg.*, **46**, 218–223

Burkitt, D.P. (1969) Etiology of Burkitt's lymphoma—an alternative hypothesis to a vectored virus. *J. Natl Cancer Inst.*, **42**, 19–28

Burkitt, D.P. (1970) General features and facial tumours. In: Burkitt, D.P. & Wright, D.H., eds, *Burkitt's Lymphoma*, Edinburgh, E. & S. Livingstone, pp. 6–15

Burkitt, D.P. & O'Conor, G.T. (1961) Malignant lymphoma in African children. I. A clinical syndrome. *Cancer*, **14**, 258–269

Burkitt, D.P. & Wright, D.H. (1966) Geographical and tribal distribution of the African lymphomas in Uganda. *Br. Med. J.*, **i**, 569–573

Cantor, K.P. & Fraumeni, J.F., Jr (1980) Distribution of non-Hodgkin's lymphoma in the United States between 1950 and 1975. *Cancer Res.*, **40**, 2645–2652

Cartwright, R.A. & McNally, R.J. (1994) Epidemiology of non-Hodgkin lymphoma. In: Armittage, J., Burnett, A., Newland, A. & Keating, A., eds, *Haematological Oncology, Vol. 3*, Cambridge, Cambridge University Press, pp. 1–34

Centers for Disease Control (1985) Revision of the case definition of acquired immunodeficiency syndrome for national reporting. *MMWR*, **34**, 373–375

Cohen, C. & Hamilton, D.G. (1980) Epidemiologic and histologic patterns of Hodgkin's disease: comparison of the black and white populations of Johannesburg, South Africa. *Cancer*, **46**, 186–189

Cool, C.D. & Bitter, M.A. (1997) The malignant lymphomas of Kenya: morphology, immunophenotype, and frequency of Epstein-Barr virus in 73 cases. *Hum. Pathol.*, **28**, 1026–1033

Correa, P. & O'Conor, G.T. (1971) Epidemiologic patterns of Hodgkin's disease. *Int. J. Cancer*, **8**, 192–201

Cozen, W., Katz, J. & Mack, T.M. (1992) Risk patterns of Hodgkin's disease in Los Angeles vary by cell type. *Cancer Epidemiol. Biomarkers Prev.*, **1**, 261–268

Dalldorf, G. (1962) Lymphomas of African children with different forms or environmental influences. *J. Am. Med. Assoc.*, **181**, 1026–1028

Dalldorf, G., Linsell, C.A., Barnhart, F.E. & Martyn, R. (1964) An epidemiological approach to the lymphomas of African children and Burkitt's sarcoma of the jaws. *Perspect. Biol. Med.*, **7**, 435–449

Delaporte, E., Peeters, M., Durand, J.P., Dupont, A., Schrijvers, D., Bedjabaga, L., Honoré, C., Ossari, S., Trebucq, A., Josse, R. & Merlin, M. (1989) Seroepidemiological survey of HTLV-I infection among randomized populations of western central African countries. *J. Acq. Immune Defic. Syndr.*, **2**, 410–413

Edington, G.M., Osunkoya, B.O. & Hendrickse, M. (1973) Histologic classification of Hodgkin's disease in the Western State of Nigeria. *J. Natl Cancer Inst.*, **50**, 1633–1637

El Bolkainy, M.N., Gad-El-Mawla, N., Tawfik, H.N. & Aboul-Enein, M.I. (1984) Epidemiology of lymphoma and leukaemia in Egypt. In: Magrath, I., O'Conor, GT. & Ramot, B., eds, *Pathogenesis of Leukemias and Lymphomas: Environmental Influences* (Progress in Cancer Research and Therapy, vol. 27), New York, Raven Press, pp. 9–16

Faggiano, F., Partanen, T., Kogevinas, M. & Boffetta, P. (1997) Socioeconomic differences in cancer incidence and mortality. In: Kogevinas, M., Pearce, N., Susser, M. & Boffetta, P., eds, *Social Inequalities and Cancer* (IARC Scientific Publications No. 138), Lyon, IARC, pp. 65–176

Fleming, A.F. (1985) The epidemiology of lymphomas and leukaemias in Africa—an overview. *Leuk. Res.*, **9**, 735–740

Fouchard, N., Mahe, A., Huerre, M., Fraitag, S., Valensi, F., Macintyre, E., Sanou, F., de The, G. & Gessain, A. (1998) Cutaneous T cell lymphomas: mycosis fungoides, Sezary syndrome and HTLV-I-associated adult T cell leukemia (ATL) in Mali, West Africa: a clinical, pathological and immunovirological study of 14 cases and a review of the African ATL cases. *Leukemia*, **12**, 578-585

Geser, A., de Thé, G., Lenoir, G., Day, N.E. & Williams, E.H. (1982) Final case reporting from the Ugandan prospective study of the relationship between EBV and Burkitt's lymphoma. *Int. J. Cancer*, **29**, 397–400

Geser, A., Brubaker, G. & Draper, C.C. (1989) Effect of a malaria suppression program on the incidence of African Burkitt's lymphoma. *Am. J. Epidemiol.*, **129**, 740–752

Gilles, H.M.J. (1963) Akeefe. *An Environmental Study of a Nigerian Village Community, Ibadan*, Ibadan University Press

Glaser, S.L. (1990) Hodgkin's disease in black populations: a review of the epidemiologic literature. *Semin. Oncol.*, **17**, 643–659

Glaser, S.L., Lin, R.J., Stewart, S.L., Ambinder, R.F., Jarrett, R.F., Brousset, P., Pallesen, G., Gulley, M.L., Khan, G., O'Grady, J., Hummel, M., Preciado, M.V., Knecht, H., Chan, J.K. & Claviez, A.. (1997) Epstein-Barr virus-associated Hodgkin's disease: epidemiologic characteristics in international data. *Int. J. Cancer*, **70**, 375–382

Haddow, A.J. (1963) An improved map for the study of Burkitt's lymphoma syndrome in Africa. *E. Afr. Med. J.*, **40**, 429–432

Hamilton-Dutoit, S.J., Raphael, M., Audouin, J., Diebold, J., Lisse, I., Pedersen, C., Oksenhendler, E., Marelle, L., Pallesen, G. (1993a) In situ demonstration of Epstein-Barr virus small RNAs (EBER 1) in acquired immunodeficiency syndrome-related lymphomas: Correlation with tumor morphology and primary site. *Blood*, **82**, 619–624

Harris, N.L., Jaffe, E.S., Stein, H., Banks, P.M., Chan, J.K., Cleary, M.L., Delsol, G., De Wolf-Peeters, C., Falini, B. & Gatter, K.C. (1994) A revised European-American classification of lymphoid neoplasms: a proposal from the International Lymphoma Study Group. *Blood*, **84**, 1361–1392

Hartge, P., Devesa, S.S., Fraumeni, J.F., Jr (1994) Hodgkin's and non-Hodgkin's lymphomas. *Cancer Surv.*, **19–20**, 423–453

Henle, G. & Henle, W. (1966) Immunofluorescence in cells derived from Burkitt's lymphoma. *J. Bacteriol.*, **91**, 1248–1256

Henle G & Henle W. (1967) Antibodies to Epstein Barr virus in Burkitt's lymphoma and in control groups. *J. Natl Cancer Inst.*, **43**, 1147–1157

Henle, G,. Henle, W., Clifford, P., Diehl, V., Kafuko, G.W., Kirya, B.G., Klein, G., Morrow, R.H., Munube, G.M.R., Pike, P., Tukei, P.M. & Ziegler, J.L. (1969) Antibodies to Epstein-Barr virus in Burkitt's lymphoma and control groups. *J. Natl Cancer Inst.*, **43**, 1147–1157

Henle, G., Henle, W., Klein, G., Gunven, P., Clifford, P., Morrow, R.H. & Ziegler, J.L. (1971) Antibodies to early Epstein-Barr virus-induced antigens in Burkitt's lymphoma. *J. Natl. Cancer Inst.*, **46**, 861–871

Hesseling, P.B., Wessels, G., Van Jaarsveld, D. & Van Riet, F.A. (1997) Hodgkin's disease in children in southern Africa: epidemiological characteristics, morbidity and long-term outcome. *Ann. Trop. Paediatr.*, **17**, 367–373

Hirshaut, Y., Cohen, M.H. & Stevens, D.A. (1973) Epstein-Barr-virus antibodies in American and African Burkitt's lymphoma. *Lancet*, **ii**, 114–116

Hunsmann, G., Bayer, H., Schneider, J., Schmitz, H., Kern, P., Dietrich, M., Buttner, D.W., Goudeau, A.M., Kulkarni, G. & Fleming, A.F. (1984) Antibodies to ATLV/HTLV-I in Africa. *Med. Microbiol. Immunol.*, **173**, 167–170

IARC (1996) *IARC Monographs on the Evaluation of Carcinogenic Risks to Humans.* Vol. 67, *Human Immunodeficiency Viruses and Human T-cell Lymphotropic Viruses*, Lyon, IARC

IARC (1997) *IARC Monographs on the Evaluation of Carcinogenic Risks to Humans.* Vol. 70, *Epstein-Barr Virus and Kaposi's Sarcoma Herpesvirus/Human Herpesvirus 8*, Lyon, IARC

Jacobs, P. (1985) Immunophenotypic classification. *Leuk. Res.*, **9**, 755

Jaffe, E.S., Harris, N.L., Stein, H. & Vardiman, J.W., eds (2001) *WHO Classification of Tumours. Pathology and Genetics of Tumours of the Haematopoietic and Lymphoid Tissues*, Lyon, IARC Press

Jones, E.H., Biggar, R.J., Nkrumah, F.K. & Lawler, S.D. (1985) HLA-DR7 association and African Burkitt's lymphoma. *Hum. Immunol.*, **13**, 211–217

Kafuko, G.W. & Burkitt, D.P. (1970) Burkitt's lymphoma and malaria. *Int. J. Cancer*, **6**, 1–9

Kitinya, J.N. & Lauren, P.A. (1982) Burkitt's lymphoma on Mount Kilimanjaro and in the inland regions of northern Tanzania. *E. Afr. Med. J.*, **59**, 256–260

Klein, E., Klein, G., Nadkarni, J.S., Nadkarni, J.J., Wigzell, H.R. & Clifford, P. (1967) Surface IgM specificity on cells derived from a Burkitt's lymphoma. *Lancet*, **ii**, 1068–1070

Klein, G., Geering, G., Old, L.J., Henle, G., Henle, W. & Clifford, P. (1970) Comparison of the anti-EBV titer and the EBV-associated membrane reactive and precipitating antibody levels in the sera of Burkitt lymphoma and nasopharyngeal carcinoma patients and controls. *Int. J. Cancer*, **5**, 185–194

Knowles, D.M. (1996) Etiology and pathogenesis of AIDS-related non--Hodgkin's lymphoma. *Hematol. Oncol. Clin. North Am.*, **10**, 1081–1109

Kusuda, M., Toriyama, K., Kamidigo, N.O. & Itakura, H. (1998) A comparison of epidemiologic, histologic, and virologic studies on Hodgkin's disease in western Kenya and Nagasaki, Japan. *Am. J. Trop. Med. Hyg.*, **59**, 801–807

La Vecchia, C., Negri, E. & Franceschi, S. (1992) Education and cancer risk. *Cancer*, **70**, 2935–2941

Ladjadj, Y., Philip, T., Lenoir, G.M., Tazerout, F.Z., Bendisari, K., Boukheloua, R., Biron, P., Brunat-Mentigny, M. & Aboulola, M. (1984) Abdominal Burkitt type lymphoma in Algeria. *Br. J. Cancer*, **48**, 503–512

Lazzi, S., Ferrari, F., Nyongo, A., Palummo, N., de Milito, A., Zazzi, M., Leoncini, L., Luzi, P. & Tosi, P. (1998) HIV-associated malignant lymphomas in Kenya (Equatorial Africa). *Hum. Pathol.*, **29**, 1285–1289

Leoncini, L., Spina, D., Nyong'o, A., Abinya, O., Minacci, C., Disanto, A., De Luca, F., De Vivo, A., Sabattini, E., Poggi, S., Pileri, S. & Tosi, P. (1996) Neoplastic cells of Hodgkin's disease show differences in EBV expression between Kenya and Italy. *Int. J. Cancer*, **65**, 781–784

Levy, L.M. (1988) Hodgkin's disease in black Zimbabweans. A study of epidemiologic, histologic, and clinical features. *Cancer*, **61**, 189–194

Magrath, I. (1990) Pathogenesis of Burkitt's lymphoma. In: van der Woude, G. & Klein, G., eds, *Advances in Cancer Research,* Vol. 55, San Diego, Academic Press, pp. 136–270

Magrath, I.T. (1991) African Burkitt's lymphoma. history, biology, clinical features and treatment. *Am. J. Pediat. Hematol./Oncol.*, **13**, 222–246

Magrath, I.T. & Ziegler, J.L. (1980) Bone marrow involvement in Burkitt's lymphoma and its relationship to acute B-cell leukemia. *Leukemia Res.*, **4**, 33–59.

Modiano, D., Luoni, G., Sirima, B.S., Simpore, J., Verra, F., Konate, A., Rastrelli, E., Olivieri, A., Calissano, C., Paganotti, G.M., D'Urbano, L., Sanou, I., Sawadogo, A., Modiano, G. & Coluzzi, M. (2001) Haemoglobin C protects against clinical Plasmodium falciparum malaria. *Nature*, **414**, 305–308

Morrow, R.H., Jr (1985) Epidemiological evidence for the role of falciparum malaria in the pathogenesis of Burkitt's lymphoma. In: Lenoir, G.M., O'Conor, G.T. & Olweny, C.L.M., eds, *Burkitt's Lymphoma: a Human Cancer Model* (IARC Scientific Publications No. 60), Lyon, IARC, pp. 177–186

Morrow, R.H., Pike, M.C., Smith, P.G., Ziegler, J.L. & Kisuule, A. (1971) Burkitt's lymphoma, a time-space cluster of cases in Biomba county of Uganda. *Br. J. Cancer*, **ii**, 491–492

Morrow, R.H., Kisuule, A. & Mafigiri, J. (1974) Socioeconomic factors in Burkitt's lymphoma. *Cancer Res.*, **34**, 1212

Morrow, R.H., Kisuule, A., Pike, M.C. & Smith, P.G. (1976) Burkitt's lymphoma in the Mengo districts of Uganda: epidemiologic features and their relationship to malaria. *J Natl Cancer Inst.*, **56**, 479–482

Morrow, R.H., Pike, M.C. & Smith, P.G. (1977) Further studies of space-time clustering of Burkitt's lymphoma in Uganda. *Br. J. Cancer*, **35**, 668–673

Mueller, N.E. (1996) Hodgkin's disease. In: Schottenfeld, D. & Fraumeni, J.F., Jr, eds, *Cancer Epidemiology and Prevention*, 2nd Ed., New York, Oxford University Press, pp. 893–919

Mueller, B.U. (1998) Cancers in human immunodeficiency virus-infected children. *J. Cancer Natl Inst. Monogr.*, **23**, 31–35

Mueller, N.E., Evans, A., Harris, N.L., Comstock, G.W., Jellum, E., Magnus, K., Orentreich, N., Polk, B.F. & Vogelman, J. (1989) Hodgkin's disease and Epstein-Barr virus. Altered antibody pattern before diagnosis. *New Engl. J. Med.*, **320**, 689–695

Ngendahayo, P. & Schmauz, R. (1992) The pattern of malignant lymphomas in Rwanda. *Bull. Cancer*, **79**, 1087–1096

Nkrumah, F.K. (1984) Changes in the presentation of Burkitt's lymphoma in Ghana over a 15-year period (1969–82). In: Williams, A.O., O'Conor, G.T., de Thé, G.B. & Johnson, C.A., eds, *Virus-associated Cancers in Africa* (IARC Scientific Publications No. 63), Lyon, IARC, pp. 665–674

Nkrumah, F.K. & Perkins, I.V. (1976) Sickle cell trait, hemoglobin C trait, and Burkitt's lymphoma. *Am. J. Trop. Med. Hyg.*, **25**, 633–636

Nkrumah, F., Henle, W., Henle, G., Herberman, R., Perkins, V. & Depue, R. (1976) Burkitt's lymphoma: its clinical course in relation to immunologic reactivities to Epstein-Barr virus and tumor-related antigens. *J. Natl Cancer Inst.*, **57**, 1051–1056

O'Conor, G. (1961) Malignant lymphoma in African children. Cancer. II. A pathological entity. *Cancer*, **14**, 270–283

O'Conor, G.T. (1970) Persistent immunologic stimulation as a factor in oncogenesis with special reference to Burkitt's tumour. *Ann.J. Med.*, **48**, 279–285

O'Conor, G.T. & Davies, J.N.P. (1960) Malignant tumors in African children with special reference to malignant lymphomas. *J. Pediatr.*, **56**, 526–535

O'Conor, G.T., Rappaport, H. & Smith, E.B. (1965) Childhood lymphoma resembling "Burkitt tumor" in the United States. *Cancer*, **18**, 411–417

Okpala, I.E., Akang, E.E. & Okpala, U.J. (1991) Lymphomas in University College Hospital, Ibadan, Nigeria. *Cancer*, **68**, 1356–1360

Olurin, O. & Williams, A.O. (1972) Orbito-ocular tumors in Nigeria. *Cancer*, **30**, 580–587

Osato, T., Mizuno, F., Imai, S., Aya, T., Koizumi, S., Kinoshita, T., Tokuda, H., Ito, Y., Hirai, N., Hirota, M., Ohigashi, H., Koshimizu, K., Kofi-Tsekpo, W.M., Were, J.B.O. & Mugambi, M. (1987) African Burkitt's lymphoma and an Epstein-Barr virus-enhancing plant Eurphorbia tirucalli (Letter to the Editor). *Lancet*, **i**, 1257–1258

Osato, T., Imai, S., Kinoshita, T., Aya, T., Sugiura, M., Koizumi, S. & Mizuno, F. (1990) Epstein Barr virus, Burkitt's lymphoma, and an African tumor promoter. *Adv. Exp. Med. Biol.*, **278**, 147–150

Pagano, J.S. (1992) Epstein-Barr virus: culprit or consort? *New Engl. J. Med.*, **327**, 1750–1751

Parkin, D.M., Sohier, R. & O'Conor, G.T. (1985) Geographic distribution of Burkitt's lymphoma. In: Lenoir, G.M., O'Conor, G.T. & Olweny, C.L.M., eds, *Burkitt's Lymphoma: a Human Cancer Model* (IARC Scientific Publications No. 60), Lyon, IARC, pp. 155–164

Pike, M.C., Williams, E.H. & Wright, B. (1967) Burkitt's tumor in the West Nile District of Uganda, 1961-63. *Br. Med. J.*, **ii**, 395–399

Pike, M.C., Morrow, R.H., Kisuule, A. & Mafigiri, J. (1970) Burkitt's lymphoma and sickle cell trait. *Br. J. Prev. Soc. Med.*, **24**, 39–41

Rappaport, H., Ramot, B., Hulu, N. & Park, J.K. (1972) The pathology of so-called Mediterranean abdominal lymphoma with malabsorption. *Cancer*, **29**, 1502–1511

Remick, S.C. (1995) Acquired immunodeficiency syndrome-related non-Hodgkin's lymphoma. *Cancer Control*, **2**, 97–103

Roithmann, S. & Andrieu, J.-M. (1992) Clinical and biological characteristics of malignant lymphomas in HIV-infected patients. *Eur. J. Cancer*, **28A**, 1501–1508

Saxinger, W., Blattner, A.W., Levine, P.H., Clark, J., Biggar, R., Hoh, M., Moghissi, J., Jacobs, P., Wilson, L., Jacobson, R., Crookes, R., Strong, M., Ansarii, A.A., Dean, A.G., Nkrumah, F.K., Mourali, N. & Gallo, R.C. (1984) Human T-cell leukaemia virus (HTLV-I) antibodies in Africa. *Science*, **225**, 1473–1476

Schmauz, R., Mugerwa, J.W. & Wright, D.H. (1990) The distribution of non-Burkitt, non-Hodgkin's lymphomas in Uganda in relation to malarial endemicity. *Int. J. Cancer*, **45**, 650–653

Siemiatycki, J., Brubaker, G. & Geser, A. (1980) Space-time clustering of Burkitt's lymphoma in East Africa: analysis of recent data and a new look at old data. *Int. J. Cancer*, **25**, 197–203

Silvestri, F., Sperotto, A. & Fanin, R. (2000) Hepatitis C and lymphoma. *Curr. Oncol. Rep.*, **2**, 172–175

Standaert, B., Kocheleff, P., Kadende, P., Nitunga, N., Guerna, T., Laroche, R. & Piot, P. (1988) Acquired immunodeficiency syndrome and human immunodeficiency virus infection in Bujumbura, Burundi. *Trans. R. Soc. Trop. Med. Hyg.*, **82**, 902–904

de-The, G., Geser, A., Day, N.E., Tukei, P.M., Williams, E.H., Beri, D.P., Smith, P.G., Dean, A.G., Bornkamm, G.W., Feorino, P. & Henle, W. (1978) Epidemiological evidence for a causal relationship between Epstein-Barr virus and Burkitt's lymphoma: results of the Ugandan prospective study. *Nature*, **274**, 756–761

Thomas, J.O., Rafindadi, A., Heyret, A., Jones, M., Gatter, K.C. & Mason, D.Y. (1991) Immunophenotyping of Nigerian cases of non Hodgkin's lymphomas on paraffin sections. *Histopathology*, **18**, 505–510

Vianna, N.J., Thind, I.S., Louria, D.B., Polan, A., Kirmss, V. & Davies, J.N. (1977) Epidemiologic and histologic patterns of Hodgkin's disease in blacks. *Cancer*, **40**, 3133–3139

Wabinga, H.R., Parkin, D.M., Wabwire-Mangen, F. & Nambooze, S. (2000) Trends in cancer incidence in Kyadondo County, Uganda, 1960-1997. *Br. J. Cancer*, **82**, 1585–1592

Weinreb, M., Day, P.J., Niggli, F., Powell, J.E., Raafat, F., Hesseling, P.B., Schneider, J.W., Hartley, P.S., Tzortzatou-Stathopoulou, F., Khalek, E.R.A., Mangoud, A., El-Safy, U.R., Madanat, F., Al Sheyyab, M., Mpofu, C., Revesz, T., Rafii, R., Tiedemann, K., Waters, K.D., Barrantes, J.C., Nyongo, A., Riyat, M.S. & Mann, J.R. (1996) The role of Epstein-Barr virus in Hodgkin's disease from different geographical areas. *Arch. Dis. Child.*, **74**, 27–31

Williams, A.O. (1966) Haemoglobin genotypes, ABO blood groups and Burkitt's tumour. *J. Med. Genet.*, **3**, 177–179

Williams, E.H. (1968) Variations in tumour distribution in the West Nile district of Uganda. In: Clifford, P., Linsell, C.A. & Timms, G.L., eds, *Cancer in Africa*, Nairobi, East African Publishing House, pp. 37–42

Williams, A.O. (1975) Tumours of children in Ibadan, Nigeria. *Cancer*, **36**, 370–378

Williams, C.K. (1988) Clustering of Burkitt's lymphoma and other high-grade malignant lymphoproliferative diseases, but not acute lymphoblastic leukaemia among socio-economically deprived Nigerians. *E. Afr. Med. J.*, **65**, 253–263

Williams, E.H., Day, N.E. & Geser, A. (1974) Seasonal variation in onset of Burkitt's lymphoma in the West Nile District of Uganda. *Lancet*, **ii**, 19–22

Williams, E.H., Smith, P.G., Day, N.E., Geser, A., Ellice, J. & Tukei, P. (1978) Space-time clustering of Burkitt's lymphoma in West Nile district of Uganda: 1961-1975. *Br. J. Cancer*, **37**, 805–809

Williams, C.K., Alexander, S.S., Bodner, A., Levine, A., Saxinger, C., Gallo, R.C. & Blattner, W.A. (1993) Frequency of adult T-cell leukaemia/lymphoma and HTLV-I in Ibadan, Nigeria. *Br. J. Cancer*, **67**, 783–786

Wood, R.E., Nortje, C.J., Hesseling, P. & Mouton, S. (1988) Involvement of maxillofacial region in African Burkitt's lymphoma in the Cape Province and Namibia. *Dentomaxillofac. Radiol.*, **17**, 57–60

Wright, D.H. (1967) The epidemiology of Burkitt's tumour. *Cancer Res.*, **27**, 2424–2438

Wright, D.H. (1973) Lympho-reticular neoplasms. *Recent Results Cancer Res.*, **41**, 270–291

Wright D.H. & Roberts, M. (1966) The geographical distribution of Burkitt's tumour compared with the geographical distribution of other types of malignant lymphoma in Uganda. *Br. J. Cancer*, **20**, 469–474

Ziegler, J.L., Bluming, A.I., Morrow, R.H., Fass, L. & Carbone, P.O. (1970) Central nervous system involvement in Burkitt's lymphoma. *Blood*, **36**, 718–728

zur Hausen, H. & Schulte-Holthausen, H. (1970) Presence of EB virus nucleic acid homology in a 'virus-free' line of Burkitt tumour cells. *Nature*, **227**, 245–248

4.11 Malignant melanoma of skin

Introduction

Malignant melanoma is a tumour of melanocytes, which are pigment-producing cells of the epidermis. There are similar densities of melanocytes in different races, and differences in skin colour reflect differences in melanocyte activity in transferring melanin granules organized into melanosomes to surrounding keratinocytes (Crombie, 1979).

Descriptive epidemiology in Africa

Malignant melanoma of skin accounts for about 1.3% of new cancer cases in Africa. The incidence is much higher in white populations of European origin than in black populations of African descent. In the United States, the incidence rate in white males is 15 times that of black males. Reports from both population-based and histology-based cancer registries in southern Africa where populations of European origin have lived for more than three generations show significant differences in the incidence of melanoma between blacks and whites (Sitas & Pacella, 1994; Bassett *et al.*, 1995).

There are also clear ethnic differences in the site distribution of melanomas. In Africans, 60% or more are reported to occur on the sole of the foot (Figure 1), compared with 6–12% in whites (Oettlé, 1966; Lewis, 1967; Giraud *et al.*, 1975; Isaacson 1978) and a similar distribution is observed in blacks and whites in the United States (Feibleman & Maize 1981). However, the difference in the actual *incidence* of plantar melanoma between black and white populations is small (Feibleman & Maize, 1981; Stevens *et al.*, 1990).

Examination of recent data from Africa confirms the low incidence rates in most populations. In southern Africa, there is an approximately 15-fold difference in incidence between black and

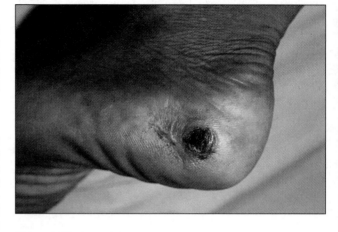

Figure 1. Plantar melanoma

white populations of South Africa and Zimbabwe (although the difference is much smaller for females in Zimbabwe, because of the relatively high incidence rate in black females (Table 1).

Table 2 shows incidence data from time periods in the 1960s and 1970s.

In white populations, the incidence of malignant melanoma increases rapidly with age, so that it is already a relatively common cancer by the age of 20–29 years. The incidence is higher in young females (under age 45 years) and in older males (Figure 2) In contrast, the increase with age is more gradual in blacks in the

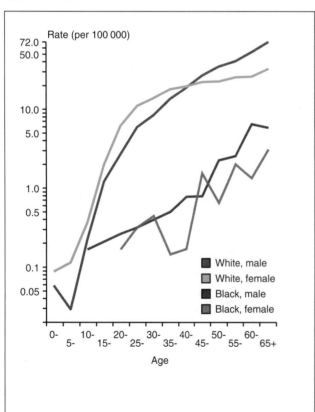

Figure 2. Age-specific incidence of melanoma of skin. USA, SEER, 1993–97

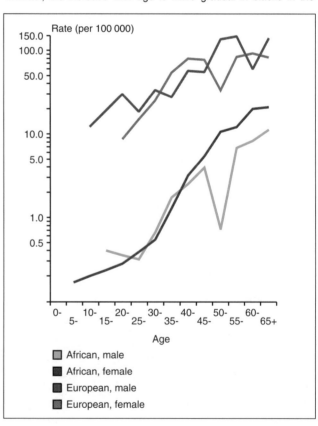

Figure 3. Age-specific incidence of melanoma of skin. Harare, Zimbabwe, 1990–97

Table 1. Age-standardized (world) and cumulative (0-64) incidence
Melanoma of skin (C43)

	MALE				FEMALE			
	Cases	CRUDE (per 100,000)	ASR(W) (per 100,000)	Cumulative (%)	Cases	CRUDE (per 100,000)	ASR(W) (per 100,000)	Cumulative (%)
Africa, North								
Algeria, Algiers (1993-1997)	22	0.4	**0.6**	0.03	19	0.3	**0.4**	0.03
Algeria, Constantine (1994-1997)	3	0.2	**0.3**	0.02	3	0.2	**0.4**	0.02
Algeria, Oran (1996-1998)	9	0.5	**0.6**	0.05	15	0.9	**1.2**	0.08
Algeria, Setif (1993-1997)	-	-	**-**	-	1	0.0	**0.1**	-
Tunisia, Centre, Sousse (1993-1997)	4	0.3	**0.5**	0.03	9	0.8	**1.0**	0.03
Tunisia, North, Tunis (1994)	8	0.4	**0.5**	0.02	12	0.6	**0.7**	0.04
Tunisia, Sfax (1997)	2	0.5	**0.6**	0.02	1	0.3	**0.2**	0.01
Africa, West								
The Gambia (1997-1998)	2	0.2	**0.3**	0.02	1	0.1	**0.1**	0.01
Guinea, Conakry (1996-1999)	18	0.8	**1.6**	0.16	14	0.6	**1.5**	0.09
Mali, Bamako (1988-1997)	9	0.2	**0.4**	0.04	16	0.4	**1.2**	0.12
Niger, Niamey (1993-1999)	3	0.2	**0.7**	0.01	4	0.2	**0.8**	0.09
Nigeria, Ibadan (1998-1999)	5	0.3	**0.7**	0.03	4	0.3	**0.4**	0.04
Africa, Central								
Congo, Brazzaville (1996-1999)	8	0.7	**1.1**	0.09	9	0.7	**1.1**	0.04
Africa, East								
France, La Reunion (1988-1994)	28	1.3	**1.6**	0.13	40	1.8	**1.8**	0.12
Kenya, Eldoret (1998-2000)	2	0.2	**0.4**	0.00	14	1.5	**3.2**	0.18
Malawi, Blantyre (2000-2001)	3	0.3	**0.6**	0.05	4	0.5	**1.4**	0.13
Uganda, Kyadondo County (1993-1997)	11	0.4	**1.3**	0.06	13	0.4	**2.0**	0.12
Zimbabwe, Harare: African (1990-1993)	18	0.8	**1.7**	0.10	17	0.8	**3.5**	0.22
Zimbabwe, Harare: African (1994-1997)	24	0.9	**2.0**	0.12	34	1.3	**4.4**	0.31
Zimbabwe, Harare: European (1990-1997)	91	59.5	**40.5**	2.91	78	46.2	**30.2**	2.34
Africa, South								
Namibia (1995-1998)	65	2.0	**3.5**	0.24	53	1.7	**2.4**	0.17
South Africa: Black (1989-1992)	349	0.6	**1.2**	0.07	475	0.8	**1.4**	0.08
South Africa: Indian (1989-1992)	13	0.7	**0.7**	0.07	13	0.7	**0.9**	0.06
South Africa: Mixed race (1989-1992)	27	0.4	**0.8**	0.05	45	0.7	**1.1**	0.07
South Africa: White (1989-1992)	1718	17.1	**15.3**	1.05	1762	17.3	**14.2**	0.99
South Africa, Transkei, Umtata (1996-1998)	-	-	**-**	-	-	-	**-**	-
South Africa, Transkei, 4 districts (1996-1998)	3	0.4	**0.9**	0.08	1	0.1	**0.2**	0.02
Swaziland (1996-1999)	6	0.3	**0.6**	0.04	10	0.5	**0.9**	0.07
Europe/USA								
USA, SEER: White (1993-1997)	9558	19.6	**15.5**	1.05	7772	15.5	**11.6**	0.85
USA, SEER: Black (1993-1997)	59	0.9	**1.0**	0.07	45	0.6	**0.6**	0.03
France, 8 registries (1993-1997)	1157	8.4	**6.5**	0.43	1543	10.7	**7.9**	0.58
The Netherlands (1993-1997)	3985	10.4	**8.0**	0.58	5710	14.6	**10.9**	0.82
UK, England (1993-1997)	9624	8.0	**5.8**	0.40	13791	10.8	**7.5**	0.54

In italics: histopathology-based registries

Table 2. Incidence of malignant melanoma of skin in Africa, 1953–74

Registry	Period	ASR (per 100 000)		Source
		Male	Female	(see Chap. 1)
Senegal, Dakar	1969–74	1.2	1.3	4
Mozambique, Lourenço Marques	1956–60	–	–	1
Nigeria, Ibadan	1960–69	0.9	2.2	3
SA, Cape Province: Bantu	1956–59	*0.7*	*3.3*	2
SA, Cape Province: Coloured	1956–59	0.2	*1.0*	2
SA, Cape Province: White	1956–59	3.1	5.2	2
SA, Johannesburg, Bantu	1953–55	*1.2*	*2.0*	1
SA, Natal Province: African	1964–66	*0.8*	*2.4*	2
SA, Natal Province: Indian	1964–66	*0.9*	*0.0*	2
Uganda, Kyadondo	1954–60	*1.4*	*0.0*	1
Uganda, Kyadondo	1960–71	*0.6*	2.2	5
Zimbabwe, Bulawayo	1963–72	*0.1*	*0.3*	6

Italics: Rate based on less than 10 cases

United States, and rates remain higher in men at all ages. In Zimbabwe, the pattern is somewhat similar, with the difference between whites and blacks narrowing with age (Figure 3).

In clinical series from hospitals in Johannesburg, South Africa, Rippey and Rippey (1984) noted a much later stage at presentation for black patients (half of the lesions 5 cm or more, compared with 6% in whites) and their poorer survival: a crude three-year survival of 28% in blacks versus 56% in whites.

Etiology
Solar and artificial ultraviolet radiation
Sun exposure accounts for more than 60% of melanomas worldwide, especially in white populations (IARC, 1992; Armstrong & Kricker, 1995). In addition, there is evidence that exposure to artificial sources of ultraviolet (UV) radiation, in particular sunlamps and sun beds, can increase the risk of melanoma (Armstrong et al., 1995). These two sources of exposure to UV irradiation and their relationship with melanoma of skin have been extensively reviewed by the International Agency for Research on Cancer (see IARC, 1992). Intermittent intense exposure to UV radiation from sunlight is associated with increased risk. Although there is a consistent and strong association between melanoma and a history of sunburn, the relationships with occupation and with total or chronic sun exposure are inconsistent (Elwood, 1996; Osterlind, 1992), which is an indication of the complexity of the relationship. Benign pigmented naevi, especially the so-called dysplastic naevi, of pale skin, are an indicator of risk. Their development is associated with sun exposure in childhood, and it seems that exposures early in life are critically important in determining lifetime risk in white populations. Thus, studies of migrants to Australia have shown that arrival in the sunny environment in childhood determines the increase in risk of melanoma later in life (Khlat et al., 1992). Other factors of possible relevance to etiology are hereditary (familial dysplastic naevi syndrome), and hormonal (as shown by associations with fertility in women), as well as diet, alcohol, medications, hair dyes, fluorescent light, petroleum and hydrocarbons (reviewed by Armstrong & Holman, 1987).

The rapid increase in the incidence of melanoma in the last 20–30 years in many Caucasian populations suggests that there has been increasing sun exposure (Coleman et al., 1993; Gallagher et al., 1989). Evidence from analytical studies implicates intermittent recreational sun exposure as responsible for these increases, which are evident in successive birth cohorts in many European countries (Osterlind, 1992). It is also possible that some of the increase is the result of increased awareness and early diagnosis of thin lesions (Armstrong, 1988); however this is not a major factor in the increasing rates (van der Esch et al., 1991). A 43% increase in mortality from melanoma of skin over a period of 10 years (1962–71) has been reported for whites living in South Africa (Rippey & Rippey, 1984). Similar increases in incidence in white populations over the past three decades have also been demonstrated in Queensland, Australia. However, no corresponding increases were observed in black populations living in these geographical areas (see Rippey & Rippey, 1984; Armstrong, 1988).

Melanin pigmentation of the skin protects against UV radiation and presumably accounts for the low risk of melanoma on the sun-exposed parts of the body in black populations. The low risk persists in migrant populations, and, in African migrants to Israel, in their offspring (Parkin & Iscovich, 1997).

Plantar melanoma
Exposure to UV radiation seems unlikely to play a major role in plantar melanoma, and etiological hypotheses have focused on other environmental and constitutional factors.

Pigmented patches and frank naevi (areas of dark pigmentation with clear-cut margins) appear to be relatively frequent in some African populations (Gordon & Henry, 1971). Lewis (1967) noted a correlation between the prevalence of such pigmented spots in different tribes of Uganda and the histological diagnosis rate of melanoma of the foot, and suggested that such ectopic, unstable collections of melanocytes may be important precursors of invasive disease. Some clinical studies have suggested that a relatively high proportion of plantar melanomas may arise from pre-existing naevi (Allen & Spitz, 1953; Lewis, 1967; Clark et al., 1978). A history of naevi preceding the occurrence of malignant melanoma was reported by 7.5% of black patients in the United States (Muelling, 1948), but Feibleman et al. (1980) found no evidence of antecedent naevi in any of a series of retrospectively examined melanoma specimens among 49 cases of plantar melanoma occurring in white patients during a 50-year period.

Trauma has often been suggested as a risk factor, in part because walking barefoot is common in populations in which plantar melanoma appears to be frequent (McDonald, 1959; Oettlé, 1966). A high proportion of melanomas are found in weight-bearing areas of the sole (Camain et al., 1972; Feibleman et al., 1980), and there are numerous clinical reports of the development of melanoma being related to trauma (e.g., arising in burn scars). According to Higginson and Oettlé (1960), the incidence decreased with urbanization (and habitual shoe-wearing) in South Africa, but others found no difference between urban and rural residents (Giraud et al., 1975; Isaacson et al., 1978). In a study of 150 rickshaw boys in Durban, whose bare feet were habitually exposed to the grossest degree of trauma, no evidence of "traumatic melanoma" was found (Bentley-Phillips & Bayles, 1972). The sole of the foot remains the most common site of melanoma for shoe-wearers in Africa and in the United States, with virtually no sex differences in incidence (Lewis, 1967; McGovern,1977).

References
Allen, A.C. & Spitz, S. (1953) Malignant melanoma: a clinicopathological analysis of the criteria for diagnosis and prognosis. Cancer, **6**, 1–45

Armstrong, B.K. (1988) Epidemiology of malignant melanoma: intermittent or total accumulated exposure to the sun? J. Dermatol. Surg. Oncol., **14**, 835–849

Armstrong, B.K. & Holman, C.D.J. (1987) Malignant melanoma of the skin. Bull. World Health Org., **65**, 245–252

Armstrong, B.K. & Kricker, A. (1995) Skin cancer. Dermatol. Clin., **13**, 583–594

Bassett, M.T., Chokunonga, E., Mauchaza, B., Levy, L., Ferlay, J. & Parkin, D.M. (1995) Cancer in the African population of Harare, Zimbabwe, 1990-1992. Int. J. Cancer, **63**, 29–36

Bentley-Phillips, B. & Bayles, M.A. (1972) Melanoma and trauma. A clinical study of Zulu feet under conditions of persistent and gross trauma. S. Afr. Med. J., 46, 535–538

Camain, R., Tuyns, A.J., Sarrat, H., Quenum, C. & Faye, I. (1972) Cutaneous cancer in Dakar. J. Natl Cancer Inst., **48**, 33–49

Clark, W., Reimer, R., Green, M., Ainsworth, A.M. & Mastrangelo, M.J. (1978) Origin of familial malignant melanomas from heritable melanocytic lesions: the B-K mole syndrome. Arch. Dermatol., **114**, 732–738

Crombie, I.K. (1979) Racial differences in melanoma incidence .Br. J. Cancer, **40**, 185–193

Elwood, J.M. (1996) Melanoma and sun exposure. Semin. Oncol., **23**, 650–666

van der Esch, E.P., Muir, C.S., Nectoux, J., Macfarlane, G., Maisonneuve, P., Bharucha, H., Briggs, J., Cooke, R.A., Dempster, A.G., Essex, W.B., Hofer, P.A., Hood, A.F., Ironside, P., Larsen, T.E., Little, J.H., Philipps, R., Pfau, R.S., Prade, M., Pozharisski, K.M., Rilke, F. & Schafler, K. (1991) Temporal change in diagnostic criteria as a cause of the increase of malignant melanoma over time is unlikely. Int. J. Cancer, **47**, 483–489

Feibleman, C.A., Stoll, H. & Maize, J.C. (1980) Melanomas of the palm, sole and nailbed: a clinicopathology study. Cancer, **46**, 2492–2504

Feibleman, C.E. & Maize, J.C. (1981) Racial differences in cutaneous melanoma incidence and distribution. In: Ackerman, A.B., ed., *Pathology of Malignant Melanoma*, New York, Masson, pp. 47–55

Giraud, R.M.A., Rippey, E. & Rippey, J.J. (1975) Malignant melanoma of the skin in black Africans. *S. Afr. Med. J.*, **49**, 665–668

Gordon, J.A. & Henry, S.A. (1971) Pigmentation of the sole of the foot in Rhodesian Africans. *S. Afr. Med. J.*, **45**, 88–91

Higginson, J. & Oettlé, A.G. (1960) Cancer incidence in the Bantu and "Cape Coloured" races of South Africa: report of a cancer survey in the Transvaal (1953–55). *J. Natl Cancer Inst.*, **24**, 589–653

IARC (1992) *IARC Monographs on the Evaluation of Carcinogenic Risks to Humans,* Vol. 55, *Solar and Ultraviolet Radiation*, Lyon, IARC

Isaacson, C., Selzer, G., Kaye, V., Greenberg, M., Woodruff, J.D., Davies, J., Ninin, D., Vetten, D. & Andrew, M. (1978) Cancer in the urban blacks of South Africa. *S. Afr. Cancer Bull.*, **22**, 49–84

Khlat, M., Vail, A., Parkin, D.M. & Green, A. (1992) Mortality from melanoma in migrants to Australia: variation by age at arrival and duration of stay. *Int. J. Cancer*, **135**, 1103–1113

Lewis, M.G. (1967) Malignant melanoma in Uganda (The relationship between pigmentation and malignant melanoma on the soles of the feet). *Br. J. Cancer*, **XXI**, 483–495

MacDonald, E.J. (1959) Malignant melanoma among Negroes and Latin Americans in Texas. In: Gordon, M., ed., *Pigment Cell Biology*, New York, Academic Press, pp. 171–181

McGovern, V.J. (1977) Epidemiological aspects of melanoma: a review. *Pathology*, **9**, 231–241

Muelling, R. (1948) Malignant melanoma: a comparative study of the incidence in Negro race. *Milit. Surg.*, **103**, 359–364

Oettlé, A.G. (1966) Epidemiology of melanomas in South Africa. In: Della Porto, G & Mulboch, O., eds, *Structure and Control of the Melanocyte*, Berlin, Springer-Verlag, pp. 292–308

Osterlind, A. (1992) Epidemiology of malignant melanoma in Europe. *Acta Oncol.*, **31**, 903–908

Parkin, D.M., Vizcaino, A.P., Skinner, M.E.G. & Ndhlovu, A. (1994) Cancer patterns and risk factors in the African population of southwestern Zimbabwe, 1963–1977. *Cancer Epidemiol. Biomarkers Prev.*, **3**, 537–547

Parkin, D.M. & Iscovich, J. (1997) Risk of cancer in migrants and their descendants in Israel: II Carcinomas and germ cell tumours. *Int. J. Cancer*, **70**, 654–660

Rippey, J.J. & Rippey, E. (1984) Epidemiology of malignant melanoma of the skin in South Africa. *S. Afr. Med. J.*, **65**, 595–598

Sitas, F. & Pacella, R. (1994) *Histologically Diagnosed Cancer in South Africa 1989*, Johannesburg, SAIMR

Stevens, N.G., Liff, J.M. & Weiss, N.S. (1990) Plantar melanoma: is the incidence of melanoma of the sole of the foot really higher in blacks than whites? *Int. J. Cancer*, **45**, 691–693

Wabinga, H.R., Parkin, D.M., Wabwire-Mangen, F. & Nambooze, S. (2000) Trends in cancer incidence in Kyadondo County, Uganda, 1960–1997. *Br. J. Cancer*, **82**, 1585–1592

4.12 Nasopharyngeal carcinoma

Introduction

Nasopharyngeal carcinoma (NPC) has been recognized for many years, and traces of the disease can be found in Egyptian mummies dating from 5000 years ago (Smith *et al.*, 1924). NPC is an epithelial neoplasm arising in the squamous epithelium overlying the nasopharyngeal lymphoid tissue. Most of the tumours are undifferentiated or poorly differentiated, comprising small cells with heavy lymphoid infiltration.

Nasopharyngeal carcinoma is a rare malignancy in most parts of the world; age-standardized incidence rates for people of either sex are generally less than 1 per 100 000 per year (Parkin *et al.*, 1997), so that NPC comprises only about 0.6% of new cancer cases. However, in several regions, rates are very much higher. The overall incidence is elevated in the southern provinces of China (Guangdong, Guanxi, Hunan and Fujian) (Li *et al.*, 1979) and in Inuit (Eskimo) populations of Alaska and northern Canada (Nielsen *et al.*, 1996). NPC occurs with moderately raised incidence in populations from south-east Asia (Parkin *et al.*, 1997).

Descriptive epidemiology in Africa

In Africa, there are about 5500 new cases of NPC annually (0.9% of new cancers), but almost half of this total is from north Africa, where NPC comprises 2.1% of new cancer cases. Incidence rates in north Africa (Algeria and Tunisia) are in the low to moderate range (3–7.5 per 100 000 in men and 1.5–2.5 per 100 000 in women) (Table 1). Reviews of hospital series indicate that the frequency of nasopharyngeal carcinoma is relatively high in the mainly Arab populations of Tunisia, Morocco, Sudan and Saudi Arabia (Muir, 1971; Cammoun *et al.*, 1974; Hidayatalla *et al.*, 1983; Al-Idrissi, 1990).

Table 2 shows incidence data from time periods in the 1960s and 1970s.

A peak in incidence is observed in adolescents of each sex in a number of populations at low to moderate risk for nasopharyngeal carcinoma, including Tunisia (Ellouz *et al.*, 1978) (Figure 2). As a result, up to a quarter of NPC cases occur before the age of 25 years in these populations. In the United States, a minor peak in the age group 10–19 years is seen in blacks (Burt *et al.*, 1992; Parkin *et al.*, 1997).

Sub-Saharan Africa is a relatively low-risk area for nasopharyngeal carcinoma, and undifferentiated nasopharyngeal carcinoma is also the predominant histopathological type (Cammoun *et al.*, 1974). In general, incidence rates are low (Table 1), with somewhat higher values in Kampala, Uganda, and especially in Eldoret, in western Kenya. The data on frequency of NPC in early case series from Africa were reviewed by Clifford (1970a). The percentage of NPC among different series from Kenya was 2–9%, but there were higher rates (of hospitalization) estimated for the inland, highland areas of the country than on the coast, irrespective of ethnic group (Clifford, 1965, 1967). The highest (crude) incidence recorded was among men of the Nandi tribe (2.8 per 100 000) (Clifford 1965). Varying rates have also been reported within Uganda (Schmauz & Templeton, 1972) and Sudan (Hidayatalla *et al.*, 1983).

Migrant studies

The risk of NPC in Chinese living in the United States is high, and, although the risk in Chinese born in the United States is about half that of migrants born in China, it remains at least ten times higher than in the white population of the United States (Buell, 1974). In Singapore, the different Chinese dialect groups preserve the ratio of risks observed in southern China, with the highest risk in Cantonese

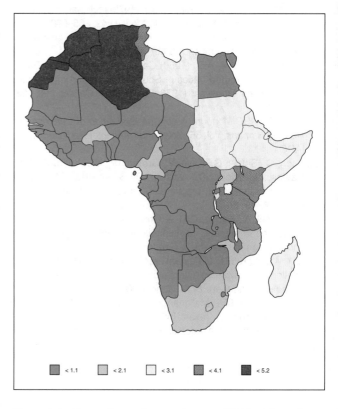

Figure 1. Incidence of nasopharyngeal cancer: ASR (world) - males

(double that in other dialect groups), and little change in incidence between the locally born and migrants from China (Lee *et al.*, 1988). Migrants to France from North African countries (Morocco, Algeria and Tunisia) have higher rates of mortality from NPC than the locally born population, and among such migrants, there is a small peak in age-specific mortality rates at ages 15–24 years (Bouchardy *et al.*, 1996). There also is a significantly higher than expected mortality from NPC among migrants to Australia from Egypt (Khlat *et al.*, 1993). Migrants to Israel from North Africa also have higher risks of NPC than the local population, and furthermore the offspring of such migrants retain their elevated risk relative to individuals with locally born parents (Parkin & Iscovich, 1997).

These findings, as for those of migrants of southern Chinese origin, suggest a strong genetic component to the increased risk in these populations. However, Jeannel *et al.* (1993) found that men of French origin who were born in North Africa also had a significantly higher rate of nasopharyngeal carcinoma than French men born in France.

Etiology

Environmental risk factors

Environmental risk factors for NPC have been extensively studied. The Epstein–Barr virus (EBV) is now generally accepted to be important in carcinogenesis at this site. The initial evidence came from serological studies, showing higher titres of antibodies to various EBV antigens in NPC cases (particularly undifferentiated NPCs) than control subjects. Klein *et al.* (1970) found higher reactivity in three assays of anti-EBV activity in sera of 26 cases of NPC (23 of them Africans) than in control subjects. Patients with advanced nasopharyngeal carcinoma, whether Cantonese Chinese in Hong Kong, Maghrebian Tunisians or Caucasians in France, had higher

Table 1. Age-standardized (world) and cumulative (0-64) incidence
Nasopharynx (C11)

	MALE				FEMALE			
	Cases	CRUDE	ASR(W) (per 100,000)	Cumulative (%)	Cases	CRUDE	ASR(W) (per 100,000)	Cumulative (%)
Africa, North								
Algeria, Algiers (1993-1997)	128	2.3	**2.7**	0.22	61	1.1	**1.2**	0.09
Algeria, Constantine (1994-1997)	51	3.3	**5.3**	0.38	26	1.7	**2.5**	0.22
Algeria, Oran (1996-1998)	103	5.8	**6.6**	0.50	50	2.8	**3.3**	0.28
Algeria, Setif (1993-1997)	134	4.5	**6.3**	0.52	51	1.7	**2.2**	0.17
Tunisia, Centre, Sousse (1993-1997)	46	4.0	**4.9**	0.36	16	1.4	**1.5**	0.12
Tunisia, North, Tunis (1994)	67	3.1	**3.7**	0.34	33	1.6	**1.8**	0.15
Tunisia, Sfax (1997)	12	3.1	**3.7**	0.27	3	0.8	**0.9**	0.05
Africa, West								
The Gambia (1997-1998)	1	0.1	**-**	-	-	-	**-**	-
Guinea, Conakry (1996-1999)	5	0.2	**0.5**	0.05	1	0.0	**0.1**	0.00
Mali, Bamako (1988-1997)	1	0.0	**0.1**	0.01	1	0.0	**0.0**	0.00
Niger, Niamey (1993-1999)	1	0.1	**0.3**	-	-	-	**-**	-
Nigeria, Ibadan (1998-1999)	12	0.8	**1.1**	0.10	6	0.4	**0.6**	0.04
Africa, Central								
Congo, Brazzaville (1996-1999)	3	0.2	**0.4**	0.04	2	0.2	**0.2**	0.01
Africa, East								
France, La Reunion (1988-1994)	11	0.5	**0.6**	0.05	4	0.2	**0.2**	0.01
Kenya, Eldoret (1998-2000)	20	2.1	**3.9**	0.32	13	1.4	**2.9**	0.24
Malawi, Blantyre (2000-2001)	1	0.1	**0.1**	0.01	1	0.1	**0.4**	0.05
Uganda, Kyadondo County (1993-1997)	33	1.2	**1.8**	0.18	30	1.0	**1.4**	0.12
Zimbabwe, Harare: African (1990-1993)	14	0.6	**1.4**	0.04	7	0.3	**0.7**	0.04
Zimbabwe, Harare: African (1994-1997)	12	0.4	**0.6**	0.05	7	0.3	**0.6**	0.04
Zimbabwe, Harare: European (1990-1997)	-	-	**-**	-	2	1.2	**1.2**	0.09
Africa, South								
Namibia (1995-1998)	22	0.7	**1.1**	0.06	14	0.4	**0.5**	0.03
South Africa: Black (1989-1992)	445	0.8	**1.4**	0.10	111	0.2	**0.3**	0.02
South Africa: Indian (1989-1992)	7	0.4	**0.6**	0.02	6	0.3	**0.4**	0.02
South Africa: Mixed race (1989-1992)	97	1.5	**2.5**	0.18	24	0.4	**0.5**	0.04
South Africa: White (1989-1992)	123	1.2	**1.1**	0.08	42	0.4	**0.3**	0.02
South Africa, Transkei, Umtata (1996-1998)	4	1.1	**2.1**	0.20	-	-	**-**	-
South Africa, Transkei, 4 districts (1996-1998)	1	0.1	**0.3**	0.04	1	0.1	**0.1**	-
Swaziland (1996-1999)	2	0.1	**0.2**	0.02	-	-	**-**	-
Europe/USA								
USA, SEER: White (1993-1997)	271	0.6	**0.5**	0.03	145	0.3	**0.2**	0.01
USA, SEER: Black (1993-1997)	57	0.9	**0.9**	0.06	23	0.3	**0.3**	0.03
France, 8 registries (1993-1997)	107	0.8	**0.6**	0.05	37	0.3	**0.2**	0.01
The Netherlands (1993-1997)	222	0.6	**0.5**	0.03	82	0.2	**0.2**	0.01
UK, England (1993-1997)	637	0.5	**0.4**	0.03	304	0.2	**0.2**	0.01

In italics: histopathology-based registries

Table 2. Incidence of nasopharyngeal carcinoma in Africa, 1953–74

Registry	Period	ASR (per 100 000)		Source (see Chap. 1)
		Male	Female	
Senegal, Dakar	1969–74	*0.3*	*0.3*	4
Mozambique, Lourenço Marques	1956–60	*2.2*	*0.0*	1
Nigeria, Ibadan	1960–69	2.5	1.8	3
SA, Cape Province: Bantu	1956–59	*0.0*	*0.0*	2
SA, Cape Province: Coloured	1956–59	*0.6*	*0.1*	2
SA, Cape Province: White	1956–59	*0.4*	*0.4*	2
SA, Johannesburg, Bantu	1953–55	*0.9*	*1.2*	1
SA, Natal Province: African	1964–66	*1.1*	*0.7*	2
SA, Natal Province: Indian	1964–66	*0.8*	*0.2*	2
Uganda, Kyadondo	1954–60	*0.0*	*0.0*	1
Uganda, Kyadondo	1960–71	*1.0*	*0.5*	5
Zimbabwe, Bulawayo	1963–72	*0.1*	*0.8*	6

Italics: Rate based on less than 10 cases

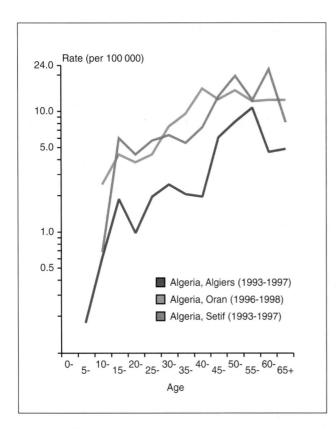

Figure 2. Age-specific incidence rates of NPC in three Algerian registries (males)

IgG and IgA titres to VCA and EA than patients with other tumours or than normal subjects (de Thé *et al.*, 1978). The viral genome is present in all NPCs, and in monoclonal form, implying that its presence antedates the tumour; it is never found in normal epithelial cells in the nasopharynx (IARC, 1997). But human infection with EBV is ubiquitous, so that it can by no means explain the striking geographical and ethnic patterns, and other agents must be involved.

Several studies strongly support the hypothesis that Cantonese-style salted fish is a nasopharyngeal carcinogen in humans. The studies suggest that age at exposure is an important co-determinant of risk, earlier age at exposure being associated with a higher risk for disease. There are also experimental data to support the carcinogenicity of Cantonese-style salted fish (IARC, 1997; Hildesheim & Levine, 1993). Jeannel *et al.* (1990) conducted a case–control study among Tunisians, who are at intermediate risk for nasopharyngeal carcinoma. Eighty histologically confirmed incident cases identified at the only cancer hospital in Tunisia and 160 population controls individually matched to the cases by age, sex and neighbourhood of residence were interviewed about dietary habits in the year preceding the cancer diagnosis and during childhood. The intake of several preserved food products during childhood and/or adulthood was significantly associated with the risk for nasopharyngeal carcinoma after adjustment for socioeconomic status. These foods were *touklia* (a stewing mixture of red and black peppers, paprika, caraway seed and/or coriander seed, salt and olive or soya-bean oil), *quaddid* (dried mutton preserved in olive oil), pickled vegetables, pickled olives and *harissa* (a mixture of red pepper, garlic, caraway seed, salt and olive oil). After adjustment for each other and for other potential confounders, only childhood exposure to *touklia*, *quaddid* and *harissa* were significant risk factors for nasopharyngeal carcinoma in Tunisia. The odds ratio for childhood consumption of *touklia* was 8.6 (95% CI 1.7–44), that for consumption of *quaddid* more than once a month was 1.9 (95% CI 1.0–3.7) and that for consumption of *harissa* more than once a month was 4.2 (95% CI 1.1–17).

Low levels of several volatile nitrosamines and directly acting genotoxic substances have been detected in Tunisian *touklia, quaddid* and *harissa* (Poirier *et al.*, 1987, 1989). In addition, samples of *harissa* and *quaddid* were shown to contain EBV-activating substances (Poirier *et al.*, 1989).

A variety of other possible etiological factors have been studied in case–control studies. Few have shown a strong or consistent association with risk (Hildesheim & Levine, 1993).

Clifford (1965) noted the presence of wood fires in chimneyless houses among tribal groups in Kenya with moderately elevated rates of nasopharyngeal carcinoma, and suggested a role for wood smoke. The same author (1972) measured serum carotene levels in 17 male African patients with nasopharyngeal carcinoma and 53 male controls and reported a significantly lower level in the cases.

Two case–control studies in US populations suggest an association with tobacco smoking (Mabuchi *et al.*, 1985; Nam *et al.*, 1992), while one was negative (Henderson *et al.*, 1976). In the US veterans cohort (Dorn, 1959), 46 deaths from NPC had occurred after 26 years; the odds ratio for smoking (ever/never) was 3.2.

Snuff has been suggested as an etiological factor; based upon chemical analysis of Zulu and Venda snuff, it appears that benzo[a]pyrene (for which a role has been proposed in China and Tunisia) is present in a considerable amount together with other carcinogenic hydrocarbons (Hubert & de Thé, 1982; Hubert *et al.*, 1993).

The results of analyses for trace quantities of six elements in maize leaf samples (iron, manganese, zinc copper, boron, molybdenum, nickel and lead) suggested that there was no association with incidence of nasopharyngeal carcinoma in Kenya (Robinson, 1967; Robinson & Clifford, 1968).

A comparison of the microflora of the nasopharyngeal area in subjects from Algeria and France suggested that the count of nitrate-reducing bacteria was higher in the former. This was suggested as a possible link to the higher risk of NPC, via the formation of nitrosamines (Charrière *et al.*, 1991).

Host factors

Observations of squamous metaplasia of the nasal mucosa following prolonged administration of estrogenic hormones appears to have stimulated several studies of sex hormone profiles in cases of NPC and controls in east Africa (Clifford & Bulbrook, 1966; Wang *et al.*, 1968). They showed a ratio of urinary estrogen to 11-deoxy-17-oxosteroids higher in NPC cases than in controls, while serum levels of dehydroepiandrosterone sulfate were lower, and no difference was observed in levels of androsterone sulfate. The significance, if any, of these observations is not clear.

Clifford (1970b) compared the ABO blood group profile of 233 patients with NPC from six Kenyan tribes with the normal distribution of blood groups in the same tribes; he observed that blood group A individuals appeared to be at reduced risk of NPC.

Several studies within populations of southern Chinese origin have identified associations between HLA locus A and B antigens and NPC risk (Chan *et al.*, 1983). It is not clear how much of the difference between populations could be attributed to HLA profiles, though Simons *et al.* (1976) did note that the frequency of the A2-B46 phenotype, associated with a relative risk of about 2, was twice as common in Cantonese relative to the Chiu Chau/Fujianese dialect groups, in parallel with the two-fold difference in NPC incidence.

A significant link with the HLA groups B5 and B17 has been observed in Algerian NPC patients (Tursz *et al.*, 1982). An investigation of HLA profiles among NPC cases and controls from Tunisia showed that at the second HLA locus, the results were similar to those found in Singapore, but the effect was less marked and did not reach statistical significance. At the first HLA locus, no association between A2 and NPC was found, in contrast to the Singapore results (Betuel *et al.*, 1975). Herait *et al.* (1983), comparing 76 cases of NPC from Algeria with a control population (with renal failure) did not observe any statistically significant difference in frequency of HLA-A and HLA-B antigens. On the other hand, Hall *et al.* (1982) in a study of 141 cases in Kenya found an elevated risk with HLA-A29 and a factor of resistance associated with Bw44 for both NPC and Burkitt lymphoma. In addition to HLA, Chaabani & Ellouz (1986) found a relationship between NPC and certain immunoglobulin allotypes (Gm (1,17; 11,15,21) and Gm (1,3; 5,11), and the Km (1) antigen), but these findings were not confirmed in a study in Malaysia (Tarone *et al.*, 1990).

A linkage study based on affected sib pairs among southern Chinese in China, Hong Kong, Singapore and Malaysia suggests that a gene (or genes) closely linked to the HLA locus is associated with a 20-fold increased risk of NPC (Lu *et al.*, 1990). Some cancers show deletions at specific regions of chromosome 9 (Lo *et al.*, 1995). However, the genetic basis of susceptibility to NPC remains largely an enigma.

References

Al-Idrissi, H.Y. (1990) Head and neck cancer in Saudi Arabia: Retrospective analysis of 65 patients. *J. Int. Med. Res.*, **18**, 515–519

Betuel, H., Cammoun, M., Comombani, J., Day, N.E., Ellouz, R. & De The, G. (1975) The relationship between nasopharyngeal carcinoma and the HLA system among Tunisians. *Int. J. Cancer*, **16**, 249–254

Bouchardy, C., Parkin, D.M., Wanner, P. & Khlat, M. (1996) Cancer mortality among North African migrants in France. *Int. J. Epidemiol.*, **25**, 5–13

Buell, P. (1974) The effect of migration on the risk of nasopharyngeal cancer among Chinese. *Cancer Res.*, **34**, 1189–1191

Burt, R.D., Vaughan, T.L. & McKnight, B. (1992) Descriptive epidemiology and survival analysis of nasopharyngeal carcinoma in the United States. *Int. J. Cancer*, **52**, 549–556

Cammoun, M., Vogt Hoerner, G. & Mourali, N. (1974) Tumors of the nasopharynx in Tunisia. An anatomic and clinical study based on 143 cases. *Cancer*, **33**, 184–192

Chaabani H., & Ellouz R. (1986) Immunoglobulin allotypes in patients with nasopharyngeal carcinoma. *Hum. Hered.*, **36**, 402–404

Chan, S.H., Day, N.E., Kunaratnam, N., Chia, K.B. & Simons, M.J. (1983) HLA and nasopharyngeal carcinoma in Chinese – a further study. *Int. J. Cancer*, **32**, 171–176

Charrière, M., Poirier, S., Calmels, S., de Montclos, H., Dubreuil, C., Poizat, R., Hamdi Cherif, M. & de Thé, G. (1991) Microflora of the nasopharynx in caucasian and maghrebian subjects with and without nasopharyngeal carcinoma. In: O'Neill, I.K., Chen, J. & Bartsch H., *Relevance to Human Cancer of N-Nitroso Compounds, Tobacco Smoke and Mycotoxins* (IARC Scientific Publications No. 105), Lyon, IARC, pp. 158–161

Clifford, P. (1965) Carcinoma of the nasopharynx in Kenya. *E. Afr. Med. J.*, **42**, 373–396

Clifford, P. (1967) Malignant disease of the nasopharynx and paranasal sinuses in Kenya. In: Muir, C.S. & Shanmugaratnam, K., eds, *Cancer of the Nasopharynx* (UICC Monograph series 1), Copenhagen, Munksgaard, pp. 82–94

Clifford, P. (1970a) On the epidemiology of nasopharyngeal carcinoma. *Int. J. Cancer*, **5**, 287–309

Clifford, P. (1970b) Blood-groups and nasopharyngeal carcinoma. *Lancet*, **2**, 48–49

Clifford, P. (1972) Carcinogens in the nose and throat: Nasopharyngeal carcinoma in Kenya. *Proc. R. Soc. Med.*, **65**, 682–686

Clifford, P. & Bulbrook, R.D. (1966) Endocrine studies in African males with nasopharyngeal cancer. *Lancet*, **1**, 1228–1231

Dorn, H. (1959) Tobacco consumption and mortality from cancer and other diseases. *Publ. Health. Rep.*, **74**, 581–593

Ellouz, R., Cammoun, M., Ben Attia, R. & Bahi, J. (1978) Nasopharyngeal carcinoma in children and adolescents in Tunisia: clinical aspects and the paraneoplastic syndrome. In: de Thé, G. & Ito, Y., eds, *Nasopharyngeal Carcinoma: Etiology and Control* (IARC Scientific Publications No. 20), Lyon, IARC, pp. 471–481

Hall, P.J., Levin, A.G., Entwistle, C.C., Knight, S.C., Wasunna, A., Kung'u, A. & Brubaker, G. (1982) HLA antigens in East African Black patients with Burkitt's lymphoma or nasopharyngeal carcinoma and in controls: a pilot study. *Hum. Immunol.*, **5**, 91–105

Henderson, B.E., Louie, E., SooHoo Jing, J., Buell, P. & Gardner, M.B. (1976) Risk factors associated with nasopharyngeal carcinoma. *New Engl. J. Med.*, **295**, 1101–1106

Herait, P., Tursz, T., Guillard, M.Y., Hanna, K., Lipinski, M., Micheau, C., Sancho-Garnier, H., Schwaab, G., Cachin, Y., Degos, L., *et al.* (1983) HLA-A, -B, and -DR antigens in North African patients with nasopharyngeal carcinoma. *Tissue Antigens*, **22**, 335–341

Hidayatalla, A., Malik, M.O.A., El Hadi, A.E., Osman, A.A. & Hutt, M.S.R. (1983) Studies on nasopharyngeal carcinoma in the Sudan. I. Epidemiology and aetiology. *Eur. J. Cancer Clin. Oncol.*, **19**, 705–710

Hildesheim, A. & Levine, P.H. (1993) Etiology of nasopharyngeal carcinoma: a review. *Epidemiol.Rev.*, **15**, 466–485

Hou-Jensen, K. (1964) On the occurrence of post nasal space tumours in Kenya. *Br. J. Cancer*, **18**, 58–68

Hubert, A. & De The, G. (1982) Comportement alimentaire, mode de vie et cancer du rhino-pharynx. *Bull. Cancer*, (Paris), **69**, 476–482

Hubert, A., Jeannel, D., Tuppin, P. & De The, G. (1993) Anthroplogy and epidémiology. Pluridisciplinary approach of environment factors of nasopharyngeal carcinoma. In: Tursz, T., Pagano, J.S., Ablashi, T.V., De The, G., Lenoir, G. & Pearson, G.R., eds, *The Epstein-Barr Virus and Associated Diseases*, Volume 225, Colloque INSERM / John Lippey Eurotext, pp. 777–790

IARC (1997) *IARC Monographs on the Evaluation of Carcinogenic Risks to Humans. Volume 70, Epstein-Barr Virus and Kaposi's Sarcoma Herpesvirus/Human Herpesvirus 8*, Lyon, IARC

Jeannel, D., Hubert, A., deVathaire, F., Ellouz, R., Camoun, M., Ben Salem, M., Sancho-Garnier, H., deThé, G. (1990) Diet, living conditions and nasopharyngeal carcinoma in Tunisia – a case-control study. *Int. J. Cancer*, **46**, 421–425

Jeannel, D., Ghnassia, M., Hubert, A., Sancho-Garnier, H., Eschwège, F., Crognier, E. & de Thé, G. (1993) Increased risk of nasopharyngeal carcinoma among males of French origin born in Maghreb (North Africa). *Int. J. Cancer*, **54**, 536–539

Khlat, M., Bouchardy, C. & Parkin, D.M. (1993) Mortalité par cancer chez les immigrés du proche orient en Australie. *Rev. Epidémiol. Santé Publique*, **41**, 208–217

Klein, G., Geering, G., Old, L.J., Henle, G., Henle, W. & Clifford, P. (1970) Comparison of the anti-EBV titer and the EBV-associated membrane reactive and precipitating antibody levels in the sera of Burkitt lymphoma and nasopharyngeal carcinoma patients and controls. *Int. J. Cancer*, **5**, 185–194

Lee, H.P., Duffy, S.W., Day, N.E. & Shanmugaratnam, K. (1988) Recent trends in cancer incidence among Singapore Chinese. *Int. J. Cancer*, **42**, 159–166

Li, J.-Y., Liu, B., Li, G., Rong, S., Cao, D. and 25 others (1979) *Atlas of Cancer Mortality in the People's Republic of China*, Shanghai, China Map Press

Lo, K.W., Huang, D.P. & Lau, K.M. (1995) p16 gene alterations in nasopharyngeal carcinoma. *Cancer Res.*, **55**, 2039–2043

Lu, S.J., Day, N.E., Degos, L., Lepage, V., Wang, P.C., Chan, S.H., Simons, M., McKnight, B., Easton, D., Zeng, Y. & de-The G. (1990) Linkage of a nasopharyngeal carcinoma susceptibility locus to the HLA region. *Nature*, **346**, 470–471

Mabuchi, K., Bross, D.S. & Kessler, I.I. (1985) Cigarette smoking and nasopharyngeal carcinoma. *Cancer*, **55**, 2874–2876

Muir, C.S. (1971) Nasopharyngeal carcinoma in non-Chinese populations with special reference to south-east Asia and Africa. *Int. J. Cancer*, **8**, 351–363

Nam, J.-M., McLaughlin, J.K. & Blot, W.J. (1992) Cigarette smoking, alcohol, and nasopharyngeal carcinoma; a case control study among US whites. *J. Natl Cancer Inst.*, **84**, 619–622

Nielsen, N.H., Storm, H.H., Gaudette, L.A. & Lanier, A.P. (1996) Cancer in circumpolar Inuit 1969–1988. A summary. *Acta Oncol.*, **35**, 621-628

Parkin, D.M. & Iscovich, J.A. (1997) The risk of cancer in migrants and their descendants in Israel: II Carcinomas and germ cell tumours. *Int. J. Cancer*, **70**, 654–660

Parkin, D.M., Whelan, S.L., Ferlay, J., Raymond, L. & Young, J., eds (1997) *Cancer Incidence in Five Continents* Vol VII (IARC Scientific Publications No 143), Lyon, IARC

Poirier, S., Ohshima, H., de Thé, G., Hubert, A., Bourgade, M.C. & Bartsch, H. (1987) Volatile nitrosamine levels in common foods from Tunisia, south China and Greenland, high-risk areas for nasopharyngeal carcinoma (NPC). *Int. J. Cancer*, **39**, 293–296

Poirier, S., Bouvier, G., Malaveille, C., Ohshima, H., Shao, Y.M., Hubert, A., Zeng, Y., de Thé, G. & Bartsch, H. (1989) Volatile nitrosamine levels and genotoxicity of food samples from high-risk areas for nasopharyngeal carcinoma before and after nitrosation. *Int. J. Cancer*, **44**, 1088–1094

Robinson, J.B.D. (1967) Notes on some chemical elements in relation to carcinoma of the nasopharynx in Kenya. In: Clifford, P., Linsell, A.C. & Timms, G.L., eds, *Cancer in Africa*, Nairobi, East African Publishing House

Robinson, J.B.D. & Clifford, P. (1968) Trace element levels and carcinoma of the nasopharynx in Kenya. *E. Afr. Med. J.*, **45**, 694–700

Schmauz, R. & Templeton, A.C. (1972) Nasopharyngeal carcinoma in Uganda. *Cancer*, **29**, 610–621

Simons, M.J., Wee, G.B., Goh, E.H., Chan, S.H., Shanmugaratnam, K., Day, N.E. & de Thé, G. (1976) Immunogenetic aspects of nasopharyngeal carcinoma. IV. Increased risk in Chinese of nasopharyngeal carcinoma associated with a Chinese-related HLA profile. *J. Natl Cancer Inst.*, **57**, 977–980

Smith, G.E., Dawson, W.R. 1924) Egyptian Mummies, London, Allan and Unwin, p. 157. Cited by: Hubert, A., De Thé, G. (1982) Comportement alimentaire, mode de vie et cancer du rhino-pharynx. *Bull. Cancer (Paris)*, **69**, 476–482

Tarone, R.E., Levine, P.H., Yadav, M. & Pandey, J.P. (1990) Relationship between immunoglobulin allotypes and susceptibility to nasopharyngeal carcinoma in Malaysia. *Cancer Res.*, **50**, 3186–3188

de Thé, G., Lavoué, M.-F. & Muenz, L. (1978) Differences in EBV antibody titres of patients with nasopharyngeal carcinoma originating from high, intermediate and low incidence areas. In: de Thé, G. & Ito, Y., eds, *Nasopharyngeal Carcinoma: Etiology and Control* (IARC Scientific Publications No. 20), Lyon, IARC, pp. 471–481

Tursz, T., Herait, P., Guillard, M.Y., Lipinski, M. & De The, G. (1982) Etudes immunologiques dans le cancer du nasopharynx. In: *Cancer du nasopharynx. Progrès cliniques, thérapeutiques et étio-pathogéniques. Actualités cancérologiques.* Paris, Institut Gustave Roussy

Wabinga, H.R., Parkin, D.M., Wabwire-Mangen, F. & Nambooze, S. (2000) Trends in cancer incidence in Kyadondo County, Uganda, 1960-1997. *Br. J. Cancer*, **82**, 1585–1592

Wang, D.Y., Bulbrook, R.D. & Clifford, P. (1968) Plasma-levels of the sulphate esters of dehydroepiandrosterone and androsterone in Kenyan men and their relation to cancer of the nasopharynx. *Lancet*, **1**, 1003–1004

4.13 Cancer of the oesophagus

Introduction

Oesophageal cancer ranks eighth in frequency of occurrence worldwide, with about 391 000 new cases each year, and 355 000 deaths. The geographical variation in risk is very large—more than for almost any other cancer. The highest-risk areas of the world are in the Asian 'oesophageal cancer belt' (stretching from northern Iran through the central Asian republics to north-central China), with incidence rates as high as 200 per 100 000 (and, in some areas, a female predominance), East and south-eastern Africa (Uganda, Zimbabwe, Natal, Transkei), eastern South America (southern Brazil, Uruguay, Paraguay, northern Argentina) and certain parts of western Europe (especially France and Switzerland). Oesophageal cancer is more common in males in most areas—for example, the sex ratio is 6.5:1 in France (Ferlay *et al.*, 2001), although in the high-risk areas of Asia, the sex ratio is much closer to unity, e.g. 1.5 in Linxian County, Henan, China (Lu *et al.*, 1985).

Descriptive epidemiology in Africa

Table 1 shows the incidence rates in the population-based data-sets in this volume. The incidence is low in North, West, and Central Africa (ASR less than 2 per 100 000 in men and 1 per 100 000 in women). However, in the African populations of eastern and southern Africa, the incidence is high (rates in white populations are similar to those in Europe and United States). Generally, the sex ratio is not very wide, 2–3:1; the exception is Reunion, which resembles metropolitan France in the large excess in men. The results from the older data in the 1950s and 60s are not dissimilar (Table 2), although the sex ratios in southern Africa seem to be rather wider in some centres (e.g., Johannesburg 10:1, Bulawayo, 7:1, Natal 3.3:1, Cape Province 2.6:1).

Cancer incidence among the Bantu of the Transkei, South Africa, has been reported in a number of surveys covering the period 1955–84 (Rose, 1967, 1973; Rose & Fellingham, 1981; Jaskiewicz *et al.*, 1987a). Age-standardized incidence (African standard) for all cancer sites combined (1965–69) was 60 and 42 per 100 000 per year for men and women, respectively (Rose & Fellingham, 1981); oesophageal cancer accounted for approximately half of the cases (35 and 17–19 per 100 000) in 1955–69, based on 5095 cases (Rose, 1973). More recently, in what was formerly Transkei, an incidence rate for males of 46.7 per 100 000 was recorded (Makaula *et al.*, 1996) and the data from the cancer registry in Umtata, Transkei, from 1996–98 (Table 1) confirm the persistence of these high rates.

In South Africa and Zimbabwe, the incidence of oesophageal cancer is higher in the black population than among whites; persons of mixed or Asian/Indian background in South Africa have rates that are intermediate between those of blacks and whites.

These various data from registries and relative frequencies from case series have been used to estimate national incidence rates (Figure 1). The estimates of age-standardized incidence in males range from less than 1 in many countries of West and Central Africa, to more than 10 per 100 000 in East and South Africa.

Transkei, South Africa

Within the Transkei, areas of high, moderate and low risk of oesophageal cancer were identified by Oettlé (1963) and Burrell (1957, 1962), with the high-risk districts being in the western part of the Transkei and the low risk ones in the eastern part.

Transkei subsequently became the focus of cancer registration and study (Rose, 1973). Between 1964 and 1969, all hospitals in the Transkei, three major referral hospitals in Natal (now KwaZulu-Natal) Province, and the major radiotherapy centre just outside the

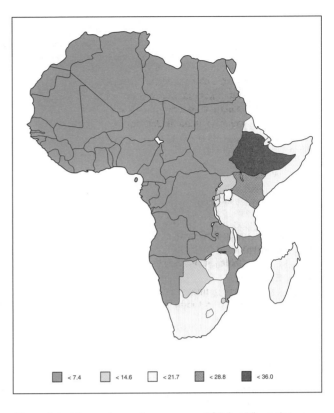

Figure 1. Incidence of oesophagus cancer: ASR (world) - males

Transkei in the Eastern Cape (East London), provided data on a total of 4247 cases of cancer (Rose & McGlashan 1975; Rose & Fellingham 1981). Overall, the age-standardized incidence rate for oesophageal cancer per 100 000 in males was 102.6 in the high-risk districts, 59.5 in the moderate-risk districts and 22.4 in the low-risk districts (Table 3). Incidence in the moderate-risk districts was similar to that observed in Durban in 1964–66 (40.7; Schonland & Bradshaw, 1968) and in Cape Town (37.5; Muir Grieve, 1967, 1970). Rates for oesophageal cancer in Johannesburg black males were lower, (12.8) (Table 2).

Cancer registration was continued by the Medical Research Council in the Transkei in two low-risk (Bizana and Lusikisiki) and two high-risk districts (Butterworth and Kentani). Data for 1981–84 (Jaskiewicz *et al.*, 1987 a) and 1985–90 (Makaula *et al.*, 1996) suggest that the incidence of oesophageal cancer has been declining in the high-risk districts and increasing in the low-risk districts. The reasons for this 'equalization' of the oesophageal cancer rates in the Transkei are unclear, but it is possible, given the high rates of migration in these areas and the large contrasts in access to diagnostic facilities, that some of the past differences in risk between the different regions may have been exaggerated.

Kenya

On the basis of hospital records, marked local variation in risk of oesophageal cancer among people of similar ethnic origin around Lake Victoria was suggested by Ahmed (1966) and Ahmed and Cook (1969), who noted that about 30% of cancers seen at the Kisumu hospital in western Kenya were oesophageal, whereas in Shirati hospital nearby in Tanzania, cancer of the oesophagus comprised only 2% of all cases, and in Uganda 1.8% of all cases. There was some evidence of variation within Nyanza province but this was inconclusive, partly because of the selective admission of

Table 1. Age-standardized (world) and cumulative (0-64) incidence
Oesophagus (C15)

	Cases	CRUDE	ASR(W) (per 100,000)	Cumulative (%)	Cases	CRUDE	ASR(W) (per 100,000)	Cumulative (%)
	MALE				**FEMALE**			
Africa, North								
Algeria, Algiers (1993-1997)	34	0.6	**0.9**	0.06	19	0.3	**0.5**	0.02
Algeria, Constantine (1994-1997)	3	0.2	**0.4**	0.01	1	0.1	**0.1**	0.02
Algeria, Oran (1996-1998)	17	1.0	**1.5**	0.08	8	0.5	**0.6**	0.02
Algeria, Setif (1993-1997)	9	0.3	**0.5**	0.02	5	0.2	**0.3**	0.02
Tunisia, Centre, Sousse (1993-1997)	3	0.3	**0.4**	0.01	3	0.3	**0.4**	0.03
Tunisia, North, Tunis (1994)	19	0.9	**1.2**	0.09	16	0.8	**1.0**	0.06
Tunisia, Sfax (1997)	2	0.5	**0.6**	-	2	0.5	**0.7**	0.04
Africa, West								
The Gambia (1997-1998)	7	0.7	**1.4**	0.10	5	0.5	**1.1**	0.05
Guinea, Conakry (1996-1999)	13	0.6	**0.9**	0.08	5	0.2	**0.5**	0.05
Mali, Bamako (1988-1997)	34	0.9	**2.0**	0.18	17	0.5	**0.9**	0.07
Niger, Niamey (1993-1999)	7	0.4	**1.0**	0.12	7	0.4	**1.3**	0.11
Nigeria, Ibadan (1998-1999)	7	0.5	**1.1**	0.03	2	0.1	**0.3**	0.03
Africa, Central								
Congo, Brazzaville (1996-1999)	4	0.3	**0.5**	0.04	1	0.1	**0.1**	-
Africa, East								
France, La Reunion (1988-1994)	362	17.3	**22.8**	1.76	36	1.7	**1.9**	0.11
Kenya, Eldoret (1998-2000)	89	9.5	**24.5**	1.66	51	5.6	**15.5**	1.36
Malawi, Blantyre (2000-2001)	72	8.0	**17.4**	1.28	38	4.4	**10.7**	0.79
Uganda, Kyadondo County (1993-1997)	106	3.8	**13.3**	0.82	91	3.1	**12.1**	0.68
Zimbabwe, Harare: African (1990-1993)	212	8.9	**27.9**	1.38	36	1.7	**8.6**	0.48
Zimbabwe, Harare: African (1994-1997)	169	6.1	**17.2**	0.89	51	1.9	**8.4**	0.37
Zimbabwe, Harare: European (1990-1997)	18	11.8	**6.3**	0.19	8	4.7	**2.3**	0.14
Africa, South								
Namibia (1995-1998)	107	3.4	**6.3**	0.36	33	1.0	**1.7**	0.07
South Africa: Black (1989-1992)	7009	12.3	**23.1**	1.61	3220	5.7	**9.1**	0.68
South Africa: Indian (1989-1992)	179	9.2	**13.1**	1.04	102	5.1	**7.3**	0.46
South Africa: Mixed race (1989-1992)	520	8.1	**16.0**	1.13	178	2.7	**4.2**	0.31
South Africa: White (1989-1992)	597	5.9	**5.5**	0.35	208	2.0	**1.6**	0.09
South Africa, Transkei, Umtata (1996-1998)	117	32.7	**62.5**	5.30	97	22.9	**34.5**	2.57
South Africa, Transkei, 4 districts (1996-1998)	134	18.5	**37.5**	2.83	173	19.2	**26.5**	2.01
Swaziland (1996-1999)	113	6.4	**14.0**	1.01	41	2.1	**4.1**	0.32
Europe/USA								
USA, SEER: White (1993-1997)	3025	6.2	**4.8**	0.26	1125	2.2	**1.3**	0.06
USA, SEER: Black (1993-1997)	593	8.9	**10.6**	0.74	252	3.4	**3.4**	0.24
France, 8 registries (1993-1997)	2045	14.9	**11.0**	0.75	346	2.4	**1.4**	0.08
The Netherlands (1993-1997)	3297	8.6	**6.3**	0.35	1640	4.2	**2.4**	0.12
UK, England (1993-1997)	16669	13.9	**8.7**	0.41	11059	8.7	**4.0**	0.14

In italics: histopathology-based registries

Table 2. Incidence of oesophageal cancer in Africa, 1953–74

Registry	Period	ASR (per 100 000) Male	Female	Source (see Chap. 1)
Senegal, Dakar	1969–74	*0.2*	*0.2*	4
Mozambique, Lourenço Marques	1956–60	*4.4*	*0.0*	1
Nigeria, Ibadan	1960–69	1.5	*1.1*	3
SA, Cape Province: Bantu	1956–59	37.5	*14.3*	2
SA, Cape Province: Coloured	1956–59	10.1	*0.0*	2
SA, Cape Province: White	1956–59	6.4	1.0	2
SA, Johannesburg, Bantu	1953–55	12.8	*1.2*	1
SA, Natal Province: African	1964–66	40.9	12.3	2
SA, Natal Province: Indian	1964–66	22.1	30.0	2
Uganda, Kyadondo	1954–60	*1.8*	*1.1*	1
Uganda, Kyadondo	1960–71	3.3	5.3	5
Zimbabwe, Bulawayo	1963–72	58.6	8.1	6

Italics: Rate based on less than 10 cases

Table 3. Oesophageal cancer incidence (age-standardized incidence, world standard) in Transkei, 1965–69 (calculated from Rose & McGlashan, 1975)

	Males	Females	MV (%)
High-risk districts	102.6	56.4	77%
Moderate-risk districts	59.5	29.9	75%
Low-risk districts	22.4	6.3	85%

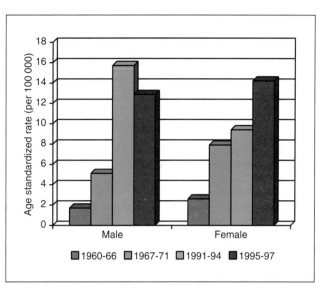

Figure 2. Trends in incidence of oesophageal cancer, Kyadondo County, Uganda, 1960–1997 (Wabinga *et al.* 2000)

cancer patients from around the main hospital (Ahmed & Cook, 1969). Using data from the histopathology register at Kenyatta National Hospital, Nairobi, Gatei *et al.* (1978) noted that 80% of oesphageal cancer cases occurred in individuals from just three tribes: the Kikuyu, Luo and Luhya. Since the first group lives in central Kenya (around Nairobi), a relative over-representation is perhaps not surprising, but the large number of cases among the Luo and Luhya, who come from western Kenya (around Lake Victoria) was considered a significant finding. Interestingly, there were few cases (< 1%) among the Kalenjin, who come from the Rift Valley region, around Eldoret, yet the most recent registry data from Eldoret, presented in this volume, show a fairly high incidence, suggesting that the area of high risk is considerably greater than implied in these publications.

Morphology
Worldwide, most oesophageal cancers are squamous-cell carcinomas, arising in the middle and lower third of the oesophagus. Recently, in developed countries an increase has been observed in relative and absolute numbers of adenocarcinomas of the lower third of the oesophagus, associated with Barrett's oesophagus (Vizcaino *et al.*, 2002). The profiles of genetic changes (mutations) are different in these two histological subtypes, implying different etiology. In Africa, oesophageal cancer is predominantly of squamous-cell origin. Adenocarcinoma of the oesophagus comprises less than 15% of oesophageal cancers in sub-Saharan African populations. In the Caucasian populations of South Africa and in North African countries, adenocarcinoma of the oesophagus comprises about a third of all cases (see Table 4).

Sex ratio
As noted earlier, the sex ratio of oesophageal cancer is quite variable, with a strong male predominance in some high-risk areas in Europe (where tobacco and alcohol are the main risk factors— see below) to near equality, or even a female predominance, in the high-risk areas of central Asia and China. In Africa, the male:female ratio is usually about 2 (Table 1), although earlier ratios of 11.8 in Kenya and 4.2 in Johannesburg were recorded (Cook Mozzaffari, 1989), while in the former Transvaal, South Africa, a ratio of 75 was reported by Oettlé (1967).

Time trends
Several pieces of evidence suggest that the high incidence of oesophageal cancer in South and East Africa is a relatively recent phenomenon. Oesophageal cancer was rare in the 1930s in South Africa (Berman, 1935), but it is now the leading cancer in black males (Higginson & Oettlé, 1962; Sitas *et al.*, 1998). Increases in the relative frequency have been noted in the rural Transvaal (now Northern Province) (Higginson & Oettlé, 1962; Sitas *et al.*, 1998) (see Chapter 3.5.4). Records from Umtata hospital (Transkei) also show a dramatic increase in the frequency of oesophageal cancer relative to all other major cancer types (liver, cervix and breast): in

1925 oesophageal cancer comprised less than 10% of all these cancers, but by 1969 this proportion had increased to just under 60% (Rose & Fellingham, 1981).

In their analysis of incidence rates of cancer among black gold miners in South Africa, Bradshaw *et al.* (1982) observed a small decrease in crude incidence rates over the period 1964–79.

Increases in the frequency of oesophageal cancer have also been noted in Kenya (0.1% in 1930 vs. 16% in the 1960s (Vint, 1935; Cook & Burkitt, 1975), in Swaziland (Keen & Martin, 1971) and in Botswana (Macrae & Cooke, 1975).

In Kampala, Uganda, the incidence of oesophageal cancer has increased progressively in both sexes over the last 30–40 years (Figure 2).

Survival
Survival of oesophageal cancer patients is poor and is strongly related to stage at presentation. In a study in South Africa, 21% of 265 patients with oesophageal cancer presented with the disease confined to the oesophagus, and only 30% of these survived over three years after oesophagotomy (Kneebone & Mannell, 1985).

Risk factors
Studies of squamous-cell carcinoma in developed countries have consistently shown the etiological importance of tobacco and alcohol, particularly in combination. However, the geographical patterns in Africa (and elsewhere) strongly imply that other factors play an important role. In general, the populations at highest risk are poorer, have limited or restricted diets, and consume certain forms of alcohol and tobacco (smoked or chewed) (Rose, 1981). McGlashan (1969a), reviewing geographical variation in oesophageal cancer in East and southern-central Africa, noted that there seemed to be a correlation between relative frequency in hospital case series and consumption of certain spirits brewed from maize husks. Polarographic analysis of these drinks suggested the presence of nitrosamines (McGlashan *et al.*, 1968; McGlashan, 1969b). However, Collis *et al.* (1971), analysing alcoholic drinks from areas near hospitals in Kenya and Uganda with different frequencies of oesophageal cancers, found no association between the suspected constituents, as indicated by polarography, and presence of nitrosamine as evaluated by gas chromatography and mass spectrometry. The nitrosamine levels were not related to the local frequency of oesophageal cancer. Cook (1971) and later van Rensburg (1981) showed a geographical correlation between incidence of oesophageal

cancer and consumption of maize-based staple diets and beer brewed from maize (replacing the traditional sorghum or millet). Several studies of the carcinogenicity of these maize-based beers (for example, nitrites, fermentation products or fungal contaminants such as fumonisins) have been conducted but none has shown, at the individual level, an association with oesophageal cancer.

Alcohol and tobacco

Numerous case–control and cohort studies have shown that both tobacco and alcohol increase the risk of oesophageal cancer, and that their joint effect is multiplicative (IARC, 1986, 1988). Several studies have been conducted in Africa.

The earliest case–control study (Bradshaw & Schonland, 1969) examined 98 cases and 341 unmatched hospital controls in Durban, South Africa. This study was re-analysed, together with a later one of 196 male cases and 1064 age-matched controls in Baragwanath Hospital, Johannesburg (Bradshaw & Schonland, 1974). In both, oesophageal cancer was strongly associated with tobacco use, particularly with the use of pipe tobacco in cigarettes (OR in Durban 5.4, in Johannesburg 7.8, relative to non-smokers). Stratified by level of tobacco consumption, there was no significant effect of alcohol (traditional beer, western type liquors, or 'concoctions') on risk.

In a subsequent hospital-based case–control study in Durban, South Africa, in 1978–81 (van Rensburg et al., 1985), 211 hospital cases (Zulu males) were compared with controls matched on age and residence (urban/rural). In a multivariate model, an association was again found with smoking of commercial cigarettes (OR = 2.6 for current smokers, 1.6 for past smokers) and pipe smoking (OR = 2.1), but data for alcohol consumption were not shown.

In a case–control analysis based on data collected in the cancer registry of Bulawayo, Zimbabwe, in 1963–77 (Vizcaino et al., 1995), 881 cases of oesophageal cancer were compared with 5238 controls (patients with cancers not related to tobacco or alcohol). In men, a dose–response relationship was found for tobacco consumption, with an OR of 3.5 for those smoking 1–14 cigarettes per day and 5.7 for those smoking over 15 g of total tobacco per day (cigarettes usually weigh about a gram). Among women who had ever smoked tobacco, the OR was 4.0 compared with those who had never smoked. No effect in relation to alcohol drinking was found (OR = 0.9) for daily consumption of either local beer or total alcohol.

In the Transkei, populations with 'high', 'medium' and 'low' incidence of oesophageal cancer were compared with respect to prevalence of tobacco smoking (particularly pipes) and consumption of different alcoholic beverages (McGlashan et al., 1982). The correlation was stronger for tobacco than for alcohol.

Also in the Transkei, a hospital-based case–control study (130 cases, controls matched by age and level of education) (Sammon, 1992) found a positive association with smoking (OR = 2.6; 95% CI 1.5–5.0), but no relationship with drinking of 'traditional' beer (OR = 1.6; 95% CI 0.9–3.0).

In contrast, a hospital-based case–control study in Soweto (Segal et al., 1988) found that both alcohol and tobacco had an independent and multiplicative effect on the risk of developing oesophageal cancer. For example, in the heaviest drinkers and smokers (more than 40 g tobacco and 91 g ethanol per day) an OR of 39 was observed. For tobacco alone (adjusted for alcohol), the OR was 3.0 for those smoking 20–39 g per day and 2.2 for those smoking over 40 g per day. By contrast, the relative risks in relation to alcohol consumption (adjusted for tobacco) were 5.4 in those consuming 31–60 g ethanol per day, 10.5 in those consuming 61–90 g and 18.3 for the highest daily consumption of ethanol (> 90 g per day).

In a study by Pacella-Norman et al. (2002), among the black population of Johannesburg and Soweto, the odds ratio associated with heavy smoking in males (15+ g of tobacco per day) was 6.0 (95% CI 3.2–11.0) for developing oesophageal cancer and in females, 6.2 (95% CI 1.9–20.2). Daily alcohol consumption was a risk factor for the development of oesophageal cancer in males (OR = 1.8, 95% CI 1.2–2.8) and females (OR = 1.7; 95% CI 1.0–2.9). For alcohol consumption in combination with smoking, males and females were at increased risk of developing oesophageal cancer (OR = 4.7; 95% CI 2.8–7.9, and 4.8; 95% CI 3.0–7.8, respectively) compared with lifelong non-smokers and non-drinkers. Increased risks of developing oesophageal cancer were noted in both males and females who reported having lived in the former Transkei for over 34 years (OR males = 3.1; 95% CI 0.9–10.8; OR females = 14.7; 95% CI 4.7–46.0).

The reason for the rather discrepant results between earlier studies and more recent ones based on urban populations, with respect to the effect of alcohol on risk, may lie in the actual amounts of alcohol consumed. In Soweto, consumption (in grams of alcohol per day) was far greater than that reported in the studies from Bulawayo and rural South Africa, where the principal alcoholic beverage was maize beer, with a low alcohol content (2–4%). In Bulawayo, for example, it was estimated that individuals in the heaviest drinking categories were consuming only about 20–40 g of alcohol per day, a quantity that is associated with only about a doubling of risk of oesophageal cancer in studies elsewhere. It is therefore possible that the early southern African studies could not detect such low relative risks.

Chewing/ingestion of tobacco

In the Transkei, swallowing of dottle from the pipe stem (i.e., tobacco pyrolysis products) was thought to be associated with increased oesophageal cancer risk (Rose, 1978). A bacterial mutagenicity assay demonstrated significant mutagenic activity in this material (Hewer et al., 1978;). However, only 2–5% of the population claimed to do this (Bradshaw et al., 1983).

Nutritional deficiencies

Many of the 'clusters' of high oesophageal cancer risk appear to occur in populations who are poor and consume restricted diets. Oesophageal cancer has been found to be associated with low social class in developed countries (e.g., USA; Brown et al., 1994) and China (Cheng et al., 1992) and with poor nutritional status. Thus in the United States, those with diets poor in nutrients and low in fruits and vegetables (particularly those rich in vitamin C) are at increased risk of developing oesophageal cancer (Brown et al., 1998). In many African populations, a restricted diet could be a major background factor associated with oesophageal cancer (Cook Mozzaffari, 1989); Burrell (1957) noted that the Transkei was an infertile area where plants had a number of mineral deficiencies. In a comparison of areas of moderate and high risk of oesophageal cancer, persons living in areas of high risk had lower levels of vitamins A and C, magnesium and riboflavin (van Rensburg et al., 1983). In the Transkei, populations with high oesophageal cancer rates appeared to eat maize as a staple, which has low levels of niacin, riboflavin, vitamin C, zinc, calcium and magnesium. Pellagra is associated with high intake of maize and acute oesophagitis is associated with this disease.

In the hospital-based case–control study of Sammon (1992) in Umtata (Transkei), cases reported more frequent use of traditional dietary staples than controls. In the case–control study in Durban, Natal (van Rensburg et al., 1985), consumption of maize meal was a risk factor for oesophageal cancer (OR for daily consumers 5.7, weekly consumers 2.4, compared with those who consumed it less often). It has been suggested that chronic oesophagitis is a precursor of oesophageal cancer, but it is unclear under what circumstances acute oesophagitis develops into chronic oesophagitis.

Table 4. Percentage distribution of microscopically verified cases by histological type
Oesophagus (C15) - Both sexes

	Squamous	Carcinoma Adeno	Other	Unspecified	Sarcoma	Other	Unspecified	Number of cases MV	Total
Algeria, Algiers	46.2	33.3	-	20.5	-	-	-	**39**	53
Algeria, Batna	92.3	7.7	-	-	-	-	-	**13**	14
Algeria, Constantine	50.0	50.0	-	-	-	-	-	**2**	4
Algeria, Oran	55.0	35.0	-	10.0	-	-	-	**20**	25
Algeria, Setif	41.7	41.7	-	16.7	-	-	-	**12**	14
Burkina Faso, Ouagadougou	-	80.0	-	20.0	-	-	-	**5**	9
Congo, Brazzaville	25.0	25.0	-	50.0	-	-	-	**4**	5
France, La Reunion	93.9	4.1	0.5	1.0	-	0.3	0.3	**392**	398
The Gambia	100.0	-	-	-	-	-	-	**1**	12
Guinea, Conakry	50.0	20.0	-	30.0	-	-	-	**10**	18
Kenya, Eldoret	75.9	1.9	-	16.7	-	-	5.6	**54**	140
Malawi, Blantyre	83.3	16.7	-	-	-	-	-	**24**	110
Mali, Bamako	85.7	10.7	-	3.6	-	-	-	**28**	51
Namibia	89.9	4.3	-	5.1	0.7	-	-	**138**	140
Niger, Niamey	77.8	22.2	-	-	-	-	-	**9**	14
Nigeria, Ibadan	100.0	-	-	-	-	-	-	**2**	9
Rwanda, Butare	-	-	-	-	-	-	-	**-**	1
South Africa: Black	88.9	1.8	0.3	2.2	0.1	0.1	6.8	**10229**	10229
South Africa: White	64.5	28.1	1.2	5.2	0.2	-	0.7	**805**	805
South Africa: Indian	79.0	6.8	-	5.3	-	-	8.9	**281**	281
South Africa: Mixed race	90.1	5.6	0.6	3.4	-	-	0.3	**698**	698
South Africa, Elim	85.7	2.4	-	11.9	-	-	-	**42**	57
South Africa, Transkei, Umtata	87.5	-	-	6.3	-	-	6.3	**64**	214
South Africa, Transkei, 4 districts	100.0	-	-	-	-	-	-	**24**	307
Swaziland	100.0	-	-	-	-	-	-	**14**	154
Tanzania, Dar Es Salaam	92.0	4.6	-	3.4	-	-	-	**87**	87
Tanzania, Kilimanjaro	65.2	13.0	-	21.7	-	-	-	**23**	100
Tunisia, Centre, Sousse	100.0	-	-	-	-	-	-	**6**	6
Tunisia, North, Tunis	65.6	31.3	-	3.1	-	-	-	**32**	35
Tunisia, Sfax	100.0	-	-	-	-	-	-	**3**	4
Uganda, Mbarara	50.0	8.3	-	41.7	-	-	-	**12**	52
Uganda, Kyadondo County	86.3	8.8	-	2.5	-	-	2.5	**80**	197
Zimbabwe, Harare: African	89.1	3.6	-	7.3	-	-	-	**220**	468
Zimbabwe, Harare: European	54.5	36.4	-	9.1	-	-	-	**11**	26

Contaminants in the diet

In a case–control study in the Transkei, 'usual consumption' of the plant *Solanum nigrum* in the previous ten years was found to be associated with oesophageal cancer. *S. nigrum* has an irritating effect on the oesophageal mucosal lining (Sammon, 1992). *Candida albicans* infection of the oesophagus (common in China; Hsia *et al.*, 1988) is thought to promote the production of nitrosamines, which are thought to be carcinogenic. This may be of particular relevance to southern Africa, especially against a background of tobacco smoking and alcohol consumption (Silber, 1985).

Mycotoxins

Fumonisin B_1, fumonisin B_2 and fusarin C are mycotoxins produced by *Fusarium* species that occur primarily on maize. These toxins occur particularly when maize is grown under warm, dry conditions. Exposure occurs through dietary consumption of contaminated maize. Populations that eat milled or ground maize as a dietary staple can be exposed to significant amounts of fumonisins and to lesser amounts of fusarin C.

An IARC (1993) working group concluded that there was sufficient evidence for the carcinogenicity to experimental animals of cultures of F. moniliforme that contain significant amounts of fumonisins, and limited evidence for the carcinogenicity of fumonisin B_1 and fusarin C.

A number of ecological studies have addressed the relationship between exposure to *Fusarium* toxins and oesophageal cancer. Most of the studies refer to mixtures of many toxins from many species of fungi on maize.

Marasas *et al.* (1979) examined the amounts of deoxynivalenol and zearalenone in samples of mouldy maize from randomly selected areas in the high-risk and low-risk oesophageal cancer regions of the Transkei, where maize is the main dietary staple. The level of contamination of maize kernels with each of these two *Fusarium* mycotoxins was apparently higher in the pooled samples from the high-risk than the low-risk region. In an extension of this study, Marasas *et al.* (1981) included an area of the Transkei with an intermediate rate of oesophageal cancer and collected visibly healthy maize samples at random from each of the three study areas. The proportion of kernels in both mouldy and healthy maize samples infected by *F. graminearum* (which was responsible for contamination of the crops with deoxynivalenol and zearalenone), was not correlated with oesophageal cancer rates.

Marasas *et al.* (1988) studied the prevalence of three *Fusarium* species and other fungi in home-grown maize harvested in 1985 by 12 households situated in a district of high incidence of oesophageal cancer in the Transkei (Kentani) and by 12 households in a low-incidence district (Bizana). Households in the high-incidence area were identified during a preliminary cytological screening for oesophageal cancer as having one or more adult occupants who showed mild to severe oesophageal abnormalities; households in the other study area were chosen at random. The ears of maize were sorted by the housewife at each domicile into 'good' ears intended for making porridge and 'mouldy' ears intended for brewing beer. No correlation was found between the occurrence of *F. graminearum* in healthy maize and risk for oesophageal cancer, but an inverse correlation was seen with the occurrence of this fungus in mouldy maize. However, the mean proportions of maize kernels infected with *F. moniliforme* in both healthy and mouldy maize samples from households in the area of high oesophageal cancer incidence were significantly higher (42% in healthy and 68% in mouldy maize) than those in the low-incidence area (8% and 35%, respectively). The same authors conducted a similar survey one year later, with the same criteria for high and low incidence but adding 24 households from a study area with an intermediate incidence of oesophageal cancer (Butterworth). Although the proportion of kernels infected with *F. moniliforme* in healthy maize from the latter area lay between those from the high- and low-incidence areas, further subdivision of households in the intermediate-incidence area into 12 situated in a low-risk zone and 12 in a high-risk zone (with an estimated six-fold difference in oesophageal cancer rates) did not reveal a difference in the proportion of infected kernels in the corresponding samples (26 and 24%, respectively). Furthermore, there was no difference in the prevalence of cytological abnormalities of the oesophagus in adult occupants of the low- and high-risk zones of the intermediate-incidence area and the sampling strategy differed between the high- and low-risk areas.

Sydenham *et al.* (1990a) found high concentrations of various *Fusarium* mycotoxins in the same samples of mouldy home-grown maize collected during 1985 and examined by Marasas *et al.* (1988). The mean levels of nivalenol and zearalenone, produced by *F graminearum*, were significantly higher in mouldy maize samples from the low-risk area than in those from the high-risk area (Sydenham *et al.*, 1990b). Significantly higher mean numbers of kernels infected with *F. moniliforme* and correspondingly higher levels of the mycotoxins fumonisin B_1 and fumonisin B_2 were found in mouldy maize samples in the high-risk oesophageal cancer area than in the low-risk area ($p < 0.01$). Fumonisin B_1 and B_2 levels in healthy maize samples from the low-risk area were approximately 20 times lower than those in healthy samples from the high-risk area, and only three out of 12 samples in the low-risk areas contained these toxins versus 12/12 in the high-risk areas, but again the sampling strategy differed between the high- and low-risk areas.

Because of the methodological difficulties encountered in these studies, the IARC (1993) working group concluded that there was inadequate evidence in humans for the carcinogenicity of toxins derived from *F. moniliforme* and that toxins derived from *F. moniliforme* were possibly carcinogenic to humans.

Human papillomaviruses

Dillner *et al.* (1994), in a study in Sweden based on serology (anti-HPV antibody), found an association between the HPV 16 subtype and oesophageal cancer (OR = 14.6); however, in a subsequent study (Lagergren *et al.*, 1999), no association was found with high serum antibody levels for either the HPV 16 (OR = 0.9) or the 18 subtypes (OR = 0.3). In South Africa, Hale *et al.* (1989) found HPV in 13/20 oesophageal cancer biopsies; no control specimens were tested. However in another South African study, no virally-induced koilocytosis was found in 513 oesophageal cancer autopsies in the western Cape and the Transkei (Jaskiewicz *et al.*, 1992). It is possible that HPV is merely an indirect measure of poorer environmental conditions, known to be risk factors for the development of oesophageal cancer.

Other exposures

In a small case–control study in Ethiopia, Astini *et al.* (1990) found that subjects with oesophageal cancer drank less water during

meals (2/26) than controls (37/52) (OR = 0.06; 95% CI 0.02–0.19). No association with intake of hot food was found.

Genetic factors

Knowledge about the molecular and genetic basis of oesophageal cancer development has increased significantly and the mechanisms of carcinogenesis have been reviewed (see, for example, Montesano *et al.*, 1996; Stemmerman *et al.*, 1994). One area of interest, largely unexplored in Africa, has been the epidemiology of aldehyde dehydrogenase 2 (ALDH2) and its mutant allele ALDH*2. ALDH2 is a key enzyme that eliminates acetaldehyde formed from alcohol. Acetaldehyde is thought to be a carcinogen and may be responsible for alcohol-related cancers in humans (Blot *et al.*, 1991). The mutation in ALDH*2 leads to inactivity of the enzyme and accumulation of acetaldehyde; this allele is common in far-eastern populations and is responsible for the 'flushing syndrome'. Increased risks for oesophageal and upper digestive tract cancers have been found in relation to the presence of the ALDH*2 mutant in Japan (Yokoyama *et al.*, 1998). The relevance of ALDH2 metabolism in the epidemiology of oesophageal cancer in Africa is, however, unclear and the distribution of these mutants in African populations is unknown.

Conclusion

While the importance of both alcohol and tobacco in the development of oesophageal cancer in Africa (and other parts of the world) is clear, much needs to be done to measure the relative importance of different alcoholic drinks in different settings. Defining the content of these drinks is notoriously difficult and it is often unclear whether they should be defined according to their alcoholic content or to a range of potential contaminants. In addition, the 'recipes' for many of the alcoholic drinks vary from place to place, seasonally and over time, often depending upon which fruits or vegetables are available. This makes any precise measurement of exposure very problematic.

Smoking data appear to be reasonably well collected retrospectively, but data on diet and alcohol, especially usual quantities consumed in the past have not been uniformly collected, especially in Africa. In addition it is also often difficult to identify a role for dietary factors in studies that are based within populations that are typically poor and consuming a relatively homogeneous diet.

The Transkei has been consistently associated with high oesophageal incidence rates, and the risks appear to increase with increasing period of residence there, even after adjustment for smoking and alcohol consumption (albeit incomplete). This suggests the influence of an environmental factor, but it remains unclear which factors are responsible (low nutritional status, exposure to mycotoxins).

References

Ahmed, N. (1966) Geographical incidence of oesophageal cancer in West Kenya. *E. Afr. Med. J.*, **43**, 235–248

Ahmed, N. & Cook, P. (1969) The incidence of cancer of the oesophagus in west Kenya. *Br. J. Cancer*, **23**, 302–312

Astini, C., Mele, A., Desta, A., Doria, F., Carrieri, M.P., Osborn, J. & Pasquini, P. (1990) Drinking water during meals and oesophageal cancer: a hypothesis derived from a case control study in Ethiopia. *Ann. Oncol.*, **1**, 447–448

Berman, C. (1935) Malignant diseases in the Bantu of Johannesburg and the Witwatersrand gold mines. *S. Afr. J. Med. Sci.*, pp. 12–30

Blot, W.J., Devesa, S.S., Kneller, R.W. & Fraumeni, J.F. (1991) Rising incidence of adenocarcinoma of the esophagus and gastric cardia. *JAMA*, **265**, 1287–1289

Bradshaw, E. & Schonland, M. (1969) Oesophageal and lung cancers in Natal African males in relation to certain socioeconomic factors. *Br. J. Cancer*, **23**, 275–284

Bradshaw, E. & Schonland, M. (1974) Smoking, drinking and oesophageal caner in African males of Johannesburg, South Africa. *Br. J. Cancer*, **30**, 157–163

Bradshaw, E., McGlashan, N.D., Fitzgerald, D. & Harington, J.S. (1982) Analyses of cancer incidence in black gold miners from Southern Africa (1964-79). *Br. J. Cancer*, **46**, 737–748

Bradshaw E, McGlashan ND, Harington JS. The use of tobacco and alcoholic beverages by male and female Xhosa in Transkei in relation to cancer of the oesophagus. Institute of Social and Economic Research, Rhodes University, 1983.

Brown, L.M., Silverman, D.T., Pottern, L.M., Schoenberg, J.B., Greenberg, R.S., Swanson, G.M., Liff, J.M., Schwartz, A.G., Hayes, R.B., Blot, W.J. & Hoover, R.N. (1994) Adenocarcinoma of the esophagus and esophagogastric junction in white men in the United States: alcohol, tobacco, and socioeconomic factors. *Cancer Causes Control*, **5**, 333–340

Brown, L.M., Swanson, C.A., Gridley, G., Swanson, G.M., Silverman, D.T., Greenberg, R.S., Hayes, R.B., Schoenberg, J.B., Pottern, L.M., Schwartz, A.G., Liff, J.M., Hoover, R. & Fraumeni, J.F., Jr (1998) Dietary factors and the risk of squamous cell esophageal cancer among black and white men in the United States. *Cancer Causes Control*, **9**, 467–474

Burrell, R.J.W. (1957) Oesophageal cancer in the Bantu. *S. Afr. Med. J.*, **31**, 401–409

Burrell, R.J.W. (1962) Oesophageal cancer among Bantu in the Transkei. *J. Natl Cancer Inst.*, **28**, 495–514

Cheng, K.K., Day, N.E., Duffy, S.W., Lam, T.H., Fok, M. & Wong, J. (1992) Pickles vegetables in the aetiology of oesophageal cancer in Hong Kong Chinese. *Lancet*, **339**, 1314–1317

Collis, C.H., Cook, P.J., Foreman, J.K. & Palframan, J.F. (1971) A search for nitrosamines in East African spirit samples from areas of varying oesophageal cancer frequency. *Gut*, **12**, 1015–1018

Cook, P. (1971) Cancer of the oesophagus in Africa. A summary and evaluation of the evidence for the frequency of occurrence and a preliminary indicator of the possible association with the consumption of alcoholic drinks made from maize. *Br. J. Cancer*, **25**, 853–880

Cook, P.J. & Burkitt, D.P. (1971) Cancer in Africa. *Br. Med Bull.*, **27**, 14–20

Cook-Mozzaffari, P. (1989) Epidemiology and predisposing factors. In: Hurt, E.L., ed., *Management of Oesophageal Cancer*, London, Springer Verlag

Dillner, J., Knekt, P., Schiller, J.T. & Hakulinen, T. (1994) Prospective seroepidemiological evidence that human papillomavirus type 16 infection is a risk factor for oesophageal squamous cell carcinoma. *Br. Med. J.*, **311**, 1346

Ferlay, J., Bray, F., Pisani, P. & Parkin, D.M. (2001) *GLOBOCAN 2000: Cancer Incidence, Mortality and Prevalence Worldwide*, Version 1.0, IARC CancerBase No. 5 [CD-ROM], Lyon, IARCPress

Gatei, D.G., Odhiambo, P.A., Orinda, D.A., Muruka, F.J. & Wasunna, A. (1978) Retrospective study of carcinoma of the oesophagus in Kenya. *Cancer Res.*, **38**, 303–307

Hale, M.J., Liptz, T.R. & Paterson, A.C. (1989) Association between human papollomavirus and carcinoma of the oesophagus in South African blacks. A histochemical and immunohistochemical study. *S. Afr. Med. J.*, **76**, 329–330

Hewer, T., Rose, E., Ghadirian, P., Castegnaro, M., Malaveille, C., Bartsch, H. & Day, N. (1978) Ingested mutagens from opium and tobacco pyrolysis products and cancer of the oesophagus. *Lancet*, **ii**, 494–496

Higginson, J. & Oettle, A.G. (1960) Cancer incidence in the Bantu and "Cape Colored" races of South Africa: Report of a cancer survey in the Transvaal (1953-55). *J. Natl Cancer Inst.*, **24**, 589–671

Hsia, C.C., Wu, J.L., Lu, X.Q. & Li, Y.S. (1988) Natural occurrence and clastogenic effects of nivalenol, deoxynivalenol, 3-acetyl-deoxynivalenol, 15-acetyl-deoxynivalenol, and zearalenone in corn from a high-risk area of esophageal cancer. *Cancer Detect. Prev.*, **13**, 79–86

IARC (1986) *IARC Monographs on the Evaluation of Carcinogenic Risk of Chemicals to Humans.* Volume 38, *Tobacco Smoking*, Lyon, IARC

IARC (1988) *IARC Monographs on the Evaluation of Carcinogenic Risks to Humans.* Volume 44, *Alcohol Drinking*, Lyon, IARC

IARC (1993) *IARC Monographs on the Evaluation of Carcinogenic Risks to Humans.* Volume 56, *Some Naturally Occurring Substances: Food Items and Constituents, Heterocyclic Aromatic Amines and Mycotoxins*, Lyon, IARC

Jaskiewicz, K., Marasas, W.F.O., Van der Walt, F.E. (1987a) Oesophageal and other main cancer patterns in four districts of Transkei 1981-1984. *S. Afr. Med. J.*, **72**, 27–30

Jaskiewicz, K., van Rensburg, S.J., Marasas, W.E. & Gelderblom, W.C. (1987b) Carcinogenicity of Fusarium moniliforme culture material in rats. *J. Natl Cancer Inst.*, **78**, 321–325

Jaskiewicz, K., Banach, L., Mafungo, V. & Knobel, J. (1992) Oesophageal mucosa in a population at risk of oesophageal cancer: Post-mortem studies. *Int. J. Cancer*, **50**, 32–35

Keen, P. & Martin P. (1971) Is aflatoxin carcinogenic in man? The evidence in Swaziland. *Trop. Geog. Med.*, **23**, 44–53

Kneebone, R.L. & Mannell, A. (1985) Cancer of the oesophagus in Soweto. *S. Afr. Med. J.*, **67**, 839–842

Lu JB, Yang WX, Liu JM, Li YS, Qin YM. Trends in morbidity and mortality for oesophageal cancer in Linxian County, 1959-1983. *Int J Cancer* 1985, **36**, 643-5.

Lagergren, J., Wang, Z., Bergstrom, R., Dillner, J. & Nyren, O. (1999) Cancer: a nationwide seroepidmiologic case-control study in Sweden. *JNCI*, **91**, 156–162

Macrae, S.M. & Cook, B.V. (1975) A retrospective study of the cancer patterns among hospital inpatients in Botswana 1960-1972. *Br. J. Cancer*, **32**, 121–133

Makaula, A.N., Marasas, W.F., Venter, F., Badenhost, C., Bradshaw, D. & Swanenvelder, S. (1996) Oesophageal and other cancer patterns in four selected districts of Transkei, Southern Africa: 1985-1990. *Afr. J. Health Sci.*, **3**, 11–15

Marasas, W.E.O., van Rensburg, S.J. & Mirocha, C.J. (1979) Incidence of *Fusarium* species and the mycotoxins deoxynivalenol and zearalenone in corn produced in esophageal cancer areas in Transkei. *J. Agric. Food Chem.*, **27**, 1108–1112

Marasas, W.E.O., Wehner, P.C., van Rensburg, S.J. & van Schalkwyk, D.J. (1981) Mycoflora of corn produced in human esophageal cancer areas in Transkei, southern Africa. *Phytopathology*, **71**, 792–796

Marasas, W.E.O., Jaskiewicz, K., Venter, F.S. & van Schalkwyk, D.J. (1988) *Fusarium moniliforme* contamination of maize in oesophageal cancer areas in Transkei. *S. Afr. Med. J.*, **74**, 110–114

McGlashan, N.D. (1969a) Oesophageal cancer and alcoholic spirits in central Africa. *Gut*, **10**, 643–650

McGlashan, N.D. (1969b) Nitrosamines in South African drinks in relation to oesophageal cancer. *S. Afr. Med. J.*, **43**, 800

McGlashan, N.D., Walters, C.L. & McLean, M.D. (1968) Nitrosamines in African alcoholic spirits and oesophageal cancer. *Lancet*, **ii**, 1017

McGlashan, N.D., Bradshaw, E. & Harington, J.S. (1982) Cancer of the oesophagus and the use of tobacco and alcoholic beverages in Transkei 1975-6. *Int. J. Cancer*, **29**, 249–256

Montesano, R., Hollstein, M. & Hainaut, P. (1996) Genetic alterations in esophageal cancer and their relevance to etiology and pathogenesis: a review. *Int. J. Cancer*, **69**, 1–11

Muir Grieve, J. (1967) *Cancer in the Cape Division of South Africa. A Demographic and Medical Survey*, Oxford, Oxford University Press

Muir Grieve, J. (1970) South Africa, Cape Province. In: Doll, R., Muir, C. & Waterhouse, J., eds, *Cancer Incidence in Five Continents*, Vol. II, Berlin, Springer Verlag, pp. 98–109

Oettlé, A.G. (1963) Regional variations in the frequency of Bantu oesophageal cancer cases admitted to hospitals in South Africa. *S. Afr. Med. J.*, **37**, 434–439

Oettlé, A.G. (1967) Primary neoplasms of the alimentary canal in Whites and Bantu of the Transvaal, 1949-1953. *National Cancer Institute Monographs*, **25**, 97–109

Pacella-Norman, R., Urban, M.I., Sitas, F., Carrara, H., Sur, R., Hale, M., Ruff, P., Patel, M., Newton, R., Bull, D. & Beral, V. (2002) Risk factors for oesophageal, lung, oral and laryngeal cancers in black South Africans. *Br. J. Cancer*, **86**, 1751–1756

Parkin, D.M., Vizcaino, A.P., Skinner, M.E.G. & Ndhlovu, A. (1994) Cancer patterns and risk factors in the African population of southwestern Zimbabwe, 1963-1977. *Cancer Epidemiol. Biomarkers Prev.*, **3**, 537–547

Rose, E.F. (1967) A study of esophageal cancer in the Transkei. *Natl Cancer Inst. Monogr.*, **25**, 83–96

Rose, E.F. (1973) Esophageal cancer in the Transkei: 1955-69. *J. Natl Cancer Inst.*, **51**, 7–16

Rose, E.F. (1973) Esophageal cancer in the Transkei: 1955-69. *J. Natl Cancer Inst.*, **51**, 7–16

Rose, E. (1978) Environmental factors associated with cancer of the esophagus in Transkei. In: Silber, W., ed., *Carcinoma of the Esophagus*, Rotterdam, Balkema, pp.91–98

Rose, E.F. & McGlashan, N.D. (1975) The spatial distribution of oesophageal carcinoma in the Transkei, South Africa. *Br. J. Cancer*, **31**, 197–206

Rose, E.F. & Fellingham, S.A. (1981) Cancer patterns inTranskei. *S. Afr. J. Sci.*, **77**, 555–561

Sammon, A.M. (1992) A case-control study of diet and social factors in cancer of the oesophagus in Transkei. *Cancer*, **69**, 860–865

Schonland, M. & Bradshaw, R. (1968) Cancer in the Natal African and Indian 1964-1966. *Int. J. Cancer*, **3**, 304–316

Segal, I., Reinach, S.G. & de Beer, M. (1988) Factors associated with oesophageal cancer in Soweto, South Africa. *Br. J. Cancer*, **58**, 681–686

Silber, W. (1985) Carcinoma of the oesophagus: aspects of epidemiology and aetiology. *Proc. Nutr. Soc.*, **44**, 101–110

Sitas, F., Blaauw, D., Terblanche, M. & Madhoo, J. (1998) *Incidence of histologically diagnosed cancer in South Africa 1992*, Johannesburg, South African Institue of Medical Research

Stemmermann, G., Heffelfinger, S.C., Noffsinger, A., Zhong Hui, Y., Miller, M.A. & Fenoglio-Preiser, C.M. (1994) The molecular biology of esophageal and gastric cancer and their precursors: Oncogenes, tumor suppressor genes, and growth factors. *Human Pathol.*, **25**, 968–981

Sydenham, E.W, Gelderblom, W.C.A., Thiel, P.O. & Marasas, W.E.O. (1990a) Evidence for the natural occurrence of fumonisin B1, a mycotoxin produced by *Fusarium moniliforme*, in corn. *J. Agric. Food Chem.*, **38**, 285–290

Sydenham, E.W, Thiel, P.G., Marasas, W.E.O., Shephard, G.S., Van Schalkwyk, D.J. & Koch, K.R. (1990b) Natural occurrence of some *Fusarium* mycotoxins in corn from low and high esophageal cancer prevalence areas of the Transkei, southern Africa. *J. Agric. Food Chem.*, **38**, 1900–1903

Van Rensburg, S.J. (1981) Epidemiologic and dietary evidence for a specific nutritional predisposition to esophageal cancer. *J. Natl Cancer Inst.*, **67**, 243–251

Van Rensburg, S.J., Ambrose, S.B., Rose, E.F. & Plessis, J.P. (1983) Nutritional status of African populations predisposed to esophageal cancer. *Nutr. Cancer*, **4**, 206–214

Van Rensburg, S.J., Bradshaw, E.S. & Rose, E.F. (1985) Oesophageal cancer in Zulu men, South Africa. A case control study. *Br. J. Cancer*, **51**, 339–405

Vint, F.W. (1935) Malignant disease in the natives of Kenya. *Lancet*, **ii**, 628–630

Vizcaino, A.P., Parkin, D.M., Skinner & M.E.G. (1995) Risk factors associated with oesophageal cancer in Bulawayo, Zimbabwe. *Br. J. Cancer*, **72**, 769–773

Wabinga, H.R., Parkin, D.M., Wabwire-Mangen, F. & Nambooze, S. (2000) Trends in cancer incidence in Kyadondo County, Uganda, 1960-1997. *Br. J. Cancer*, **82**, 1585–1592

Yokoyama, A., Muramatsu, T., Ohmori, T., Yokoyama, T., Okuyama, K., Takahashi, H., Hasegawa, Y., Higushi, S., Maruyama, K., Shirakura, K. & Ishii H. (1998) Alcohol related cancers and aldehyde dehydrogenase-2 in Japanese alcoholics. *Carcinogenesis*, **19**, 1383–1387

4.14 Oral cavity and pharynx

Introduction

This chapter considers cancers of the oral cavity (ICD-10 codes C00–C06, including lip, tongue and mouth cancers), cancers of the pharynx, excluding nasopharynx (ICD-10 codes C09–C10 and C12–C14) and tumours of the salivary glands (ICD-10 codes C07–C08).

Cancers of this group were responsible for an estimated 390 000 new cases worldwide in 2000 (3.9% of the total). They are more common in men (70% of cases), in whom they account for 5.1% of new cancer cases, being the seventh most common form of cancer.

Cancers of the oral cavity, and those of the pharynx, are mainly squamous-cell carcinomas arising in the mucosa of the mouth (including cheek, lips and palate), gums, tongue and the oropharynx (including tonsil) and hypopharynx (including the pyriform fossa). There is a great deal of geographical variation in their incidence. High incidence rates are seen particularly in the Indian subcontinent and in Papua New Guinea (related to chewing of tobacco/betel, as described below). Rates are also high in some parts of western (France and Switzerland) and eastern (Hungary, Slovakia) Europe, where the important factors are tobacco and alcohol. The distributions of sites within the oral cavity and pharynx also differ considerably. Lip cancers are generally uncommon, except in white populations exposed to high levels of ultraviolet radiation, as in Australia; the lower lip is involved in some 80% of cases. In France, pharyngeal cancers predominate, while in most series from India, most cancers occur in the mouth (gum or floor of mouth).

Carcinomas of the salivary glands are relatively rare. They comprise less than 10% of cancers of the oral cavity and pharynx, and are mainly adenocarcinomas.

Precancerous lesions

Oral leukoplakia is defined as a white patch or plaque occurring on the oral mucosal surface that cannot be characterized clinically or pathologically as any other disease (WHO, 1978). Leukoplakias are considered to be precancerous lesions, since a proportion will progress to dysplasia, carcinoma *in situ* and invasive cancer. The overall risk of malignancy is some 1–5%, but varies with clinical subtype, with non-homogeneous leukoplakias, particularly nodular, being more prone to progression than homogeneous lesions. Oral erythroplakia refers to red patches on the mucosa, indicating epithelial atrophy and inflammation; these lesions are much rarer than leukoplakia, but have a much higher probability of malignant transformation (tenfold in some series). Oral submucous fibrosis has been more recently characterized and appears to be specifically linked to areca nut use. It manifests as mucosal rigidity and fibrous bands, with restricted mouth opening and tongue mobility; malignant transformation is common.

Descriptive epidemiology in Africa

In Africa, the frequency of cancers of the oral cavity and pharynx is rather lower than their worldwide frequency. The estimated 19 500 new cases in 2000 represent 3.1% of new cancers (3.9% in men, 2.4% in women). Worldwide, cancers of the pharynx (excluding nasopharynx) represent less than one third of such cancers, but they are apparently more rare in Africa, where they make up only 17% of the total.

Table 1 shows age-standardized incidence rates from different centres, as reported in this volume, with data from Europe, North America and India for comparison. Table 2 shows incidence data from time periods in the 1960s and 1970s.

The incidence rates in Africa are generally lower than in the European and US populations in Table 1. For cancers of the oral cavity, the highest recorded incidence is in white males from Harare, Zimbabwe. Only 5 of the 19 cases upon which this rate is based were cancers of the lip. A high incidence is observed also in South African white males. In Reunion, only 2 of the 142 cancers in men were lip cancers, the remainder being equally divided between the oral cavity and pharynx, with the most common sites being mouth (30%), pyriform sinus (19%), tongue (17%) and tonsil (13%).

The data from the 1960s suggest that rates of oral cancer were lower in the Indian population of Natal province than in India, with a small excess in females (Table 2). The incidence of histologically diagnosed cancers from the South African National Registry (Table 1) suggests that the rates have remained moderate, and that the female predominance remains. Schonland and Bradshaw (1968) provided a commentary on the three South African series in Table 2. They noted that a relatively high proportion of oral–pharyngeal cancers in the white population of Cape Town were lip cancers (52.6% of male cases, 21.6% of female cases). There was a relatively high incidence of mouth cancers among Indian females in Durban. Altini and Kola (1985) estimated incidence rates of oral squamous cell cancers from pathology laboratory data in the Witwatersrand of South Africa for the period 1970–80. The age-standardized rates were 5.1 in men and 0.9 in women, with the most common sites involved being the tongue (51.4% cases) and floor of the mouth (32.7%).

Relative frequency data from pathology-based series frequently give the impression that oral cancers, in particular, are more common than the incidence data in Tables 1 and 2 suggest. Thus, the frequency of oral cancers in men in the series from Gabon was 10.5%, from Namibia 10.3% and from Swaziland 9.8%. These high frequencies probably relate, at least in part, to ease of biopsy. The same phenomenon can be observed in the frequency data in published series reported elsewhere in this volume. Nevertheless, the high frequency of oral cancers consistently reported in series from Sudan (see Chapter 3.1.5; Idris *et al.*, 1995a) is particularly noteworthy, in view of what is known of the prevalence of risk factors in the Sudanese population.

Most published data from Africa comprise descriptions of case series, from various clinical settings, such as those from Kenya (Onyango *et al.*, 1995 a, b) and Nigeria (Ogunbodede & Ugboko, 1997).

Migrant studies

Templeton and Viegas (1970) noted that oral cancer comprised a greater proportion of cancers in the population of Indian origin in Uganda, and recorded by the Kampala Cancer Registry (mainly histology-based) in 1959–68 (5.7%) than among the black (1.4%) or European (0.8%) populations, and ascribed this to chewing of betel nut. They noted, however, that the habit was much less frequent in this population than in India. Chopra *et al.* (1975) made equivalent observations in Kenya, where cancers of the tongue and mouth comprised 7% of cancers in Asian males and 2.4% in females, compared with 0.9% in African males and 1.7% in females. They noted that these frequencies were far below those in Indian data (from Baroda) and that chewing and bidi smoking are relatively uncommon in Kenyan Asians (perhaps due to their relatively high social status). Some data on Indian populations resident in South Africa are described below.

Risk factors

Tobacco is a major risk factor for cancers of the tongue, mouth and pharynx, whether smoked (IARC, 1986) or chewed (IARC, 1985).

Table 1a. Age-standardized (world) and cumulative (0-64) incidence
Mouth (C00-06)

	MALE				FEMALE			
	Cases	CRUDE	ASR(W)	Cumulative	Cases	CRUDE	ASR(W)	Cumulative
		(per 100,000)		(%)		(per 100,000)		(%)
Africa, North								
Algeria, Algiers (1993-1997)	49	0.9	**1.3**	0.08	29	0.5	**0.7**	0.05
Algeria, Constantine (1994-1997)	21	1.4	**2.5**	0.16	9	0.6	**1.0**	0.04
Algeria, Oran (1996-1998)	26	1.5	**2.3**	0.14	10	0.6	**0.9**	0.07
Algeria, Setif (1993-1997)	46	1.5	**2.8**	0.14	16	0.5	**0.9**	0.05
Tunisia, Centre, Sousse (1993-1997)	31	2.7	**3.7**	0.19	8	0.7	**1.0**	0.08
Tunisia, North, Tunis (1994)	48	2.2	**2.8**	0.23	16	0.8	**1.0**	0.05
Tunisia, Sfax (1997)	13	3.3	**4.2**	0.26	2	0.5	**0.6**	0.06
Africa, West								
The Gambia (1997-1998)	4	0.4	**0.9**	0.07	7	0.7	**1.2**	0.07
Guinea, Conakry (1996-1999)	33	1.4	**2.9**	0.21	14	0.6	**1.3**	0.10
Mali, Bamako (1988-1997)	14	0.4	**0.8**	0.07	11	0.3	**0.6**	0.02
Niger, Niamey (1993-1999)	10	0.5	**1.8**	0.09	9	0.5	**0.8**	0.07
Nigeria, Ibadan (1998-1999)	9	0.6	**1.1**	0.05	2	0.1	**0.3**	0.02
Africa, Central								
Congo, Brazzaville (1996-1999)	9	0.7	**1.2**	0.10	13	1.1	**1.6**	0.12
Africa, East								
France, La Reunion (1988-1994)	205	9.8	**12.5**	1.00	17	0.8	**0.9**	0.06
Kenya, Eldoret (1998-2000)	16	1.7	**3.7**	0.31	5	0.5	**1.4**	0.11
Malawi, Blantyre (2000-2001)	4	0.4	**0.8**	0.08	7	0.8	**1.3**	0.13
Uganda, Kyadondo County (1993-1997)	23	0.8	**2.1**	0.14	16	0.6	**1.8**	0.11
Zimbabwe, Harare: African (1990-1993)	17	0.7	**1.7**	0.10	5	0.2	**1.0**	0.03
Zimbabwe, Harare: African (1994-1997)	23	0.8	**1.9**	0.10	10	0.4	**1.2**	0.03
Zimbabwe, Harare: European (1990-1997)	24	15.7	**9.4**	0.58	17	10.1	**5.4**	0.38
Africa, South								
Namibia (1995-1998)	265	8.3	**15.4**	0.97	130	4.1	**6.5**	0.42
South Africa: Black (1989-1992)	2545	4.5	**8.7**	0.58	598	1.1	**1.7**	0.11
South Africa: Indian (1989-1992)	65	3.3	**4.8**	0.38	83	4.2	**5.5**	0.45
South Africa: Mixed race (1989-1992)	449	7.0	**13.5**	0.87	143	2.1	**3.3**	0.22
South Africa: White (1989-1992)	1294	12.9	**11.8**	0.77	559	5.5	**4.3**	0.26
South Africa, Transkei, Umtata (1996-1998)	14	3.9	**7.9**	0.64	2	0.5	**0.6**	-
South Africa, Transkei, 4 districts (1996-1998)	11	1.5	**2.9**	0.25	2	0.2	**0.3**	0.02
Swaziland (1996-1999)	18	1.0	**2.2**	0.15	12	0.6	**1.2**	0.07
Europe/USA								
USA, SEER: White (1993-1997)	4309	8.9	**6.9**	0.43	2298	4.6	**2.9**	0.18
USA, SEER: Black (1993-1997)	476	7.1	**8.4**	0.67	206	2.8	**2.8**	0.20
France, 8 registries (1993-1997)	2348	17.1	**13.1**	1.01	468	3.2	**2.1**	0.14
The Netherlands (1993-1997)	2738	7.2	**5.3**	0.35	1518	3.9	**2.5**	0.17
UK, England (1993-1997)	5845	4.9	**3.4**	0.22	3550	2.8	**1.6**	0.09
India								
Ahmedabad (1993-1997)	1075	10.8	**15.9**	1.16	268	3.0	**4.6**	0.33
Mumbai (Bombay) (1993-1997)	2248	7.6	**11.7**	0.76	1048	4.3	**6.9**	0.45

In italics: histopathology-based registries

The association has been demonstrated in case–control and cohort studies in a variety of populations. Alcohol drinking is also an important risk factor (IARC, 1988), and acts multiplicatively with smoking with respect to cancers of both the oral cavity and pharynx. Differences in the prevalence and use of tobacco and alcohol are thought to explain the differences in incidence between men and women, and between blacks and whites in the USA (Day et al., 1993). Diet may also be important in etiology, and diets low in fruit and vegetables have been found to increase risk, possibly due to low intake of micronutrients, especially vitamin C (WCRF, 1997). More recently, the role of human papillomaviruses has received attention, following detection of HPV DNA in tumour tissue (IARC, 1995).

Tobacco smoking/alcohol drinking
In a case–control study based upon cancer patients admitted to two hospitals in Johannesburg and Soweto, Pacella-Norman et al. (2002) compared 124 cases of oral cancer (87 men, 37 women)

with control subjects (2174) with cancers not associated with tobacco or alcohol consumption. The odds ratio associated with heavy smoking in males (15+ g of tobacco per day) was 12.5 (95% CI 4.6–33.5) and in females, 6.2 (95% CI 0.9–44.2). Daily alcohol consumption, adjusted for smoking, was a not risk factor for the development of oral cancer in either sex.

Tobacco/betel chewing
The relatively high incidence of oral cancer, especially cancers of the tongue and mouth, among Indian females in Durban, Natal, has been noted above. Schonland and Bradshaw (1969) investigated chewing habits in a special survey of 500 households in Durban. They noted that the habit was more frequent in females (30.7%) than in males (5.5%), increased in prevalence with age, and decreased with level of educational attainment. The quid used in Durban rarely contained tobacco (7.8% male chewers, 2.8% females), comprising betel nut and/or leaf, usually with lime and flavouring. The authors considered that the habit was slowly dying out in this community.

Table 1b. Age-standardized (world) and cumulative (0-64) incidence
Salivary gland (C07-08)

	MALE				FEMALE			
	Cases	CRUDE	ASR(W) (per 100,000)	Cumulative (%)	Cases	CRUDE	ASR(W) (per 100,000)	Cumulative (%)
Africa, North								
Algeria, Algiers (1993-1997)	18	0.3	0.4	0.03	9	0.2	0.2	0.01
Algeria, Constantine (1994-1997)	2	0.1	0.2	0.02	2	0.1	0.2	0.00
Algeria, Oran (1996-1998)	3	0.2	0.3	-	5	0.3	0.3	0.02
Algeria, Setif (1993-1997)	7	0.2	0.4	0.01	8	0.3	0.4	0.04
Tunisia, Centre, Sousse (1993-1997)	3	0.3	0.3	0.01	4	0.4	0.4	0.01
Tunisia, North, Tunis (1994)	3	0.1	0.2	0.01	5	0.2	0.3	0.02
Tunisia, Sfax (1997)	1	0.3	0.3	0.02	-	-	-	-
Africa, West								
The Gambia (1997-1998)	2	0.2	0.1	0.01	2	0.2	-	-
Guinea, Conakry (1996-1999)	3	0.1	0.2	0.01	4	0.2	0.3	0.02
Mali, Bamako (1988-1997)	-	-	-	-	3	0.1	0.2	0.01
Niger, Niamey (1993-1999)	5	0.3	0.7	0.04	3	0.2	0.3	0.02
Nigeria, Ibadan (1998-1999)	5	0.3	0.6	0.06	4	0.3	0.4	0.04
Africa, Central								
Congo, Brazzaville (1996-1999)	5	0.4	0.5	0.05	5	0.4	0.5	0.04
Africa, East								
France, La Reunion (1988-1994)	8	0.4	0.4	0.03	5	0.2	0.2	0.03
Kenya, Eldoret (1998-2000)	3	0.3	0.4	0.03	3	0.3	0.7	0.04
Malawi, Blantyre (2000-2001)	2	0.2	0.9	0.11	-	-	-	-
Uganda, Kyadondo County (1993-1997)	4	0.1	0.3	0.01	9	0.3	0.8	0.07
Zimbabwe, Harare: African (1990-1993)	7	0.3	0.7	0.02	6	0.3	0.5	0.01
Zimbabwe, Harare: African (1994-1997)	13	0.5	1.0	0.07	14	0.5	0.7	0.04
Zimbabwe, Harare: European (1990-1997)	2	1.3	0.7	0.05	2	1.2	0.8	0.09
Africa, South								
Namibia (1995-1998)	18	0.6	0.9	0.07	16	0.5	0.8	0.06
South Africa: Black (1989-1992)	149	0.3	0.4	0.03	124	0.2	0.3	0.02
South Africa: Indian (1989-1992)	10	0.5	0.8	0.05	8	0.4	0.5	0.05
South Africa: Mixed race (1989-1992)	19	0.3	0.5	0.02	12	0.2	0.3	0.02
South Africa: White (1989-1992)	132	1.3	1.2	0.07	60	0.6	0.5	0.03
South Africa, Transkei, Umtata (1996-1998)	-	-	-	-	-	-	-	-
South Africa, Transkei, 4 districts (1996-1998)	1	0.1	0.3	0.04	-	-	-	-
Swaziland (1996-1999)	2	0.1	0.3	0.03	4	0.2	0.3	0.02
Europe/USA								
USA, SEER: White (1993-1997)	679	1.4	1.1	0.06	538	1.1	0.8	0.05
USA, SEER: Black (1993-1997)	60	0.9	1.0	0.06	51	0.7	0.6	0.05
France, 8 registries (1993-1997)	138	1.0	0.7	0.04	112	0.8	0.5	0.03
The Netherlands (1993-1997)	294	0.8	0.6	0.03	231	0.6	0.4	0.03
UK, England (1993-1997)	1061	0.9	0.6	0.03	883	0.7	0.4	0.03
India								
Ahmedabad (1993-1997)	38	0.4	0.6	0.04	24	0.3	0.4	0.03
Mumbai (Bombay) (1993-1997)	100	0.3	0.5	0.03	59	0.2	0.3	0.02

In italics: histopathology-based registries

In a later study in Durban, Seedat and van Wyk (1988) investigated betel-nut chewing habits and the intake of chillies in the diet in 178 chewers and 124 hospital patients suffering from submucous fibrosis (SF). In the survey of chewers, 63 subjects were found to have features of impending or established SF. Those suffering from SF had practised the habit for a significantly *shorter* period than chewers without SF, and were significantly younger. A significantly larger proportion of this group preferred the boiled nut by itself and not as part of a betel quid (pan). No relationship was established between SF and the use of tobacco, lime or chillies.

van Wyk *et al.* (1993) studied 143 cases of oral squamous-cell carcinoma diagnosed in Indian patients in Natal in 1983–89. Information on smoking and chewing habits was obtained by interview of the patients (52%) or their relatives (29%) or from hospital records (18%). There were 89 women and 54 men. Squamous-cell carcinomas of the cheek (buccal mucosa, alveolar sulcus and gingiva) occurred most frequently, especially in women (64%), while in men tongue cancer predominated (41%). 93% of women (83/89) and 17%

of men (9/54) habitually chewed the areca nut. Most female chewers used only the areca nut (53%), with 13% using betel quids, and 34% both. In contrast, most of the male cases (87%) were smokers, while only 7% of female cases smoked. The cases were compared with a group of "controls": Indian-origin subjects who had been interviewed during a community survey in 1983. From the data on distribution of female cases and "controls" by age stratum and areca nut chewing habit, one can estimate age-stratified (Mantel–Haenszel) odds ratios of 38.7 (95% CI 15.8–104.1) for areca nut alone, and 52.9 (95% CI 11.1–56.8) for areca nut with tobacco, versus no use.

Toombak

The sparse information on the cancer profile in Sudan suggests a relatively high frequency of oral cancer in data from the pathology-based Sudan Cancer Registry (SCR), and from the hospital-based registry in the Radiation and Isotope Centre, Khartoum (RICK) (see Chapter 3.1.5). Idris *et al.* (1995a) confirmed that the frequencies of oral neoplasms in 1970–85 were 12.6% from SCR

Table 1c. Age-standardized (world) and cumulative (0-64) incidence
Pharynx (excl. nasopharynx) (C09-10,C12-14)

	MALE				FEMALE			
	Cases	CRUDE	ASR(W) (per 100,000)	Cumulative (%)	Cases	CRUDE	ASR(W) (per 100,000)	Cumulative (%)
Africa, North								
Algeria, Algiers (1993-1997)	31	0.6	**0.8**	0.05	10	0.2	**0.2**	0.02
Algeria, Constantine (1994-1997)	7	0.5	**0.8**	0.06	1	0.1	**0.1**	0.02
Algeria, Oran (1996-1998)	15	0.8	**1.3**	0.10	6	0.3	**0.5**	0.04
Algeria, Setif (1993-1997)	58	1.9	**3.8**	0.30	9	0.3	**0.5**	0.04
Tunisia, Centre, Sousse (1993-1997)	6	0.5	**0.8**	0.06	2	0.2	**0.2**	0.02
Tunisia, North, Tunis (1994)	16	0.7	**0.9**	0.09	6	0.3	**0.3**	0.03
Tunisia, Sfax (1997)	4	1.0	**1.3**	0.09	4	1.1	**1.4**	0.06
Africa, West								
The Gambia (1997-1998)	-	-	**-**	-	-	-	**-**	-
Guinea, Conakry (1996-1999)	18	0.8	**1.6**	0.11	5	0.2	**0.3**	0.02
Mali, Bamako (1988-1997)	10	0.3	**0.5**	0.02	2	0.1	**0.1**	0.01
Niger, Niamey (1993-1999)	7	0.4	**0.9**	0.05	2	0.1	**0.2**	0.02
Nigeria, Ibadan (1998-1999)	3	0.2	**0.4**	0.05	1	0.1	**0.1**	-
Africa, Central								
Congo, Brazzaville (1996-1999)	13	1.1	**1.7**	0.13	5	0.4	**0.5**	0.04
Africa, East								
France, La Reunion (1988-1994)	228	10.9	**13.9**	1.16	16	0.7	**0.8**	0.08
Kenya, Eldoret (1998-2000)	5	0.5	**0.9**	0.05	-	-	**-**	-
Malawi, Blantyre (2000-2001)	-	-	**-**	-	-	-	**-**	-
Uganda, Kyadondo County (1993-1997)	17	0.6	**1.8**	0.16	6	0.2	**0.7**	0.08
Zimbabwe, Harare: African (1990-1993)	6	0.3	**0.8**	0.03	4	0.2	**0.9**	0.06
Zimbabwe, Harare: African (1994-1997)	15	0.5	**1.3**	0.11	2	0.1	**0.1**	0.01
Zimbabwe, Harare: European (1990-1997)	5	3.3	**1.8**	0.10	5	3.0	**1.6**	0.09
Africa, South								
Namibia (1995-1998)	74	2.3	**4.4**	0.28	26	0.8	**1.3**	0.10
South Africa: Black (1989-1992)	361	0.6	**1.2**	0.09	64	0.1	**0.2**	0.01
South Africa: Indian (1989-1992)	14	0.7	**1.2**	0.06	7	0.4	**0.4**	0.02
South Africa: Mixed race (1989-1992)	64	1.0	**1.8**	0.13	18	0.3	**0.4**	0.04
South Africa: White (1989-1992)	84	0.8	**0.8**	0.05	26	0.3	**0.2**	0.01
South Africa, Transkei, Umtata (1996-1998)	10	2.8	**4.6**	0.36	5	1.2	**1.8**	0.14
South Africa, Transkei, 4 districts (1996-1998)	2	0.3	**0.5**	0.04	-	-	**-**	-
Swaziland (1996-1999)	24	1.4	**3.0**	0.26	5	0.3	**0.4**	0.03
Europe/USA								
USA, SEER: White (1993-1997)	1982	4.1	**3.3**	0.23	715	1.4	**0.9**	0.06
USA, SEER: Black (1993-1997)	417	6.2	**7.4**	0.62	115	1.5	**1.6**	0.14
France, 8 registries (1993-1997)	4438	32.3	**24.4**	1.78	564	3.9	**2.5**	0.17
The Netherlands (1993-1997)	9549	25.0	**18.1**	0.92	2326	6.0	**3.7**	0.24
UK, England (1993-1997)	8499	7.1	**4.7**	0.27	3234	2.5	**1.4**	0.08
India								
Ahmedabad (1993-1997)	736	7.4	**12.1**	0.79	132	1.5	**2.1**	0.14
Mumbai (Bombay) (1993-1997)	1660	5.6	**9.7**	0.56	379	1.6	**2.5**	0.15

In italics: histopathology-based registries

Table 2. Incidence of cancer of the oral cavity in Africa, 1953–74

Registry	Period	Oral cavity		Salivary gland		Pharynx*		Source
		Male	Female	Male	Female	Male	Female	(see Chap. 1)
Senegal, Dakar	1969–74	2.1	2.0	*0.5*	*0.0*	*0.6*	0.0	4
Mozambique, Lourenço Marques	1956–60	*3.0*	*3.1*	*0.0*	*3.8*	*2.2*	*0.0*	1
Nigeria, Ibadan	1960–69	2.2	1.6	1.9	1.4	0.8	*0.4*	3
SA, Cape Province: Bantu	1956–59	*13.7*	–			*6.8*	*1.3*	2
SA, Cape Province: Coloured	1956–59	8.0	*0.9*			*5.4*	*0.2*	2
SA, Cape Province: White	1956–59	28.5	3.4			13.6	*0.8*	2
SA, Johannesburg, Bantu	1953–55	5.5	*1.1*	*0.3*	*0.8*	*0.1*	*0.0*	1
SA, Natal Province: African	1964–66	5.8	*1.5*	*0.8*	*0.8*	4.0	*0.2*	2
SA, Natal Province: Indian	1964–66	*6.7*	11.7	*0.7*	*0.4*	*1.0*	*2.1*	2
Uganda, Kyadondo	1954–60	–	*1.0*	*0.2*	*0.9*	*0.4*	*0.5*	1
Uganda, Kyadondo	1960–71	1.0	1.2	*0.1*	*0.1*	*0.6*	*0.4*	5
Zimbabwe, Bulawayo	1963–72	2.2	–	*0.6*	*0.2*	*1.3*	–	6

Italics: Rate based on less than 10 cases

* Excluding nasopharynx

and 8.1% from RICK. In the SCR series, squamous-cell carcinoma was the most common malignancy (66.5%), followed by tumours of the salivary gland (14.7%), neoplasms of non-epithelial origin (9.6%) and odontogenic neoplasms (8.6%). Men had a higher frequency than women. A large proportion of cases of squamous-cell carcinoma were among patients from northern Sudan. It was noted that 58% of subjects with squamous-cell cancers of the lip and mouth were users of 'toombak', compared with 11% of subjects with salivary or non-epithelial cancers. Toombak is a form of snuff prepared locally in pats of north, central and eastern Sudan from *Nicotiana rustica*, an indigenous tobacco species with high levels of nicotine and nornicotine. The finely ground tobacco leaves are mixed with sodium bicarbonate, water is added, and a paste is made. The resulting 'saffa' is placed in the oral vestibule where it remains for up to several hours. In general, a saffa is replaced 10–30 times per day. In a survey in Nile province, northern Sudan (Idris *et al.*, 1994), the toombak habit was found to be especially prevalent (> 45%) among males aged 40 years or older. Among women, toombak use is popular only in the older age groups, where up to 10% engage in the habit, while cigarette smoking is uncommon (< 1.5%).

Chemical analytical studies have shown that toombak contains at least 100-fold higher concentrations of tobacco-specific *N*-nitrosamines than Swedish commercial snuff and a US brand. These nitrosamines are by far the most powerful and most abundant carcinogens in snuff (Idris *et al.*, 1991). Mucosal lesions characterized by parakeratosis, pale surface staining of the epithelium and basal-cell hyperplasia, similar to those observed in Swedish snuff-dippers, are observed in long-term users, although epithelial dysplasia seems to be infrequent (Idris *et al.*, 1996).

Early studies suggested a link between use of toombak and oral cancers, and noted that the majority of tumours were at the site of contact with the tobacco or in adjacent areas (Elbeshir *et al.*, 1989). In a curious case–control study, Idris *et al.* (1995b) compared 375 cases with cancers of the lip and mouth with a group of 204 controls from the same hospital with non-epithelial oral and head and neck cancers, and salivary neoplasms, and 2840 "population controls" attending health education programmes in various parts of the country. Subjects were interviewed about their smoking habits and use of toombak. The groups were very different with respect to every variable measured— age, sex, tribe, region of residence, so an adjustment was made to the estimated odds ratios. Toombak use was associated with a significant increase in risk (OR ever/never 7.3; 95% CI 4.3–12.4) for hospital controls, 3.9 (95% CI 2.9–5.3) for population controls). The effect was entirely confined to long-term (> 10 years) users. Cigarette smoking did not increase risk of these cancers. When a different group of oral cancers (tongue, palate, maxillary sinus) was compared with the two control groups, there was no significant effect of either toombak or of cigarette smoking. The authors ascribed this to these sites not being in direct contact with the toombak quid during its use.

The squamous-cell tumours from toombak users appear to have a rather different profile of mutations in the p53 gene from those in non-users (Ibrahim *et al.*, 1999).

Oral leukoplakia, tobacco and alcohol
Macigo *et al.* (1995a) carried out a population survey for oral mucosal lesions in a rural population in Meru district, north-central Kenya. 48.6% of the population aged 15 years or more had some type of lesion; the prevalence of oral leukoplakia was 10.6%. This was significantly more frequent in males; 80/85 were homogeneous lesions and 67/85 were noted to be associated with tobacco use. Tobacco use in this population is predominantly a male habit, and takes the form of smoking of cigarettes or of kiraiku (hand-rolled traditionally processed tobacco). These observations prompted a case–control comparison of the 85 leukoplakia cases, who were matched with 141 controls form the same survey (by sex, age ± 3 years and neighbourhood) without oral lesions; both groups were

interviewed about tobacco and alcohol habits. The OR associated with cigarette smoking (never/current) was 8.4 (95% CI 4.1–17.4) and with kiraiku smoking (never/current) was 10.0 (95% CI 2.9–43.4). The OR associated with smoking cigarettes alone was 4.5 (95% CI 1.9–10.8), smoking of both products (OR = 15.2) suggested probable synergy or additive effects. Commercial beer, wines and spirits were relatively weak, but statistically significant, risk factors. The independent effects of these various risk factors were not evaluated (Macigo *et al.*, 1995b). A further analysis (Macigo *et al.*, 1996) suggested a dose-dependent association between oral leukoplakia and the use of tobacco and alcohol, in which the number of cigarettes smoked, the quantity of beer consumed and the frequency of consumption were more important than the duration of use of these products.

Viruses
Van Rensburg *et al.* (1996) examined 146 fixed tissue blocks from South African cases of oral squamous-cell carcinoma for four types of human papillomavirus (HPV) (6,11,16,18) using a polymerase chain reaction (PCR)-based method. Only two cases were positive (one for HPV 11, one for HPV 16). In a different study (van Rensburg *et al.*, 1995), using the same materials, DNA of Epstein–Barr virus was found in 26% of tumours and in 42% of blocks from non-malignant, non-viral-associated lesions.

Other factors
Badawi *et al.* (1998) found higher levels of salivary nitrate, nitrite and the enzyme nitrate reductase in oral cancer patients than in healthy individuals in Egypt; this could simply reflect the presence of the tumour rather than an antecedent risk pattern.

References
Altini, M. & Kola, A.H. (1985) Age-specific and age-standardised incidence rates for intra-oral squamous cell carcinoma in Blacks on the Witwatersrand, South Africa. *Community Dent. Oral Oncol.*, **13**, 334–339

Badawi, A.F., Hosny, G., el-Hadary, M. & Mostafa, M.H. (1998) Salivary nitrate, nitrite and nitrate reductase in relation to risk of oral cancer in Egypt. *Dis. Markers*, **14**, 91–97

Chopra, S.A., Linsell, C.A., Peers, F.G. & Chopra, F.S. (1975) Cancer in Asians in Kenya. *Int. J. Cancer*, **15**, 684–693

Day, G.L., Blot, W.J., Austin, D.F., Bernstein, L., Greenberg, R.S., Silverman, D.T., Schwartz, A.G., Swanson, G.M., Liff, J.M. & Pottern, L.M. (1993) Racial differences in risk of oral and pharyngeal cancer. *J. Natl Cancer Inst.*, **85**, 465–473

Elbeshir, E.I., Abeen, H.A., Idris, A.M. & Abbas, K. (1989) Snuff dipping and oral cancer in Sudan: a retrospective study. *Br. J. Oral Maxillofacial Surg.*, **27**, 243–248

Ibrahim, S.O., Vasstrand, E.N., Johannessen, A.C., Idris, A.M., Magnusson, B., Nilsen, R. & Lillehaugh, J.R. (1999) Mutations of the p53 gene in oral squamous-cell carcinomas from Sudanese dippers of nitrosamine-rich toombak and non-snuff-dippers from the Sudan and Scandinavia. *Int. J. Cancer*, **81**, 527–534

Idris, A.M., Nair, J., Ohshima, H., Friesen, M., Brouet, I., Faustman, E.M. & Bartsch, H. (1991) Unusually high levels of carcinogenic tobacco-specific nitrosamines in Sudan snuff (toombak). *Carcinogenesis*, **12**, 1115–1118

Idris, A.M., Prokopczyk, B. & Hoffmann, D. (1994) Toombak: a major risk factor for cancer of the oral cavity in Sudan. *Prev. Med.*, **23**, 832–839

Idris, A.M., Ahmed, H.M., Mukhtar, B.I., Gadir, A.F., el-Beshir, E.I. (1995a) Descriptive epidemiology of oral neoplasms in Sudan 1970-1985 and the role of toombak. *Int. J. Cancer*, **61**, 155–158

Idris, AM, Ahmed, H.M. & Malik, M.O.A. (1995b) Toombak dipping and cancer of the oral cavity in the Sudan: a case-control study. *Int. J. Cancer*, **63**, 477–480

Idris, A.M., Warnakulasuriya, K.A., Ibrahim, Y.E., Nielsen, R., Cooper, D. & Johnson, N.W. (1996) Toombak-associated oral mucosal lesions in Sudanese show a low prevalence of epithelial dysplasia. *J. Oral Pathol. Med.*, **25**, 239–244

IARC (1985) *IARC Monographs on the Evaluation of Carcinogenic Risks to Humans, Volume 37, Tobacco Habits other than Smoking; Betel Quid and Areca Nut Chewing; and some Related Nitrosamines*, Lyon, IARC

IARC (1986) *IARC Monographs on the Evaluation of Carcinogenic Risks to Humans, Volume 38, Tobacco Smoking*, Lyon, IARC

IARC (1988) *IARC Monographs on the Evaluation of Carcinogenic Risks to Humans, Volume 44. Alcohol Drinking*, Lyon, IARC

IARC (1995) *IARC Monographs on the Evaluation of Carcinogenic Risks to Humans, Volume 64. Human Papillomaviruses*, Lyon, IARC

Macigo, F.G., Mwaniki, D.L. & Guthua, S.W. (1995a) Prevalence of oral mucosal lesions in Kenyan population with special reference to oral leukoplakia. *E. Afr. Med. J.*, **72**, 778–782

Macigo, F.G., Mwaniki, D.L. & Guthua, S.W. (1995b) The association between oral leukoplakia and use of tobacco,alcohol and khat based on relative risks assessment in Kenya. *Eur. J. Oral Sci.*, **103**, 268–273

Macigo, F.G., Mwaniki, D.L. & Guthua, S.W. (1996) Influence of dose and cessation of kiraiku, cigarettes and alcohol use on the risk of developing oral leukoplakia. *Eur. J. Oral Sci.*, **104**, 498–502

Ogunbodede, E.O., Ugboko, V.I. & Ojo, M.A. (1997) Oral malignancies in Ile-Ife, Nigeria. *E. Afr. Med. J.*, **74**, 33–36

Onyango, J.F., Awange, D.O. & Wakiaga, J.M. (1995a) Oral tumours and tumour-like conditions in Kenya: I. Histological distribution. *E. Afr. Med. J.*, **72**, 560–563

Onyango, J.F., Awange, D.O. & Wakiaga, J.M. (1995b) Oral tumours and tumour-like conditions in Kenya: II. Age, sex and site distribution. *E. Afr. Med. J.*, **72**, 568–576

Pacella-Norman, R., Urban, M.I., Sitas, F., Carrara, H., Sur, R., Hale, M., Ruff, P., Patel, M., Newton, R., Bull, D. & Beral, V. (2002) Risk factors for oesophageal, lung, oral and laryngeal cancers in black South Africans. *Br. J. Cancer*, **86**, 1751–1756

Schonland, M. & Bradshaw, E. (1968) The incidence of oral and oropharyngeal cancer in various racial groups. *J. Dent. Assoc. S. Afr.*, **23**, 291–295

Schonland, M. & Bradshaw, E. (1969) Upper alimentary tract cancer in Natal Indians with special reference to the betel-chewing habit. *Br. J. Cancer*, **23**, 670-682

Seedat, H.A. & van Wyk, C.W. (1998) Betel chewing and dietary habits of chewers without and with submucous fibrosis and with concomitant oral cancer. *S. Afr. Med. J.*, **74**, 572–575

Templeton, A.C. & Viegas, O.A. (1970) Racial variations in tumour incidence in Uganda. *Trop. Geogr. Med.*, **22**, 431–438

Van Rensburg, E.J., Engelbrecht, S., van Heerden, W., Raubenheimer, F. & Schoub, B.D. (1995) Detection of EBV DNA in oral squamous cell carcinomas in a black African population sample. *In Vivo*, **9**, 199–202

Van Rensburg, E.J., Engelbrecht, S., van Heerden, W., Raubenheimer, F. & Schoub, B.D. (1996) Human papillomavirus DNA in oral squamous cell carcinomas from an African population sample. *Anticancer Res.*, **16**, 969–973

Van Wyk, C.W., Stander, I., Padayachee, A. & Grobler-Rabie, A.F. (1993) The areca nut chewing habit and oral squamous cell carcinoma in South African Indians. A retrospective study. *S. Afr. Med. J.*, **83**, 425–429

World Cancer Research Fund (WCRF) (1997) *Diet, Nutrition and the Prevention of Cancer: A Global Perspective*. Washington, DC, World Cancer Research Fund

World Health Organization (WHO) (1978) Definition of leukoplakia and related lesions: an aid to studies of oral precancer. *Oral Surg.*, **46**, 318–338

4.15 Cancer of the penis

Introduction

On a global basis, cancer of the penis is a rare cancer, accounting for less than 1% of cancers in men. In western countries, the age-standardized incidence is less than 1 per 100 000. Incidence rates greater than 1.5 per 100 000 are observed in cancer registries in India, south-east Asia (Thailand and Viet Nam), Latin America (Paraguay, Puerto Rico, Peru, Brazil) and the Caribbean (Martinique), as well as in sub-Saharan Africa. In India, the incidence in non-Muslims (Hindus, Buddhists) is significantly higher than reported in Muslims and Parsis (Muir & Nectoux, 1979). Incidence in Jewish populations is particularly low – 0.05 per 100 000 in the Jewish population of Israel in 1988–92, for example (Parkin et al., 1997).

Descriptive epidemiology in Africa

Table 1 shows age-standardized incidence rates from different centres, as reported in this volume, with comparison data from Europe and North America.

Table 2 shows incidence data from time periods in the 1960s and 1970s.

The incidence of cancer of the penis in Africa is generally not very high compared with that of liver, Kaposi sarcoma and cervical carcinoma, but there is considerable variation between countries. From Tables 1 and 2, it is clear that the incidence is low in northern and western Africa and considerably higher in eastern and southern Africa. Frequency data in this volume show relatively high percentages of penile cancers in Swaziland (4.4% of all male cancers, 1990–95) and Rwanda (2.9% of male cancers in 1991–93). The highest recently recorded incidence is in Uganda with an estimated rate from Kampala Cancer Registry for Kyadondo county of 4.1 per 100 000. The incidence reported by this registry in the 1990s is lower than that in the 1960s (Figure 1).

In addition to the international variation of incidence, there is considerable variation within countries, regionally, and by ethnic group. This has been widely discussed within the context of the etiological importance of circumcision (see below).

Risk factors

The importance of circumcision in determining the risk of penile cancer has been evident for many years on the basis of the clinical observation that it occurs very rarely in men who have been circumcised at birth. The observation has been confirmed in case–control studies in the United States, which suggest that the risk is reduced about threefold (Maden et al., 1993; Tseng et al., 2001). Phimosis is also clearly an important risk factor; a large proportion of cases (in western countries) are preceded by a history of phimosis, and the association has been confirmed in several case–control studies (Widerhoff & Schottenfeld, 1996).

The mechanisms underlying these findings have been a subject of much debate. Originally, it was thought that exposure to chemical carcinogens in smegma were important, and that the adverse consequences of possession of a foreskin, and of phimosis, could be countered by penile hygiene. More recently, it has been suggested that the prepuce could predispose to sexually transmitted infections, by permitting accumulation of infected vaginal secretions, or by simply providing an increased surface of non-keratinized epithelium. Studies in Kenya have shown that lack of circumcision predisposes to infection with HIV (Cameron et al., 1989). The role of infectious agents has been suspected for many years, based upon the frequent history of sexually transmitted diseases, including genital warts, in cases of penile cancer. The concordance of cancer of cervix and cancer of the penis in married

couples suggested a possible common etiology. This link has since been refined by detection of HPV DNA in about 40–50% of all penile cancers and by cross-sectional and prospective serological studies that have confirmed the role of, especially, HPV 16 and 18 (Dillner et al., 2000).

Studies in Africa

The clinical observations with respect to the protective effect of circumcision resulted in many ecological studies comparing risk of penis cancer and prevalence of circumcision in different populations. Africa was a particularly fruitful location for this type of study.

Dodge et al. (1973), in an analysis of histopathology data for the whole of Uganda for the period 1964–68, found penile cancer to be the commonest tumour in males, accounting for 12% of the total. However the frequency of penile cancer as a percentage of all cancers in the series varied in different ethnic groups. As already reported by Schmauz and Jain (1971), the frequency was highest among the Banyoro, Toro and Iteso, while lowest rates were reported among the Gishu, Bakonjo Lugbara and Kiga. Similar observations had been made by Hutt and Burkitt (1965), who showed that cancer of the penis accounted for 17% and 20% of all malignant tumours in Teso and Bunyoro, respectively, whereas in Lango and West Nile/Madi the figures were only 1.4% and 0.0%, respectively.

The low frequency of penile cancer among the Gishu and Bakonjo has been ascribed to the circumcision carried out on young adults as a cultural practice (Dodge & Kaviti, 1965). However, there was clearly some variability in frequency between tribes which do not practice circumcision (Schmauz & Jain, 1971). Kyalwazi (1966) had earlier reported that genital cleansing may be responsible for the variation of frequency of this tumour among those ethnic groups which do not practice circumcision.

A recent study of cancer patterns in Mbarara, western Uganda, found that penile cancer accounted for 17% of male cancer and this was thought to be due to the rural setting with perhaps lack of hygiene; circumcision is not practiced by the majority of males in this area (Wabinga, 2002).

Dodge and Linsell (1963) examined the records of the Medical Research Laboratory, Nairobi, for the period 1957–61. There were 27 penile cancers diagnosed, 1.9% of cancers in men. The Kikuyu, the largest tribal group, who practise circumcision, contributed only one case, but the frequency was much higher among the Luo and Turkan ethnic groups, who do not practice circumcision (Dodge & Kaviti 1965). In the recent results from the new population-based cancer registry in Eldoret, western Kenya, there was no case of penile cancer in a series of 254 cancer cases (see Chapter 3.4.6).

In Tanzania also, the prevalence of penile cancer is very low in ethnic groups which culturally practice circumcision—mainly the Masai in the north-eastern part of Tanzania and those in the coastal area, with a cultural influence from the Arabs (Dodge & Kaviti, 1965). Zanzibar and Pemba Islands, which were predominantly Islamic, recorded a low frequency of penile cancer. In northern Tanzania, records from Shirati Hospital indicate that penile cancer was more common in the Luo ethnic group and low in the Bantu ethnic groups in that region; all the Bantu ethnic groups in this region practise circumcision, unlike the Luo (Eshleman, 1960).

Prates and Torres (1965) reported a low frequency of penile cancer in their survey in Lourenço Marques, Mozambique; it accounted for only 0.8% of all tumours in this population. They also observed that the

Table 1. Age-standardized (world) and cumulative (0-64) incidence
Penis (C60)

	MALE				FEMALE			
	Cases	CRUDE	ASR(W) (per 100,000)	Cumulative (%)	Cases	CRUDE	ASR(W) (per 100,000)	Cumulative (%)
Africa, North								
Algeria, Algiers (1993-1997)	-	-	-	-	-	-	-	-
Algeria, Constantine (1994-1997)	-	-	-	-	-	-	-	-
Algeria, Oran (1996-1998)	-	-	-	-	-	-	-	-
Algeria, Setif (1993-1997)	1	0.0	**0.1**	-	-	-	-	-
Tunisia, Centre, Sousse (1993-1997)	1	0.1	**0.1**	-	-	-	-	-
Tunisia, North, Tunis (1994)	1	0.0	**0.1**	0.01	-	-	-	-
Tunisia, Sfax (1997)	-	-	-	-	-	-	-	-
Africa, West								
The Gambia (1997-1998)	4	0.4	**0.7**	0.04	-	-	-	-
Guinea, Conakry (1996-1999)	-	-	-	-	-	-	-	-
Mali, Bamako (1988-1997)	3	0.1	**0.2**	0.01	-	-	-	-
Niger, Niamey (1993-1999)	-	-	-	-	-	-	-	-
Nigeria, Ibadan (1998-1999)	-	-	-	-	-	-	-	-
Africa, Central								
Congo, Brazzaville (1996-1999)	-	-	-	-	-	-	-	-
Africa, East								
France, La Reunion (1988-1994)	14	0.7	**0.9**	0.05	-	-	-	-
Kenya, Eldoret (1998-2000)	2	0.2	**0.7**	0.05	-	-	-	-
Malawi, Blantyre (2000-2001)	4	0.4	**0.3**	0.02	-	-	-	-
Uganda, Kyadondo County (1993-1997)	34	1.2	**4.1**	0.12	-	-	-	-
Zimbabwe, Harare: African (1990-1993)	17	0.7	**2.3**	0.10	-	-	-	-
Zimbabwe, Harare: African (1994-1997)	17	0.6	**1.6**	0.07	-	-	-	-
Zimbabwe, Harare: European (1990-1997)	1	0.7	**0.3**	-	-	-	-	-
Africa, South								
Namibia (1995-1998)	14	0.4	**0.8**	0.06	-	-	-	-
South Africa: Black (1989-1992)	404	0.7	**1.3**	0.08	-	-	-	-
South Africa: Indian (1989-1992)	23	1.2	**2.1**	0.09	-	-	-	-
South Africa: Mixed race (1989-1992)	43	0.7	**1.2**	0.07	-	-	-	-
South Africa: White (1989-1992)	75	0.7	**0.7**	0.04	-	-	-	-
South Africa, Transkei, Umtata (1996-1998)	1	0.3	**0.7**	0.07	-	-	-	-
South Africa, Transkei, 4 districts (1996-1998)	-	-	-	-	-	-	-	-
Swaziland (1996-1999)	31	1.8	**3.2**	0.22	-	-	-	-
Europe/USA								
USA, SEER: White (1993-1997)	307	0.6	**0.5**	0.02	-	-	-	-
USA, SEER: Black (1993-1997)	39	0.6	**0.6**	0.03	-	-	-	-
France, 8 registries (1993-1997)	145	1.1	**0.7**	0.03	-	-	-	-
The Netherlands (1993-1997)	378	1.0	**0.7**	0.03	-	-	-	-
UK, England (1993-1997)	1487	1.2	**0.8**	0.05	-	-	-	-

In italics: histopathology-based registries

Table 2. Incidence of penis cancer in Africa, 1953–74

Registry	Period	ASR (per 100 000) Male	Source (see Chap. 1)
Senegal, Dakar	1969–74	*0.4*	4
Mozambique, Lourenço Marques	1956–60	2.7	1
Nigeria, Ibadan	1960–69	*0.2*	3
SA, Cape Province: Bantu	1956–59	4.6	2
SA, Cape Province: Coloured	1956–59	2.5	2
SA, Cape Province: White	1956–59	0.8	2
SA, Johannesburg, Bantu	1953–55	1.5	1
SA, Natal Province: African	1964–66	6.9	2
SA, Natal Province: Indian	1964–66	*2.8*	2
Uganda, Kyadondo	1954–60	–	1
Uganda, Kyadondo	1967–71	5.9	5
Zimbabwe, Bulawayo	1963–72	5.9	6

Italics: Rate based on less than 10 cases

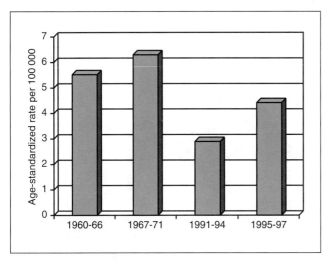

Figure 1. Trends in incidence of penile cancer, Kampala Uganda (Wabinga *et al*, 2000)

frequency of circumcision in their penile cancer cases (20%) was the same as in patents with cancer at other sites (26%), and noted that the lack of effect may be ascribed to circumcision being performed relatively late, generally in adulthood.

In South Africa, penile cancer is less prevalent in the Zulu community, who also practice circumcision (Krige, 1936), than in the Bantu of Natal province who do not circumcise, and in whom the frequency of penile cancer is relatively high (8%) (Wainwright & Roach, 1957).

As noted above, penile cancer is rare in West Africa. Edington and MacLean (1965) reported only one cases in a period of three years among residents of Ibadan, western Nigeria (0.3%) and Gueye *et al.* (1992) found it to comprise less than 1% of cancers in men in their series from Senegal. In these areas, circumcision is routinely practised.

The association of penile cancer with an infective agent was supported by the observations of Schmauz and Owor (1984), who demonstrated a relationship between cervical cancer and penile cancer in the 18 districts of Uganda, and also between condylomata acuminata and penile cancer. HPV DNA has been isolated from a high proportion of specimens of penile cancers from Uganda (Durst *et al.*, 1983; Tornesello *et al.*, 1992), and a HPV variant (Af1-u) has been particularly implicated (Buonaguro *et al.*, 2000).

References

Buonaguro, F.M., Tornesello, M.L., Salatiello, I., Okong, P., Buonaguro, L., Beth-Giraldo, E., Biryahwaho, B., Sempala, S.D. & Giraldo, G. (2000) The Uganda study on HPV variants and genital cancers. *J. Clin. Virol.*, **19**, 31–41

Cameron, D.W., Simonsen, J.N., D'Costa, L.J., Ronald, A.R., Maitha, G.M. Gakinya, M.N., Cheang, M., Ndinya-Achola, J.O., Piuot, P, Brunham, R.C. & Plummer, F.A. (1989) Female to male transmission of human immunodeficiency virus type-I: risk factors for seroconversion in men. *Lancet*, **ii**, 403–407

Dillner. J., von Krogh, G., Horenblas, S. & Meijer, C.J.L.M. (2000) Etiology of squamous cell carcinoma of penis. *Scand. J. Urol. Nephrol.*, Suppl. **205**, 189–193

Dodge, O.G. & Kaviti, J.N. (1965) Male circumcision among the peoples of East Africa and the incidence of genital cancer. *E. Afr. Med. J.*, **42**, 98–105

Dodge, O.G. & Linsell, C.A. (1963) Carcinoma of the penis in Uganda and Kenya Africans. *Cancer*, **16**, 1255–1263

Dodge, O.G., Owor, R. & Templeton, A.C. (1973) Tumours of the male genitalia. In: Templeton, A.C., ed., Tumours in a Tropical Country. Recent Results *Cancer Res.*, **41**, 132–144

Durst, M., Gissmann, L., Ikenberg, H. & zur Hausen, H. (1983) A papillomavirus DNA from a cervical carcinoma and its prevalence in cancer biopsy samples from different geographic regions. *Proc. Natl Acad. Sci. USA*, **80**, 3812–3815

Edington, G.M. & MacLean, C.M.V. (1965) A cancer rate survey in Ibadan, western Nigeria 1960-1963. *Br. J. Cancer*, **19**, 471–481

Eshleman, J C. (1960) A study of relative incidence of malignant tumours seen at Shirati Hospital, Tanzania. *E. Afr. Med. J.*, **43**, 273–283

Gueye, S.M., Diagne, B.A., Ba, M., Sylla, C. & Mensah, A. (1992) Le cancer de la verge. Aspects épidémiologiques et problèmes thérapeutiques au Sénégal. *J. Urol. (Paris)*, **98**, 159–161

Hutt, M.R.S. & Burkitt, D. (1965) Geographical distribution of cancer in East Africa: A new clinicopathological approach. *Br. Med. J.*, **2**, 719–722

Krige, W.J. (1936) *The Social System of the Zulus*, London, Longmans, Green, p. 420

Kyalwazi, S.K. Carcinoma of the penis: a review of 153 patients admitted to Mulago Hospital, Kla, Uganda. *E. Afr. Med. J.*, **43**, 415–425

Maden, C., Sherman, K.J., Beckmann, A.M., Hislop, T.G., Teh, C.Z., Ashley, R.L. & Daling, J.R. (1993) History of circumcision, medical conditions, and sexual activity and risk of penile cancer. *J. Natl Cancer Inst.*, **85**, 19–24

Parkin, D.M., Whelan, S.L., Ferlay, J., Raymond, L., & Young, J. (1997) *Cancer Incidence in Five Continents*, Vol. VII (IARC Scientific Publications No. 143), Lyon, IARC

Prates, M.D. & Torres, O. (1965) A cancer survey in Lourenço Marques, Portuguese East Africa. *J. Natl Cancer Inst.*, **35**, 729–757

Schmauz, R. & Jain, D.K. (1971) Geographical variation of carcinoma of the penis in Uganda. *Br. J. Cancer*, **25**, 25–32

Schmauz, R. & Owor, R. (1984) Epidemiological aspects of cervical cancer in tropical Africa. In: Williams, A.O., O'Conor, G.T., De Thé, G.T. & Johnson, C.A., eds, *Virus-Associated Cancers in Africa* (IARC Scientific Publications No. 63), Lyon, IARC, pp. 413–431

Tornesello, M.L., Buonaguro, F.M., Beth-Giraldo, E., Kyalwazi, S.K. & Giraldo, G. (1992) Human papillomavirus (HPV) DNA in penile carcinomas and in two cell lines from high-incidence areas for genital cancers in Africa. *Int. J. Cancer*, **51**, 587–592

Tseng, H.-F., Morgenstern, H., Mack, T. & Peters, R. (2001) Risk factors for penile cancer: results of a population-based case-control study in Los Angeles County (United States). *Cancer Causes Control*, **12**, 267–277

Wabinga, H.R. (2002) Pattern of cancer in Mbarara, Uganda. *E. Afr. Med. J.*, **79**, 22–26

Wabinga, H.R., Parkin, D.M., Wabire-Mangen, F. & Nambooze, S. (2000) Trends in cancer incidence in Kyadondo county Uganda, 1960-1997. *Br. J. Cancer*, **8**, 1585–1592

Wainwright, J. & Roach, C.G. (1957) Malignant neoplastic disease in Europeans. Africans and Indians in *Natal. S. Afr. Cancer Bull.*, **1**, 162–170

Widerhoff, L. & Schottenfeld, D. (1996) Penile cancer. In: Schottenfeld, D. & Fraumeni, J.F., Jr, *Cancer Epidemiology and Prevention*, second edition, Oxford, New York, Oxford University Press, pp. 1220–1230

4.16 Prostate cancer

Introduction

On a global basis, prostate cancer is the third most common cancer of men, with an estimated 543 000 new cases diagnosed each year (about 10.2% of all new cancers in men). More than 74% of these occur in the populations in Europe and North America. In Africa, there were an estimated 27 400 new cases in 2000 (9.1% of cancers in men).

Incidence rates are now influenced by the diagnosis of latent cancers both by screening of asymptomatic individuals and by detection of latent cancer in tissue removed during prostatectomy operations or at autopsy. Thus, especially where screening examinations are prevalent, recorded 'incidence' may be very high (in the United States, for example, where this is now by far the most commonly diagnosed cancer in men). The distribution of mortality rates is less affected by the effects of early diagnosis of asymptomatic cancers.

More than any other, this is a cancer of the elderly. About three quarters of cases worldwide occur in men aged 65 years or more.

Descriptive epidemiology in Africa

Comparability of statistics on the incidence of prostate cancer between populations is hampered by different practices concerning biopsy of lesions, the extent of histological examination of biopsy material and the use of prostate-specific antigen (PSA) testing for diagnosis. The problems introduced in the use of incidence data when latent cancers discovered through PSA screening are included in cancer registry data are likely to be rather minimal in most of Africa, where an incident case almost always implies a clinically evident, frankly invasive, relatively advanced tumour.

Table 1 shows age-standardized incidence rates from different centres, as reported in this volume, with data from Europe and North America for comparison. Table 2 shows incidence data from time periods in the 1960s and 1970s.

Figure 1 shows estimated incidence rates by country, based on these data and other information reported in this volume.

It is clear that incidence is moderately high in many of the countries of sub-Saharan Africa, and it is difficult to be sure whether the regional variations seen in Table 1 and Figure 1 are real or simply reflect awareness of the disease and diagnostic capabilities. Rates appear to be higher in urban populations than in rural settings. Thus, current incidence rates are highest in cities such as Abidjan (Côte d'Ivoire) and Harare (Zimbabwe). It also seems that incidence rates in the more recent registry series are higher than those reported in the past. In contrast, incidence rates appear to be low in all of the countries of North Africa.

Dodge *et al.* (1973) noted that there was little evidence for any significant difference in incidence of prostate cancer between the different tribal groups in Uganda, with frequency of recording paralleling the frequency of cancer diagnoses overall.

The relatively high incidence (and mortality) recorded in African populations is reflected in populations of African descent elsewhere. Thus, within the United States, the black population has the highest incidence (and mortality) rates, some 72% higher than in whites (Table 1), who in turn have rates considerably higher than populations of Asian origin (e.g., Chinese, Japanese and Korean males). In the islands of the Caribbean, largely populated by descendants of persons from West Africa, mortality rates are some of the highest in the world (ASR 55.3 per 100 000 in Barbados, 33.3 in the Bahamas, and 32.3 in Trinidad, for example). In São Paulo, Brazil, the risk of prostate cancer in black males was 1.8 (95% CI 1.4–2.3) times that of white men, with an intermediate risk (1.4) among men of mixed race ('mulatto') (Bouchardy *et al.*, 1991).

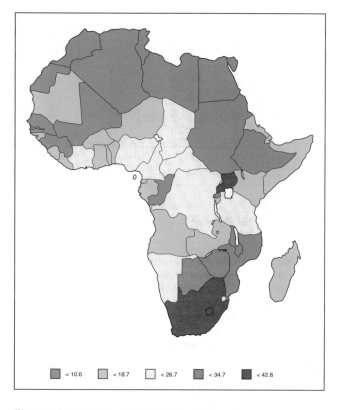

Figure 1. Incidence of prostate cancer: ASR (world)

Legend: ▨ < 10.6   ▨ < 18.7   ☐ < 26.7   ▨ < 34.7   ■ < 42.8

In the recent African series reported in Table 1, incidence rates were higher in white populations than in black. This probably represents their more ready access to modern diagnostic and treatment methods, as well as testing for PSA (Bassett *et al.*, 1995). It is notable that in the old data (1956–59) from the registry in Cape Province, South Africa, the incidence in blacks was double that in whites (Table 2).

Migrants from West Africa to England & Wales have mortality rates 3.5 times (95% CI 2.4–5.1) those of the local-born population, and mortality is significantly higher also among migrants from the Caribbean (RR 1.7; 95% CI 1.5–2.0); in contrast, mortality among migrants from East Africa, of predominantly Asian (Indian) ethnicity, are not high (Grulich *et al.*, 1992). The risk of prostate cancer mortality among migrants from sub-Saharan Africa to France was not, however, significantly different from that of the local-born population (Bouchardy *et al.*, 1995). Migrants to France from North Africa (Morocco, Algeria, Tunisia) had significantly lower mortality rates (OR 0.7–0.8), in keeping with the low rates of prostate cancer in their countries of origin (Bouchardy *et al.*, 1996).

Many elderly men are found to harbour latent cancers in their prostate, the prevalence of which greatly exceeds the cumulative incidence in the same population. Two international studies have looked at prevalence of latent prostate cancer at autopsy in different populations. Breslow *et al.* (1977) studied seven populations, two of them (Uganda and Jamaica) black. Prevalence of latent cancer increased steeply with age; allowing for this factor, it was highest in Sweden, Jamaica and Germany (28–32%), with Uganda in the middle of the range (20%), significantly above the Asian populations of Hong Kong and Singapore (13–16%). Drury and Owor (1981) reported separately on the 150 Ugandan cases in this study; prevalence increased from 12% at ages 45–54 years to 36% at ages 65 years and over. Yatani *et al.* (1982) found the highest

Table 1. Age-standardized (world) and cumulative (0-64) incidence
Prostate (C61)

	MALE				FEMALE			
	Cases	CRUDE	ASR(W) (per 100,000)	Cumulative (%)	Cases	CRUDE	ASR(W) (per 100,000)	Cumulative (%)
Africa, North								
Algeria, Algiers (1993-1997)	194	3.5	**5.4**	0.18	-	-	-	-
Algeria, Constantine (1994-1997)	46	3.0	**5.8**	0.15	-	-	-	-
Algeria, Oran (1996-1998)	74	4.2	**7.2**	0.20	-	-	-	-
Algeria, Setif (1993-1997)	71	2.4	**4.3**	0.16	-	-	-	-
Tunisia, Centre, Sousse (1993-1997)	79	6.8	**9.3**	0.11	-	-	-	-
Tunisia, North, Tunis (1994)	132	6.1	**7.9**	0.18	-	-	-	-
Tunisia, Sfax (1997)	41	10.4	**12.4**	0.22	-	-	-	-
Africa, West								
The Gambia (1997-1998)	20	2.0	**4.7**	0.10	-	-	-	-
Guinea, Conakry (1996-1999)	62	2.7	**9.7**	0.46	-	-	-	-
Mali, Bamako (1988-1997)	73	1.9	**5.7**	0.22	-	-	-	-
Niger, Niamey (1993-1999)	41	2.2	**10.8**	0.33	-	-	-	-
Nigeria, Ibadan (1998-1999)	115	7.7	**19.8**	0.84	-	-	-	-
Africa, Central								
Congo, Brazzaville (1996-1999)	45	3.7	**6.4**	0.36	-	-	-	-
Africa, East								
France, La Reunion (1988-1994)	353	16.8	**24.5**	0.50	-	-	-	-
Kenya, Eldoret (1998-2000)	54	5.8	**16.8**	0.77	-	-	-	-
Malawi, Blantyre (2000-2001)	30	3.3	**10.7**	0.57	-	-	-	-
Uganda, Kyadondo County (1993-1997)	215	7.6	**38.6**	1.19	-	-	-	-
Zimbabwe, Harare: African (1990-1993)	161	6.8	**26.9**	0.88	-	-	-	-
Zimbabwe, Harare: African (1994-1997)	209	7.5	**28.5**	0.78	-	-	-	-
Zimbabwe, Harare: European (1990-1997)	210	137.4	**70.1**	1.99	-	-	-	-
Africa, South								
Namibia (1995-1998)	352	11.1	**21.8**	0.87	-	-	-	-
South Africa: Black (1989-1992)	3432	6.0	**14.3**	0.44	-	-	-	-
South Africa: Indian (1989-1992)	121	6.2	**13.0**	0.31	-	-	-	-
South Africa: Mixed race (1989-1992)	681	10.6	**25.4**	0.67	-	-	-	-
South Africa: White (1989-1992)	4455	44.3	**41.1**	1.33	-	-	-	-
South Africa, Transkei, Umtata (1996-1998)	11	3.1	**3.7**	-	-	-	-	-
South Africa, Transkei, 4 districts (1996-1998)	12	1.7	**2.9**	0.15	-	-	-	-
Swaziland (1996-1999)	153	8.7	**21.5**	1.07	-	-	-	-
Europe/USA								
USA, SEER: White (1993-1997)	71146	146.1	**108.7**	4.74	-	-	-	-
USA, SEER: Black (1993-1997)	10337	154.4	**185.7**	9.12	-	-	-	-
France, 8 registries (1993-1997)	12274	89.3	**57.6**	1.61	-	-	-	-
The Netherlands (1993-1997)	31479	82.4	**56.6**	1.48	-	-	-	-
UK, England (1993-1997)	89532	74.6	**42.8**	0.99	-	-	-	-

In italics: histopathology-based registries

Table 2. Incidence of prostate cancer in Africa, 1953–74

Registry	Period	ASR (per 100 000) Male	Source (see Chap. 1)
Senegal, Dakar	1969–74	4.3	4
Mozambique, Lourenço Marques	1956–60	9.2	1
Nigeria, Ibadan	1960–69	9.7	3
SA, Cape Province: Bantu	1956–59	20.2	2
SA, Cape Province: Coloured	1956–59	18.5	2
SA, Cape Province: White	1956–59	10.9	2
SA, Johannesburg, Bantu	1953–55	9.4	1
SA, Natal Province: African	1964–66	23.2	2
SA, Natal Province: Indian	1964–66	9.4	2
Uganda, Kyadondo	1954–60	4.4	1
Uganda, Kyadondo	1960–71	4.5	5
Zimbabwe, Bulawayo	1963–72	21.9	6

Italics: Rate based on less than 10 cases

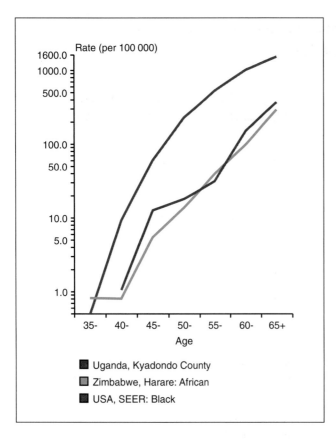

Figure 2. Age-specific incidence of prostate cancer

prevalence in US blacks (23.5%), and the differences between populations (US whites, Colombia, Japanese) were largely due to variations in prevalence of the infiltrative type of latent cancer.

The risk of prostate cancer increases very steeply with age, at approximately the 9th–10th power of age, compared with the 5th–6th power for other epithelial cancers (Cook et al., 1969). The young age structure of African populations means that the average age at diagnosis of cases in Africa is lower than in European and American populations. This is often remarked upon in clinical series from Africa (e.g., Jackson et al, 1977; Udeh, 1981), although the curves of incidence versus age are very similar to those observed elsewhere. Figure 2 shows age-specific incidence rates from two of the registry series in this volume (Kampala, Uganda, and Harare, Zimbabwe) in comparison with the black population covered by the SEER program of the United States.

Stage at presentation of tumours in Africa is generally very advanced (Jackson et al., 1977; Kehinde, 1995), with correspondingly poor prognosis.

Time trends
In almost all developing countries with relatively low rates of prostate cancer incidence, the risk appears to be increasing (Hsing et al., 2000). There are very few data from Africa. In South Africa, Bradshaw and Harington (1985) observed that mortality rates in the white population were not rising very rapidly in the period 1949–79, although the rates the 'coloured' population approximately doubled during the period, so that, by the mid-1970s, mortality was similar to that in whites; the rates in the black population were, of course, considerably underestimated. In cancer registry data, rates appear to be rather higher in more recent data than in older series. In Ibadan, Nigeria, incidence in 1998–99 was 19.8 per 100 000, compared with 9.7 per 100 000 in 1960–69 (Table 2), and Ogunbiyi and Shittu (1999) noted the increase in frequency of prostate cancer in the same registry, where it increased from 4.5% cancers in men (aged > 17 years) in the 1960s to become, with 11% of the

total, the most common cancer of men in the 1990s. In Kampala, Uganda, there has been a significant increase in incidence since the 1960s (Figure 3) (Wabinga et al., 2000). This observed increase is certainly not due to screening but may be due to increased awareness and greater readiness to perform prostatectomy for urinary symptoms in elderly men.

Mortality rates in Mauritius have also been increasing since the 1960s (Figure 4).

Risk factors
Despite extensive research, the environmental risk factors for prostate cancer are not well understood, although the fact that they do play a role is shown by the changes of risk observed in many migrant populations and their offspring. Evidence from ecological, case–control and cohort studies implicates dietary fat in the etiology of prostate cancer, although few studies have adjusted the results for caloric intake, and no particular fat component has been consistently implicated. There is a strong positive association with intake of animal products, especially red meat. The evidence from these studies for a protective effect of fruits and vegetables on prostate cancer is, unlike many other cancer sites, not convincing. There is little evidence for anthropometric associations with prostate cancer, or for a link with obesity (Kolonel, 1996; WCRF, 1997).

Walker et al. (1992) studied 166 cases of mainly advanced prostate cancer and 166 neighbourhood controls from Soweto, South Africa, using a questionnaire that included a 24-hour dietary recall. They observed a positive association of risk with high fat consumption (≥ 25% energy) and high intake of meat and eggs (≥ 5 times per week), and a reduced risk in high consumers of vegetables (carrots). These were noted to be features of a western-style diet, consumed by persons taking regular meals away from home, in canteens, or while in domestic service, so that this variable (outside meals > 10 years) emerged as the strongest risk factor (OR 3.2, 95% CI 2.0–5.1). No association was seen with anthropometry, education, social class, smoking or alcohol drinking.

Platz et al. (2000), in a cohort study of health professionals in the United States, found that differences in the distribution of possible dietary and lifestyle risk factors did not explain the higher risk (RR 1.81) of prostate cancer in blacks versus whites. Genetic factors appear therefore to play a major role in explaining the observed racial differences, and findings of elevated risk in men with a family history of the disease support this. Steinberg et al. (1990) demonstrated a 5–11-fold increased risk among men with two or more affected first-degree relatives. A similar study involving a population-based case–control study of prostate cancer among blacks, whites and Asians in the United States and Canada found the prevalence of positive family histories somewhat lower among the Asian Americans than among blacks or whites (Whittemore et al., 1995).

It is clear that male sex hormones play an important role in the development and growth of prostate cancers. Testosterone diffuses into the gland, where it is converted by the enzyme steroid 5-alpha reductase type II (SRD5A2) to the more metabolically active form dihydrotestosterone (DHT). DHT and testosterone bind to the androgen receptor (AR), and the receptor/ligand complex translocates to the nucleus for DNA binding and transactivation of genes which have androgen-responsive elements, including those controlling cell division. Much research has concentrated on the role of polymorphisms of the genes regulating this process and how inter-ethnic variations in such polymorphisms might explain the higher risk of prostate cancer in men of African descent (Ross et al., 1998). Polymorphisms in the *SRD5A2* genes may provide at least part of the explanation (Shibata & Whittemore, 1997), but more interest is focused on the *AR* gene, located on the long arm of chromosome X. The *AR* gene contains a highly polymorphic region of CAG repeats in exon 1, the normal range being 6–39 repeats. Several studies suggest that men with a lower number of AR CAG repeat lengths are at higher risk of prostate cancer (Chan et al.,

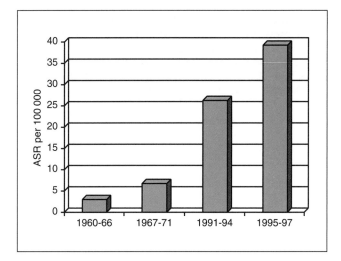

Figure 3. Trends in incidence of prostate cancer, Kampala, Uganda (Wabinga *et al.*, 2000)

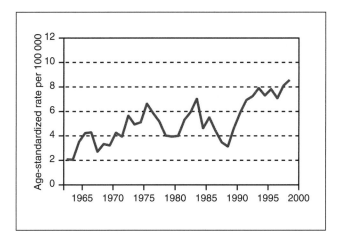

Figure 4. Mauritius: Prostate cancer mortality 1964–1998 (3-year moving average)

1998). Blacks in the United States have fewer CAG repeats than whites, which has been postulated to partly explain their susceptibility to prostate cancer (Ross *et al.*, 1998; Platz *et al.*, 2000). Other genetic mechanisms possibly related to prostate cancer risk are polymorphisms in the vitamin D receptor gene (Ingles *et al.*, 1997, 1998) or in the insulin-like growth factor (IGF) signalling pathway (Chan *et al.*, 1998b), but there is no evidence for significant inter-ethnic differences in these systems.

There have been no studies of these aspects of prostate cancer etiology in African populations.

References

Bassett, M.T., Chokunonga, E., Mauchaza, B., Levy, L., Ferlay, J. & Parkin, D.M. (1995b) Cancer in the European population of Harare, Zimbabwe 1990-1992. *Int. J. Cancer*, **63**, 24–28

Bouchardy, C., Mirra, A.P., Khlat, M., Parkin, D.M., de Souza, J.M. & Gotlieb, S.L. (1991) Ethnicity and cancer risk in São Paulo, Brazil. *Cancer Epidemiol. Biomarkers Prev.*, **1**, 21–27

Bouchardy, C., Wanner, P. & Parkin, D.M. (1995) Cancer mortality among sub-Saharan African migrants in France. *Cancer Causes Control*, **6**, 539–534

Bouchardy, C., Parkin, D.M., Wanner, P. & Khlat, M. (1996) Cancer mortality among North African migrants in France. *Int. J. Epidemiol.*, **25**, 5–13

Bradshaw, E. & Harington, J.S. (1985) The changing pattern of cancer mortality in South Africa, 1949-1979. *S. Afr. Med. J.*, **68**, 455–465

Breslow, N., Chan, C.W., Dhom, G., Drury, R.A., Franks, L.M., Gellei, B., Lee, Y.S., Lundberg, S., Sparke, B., Sternby, N.H. & Tulinius, H. (1977) Latent carcinoma of prostate at autopsy in seven areas. The International Agency for Research on Cancer, Lyons, France. *Int. J. Cancer*, **20**, 680–688

Chan, J.M., Stampfer, M.J. & Giovannucci, E.L. (1998a) What causes prostate cancer? A brief summary of the epidemiology. *Semin. Cancer Biol.*, **8**, 263–273

Chan, J.M., Stampfer, M.J., Giovannucci, E., Gann, P.H., Ma, J., Wilkinson, P., Hennekens, C.H., & Pollak, M. (1998b) Plasma insulin-like growth factor-I and prostate cancer risk: a prospective study. *Science*, **279**, 563–566

Cook, P.J., Doll, R. & Fellingham, S.A. (1969) A mathematical model for the age distribution of cancer in man. *Int. J. Cancer*, **4**, 93–112

Dodge, O.G., Owor, R. & Templeton, A.C. (1973) Tumours of the male genitalia. In Templeton, A.C., ed., *Tumours in a Tropical Country. Recent Results in Cancer Research,* Vol. 41, Berlin, Heidelberg, New York, Springer Verlag

Drury, R.A. & Owor, R. (1981) Latent carcinoma of the prostate in Uganda. *E. Afr. Med. J.*, **58**, 732–737

Grulich, A.E., Swerdlow, A.J., Head, J. & Marmot, M.G. (1992) Cancer mortality in African and Caribbean migrants to England and Wales. *Br. J. Cancer*, **66**, 905–911

Hsing, A.W., Tsao, L. & Devesa, S.S. (2000) International trends and patterns of prostate cancer incidence and mortality. *Int. J. Cancer*, **85**, 60–67

Ingles, S.A., Ross, R.K., Yu, M.C., Irvine, R.A., La Pera, G., Haile, R.W. & Coetzee, G.A. (1997) Association of prostate cancer risk with genetic polymorphisms in vitamin D receptor and androgen receptor. *J. Natl Cancer Inst.*, **89**, 166–170

Ingles, S.A., Coetzee, G.A., Ross, R.K., Henderson, B.E., Kolonel, L.N., Crocitto, L., Wang, W. & Haile, R.W. (1998) Association of prostate cancer with vitamin D receptor haplotypes in African-Americans. *Cancer Res.*, **58**, 1620–1623

Jackson, M.A., Ahluwalia, B.S., Herson, J., Heshmat, M.Y., Jackson, A.G., Jones, G.W., Kapoor, S.K., Kennedy, J., Kovi, J., Lucas, A.O., Nkposong, E.O., Olisa, E. & Williams, A.O. (1977) Characterization of prostatic carcinoma among blacks: a continuation report. *Cancer Treat Rep.*, **61**, 167–172

Kehinde, E.O. (1995) The geography of prostate cancer and its treatment in Africa. *Cancer Surv.*, **23**, 281–286

Kolonel, L.N. (1996) Nutrition and prostate cancer. *Cancer Causes Control*, **7**, 83–94

Ogunbiyi, J.O. & Shittu, O.B. (1999) Increased incidence of prostate cancer in Nigerians. *J. Natl Med. Assoc.*, **91**, 159–164

Platz, E.A., Rimm, E.B., Willett, W.C., Kantoff, P.W. & Giovannucci, E. (2000) Racial variation in prostate cancer incidence and in hormonal system markers among male health professionals. *J. Natl Cancer Inst.*, **92**, 2009–2017

Ross, R.K., Pike, M.C., Coetzee, G.A., Reichardt, J.K., Yu, M.C., Feigelson, H., Stanczyk, F.Z., Kolonel, L.N. & Henderson, B.E. (1998) Androgen metabolism and prostate cancer: establishing a model of genetic susceptibility. *Cancer Res.*, **58**, 4497–4504

Shibata, A. & Whittemore, A.S. (1997) Genetic predisposition to prostate cancer: possible explanations for ethnic differences in risk. *Prostate*, **32**, 65–72

Steinberg, G.D., Carter, B.S., Beaty, T.H., Childs, B. & Walsh, T.C. (1990) Family history and the risk of prostate cancer. *Prostate*, **17**, 337–347

Udeh, F.N. (1981) Prostatic carcinoma in Nigeria: a 10-year retrospective study. *Int. Urol. Nephrol.*, **13**, 159–166

Wabinga, H.R., Parkin, D.M., Wabwire-Mangen, F. & Nambooze, S. (2000) Trends in cancer incidence in Kyadondo county, Uganda, 1960-1997. *Br. J. Cancer*, **82**, 1585–1592

Walker, A.R.P., Walker, B.F., Tsotetsi, N.G., Sebitso, C., Siwedi, D. & Walker, A.J. (1992) Case-control study of prostate cancer in black patients in Soweto, South Africa. *Br. J. Cancer*, **65**, 438–441

Whittemore, A.S., Wu, A.H., Kolonel, L.N., John, E.M., Gallagher, R.P., Howe, G.R., West, D.W., The, C.Z. & Stamey, T. (1995) Family history and prostate cancer risk in black, white, and Asian men in the United States and Canada. *Am. J. Epidemiol.*, **141**, 732–740

World Cancer Research Fund (WCRF) (1997) *Diet, nutrition and the prevention of cancer: a global perspective*. Washington, DC, World Cancer Research Fund

Yatani, R., Chigusa, I., Akazaki, K., Stemmermann, G.N., Welsh, R.A. & Correa, P. (1982) Geographic pathology of latent prostatic carcinoma. *Int. J. Cancer*, **29**, 611–616

4.17 Skin cancer (non-melanoma)

Introduction

The incidence of non-melanoma skin cancer (NMSC) is difficult to assess. These cancers are very common but rarely fatal, and completeness of registration varies widely depending on access to out-patient records and general practitioners. Some cancer registries record basal-cell carcinomas (BCC) only, others register squamous-cell (SCC) only, and many do not collect data on either form. It has been estimated that 2.75 million new cases are diagnosed annually worldwide (Armstrong & Kricker, 1995). Some 75% are of basal-cell origin and around 25% squamous-cell (Strom & Yamamura, 1997). Other skin cancers are rare.

BCCs are generally found on the head and neck, and although they grow slowly and metastasize very rarely, can result in large (maignant-type) ulcers if neglected. SCCs can occur on any part of the body and are more frequent on the back of the hand and on the legs (particularly in Africa). In a large case series from the Sudan, 73.0% of BCC occurred on the head and neck, compared with 40% of SCC (Malik *et al.*, 1974).

NMSC increases in frequency with increasing proximity to the equator (IARC, 1992), and white-skinned populations exposed to UV radiation are particularly at risk. Susceptibility to skin cancer is inversely related to degree of melanin pigmentation. The highest rates ever reported are those from the European population of Harare, Zimbabwe, in this volume, with a standardized incidence per 100 000 of 635.3 in males and 363.3 in females (Figure 1). The lowest incidence is found in China and India, where standardized rates are generally less than 2.

Descriptive epidemiology in Africa

In Africa, incidence rates are low, except in white populations and in areas where there is a high proportion of non-black residents.

Incidence is higher in lighter-skinned North Africans than in sub-Saharan Africa. Table 1 presents the incidence data from registries in this volume, with European data for comparison. Earlier data are presented in Table 2.

Histological type

While worldwide, the frequency of BCC is much higher than that of SCC, the majority of malignant epithelial tumours in the black populations of sub-Saharan Africa are SCC (Hutt, 1991), an observation confirmed in numerous studies. The distribution of NMSC by histological type in the series from cancer registries reported in this volume is shown in Table 3. BCC is generally elevated in North Africa and in sub-Saharan populations where there are a high proportion of whites. Elsewhere SCC is predominant.

A pathology series of 24 900 specimens in Mashonaland (then in Southern Rhodesia, now Zimbabwe) yielded 4124 malignant tumours in Africans for the ten-year period from October 1955. 75.9% of skin tumours were SCC, 5.5% BCC, 0.4% sebaceous epithelioma, 0.1% sweat gland carcinoma and 17.9% melanoma. In the European population, 34.4% of skin cancers were SCC and 56.7% BCC, a ratio very different to that of the African population (Ross, 1967).

Between 1969 and 1978, SCC accounted for 59% of NMSC diagnoses reported to the pathology-based Tanzanian Cancer Registry, while only 5% were BCC. The corresponding percentages in US Blacks were 39% and 35%. In the period 1978–88, SCC still accounted for 59% of total skin malignancies (including Kaposi sarcoma and melanoma) (Amir *et al.*, 1992a).

Munyao and Othieno-Abinya (1999), using data collected in 1968–97 by the pathology-based Kenya Cancer Registry, estimated that the incidence of BCC in Africans was almost one hundred times less than that in Caucasians.

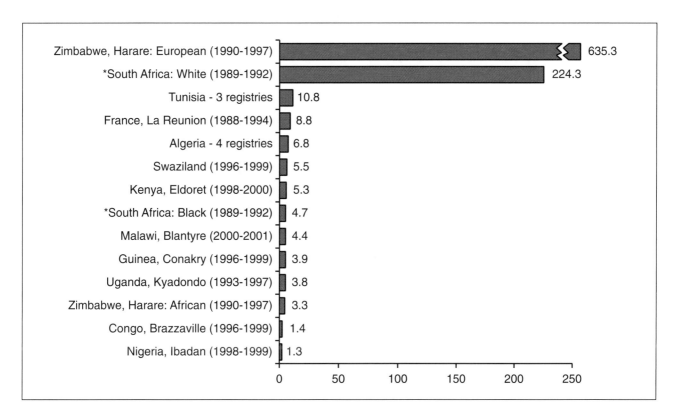

Figure 1. Age-standardized incidence rates (per 100 000) of non-melanoma skin cancer in Africa, male (all ages)

Table 1. Age-standardized (world) and cumulative (0-64) incidence
Other skin (C44)

	MALE				FEMALE			
	Cases	CRUDE	ASR(W)	Cumulative	Cases	CRUDE	ASR(W)	Cumulative
		(per 100,000)		(%)		(per 100,000)		(%)
Africa, North								
Algeria, Algiers (1993-1997)	292	5.3	**7.8**	0.44	142	2.6	**3.5**	0.17
Algeria, Constantine (1994-1997)	27	1.7	**3.2**	0.15	15	1.0	**1.5**	0.10
Algeria, Oran (1996-1998)	130	7.3	**11.7**	0.53	89	5.1	**7.1**	0.41
Algeria, Setif (1993-1997)	55	1.8	**3.0**	0.17	24	0.8	**1.3**	0.07
Tunisia, Centre, Sousse (1993-1997)	109	9.4	**12.4**	0.70	82	7.3	**8.9**	0.32
Tunisia, North, Tunis (1994)	138	6.4	**8.1**	0.44	91	4.3	**5.7**	0.30
Tunisia, Sfax (1997)	65	16.5	**20.2**	0.95	38	10.1	**12.0**	0.66
Africa, West								
The Gambia (1997-1998)	6	0.6	**1.0**	0.05	12	1.2	**2.4**	0.14
Guinea, Conakry (1996-1999)	40	1.7	**3.8**	0.30	33	1.5	**3.2**	0.26
Mali, Bamako (1988-1997)	63	1.6	**3.3**	0.27	42	1.2	**2.7**	0.20
Niger, Niamey (1993-1999)	30	1.6	**4.4**	0.38	24	1.3	**4.4**	0.42
Nigeria, Ibadan (1998-1999)	12	0.8	**1.3**	0.10	9	0.6	**1.1**	0.07
Africa, Central								
Congo, Brazzaville (1996-1999)	12	1.0	**1.4**	0.12	17	1.4	**1.8**	0.10
Africa, East								
France, La Reunion (1988-1994)	136	6.5	**8.8**	0.48	127	5.9	**6.3**	0.29
Kenya, Eldoret (1998-2000)	19	2.0	**5.3**	0.36	8	0.9	**1.6**	0.13
Malawi, Blantyre (2000-2001)	16	1.8	**4.4**	0.29	17	2.0	**4.9**	0.46
Uganda, Kyadondo County (1993-1997)	32	1.1	**3.8**	0.19	12	0.4	**1.0**	0.07
Zimbabwe, Harare: African (1990-1993)	28	1.2	**3.4**	0.11	21	1.0	**4.4**	0.16
Zimbabwe, Harare: African (1994-1997)	50	1.8	**3.3**	0.20	33	1.3	**2.5**	0.22
Zimbabwe, Harare: European (1990-1997)	1584	1036.5	**635.3**	42.34	1036	614.2	**363.3**	25.68
Africa, South								
Namibia (1995-1998)	588	18.5	**32.5**	2.05	438	13.7	**21.1**	1.27
South Africa: Black (1989-1992)	1446	2.5	**4.7**	0.25	1174	2.1	**3.2**	0.20
South Africa: Indian (1989-1992)	65	3.3	**5.4**	0.25	60	3.0	**4.2**	0.19
South Africa: Mixed race (1989-1992)	227	3.5	**6.8**	0.34	256	3.8	**5.9**	0.31
South Africa: White (1989-1992)	24620	244.6	**224.3**	12.58	16448	161.6	**125.1**	7.27
South Africa, Transkei, Umtata (1996-1998)	4	1.1	**1.9**	0.16	3	0.7	**1.0**	0.08
South Africa, Transkei, 4 districts (1996-1998)	3	0.4	**1.0**	0.10	1	0.1	**0.1**	-
Swaziland (1996-1999)	46	2.6	**5.5**	0.39	37	1.9	**3.2**	0.27
Europe/USA								
France, 8 registries (1993-1997)	6431	46.8	**31.6**	1.29	5552	38.4	**21.0**	0.97
The Netherlands (1993-1997)	8985	23.5	**16.3**	0.52	5739	14.7	**7.8**	0.29
UK, England (1993-1997)	93990	78.3	**48.9**	2.16	84431	66.1	**33.9**	1.67

In italics: histopathology-based registries

Table 2. Non-melanoma skin cancer 1953–74. Age-standardized incidence (all ages)

Registry	Period	ASR (per 100 000)		Source
		Male	Female	(see Chap. 1)
Senegal, Dakar	1969–74	10.3	7.9	4
Mozambique, Lourenço Marques	1956–60	7.9	*7.7*	1
Nigeria, Ibadan	1960–69	1.2	1.6	3
SA, Cape Province: Bantu	1956–59	*0.9*	*0.8*	2
SA, Cape Province: Coloured	1956–59	4.2	2.8	2
SA, Cape Province: White	1956–59	133.0	72.2	2
SA, Johannesburg, Bantu	1953–55	1.4	2.8	1
SA, Natal Province: African	1964–66	3.0	*1.3*	2
SA, Natal Province: Indian	1964–66	*2.5*	3.4	2
Uganda, Kyadondo	1954–60	6.6	3.0	1
Uganda, Kyadondo	1960–71	3.9	3.2	5
Zimbabwe, Bulawayo	1963–72	6.5	*2.5*	6

Italics: Rate based on less than 10 cases

Table 3. Percentage distribution of microscopically verified cases by histological type
Skin (C43+C44) - Both sexes

	Carcinoma		Melanoma	Other	Unspecified	Number of cases	
	Basal cell	Squamous cell				MV	Total
Algeria, Algiers	51.5	28.2	9.0	6.3	5.0	**458**	475
Algeria, Batna	53.9	33.0	1.9	9.7	1.5	**206**	223
Algeria, Constantine	8.5	53.2	12.8	19.1	6.4	**47**	48
Algeria, Oran	51.5	23.0	10.0	0.8	14.6	**239**	243
Algeria, Setif	3.8	78.8	1.3	11.3	5.0	**80**	80
Burkina Faso, Ouagadougou	40.0	-	20.0	20.0	20.0	**5**	12
Congo, Brazzaville	3.8	15.4	57.7	3.8	19.2	**26**	46
France, La Reunion	-	73.0	20.6	3.6	2.7	**330**	331
The Gambia	23.5	58.8	5.9	-	11.8	**17**	21
Guinea, Conakry	2.6	22.1	41.6	13.0	20.8	**77**	105
Kenya, Eldoret	11.1	41.7	41.7	5.6	-	**36**	43
Malawi, Blantyre	30.8	41.0	17.9	5.1	5.1	**39**	40
Mali, Bamako	7.6	61.9	21.2	0.8	8.5	**118**	130
Namibia	51.0	37.2	10.3	1.3	0.3	**1141**	1144
Niger, Niamey	11.6	37.2	16.3	23.3	11.6	**43**	61
Nigeria, Ibadan	11.1	33.3	25.9	22.2	7.4	**27**	30
Rwanda, Butare	3.1	37.5	18.8	15.6	25.0	**32**	32
South Africa: Black	16.9	43.0	23.9	10.1	6.0	**3444**	3444
South Africa: White	70.8	20.1	7.8	0.8	0.5	**44548**	44548
South Africa: Indian	37.1	25.8	17.2	12.6	7.3	**151**	151
South Africa: Mixed race	41.8	36.2	13.0	6.5	2.5	**555**	555
South Africa, Elim	23.3	26.7	43.3	3.3	3.3	**30**	30
South Africa, Transkei, Umtata	80.0	20.0	-	-	-	**5**	7
South Africa, Transkei, 4 districts	-	40.0	60.0	-	-	**5**	8
Swaziland	44.4	31.7	15.9	7.9	-	**63**	99
Tanzania, Dar Es Salaam	9.8	68.8	9.8	8.9	2.7	**112**	113
Tanzania, Kilimanjaro	14.3	48.6	25.7	11.4	-	**35**	35
Tunisia, Centre, Sousse	68.6	17.2	6.4	7.8	-	**204**	204
Tunisia, North, Tunis	69.5	18.5	8.0	4.0	-	**249**	249
Tunisia, Sfax	68.9	25.5	2.8	2.8	-	**106**	106
Uganda, Mbarara	-	38.9	16.7	22.2	22.2	**18**	22
Uganda, Kyadondo County	18.9	39.6	34.0	-	7.5	**53**	68
Zimbabwe, Harare: African	10.7	34.0	38.6	10.7	6.1	**197**	225
Zimbabwe, Harare: European	68.5	24.9	5.9	0.5	0.3	**2773**	2789

Table 4. Site distribution of SCCs in the Gold Coast (Ghana), 1942–55 From Edington (1956)

Site	Number
Lower leg and foot	24
Orbital area	16
Penis	16
Mouth and tongue	13
Vulva	10
Scrotum	6
Hand and forearm	6
Face	5
Neck	4
Arms	3
Other	6

Skin cancer was the most common site in a ten-year biopsy series in Yirga Alem Hospital, Ethiopia (1986–95), 46.6% of them SCC and 34.8% melanomas. Most of the cancers were located on the lower limbs and, as in other East African countries, were often associated with old tropical ulcers and scars (Ashine & Lemma, 1999).

Site distribution

Biopsy specimens for the years 1942–55 in the Gold Coast were analysed by Edington (1956). The site distribution recorded for 109 SCCs (57 were of unknown site) is shown in Table 4.

A review of SCC of skin in non-Albino black Tanzanians found that the most affected site was the lower limb, with 40% of diagnoses, followed by head and neck. The penis in males and the vulva in females were the third most affected sites (Amir *et al.*, 1992a). 30% of BCC cases arose on the face. The scalp, ear, nose and eyelid each had 9–11% of the BCC cases, and site was not specified for 17% of cases (Amir *et al.*, 1992b).

In 524 cases of SCC seen in a hospital series in Zaria, Nigeria, 54% were on the lower limb, followed by the head and neck region. Chronic leg ulcer was the most common predisposing factor (Yakubu & Mabogunje, 1995).

Risk factors

Burkitt (1973) described scar epithelioma as 'ubiquitous' throughout Uganda, Kenya, Tanzania and Malawi in the 1970. This epithelioma usually arose from a chronic ulcer, was more common in men and was usually located on the lower limb. Some cases had had an ulcer for 35–40 years. It was suggested that women might be protected by their long dresses (Davies, 1957).

Tropical ulcers were found to be frequent in East Africa and much of West Africa, but rare among the Bantu of South Africa. The tumours (mostly SCC) normally arise many years after the initial ulcer develops and often after complete healing, in the depigmented scar tissue (Cook & Burkitt, 1971). SCC was the commonest diagnosis in a biopsy series from north-eastern Zaire during the period 1971–83 and 43% of these tumours arose in a chronic (tropical) ulcer or the site of previous trauma (Oates et al., 1984).

Skin cancer reported in Ugandan Africans from the Kampala cancer registry for 1964–68 arose almost entirely in association with scars, often as a result of a tropical ulcer, and at least 80% occurred in the lower leg. The majority were well differentiated SCC and the underlying connective tissue never showed evidence of solar damage, even under depigmented scars. The picture in the Kampala Europeans was very different, with most skin tumours seen on the face and ears. Albino Africans showed a similar pattern to Europeans, but incidence was higher and the cancer occurred at an earlier age (Templeton & Viegas, 1970).

Hutt (1991) agreed that the great majority of SCCs of the skin arise in areas of damaged skin, particularly at the site of old tropical ulcers on the lower leg, and – less commonly – because of burn scars and chronic sinuses. He noted that the highest frequency of skin cancers was generally found in very poor areas with few health facilities, and occurrence could be reduced by better management of tropical ulcers and other chronic skin lesions. A report from Tanzania noted that SCC following leg ulcers had become less common because of improved treatment of tropical ulcers and better nutrition (Samitz, 1980).

References

Amir, H. Kwesigabo, G. & Hirji, K. (1992a) Comparative study of superficial cancer in Tanzania. *E. Afr. Med. J.*, **69**, 88–93

Amir, H., Mbonde, M.P. & Kitinya, J.N. (1992b) Cutaneous squamous cell carcinoma in Tanzania. *Cent. Afr. J. Med.*, **38**, 439–443

Armstrong, B.K. & Kricker, A. (1995) Skin cancer. *Dermatoepidemiology*, **13**, 583–594

Ashine, S. & Lemma, B. (1999) Malignant tumours at Yirga Alem Hospital. *Ethiop. Med. J.*, **37**, 163–172

Burkitt, D.P. (1973) Distribution of cancer in Africa. *Proc. Roy. Soc. Med.*, **66**, 312–314

Cook, P.J. & Burkitt, D.P. (1971) Cancer in Africa. *Br. Med. Bull.*, **27**, 14–20

Davies, J.N.P. (1957) Cancer in relation to other diseases in Africa. *Acta Unio int. Cancr.*, **13**, 398–903

Edington, G.M. (1956) Malignant disease in the Gold Coast. *Br. J. Cancer*, **10**, 595–609

Hutt, M.S.R. (1991) Cancer and cardiovascular diseases. In: Feachem, R.G. & Jamison, D.T., eds, *Disease and Mortality in Sub-Saharan Africa*, Oxford, Oxford University Press, pp. 221–240

IARC (1992) *IARC Monographs on the Evaluation of Carcinogenic Risks to Humans. Vol. 55, Solar and Ultraviolet Radiation*, Lyon, IARC

Malik, M.O.A., Hidayatalla, A., Daoud, E.H. & El Hassan, A.M. (1974) Superficial cancer in the Sudan. A study of 1225 primary malignant superficial tumours. *Br. J. Cancer*, **30**, 355–364

Munyao, T.M. & Othieno-Abinya, N.A. (1999) Cutaneous basal cell carcinoma in Kenya. *E. Afr. Med. J.*, **76**, 97–100

Oates, K., Dealler, S., Dickey, R. & Wood, P. (1984) Malignant neoplasms 1971-1983 in northeastern Zaire, with particular reference to Kaposi's sarcoma and malignant melanoma. *Ann. Soc. belge Méd. trop.*, **64**, 373–378

Ross, M.D. (1967) Tumours in Mashonaland Africans. *Cent. Afr. J. Med.*, **13**, 107–116 and 139–145

Samitz, M.H. (1980) Dermatology in Tanzania. Problems and solutions. *Int. J. Dermatol.*, **19**, 102–106

Strom, S.S. & Yamamura, Y. (1997) Epidemiology of nonmelanoma skin cancer. *Clinics Plastic Surg.*, **24**, pp. 627–636

Templeton, A.C. & Viegas, O.A. (1970) Racial variations in tumour incidence in Uganda. *Trop. Geogr. Med.*, **22**, 431–438

Yakubu, A. & Mabogunje, O. (1995) Skin cancer of the head and neck in Zaria, Nigeria. *Acta Oncol.*, **34**, 469–471

4.18 Stomach cancer

Introduction

In 1980, stomach cancer was still reckoned to be the most common cancer in the world (Parkin *et al.*, 1988). However, at least in developed countries with reliable data, incidence and mortality have progressively declined – a phenomenon referred to as 'an unplanned triumph' (Howson *et al.*, 1986). Stomach cancer now ranks only fourth in frequency, accounting for some 876 000 new cases (8.7% of all cancers) worldwide in the year 2000 (Ferlay *et al.*, 2001). Internationally, the world age-standardized incidence (ASR) of stomach cancer in males varies from a high of about 80 cases per 100 000 in Japan to less than 10 per 100 000 in places in India, Thailand and Africa.

Overall, stomach cancer is less common in Africa: it accounted for an estimated 28 000 new cancers in 2000, some 4.5% of the total. However, there was certainly until recently considerable underreporting because of the rapid fatality rate and lack of diagnostic facilities. This was noted in Tanzania by Burkitt *et al.* (1968); in a gastric cancer series of about 250 cases, only 25% were histologically verified. Stomach cancer diagnoses were reviewed in a rural hospital in Chogoria, Kenya, between 1960 and 1986 (MacFarlane *et al.*, 2001a). The age-standardized 'incidence' of stomach cancer increased from a low of about 3 per 100 000 before 1983 to 14 per 100 000 in 1986 (similar to rates observed in eastern Europe) after an endoscope was purchased in 1984.

Descriptive epidemiology in Africa

Table 1 shows the incidence rates of stomach cancer in Africa from cancer registries reported in this volume. The geographical patterns are not obvious; there are moderately high rates in both West Africa (Bamako, Mali – ASR 18.5 per 100 000 in men and 15.0 per 100 000 in women) and in the island of Reunion (25.3 per 100 000 for males and 9.1 per 100 000 for females). Rates are also moderately high in East Africa (Eldoret, Kenya – ASR 11.3 and 7.6 per 100 000; Harare, Zimbabwe – 13.0 and 11.5 per 100 000 for males and females, respectively). In contrast, Abidjan (Côte d'Ivoire), Niamey (Niger), Ibadan (Nigeria) and the Gambia all reported stomach cancer incidence rates less than ~3 per 100 000. In South Africa, the ASR (derived from the pathology-only National Cancer Registry) was 3.6 for males and 1.9 for females.

Data from cancer registries between the 1950s and 1970s showed marked variation in stomach cancer incidence in Africans, ranging from 2.3 per 100 000 in Kyadondo (Uganda) to a high of 37.5 per 100 000 in Cape Province, South Africa (Table 2). Corresponding rates in females were 0.9 in Uganda and 18.4 per 100 000 in Cape Province. The South African coloured (mixed race) population showed even higher rates (53.4 in males and 25.5 per 100 000 in females) in the 1950s. This high rate in the western Cape coloured population of South Africa persisted until at least the 1970s (mortality rate in 1968–72 of 49.9 per 100 000; Bradshaw *et al.*, 1983). In 1989 (the last year for which mortality statistics were available by ethnic group in South Africa), national age-standardized stomach cancer mortality rates in coloured males increased to 98 per 100 000 in males and 49 per 100 000 in females.

High stomach cancer rates were recorded between 1956 and 1960 in the Kivu province of the Democratic Republic of the Congo (former Zaire), with age-standardized rates of 9.3 per 100 000 person years among males and 15.1 per 100 000 among females (Clemmesen *et al.*, 1962). In the 'zone de santé' of Katana hospital in Kivu province during the period 1983–86, stomach cancer was the third most common cancer among males, accounting for 14.7% of all cancers, and the leading cancer in females, accounting for 17.8% of all cancers (Bourdeaux, 1988). By contrast, Oates *et al.* (1984)

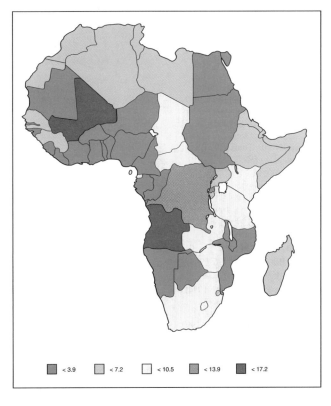

Figure 1. Incidence of stomach cancer: ASR (world) - males (all ages)

Legend: < 3.9 | < 7.2 | < 10.5 | < 13.9 | < 17.2

analysed pathological data from north-east of the country and found that between 1971 and 1983, among 794 cancers, cancer of the stomach comprised only 3%. However, in areas lacking endoscopic biopsy facilities, stomach cancers are likely to be under-reported. In Rwanda, which neighbours Kivu province of the Democratic Republic of the Congo, the age-standardized incidence rate of stomach cancer was 13 per 100 000 in males and 15 per 100 000 in females; the stomach was the third commonest tumour site in males and second commonest in females in the prefecture of Butare, southern Rwanda (Newton *et al.*, 1996). Burundi also seems to have a moderately high incidence of stomach cancer, particularly in males (8 and 5 per 100 000 in males and females, respectively) (Hamber & von Bergen, 1971).

The relative frequency of stomach cancer appears to decrease as one moves away from the province of Kivu eastward into Uganda. Hutt *et al.* (1965) reported the incidence of stomach cancer in Kampala Cancer Registry (Uganda) to be highest among the Ankole ethnic group and Rwandan immigrants, compared with other Ugandan tribes. Both groups inhabit an area to the south-west of Kampala which borders the Democratic Republic of the Congo's Kivu province.

Burkitt *et al.* (1969) reported data from hospitals in western Kenya and north-west Tanzania; stomach cancer accounted for 15% of all malignancies in Ndolage Hospital, which is near the border with Rwanda, but only 4.3% at Shirati Hospital on the eastern shore of Lake Victoria.

Further south, in Swaziland, stomach cancer rates of 1.8 per 100 000 in males and 0.2 in females have been reported (Peers & Keen, 1986).

Most of the stomach cancer data reported by Parkin (1986) were derived from either pathology-based cancer registries, which

Table 1. Age-standardized (world) and cumulative (0-64) incidence
Stomach (C16)

	MALE				FEMALE			
	Cases	CRUDE	ASR(W) (per 100,000)	Cumulative (%)	Cases	CRUDE	ASR(W) (per 100,000)	Cumulative (%)
Africa, North								
Algeria, Algiers (1993-1997)	211	3.8	**5.6**	0.35	155	2.8	**3.7**	0.25
Algeria, Constantine (1994-1997)	32	2.1	**3.6**	0.20	21	1.4	**2.2**	0.16
Algeria, Oran (1996-1998)	91	5.1	**7.6**	0.42	52	3.0	**4.0**	0.24
Algeria, Setif (1993-1997)	131	4.4	**7.8**	0.51	56	1.9	**3.1**	0.26
Tunisia, Centre, Sousse (1993-1997)	42	3.6	**5.0**	0.26	24	2.1	**2.7**	0.15
Tunisia, North, Tunis (1994)	102	4.7	**6.1**	0.37	61	2.9	**3.5**	0.25
Tunisia, Sfax (1997)	10	2.5	**3.1**	0.18	9	2.4	**2.9**	0.19
Africa, West								
The Gambia (1997-1998)	11	1.1	**2.5**	0.12	8	0.8	**2.1**	0.19
Guinea, Conakry (1996-1999)	59	2.6	**6.1**	0.38	34	1.5	**3.6**	0.26
Mali, Bamako (1988-1997)	290	7.5	**17.3**	1.25	216	6.0	**14.6**	1.16
Niger, Niamey (1993-1999)	13	0.7	**2.7**	0.28	15	0.8	**3.3**	0.34
Nigeria, Ibadan (1998-1999)	9	0.6	**1.2**	0.09	11	0.7	**1.4**	0.13
Africa, Central								
Congo, Brazzaville (1996-1999)	15	1.2	**2.0**	0.15	11	0.9	**1.3**	0.10
Africa, East								
France, La Reunion (1988-1994)	340	16.2	**21.8**	1.21	158	7.3	**7.8**	0.36
Kenya, Eldoret (1998-2000)	36	3.8	**10.4**	0.58	26	2.8	**7.8**	0.59
Malawi, Blantyre (2000-2001)	9	1.0	**2.3**	0.12	3	0.3	**0.9**	0.10
Uganda, Kyadondo County (1993-1997)	57	2.0	**7.2**	0.39	47	1.6	**5.6**	0.51
Zimbabwe, Harare: African (1990-1993)	90	3.8	**12.6**	0.44	67	3.1	**15.1**	0.58
Zimbabwe, Harare: African (1994-1997)	105	3.8	**10.6**	0.57	70	2.7	**10.3**	0.61
Zimbabwe, Harare: European (1990-1997)	41	26.8	**15.8**	1.06	18	10.7	**5.0**	0.23
Africa, South								
Namibia (1995-1998)	49	1.5	**2.7**	0.15	37	1.2	**1.8**	0.08
South Africa: Black (1989-1992)	1085	1.9	**3.6**	0.22	702	1.2	**2.0**	0.13
South Africa: Indian (1989-1992)	140	7.2	**11.7**	0.68	91	4.6	**6.4**	0.31
South Africa: Mixed race (1989-1992)	534	8.3	**16.1**	0.95	281	4.2	**6.4**	0.40
South Africa: White (1989-1992)	1110	11.0	**10.1**	0.53	638	6.3	**4.8**	0.26
South Africa, Transkei, Umtata (1996-1998)	5	1.4	**2.0**	0.05	4	0.9	**1.3**	0.05
South Africa, Transkei, 4 districts (1996-1998)	7	1.0	**1.8**	0.13	2	0.2	**0.3**	0.01
Swaziland (1996-1999)	36	2.0	**4.5**	0.29	24	1.2	**2.2**	0.19
Europe/USA								
USA, SEER: White (1993-1997)	4546	9.3	**6.9**	0.31	2618	5.2	**3.0**	0.12
USA, SEER: Black (1993-1997)	792	11.8	**13.6**	0.66	482	6.5	**5.8**	0.26
France, 8 registries (1993-1997)	2228	16.2	**11.1**	0.50	1339	9.3	**4.7**	0.17
The Netherlands (1993-1997)	7324	19.2	**13.6**	0.56	4165	10.7	**5.8**	0.23
UK, England (1993-1997)	27209	22.7	**13.8**	0.52	16159	12.6	**5.7**	0.19

In italics: histopathology-based registries

Table 2. Incidence of stomach cancer in Africa, 1953–74

Registry	Period	ASR (per 100 000)		Source
		Male	Female	(see Chap. 1)
Senegal, Dakar	1969–74	3.7	2.0	4
Mozambique, Lourenço Marques	1956–60	*3.0*	*2.4*	1
Nigeria, Ibadan	1960–69	7.2	6.4	3
SA, Cape Province: Bantu	1956–59	37.5	18.4	2
SA, Cape Province: Coloured	1956–59	53.4	25.5	2
SA, Cape Province: White	1956–59	32.4	13.8	2
SA, Johannesburg, Bantu	1953–55	10.2	6.2	1
SA, Natal Province: African	1964–66	12.1	8.3	2
SA, Natal Province: Indian	1964–66	22.1	30.0	2
Uganda, Kyadondo	1954–60	2.3	0.9	1
Uganda, Kyadondo	1960–71	3.7	2.0	5
Zimbabwe, Bulawayo	1963–72	10.6	7.3	6

Italics: Rate based on less than 10 cases

are likely to under-report the relative frequency of deep-seated tumours such as stomach cancer, or hospital-based registries that may distort rates depending on specialist interest in different conditions. In most of these registries, the male to female ratio was around 2:1 (Table 3).

These various data from registries and relative frequencies from case series have been used to estimate national incidence rates (Figure 1). The estimates of age-standardized incidence in males range from less than 3 per 100 000 in Burkina Faso, Gambia, Republic of the Congo (Brazzaville), Niger, Gabon and Tanzania, to over 15 per 100 000 in Angola, Democratic Republic of Congo, Mali and Reunion.

Gastric cancer morphology
In areas of high gastric cancer incidence, there appear to be higher proportions of the intestinal type of gastric cancer versus the diffuse type. Oettlé (1967), reviewing South African histological material from 1949–53, reported a proportion of intestinal-type gastric cancers in Africans of 54%, compared with 73% in whites. Isaacson *et al.* (1978) found 45% of gastric cancers among urban Africans to be of the intestinal type, whereas in Zimbabwe (Nkanza, 1988) the corresponding proportion was 77%. Kitinya *et al.* (1988) reported 82% intestinal-type gastric cancers in the Mount Kilimanjaro area of Tanzania, whereas the proportion in other regions of the country was 70%. In contrast, Templeton (1973) found that in Uganda 55% of gastric cancers were of the intestinal type. The reasons for these variations in the distribution of morphological types of gastric cancer are poorly understood.

Time trends
In the cancer registry of Uganda (Kyadondo), the age-standardized incidence of gastric cancer in males increased from 2.7 per 100 000 in 1960–66 to 7.6 per 100 000 in 1995–97 (Table 4); however the trend was not statistically significant (Wabinga *et al.*, 2000).

In 1949, stomach cancer was the most common cause of cancer death among whites, coloured and Asians of both sexes in South Africa. By 1969, the mortality rates had dropped for whites and Asians but not for the coloured population, who still maintained the fourth highest rate in the world (Bradshaw & Harington, 1982). However, mortality rates have subsequently fallen in all ethnic groups (see Figure 2 of Chapter 3.5.4). In a review of records at Baragwanath hospital (near Soweto, South Africa), covering 17 years (1948–64), Robertson (1969) found that stomach cancer comprised about 2.2% of all cancers in males and 1.1% in females and Isaacson *et al.* (1978) reported similar figures for the same hospital between 1966 and 1975. In the National Cancer Registry's national pathology data, stomach cancer comprised 2.8% of male and 1.7% of female cancers in 1989–92 (see Table 10 of Chapter 3.5.4).

Risk factors
Diet, tobacco, alcohol
There is convincing evidence that diets high in vegetables and fruit protect against stomach cancer. Diets high in salt probably increase risk. There is good evidence that refrigeration of food also protects against this cancer by facilitating year-round consumption of fruit and vegetables and probably by reducing the need for salt as a preservative. Vitamin C, contained in vegetables, fruits and other foods of plant origin, is probably protective, and so too are diets high in whole-grain cereals, carotenoids and also green tea (World Cancer Research Fund, 1997). Many studies suggest a small increase in risk (about two-fold) in smokers (Tredaniel *et al.*, 1997), but alcohol does not affect risk except at the gastric cardia.

In Africa, there have been no studies on the relation of diet, salt or pickled foods on the risk of developing stomach cancer. A geographical study in western Uganda suggested that most of the ethnic groups with high risk of developing stomach cancer are cattle-keepers who consume plenty of milk (Cook & Kajubi, 1966).

No studies have been conducted to measure the association between alcohol consumption or other environmental risk factors and gastric cancer. However Kitinya *et al.* (1988) noted that in the Mount Kilimanjaro area, with high frequency of stomach cancer, the alcohol commonly consumed is brewed from bananas, whereas in low-risk areas, the alcohol is made from grains. Similarly, people of western Uganda and the Gishu also brew alcohol from bananas, while the rest of the country consumes alcohol made from millet.

Helicobacter pylori
H. pylori, isolated in 1984 (Marshall & Warren, 1984), has been shown to be associated with a number of gastroduodenal diseases, including duodenal and gastric ulcers (Blaser, 1990), chronic active gastritis, chronic atrophic gastritis, intestinal metaplasia (the latter two lesions being important precursors of stomach cancer; Correa, 1988) and finally stomach cancer (IARC, 1994).

H. pylori infection is particularly prevalent among third-world populations, and in western countries, those of a lower socio-economic status have higher infection rates (Sitas *et al.*, 1991). Crowding at a young age seems to be a risk factor (Sitas *et al.*, 1992). In Africa, prevalence of infection with *H. pylori* is about 50% in children under 15 years of age (Sitas, 1990; Sathar *et al.*, 1994) and reaches over 70% in most adult populations studied (Table 5). However, in South African whites, adult infection rates resemble those in western countries (40%) (Sathar *et al.*, 1994). In Africa, *H. pylori* infection is associated with markers of hepatitis A infection (Sathar *et al.*, 1994), premastication of food in Burkina Faso (Albengue *et al.*, 1990), race (Sathar *et al.*, 1994), social class and educational standard in South Africa, but not with number of persons sharing current accommodation (Louw *et al.*, 1993). However, other population studies of seroprevalence in South Africa found no association with any index of social class (Sitas *et al.*, 1997). Virtually no studies have looked at the distribution of intestinal metaplasia in the stomach in Africa. In a follow-up endoscopic series of 51 *H. pylori*-positive patients in Kenya by McFarlane *et al.* (2001b), 61% had atrophic gastritis and 24% both atrophic gastritis and intestinal metaplasia. After a year's follow-up, the proportion of those with atrophic gastritis increased to 70% but the proportion of those with intestinal metaplasia remained the same (22%). The progression from moderate to severe atrophy was 1.8%, as in other regions of the world. Given the slow progression from atrophic gastritis to gastric cancer, the authors speculated that other factors may modulate this process. CagA-positive strains of *H. pylori* predominate in Africa (Ally *et al.*, 1998) but their role in modulating the progression of gastritis to gastric cancer remains speculative (Kuipers & Meijer, 2000).

In a number of endoscopic studies, *H. pylori* was observed microscopically or was cultured from gastric biopsies more frequently in patients diagnosed with gastritis (of varying forms). For example, Rouvroy (1987) found *H. pylori* to be present in 33% of biopsies with normal gastric mucosa, in 83% of those with gastric atrophy and in 43% with gastric cancer.

It appears that, even in a continent where the prevalence of *H. pylori* infection is high, differences in prevalence exist between those who have a 'normal' gastric mucosa (0–40%) and those with gastritis (80–100%) (Table 6). Very few data exist on the prevalence of gastritis in asymptomatic populations. In a group of 40 hospital volunteers in Kenya, 23 (58%) were found to have mild or moderate atrophic gastritis, but none had severe gastritis or intestinal metaplasia. In this group the seroprevalence of *H. pylori* was 95%, but 70% had organisms detected microscopically. This may indicate that while most adults have been infected with the organism sometime during their lives, and show elevated antibody levels, active colonization may be associated with gastritis.

Only one study in Africa has found a positive association between *H. pylori* and gastric cancer. In a series of 176 patients, the prevalence of *H. pylori* detected by microscopy was 34% in those with a normal mucosa, 79% in those with superficial

Table 3. Stomach cancer in various cases series (from Parkin, 1986)

Country	Place	Dates	%		ASR	
			male	female	male	female
Algeria	Algiers, Oran, Constantine (pathology)	1966–75	4.4	1.7	3.6	1.4
Angola	Luanda: Pathology Dept	1977–80	9.8	4.7	–	–
Egypt	Cairo	1978–79	7.3	5.5		
Gabon	Libreville: Pathogy Dept	1978–84	1.1	1.8		
Kenya	National Cancer Registry (Pathology)	1968–78	4.3	2.4		
	Coast General Hospital, Mombasa	1981	3.6	2.8		
Liberia	Cancer registry	1976–80	3.5	1.3		
Madagascar	Pathology series	1979–81	1.3	0.5		
Malawi	Pathology	1976–80	2.1	0.4		
Nigeria	Ibadan	1970–76	6.0	2.2	7.1	4.0
	Zaria (Pathology)	1976–78	1.5	1.1		
Rwanda	Pathology series	1982–84	9.9	6.5		
Sudan	Hospital (Radiotherapy) Cancer Registry	1978	2.7	1.5		
Swaziland	Cancer Registry	1979–83	2.3	0.3	1.8	0.2
Tanzania	Tanzania Cancer Registry (Pathology)	1980–81	1.7	1.5		
	Mwanza Hospital	1980–81	1.6	0.9		
	Kilimanjaro Hospital	1975–79	8.6	9.9	5.6	4.6
Tunisia	Hospital Registry	1976–80	2.1	1.5		
Uganda	Kuluva Hospital W. Nile	1961–78	0.5	–		
Zambia	Zambian Cancer Registry	1981–83	5.0	4.9		
	Ndola (Pathology)	1976–79	2.8	1.4		
Zimbabwe	Bulawayo Cancer Registry	1973–77	4.5	2.6		
	Harare (Pathology)	1973–77	4.6	2.7		

Table 4. Trends in gastric cancer incidence, Kyadondo Cancer Registry, 1960–97 (Wabinga et al., 2000)

Time period	ASR (per 100 000)	
	Males	Females
1960–66	2.7	0.8
1967–71	4.7	3.4
1991–94	4.7	3.2
1995–97	7.6	5.6

Table 5. Population seroprevalence of *H. pylori* antibodies in African adults

Population	Prevalence	Reference
Algeria	79%	Megraud et al., 1989
Côte d'Ivoire	71%	Megraud et al., 1989
Dem. Rep. Congo (Zaire)	79%	Glupczynski et al., 1992
Nigeria	85%	Holcombe et al., 1992
South Africa	86%	Sitas et al., 1997
South Africa		Sathar et al., 1994
Africans	93%	
Indians	83%	
Mixed race	81%	
Whites	42%	

gastritis, 89% in those with chronic atrophic gastritis and 100% (6/6) in those with stomach cancer (Jaskiewicz et al., 1989). In this study, *H. pylori* status in those with stomach cancer was assessed microscopically in tissue from the adjoining gastric mucosa, rather than the cancer itself (Rouvroy et al., 1987). In a review of all African studies on *H. pylori* and gastroduodenal pathology, the prevalence of *H. pylori* was 78% in six studies in relation to gastric atrophy, 78% in six studies that recorded intestinal metaplasia and 69% in studies recording stomach cancer (Kidd et al., 1999b). Wabinga (1996) studied gastric endoscopic biopsies of patients with upper gastrointestinal symptoms and demonstrated a high frequency of colonization by *H. pylori* in populations with high risk of stomach cancer development. Using a commercial kit to detect anti-HP IgG antibody in a small case–control study in South Africa (48 gastric cancer cases, 48 controls), Louw et al. (2001) found a high prevalence of infection in the control subjects with non-ulcer dyspepsia (79%), but a non-significant association with cancer (OR estimated from authors' data 1.5, 95% CI 0.5–4.9).

H. pylori strain differences may be important in the development of gastric cancer. For example, the vacA s1 genotype to be more common in patients with gastric cancer (Kidd et al., 1999a; Louw et al., 2001).

Volcanic soils

The relative frequency of gastric cancer in highland areas of East and Central Africa has led to a hypothesis of an association with exposure to volcanic soils. High relative frequencies have been recorded in the Gishu ethnic group on the slopes of Mount Elgon in eastern Uganda and among residents of the slopes of Mount Kenya (Templeton, 1973). Kitinya (1988) reported high proportions of stomach cancer in persons living on the slopes of Mount Kilimanjaro. All these mountain areas are volcanic. Ethiopia, another particularly volcanic country, has reported relatively high incidence rates of gastric cancer (Madebo et al., 1994). However, some populations living in volcanic areas have low occurrence. The

Table 6. Presence of *H. pylori* in biopsy specimens of gastric mucosa

Place	Normal	Gastritis	Atrophic gastritis	Intestinal metaplasia	Gastric cancer	Reference
Ghana		100				Wyatt *et al.*, 1987
Nigeria	33 (1/3)	87			0/1	Holcombe *et al.*, 1990
Kenya	10	80				Lachlan *et al.*, 1988
Uganda	–	100				Weir *et al.*, 1988
Zimbabwe		96				Weir *et al.*, 1988
Tunisia	24	86				Fendri *et al.*, 1988
Rwanda	33	46–96	83		43%	Rouvroy *et al.*, 1987
South Africa	38		52		100 (6/6)	Jaskiewicz *et al.*, 1989
Kenya	0 (0/9)		82			Sitas, 1990
Malawi		90–100*				Harries *et al.*, 1992

*Gastritis 'score >2'

Kiga tribe, for example, lives on slopes of the volcanic Mount Muhavura, but has low incidence rates (Templeton, 1973). Therefore, volcanic soil is unlikely to be the only factor responsible for high incidence of stomach cancer; no known carcinogens have been found in these soils (Ilnilsky *et al.*, 1976).

Blood group A

The risk of developing gastric cancer has been reported to be higher in those of blood group A (Correa, 1988). However in Africa, areas with high incidence of stomach cancer appear to have the lowest frequency of blood group A (Ssebabi, 1975).

References

Albengue, M., Tall, F., Dabis, F. *et al.* (1990) Epidemiological study of Helicobacter pylori transmission from mother to child in Africa. Abstract. *Rev. Esp. Enferm. Apar. Dig.*, **78**, 48

Ally, R., Hale, M., Morton, D., Hadjinicolou, C., Sonnendecker, H.E.M., Bardhan, K.D. & Segal, I. (1998) *Helicobacter pylori* (HP) in Soweto, South Africa. CagA status and histopathology in children (abstract). *Gastroenterology*, **114**, A55

Blaser, M.J. (1990) Epidemiology and pathophysiology of Campylobacter pylori infections. *Rev. Infect. Dis.*, **12** (suppl. 1), S99–106

Bourdeaux, L., Renard, F., Gigase, P.L., Mukolo-Ndjolo., Maldague, P. & De Muynck, A. (1988) L'incidence des cancers à l'hôpital de Katana, Kivu, Est Zaire, de 1983 à 1986. *Ann. Soc. Belg. Méd. Trop.*, **68**, 141–156

Bradshaw, E. & Harington, J.S. (1982) A comparison of cancer mortality rates in South Africa with those in other countries. *S. Afr. Med. J.*, **61**, 943–946

Burkitt, D.P., Hutt, M.S.R. & Slavin, G. (1968) Clinicopathological studies of cancer distribution in Africa. *Br. J. Cancer*, **22**, 1–6

Burkitt, D.P., Bundschuh, M., Dahlin, K., Dahlin, L. & Neale, R. (1969) Some cancer patterns in western Kenya and Northwest Tanzania. *E. Afr. Med. J.*, **46**, 188–193

Clemmesen, J., Maisin, J. & Gigase, P. (1962) Preliminary Report on Cancer in Kivu and Rwanda-Urundi, Louvain, University of Louvain, Institut de Cancer

Cook, G.C. & Kajubi, S.K. (1966) Tribal incidence of lactase deficiency in Uganda. *Lancet*, **i**, 726–729

Correa, P. (1988) A human model of gastric carcinogenesis. *Cancer Res.*, **48**, 3554–3560

Fendri, C., Ben Jilani, S., Fauchere, J.L., Kervella, M., Bonnevielle, F., Boujnah, A., Kechrid, A., Ennaifar, M. & Ben Redjeb, S. (1989) [Diagnosis of gastritis caused by Campylobacter pylori. Presentation of 3 methods: bacteriology, histology and immunoblotting]. *Tunis Med.*, **67**, 151–154

Ferlay, J., Bray, F, Pisani, P. & Parkin, D.M. (2001) *GLOBOCAN 2000: Cancer Incidence, Mortality and Prevalence Worldwide*, Version 1.0 (CD-ROM) (IARC CancerBase No. 5), Lyon, IARCPress

Glupczynski, Y., Bourdeaux, L., Verhas, M., DePrez, C., DeVos, D. & Devreker, T. (1992) Use of a urea breath test versus invasive methods to determine the prevalence of *Helicobacter pylori* in Zaire. *Eur. J. Clin. Microbiol. Infect. Dis.*, **11**, 322–327

IARC (1994) *IARC Monographs on the Evaluation of Carcinogenic Risks to Humans*, Volume 61, *Schistosomes, Liver Flukes and Helicobacter pylori*, Lyon, IARC

Hamber, G. & von Bergen, M. (1971) Peptic ulcer in the Burundi Republic and Nile-Congo watershed. *Trop. Geogr. Med.*, **23**, 213–219

Harries, A.D., Stewart, M., Deegan, K.M., Mughoho, G.K., Wirima, J.J., Hommel, M. & Hart, C.A. (1992) *Helicobacter pylori* in Malawi, central Africa. *J. Infect.*, **24**, 269–276

Holcombe, C., Lucas, S.B., Umar, H. & Abba, A. (1990) *Helicobacter (=Campylobacter) pylori* in Africa. *Trans. R. Soc. Trop. Med.*, **84**, 294–296

Holcombe, C., Omotara, B.A., Eldridge, J., Jones, D.M. (1992) *H. pylori*, the most common bacterial infection in Africa: a random serological study. *Am. J. Gastroenterol.*, **87**, 28–30

Howson, C.P., Hiyama, T. & Wynder, E.L. (1986) The decline in gastric cancer: epidemiology of an unplanned triumph. *Epidiemiol. Rev.*, **8**, 1–27

Hutt, M.S.R., Burkitt, D.P., Shepherd, B., Wright, B., Mati, J.K.G. & Auma, S. (1965) Malignant tumours of the gastrointestinal tract in Uganda. *Natl Cancer Inst. Monogr.*, **25**, 41–47

Ilnilsky, A.P., Beletsky, G.A. & Shabad, L.M. (1976) On the carcinogenic polycyclic aromatic hydrocarbon benzo(a)pyrene in volcano exhausts. *Cancer Lett.*, **1**, 291–294

Isaacson, C. (1978) The changing pattern of liver disease in South African Blacks. *S. Afr. Med. J.*, **53**, 365–368

Isaacson, C., Selzer, G., Kaye, V., Greenberg, M., Woodruff, D., Davies, J., Ninin, D., Vetten, D. & Andrew, M. (1978) Cancer in the urban blacks of South Africa. *S. Afr. Cancer Bull.*, **22**, 49–84

Jaskiewicz, K., Lowrens, H.D., Woodroof, C.W., van Wyk, M.J. & Price, S.K. (1989) The association of Campylobacter pylori with mucosal pathological changes in a population at risk of gastric cancer. *S. Afr. Med. J.*, **75**, 417–419

Kidd, M., Lastovica, A.J., Atherton, J.C. & Louw, J.A. (1999a) Heterogeneity in the Helicobacter pylori vacA and cagA genes: association with gastroduodenal disease in South Africa? *Gut*, **45**, 499-502

Kidd, M., Louw, J. & Marks, I.N. (1999b) *Helicobacter pylori* in Africa. Observations on an 'enigma within an enigma'. *J Gastroenterol. Hepatol.*, **14**, 851–858

Kitinya, J.N., Lauren, P.A., Jones, M.E., Paljarvi, L. (1988) Epidemiology of intestinal and diffuse types of gastric cancer in the Mount Kilimanjaro area, Tanzania. *Afr. J. Med. Sci.*, **17**, 89–95

Kuipers, E.J. & Meijer, G.A. (2000) *Helicobacter pylori* gastritis in Africa. *Eur. J. Gastroenterol. Hepatol.*, **12**, 601–603

Lachlan, G.W., Gilmour, H.M. & Jass, J.J. (1988) *Campylobacter pylori* in central Africa. *Br. Med. J.*, **296**, 66

Louw, J.A., Jaskiewicz, K., Girdwood, A.H., Zak, J., Trey, G., Lucke, W., Truter, H. & Kotze, T.J. (1993) *H. pylori* prevalence in non-ulcer dyspepsia-ethnic and socio-economic differences. *S. Afr. Med. J.*, **83**, 169–171

Louw, J.A., Kidd, M.S.G., Kummer, A.F., Taylor, K., Kotze, U. & Hanslo, D. (2001) The relationship between *Helicobacter pylori* infection, the virulence genotypes of the infecting strain and gastric cancer in the African setting. *Helicobacter*, **6**, 268–273

Madebo, T., Lindtjorn, B. & Henriksen, T.-H. (1994) High incidence of oesophagus and stomach cancers in the Bale highlands of south Ethiopia. *Trans. R. Soc. Trop. Med. Hyg.*, **88**, 415

McFarlane, G., Forman, D., Sitas, F. & Lachlan, G. (2001a) A minimum estimate for the incidence of gastric cancer in Eastern Kenya. *Br. J. Cancer*, **85**, 1322–1325

McFarlane, G.A., Wyatt, J., Forman, D. & Lachlan, G.W. (2001b) Trends over time in *Helicobacter pylori* gastritis in Kenya. *Eur. J. Gastroenterol. Hepatol.*, **12**, 617–621

Megraud, F., Brassens-Rabbe, M.P., Denis, F., Belbouri, A. & Hoa, D.Q. (1989) Seroepidemiology of *Campylobacter pylori* infection in various populations. *J. Clin. Microbiol.*, **27**, 1870–1873

Newton, R., Ngilimana, P., Grulich, A., Beral, V., Sindikubwabo, B., Nganyira, A. & Parkin, D.M. (1996) Cancer in Rwanda. *Int. J. Cancer*, **66**, 75–81

Nkanza, N.K. (1988) The histopathology of carcinoma of the stomach in Zimbabwe. *Cent. Afr. Med. J.*, **34**, 207–211

Oates, K., Dealler, S., Dickey, R. & Wood, P. (1984) Malignant neoplasms 1971-1983 in Northeastern Zaire, with particular reference to Kaposi's sarcoma and malignant Melanoma. *Ann. Soc. Belge Med. Trop.*, **64**, 373–378

Oettle, A.G. (1964) Cancer in Africa, especially in regions south of the Sahara. *J. Natl Cancer Inst.*, **33**, 383–439

Oettle, A.G. (1967) Primary neolasms of the alimentary canal in Whites and Bantu of the Tranvaal, 1949-1953. A histopathological series. *Natl Cancer Inst. Monogr.*, **25**, 97–109

Parkin, D.M., ed. (1986) *Cancer Occurrence in Developing Countries* (IARC Scientific Publications No. 75), Lyon, IARC

Parkin, D.M., Läärä, E. & Muir, C.S. (1988) Estimates of the worldwide frequency of sixteen major cancers in 1980. *Int. J. Cancer*, **41**, 184–187

Peers, F. & Keen, P. (1986) Swaziland. In: Parkin, D.M., ed., *Cancer Occurrence in Developing Countries* (IARC Scientific Publications No. 75), Lyon, IARC, pp. 89–92

Robertson, M.A. (1969) Clinical observation on cancer patterns at the non-white hospital Baragwanath, Johannesburg, 1948-1964. *S. Afr. Med. J.*, **26**, 915–931

Rouvroy, D., Bogaerts, J., Nsengiumwa, O., Omar, M., Versailles, L. & Haot, J. (1987) *Campylobacter pylori*, gastritis and peptic ulcer disease in central Africa. *Br. Med. J.*, **295**, 1174

Sathar, M.A., Simjee, A.E., Wittenberg, D.F. & Mayat, A.M. (1994) Seroprevalence of *Helicobacter pylori* infection in Natal/KwaZulu, South Africa. *Eur. J. Gastroenterol. Hepatol.*, **6**, 37–41

Sitas, F. (1990) The seroepidemiology of Helicobacter pylori and its relationship to chronic atrophic gastritis. D.Phil. Thesis, Green College, University of Oxford

Sitas, F., Forman, D., Yarnell, J.W., Burr, M.L., Elwood, P.C., Pedley, S. & Marks, K.J. (1991) *Helicobacter pylori* infection rates in relation to age and social class in a population of Welsh men. *Gut*, **32**, 25–28

Sitas, F., Yarnell, J. & Forman, D. (1992) *Helicobacter pylori* infection rates in relation to age and social class in a population of Welsh men. *Gut*, **33**, 1582

Sitas, F., Sathar, M.A., Simjee, A.E., Lombard, C.J., Steyn, K., Badenhorst, C.J., Jooste, P.L. & Bourne, L. (1997) *Helicobacter pylori* seroprevalence in the African adult population of the Cape Peninsula. *S. Afr. J. Epidemiol. Infect.*, **12**, 111–114

Ssebabi, E.C.T. (1975) *Characteristic of African blood. CRC Critical Reviews in Clinical Laboratory Sciences*, 19–45

Templeton, A.C. (1973) Tumour of the alimentary canal. In: Templeton, A.C., ed., *Tumours in a Tropical Country.* (Recent Results in Cancer Research Vol. 41), Berlin, Heidelberg, Springer-Verlag, pp. 23–56

Tredaniel, J., Boffetta, P., Buiatti, E., Saracci, R. & Hirsch, A. (1997) Tobacco smoking and gastric cancer: review and meta-analysis. *Int. J. Cancer*, **72**, 565–573

Wabinga, H.R. (1996) Frequency of *Helicobacter pylori* in gastroscopic biopsy of Ugandan African. *E. Afr. Med. J.*, **71**, 691–693

Wabinga, H.R., Parkin, D.M., Wabwire-Mangen, F. & Nambooze, S. (2000) Trends in cancer incidence in Kyadondo County, Uganda, 1960-1997. *Br. J. Cancer*, **82**, 1585–1592

Weir, W.R., Goodgame, R., Kiire, C.F. & Lucas, S.B. (1988) Campylobacter-like organisms and gastritis in Africa. *Trans. R. Soc. Trop. Med. Hyg.*, **82**, 172

World Cancer Research Fund (1997) *Diet, Nutrition and the Prevention of Cancer: A Global Perspective*, Washington, DC, World Cancer Research Fund

Wyatt, J., de Caestecker, J.S., Rathbone, B.J. & Heatley, R.V. (1987) *Campylobacter pyloridis* in tropical Africa. Abstract. *Gut*, **28**, A1357

4.19 Thyroid cancer

Introduction

Cancer of the thyroid is not particularly common; worldwide, the estimated 123 000 new cases annually comprise 1.2% of all cancers (0.6% of cases in men and 1.9% in women). In Africa, it is proportionately a little more common, with 6300 new cases accounting for 1.4% of new cancers (0.8% in men and 2.0% in women). The large majority of cases are carcinomas, which are classified as papillary, follicular, medullary and undifferentiated (anaplastic). In most series, papillary carcinoma is the most common, with follicular carcinomas representing about one quarter, and medullary/anaplastic tumours some 5–15% (Ron, 1996). The sex ratio is about 3:1 (except for medullary carcinomas, which occur equally in the two sexes).

It is known that diagnostic practices (for example, with respect to histological examination of resected goitres, or at autopsy) can influence apparent rates of incidence. This may account for the particularly high rates observed in the US white population. In the United States, the higher incidence of thyroid cancer among whites is confined to papillary carcinomas (Correa & Chen, 1995).

Descriptive epidemiology in Africa

Table 1 shows age-standardized incidence rates from different centres, as reported in this volume, with data from Europe and North America for comparison. Table 2 shows incidence data from time periods in the 1960s and 1970s.

In Africa, it appears that the incidence rates are similar to those elsewhere in the world (except in North American white populations). In most series, papillary carcinomas are the predominant histological subtype (Table 3). Templeton (1973) described 82 cases from the pathology department in Kampala, Uganda. Follicular tumours were more numerous than papillary (as appears to be the case today – Table 3), all types having a female excess (F:M ratio 2:1). Incidence of papillary tumours was highest in the fourth decade and declined thereafter, with the risk of follicular cancers continuing to increase with age. There did not seem to be any increased frequency in ethnic groups from goitrous areas, or regions with volcanic soils.

McGill (1978) described 63 thyroid cancers in Kenyans; papillary carcinoma predominated in lowland tribal groups, follicular carcinoma in highland groups, and a possible link between follicular carcinoma and endemic goitre was postulated. In Khartoum, Sudan (Omran & Ahmed, 1993), in a series of 112 cases, follicular carcinoma predominated (42%), followed by papillary (22.3%) and

anaplastic tumours (21.4%). In Ibadan, Nigeria (Thomas & Ogunbiyi, 1995), papillary and follicular tumours occurred in equal numbers, with a sex ratio of about 2:1; medullary carcinoma comprised 5%. Kalk et al. (1997) studied data from the histopathology register of South Africa and noted an excess of follicular carcinomas in black women. Follicular morphology predominated in blacks resident in rural areas of the former Transvaal (58%), while papillary histology predominated in urban areas, irrespective of race. The authors attributed these patterns to regional differences in iodine deficiency.

Etiology

Risk factors for thyroid cancer include radiation and possibly diet, with cruciferous vegetables being protective and seafood a possible risk factor. Areas of endemic goitre (deficiency in dietary iodine) appear to be associated with elevated risk of follicular (and perhaps anaplastic) thyroid cancer, whereas iodine rich-areas have been associated with enhanced risk of papillary carcinoma (Ron, 1996). Attention has also been drawn to the frequency of thyroid cancer in areas with volcanic activity (Hawaii and Iceland) (Kung et al., 1981).

References

Correa, P. & Chen, V.W. (1995) Endocrine gland cancer. *Cancer*, **75**, 338–352

Kalk WJ, Sitas F, Patterson AC. (1997) Thyroid cancer in South Africa – an indicator of regional iodine deficiency. *S. Afr. Med. J.*, **87**, 735–738

Kung, T.M., Ng, W.L. & Gibson, J.B. (1981) Volcanoes and carcinoma ot the thyroid: a possible association. *Arch. Environ. Health*, **36**, 265–267

McGill, P.E. (1978) Thyroid carcinoma in Kenya. *Trop. Geogr. Med.*, **30**, 81–86

Omran, M. & Ahmed, M.E. (1993) Carcinoma of the thyroid in Khartoum. *E. Afr. Med. J.*, **70**, 159–162

Ron, E. (1996) Thyroid cancer. In: Schottenfeld, D. & Fraumeni, J.F., Jr, eds, *Cancer Epidemiology and Prevention* (second edition), New York, Oxford University Press

Templeton, A.C. (1973) Tumours of endocrine glands. In: Templeton, A.C., ed., *Tumours in a Tropical Country. Recent Results in Cancer Research*, **41**, 215–221

Thomas, J.O. & Ogunbiyi, J.O. (1995) Thyroid cancers in Ibadan, Nigeria. *E. Afr. Med. J.*, **72**, 231–233

Table 1. Age-standardized (world) and cumulative (0-64) incidence
Thyroid (C73)

	MALE				FEMALE			
	Cases	CRUDE	ASR(W)	Cumulative	Cases	CRUDE	ASR(W)	Cumulative
		(per 100,000)		(%)		(per 100,000)		(%)
Africa, North								
Algeria, Algiers (1993-1997)	52	0.9	**1.2**	0.08	192	3.5	**4.2**	0.33
Algeria, Constantine (1994-1997)	11	0.7	**1.1**	0.07	31	2.0	**2.8**	0.20
Algeria, Oran (1996-1998)	7	0.4	**0.4**	0.04	62	3.5	**4.0**	0.28
Algeria, Setif (1993-1997)	7	0.2	**0.3**	0.02	36	1.2	**1.7**	0.12
Tunisia, Centre, Sousse (1993-1997)	7	0.6	**0.8**	0.04	27	2.4	**2.5**	0.16
Tunisia, North, Tunis (1994)	12	0.6	**0.6**	0.05	55	2.6	**2.9**	0.18
Tunisia, Sfax (1997)	1	0.3	**0.3**	0.02	7	1.9	**2.1**	0.11
Africa, West								
The Gambia (1997-1998)	-	-	**-**	-	4	0.4	**1.0**	0.12
Guinea, Conakry (1996-1999)	6	0.3	**0.5**	0.02	17	0.8	**1.3**	0.13
Mali, Bamako (1988-1997)	4	0.1	**0.1**	0.01	28	0.8	**1.5**	0.10
Niger, Niamey (1993-1999)	3	0.2	**0.3**	0.03	13	0.7	**1.4**	0.10
Nigeria, Ibadan (1998-1999)	6	0.4	**0.8**	0.04	9	0.6	**1.0**	0.04
Africa, Central								
Congo, Brazzaville (1996-1999)	2	0.2	**0.2**	0.02	5	0.4	**0.5**	0.04
Africa, East								
France, La Reunion (1988-1994)	12	0.6	**0.7**	0.05	33	1.5	**1.6**	0.12
Kenya, Eldoret (1998-2000)	2	0.2	**0.6**	0.07	7	0.8	**1.5**	0.05
Malawi, Blantyre (2000-2001)	1	0.1	**0.2**	0.02	6	0.7	**1.5**	0.12
Uganda, Kyadondo County (1993-1997)	6	0.2	**0.6**	0.06	47	1.6	**4.5**	0.41
Zimbabwe, Harare: African (1990-1993)	11	0.5	**1.2**	0.08	31	1.5	**5.4**	0.35
Zimbabwe, Harare: African (1994-1997)	12	0.4	**0.8**	0.04	21	0.8	**3.2**	0.11
Zimbabwe, Harare: European (1990-1997)	1	0.7	**0.9**	0.05	7	4.1	**2.5**	0.13
Africa, South								
Namibia (1995-1998)	9	0.3	**0.4**	0.02	37	1.2	**1.7**	0.10
South Africa: Black (1989-1992)	171	0.3	**0.5**	0.03	476	0.8	**1.2**	0.10
South Africa: Indian (1989-1992)	21	1.1	**1.5**	0.10	53	2.7	**2.9**	0.22
South Africa: Mixed race (1989-1992)	19	0.3	**0.5**	0.03	38	0.6	**0.7**	0.05
South Africa: White (1989-1992)	177	1.8	**1.6**	0.10	560	5.5	**4.7**	0.35
South Africa, Transkei, Umtata (1996-1998)	-	-	**-**	-	2	0.5	**0.8**	0.10
South Africa, Transkei, 4 districts (1996-1998)	-	-	**-**	-	3	0.3	**0.5**	0.04
Swaziland (1996-1999)	9	0.5	**0.9**	0.09	17	0.9	**1.3**	0.07
Europe/USA								
USA, SEER: White (1993-1997)	1664	3.4	**2.8**	0.21	4658	9.3	**7.7**	0.59
USA, SEER: Black (1993-1997)	86	1.3	**1.4**	0.09	323	4.4	**4.0**	0.31
France, 8 registries (1993-1997)	322	2.3	**1.9**	0.15	1115	7.7	**6.3**	0.51
The Netherlands (1993-1997)	499	1.3	**1.0**	0.07	1137	2.9	**2.2**	0.16
UK, England (1993-1997)	1262	1.1	**0.8**	0.05	3383	2.6	**2.0**	0.14

In italics: histopathology-based registries

Table 2. Incidence of thyroid cancer in Africa, 1953–74

Registry	Period	ASR (per 100 000)		Source
		Male	Female	(see Chap. 1)
Senegal, Dakar	1969–74	*0.6*	1.1	4
Mozambique, Lourenço Marques	1956–60	*1.8*	*2.3*	1
Nigeria, Ibadan	1960–69	0.8	*1.7*	3
SA, Cape Province: Bantu	1956–59	*0.0*	2.7	2
SA, Cape Province: Coloured	1956–59	*0.6*	*1.1*	2
SA, Cape Province: White	1956–59	*1.2*	3.0	2
SA, Johannesburg, Bantu	1953–55	*0.1*	1.7	1
SA, Natal Province: African	1964–66	*0.2*	*3.3*	2
SA, Natal Province: Indian	1964–66	*1.0*	*3.0*	2
Uganda, Kyadondo	1954–60	*0.1*	2.6	1
Uganda, Kyadondo	1960–71	*0.4*	2.1	5
Zimbabwe, Bulawayo	1963–72	*2.0*	*1.8*	6

Italics: Rate based on less than 10 cases

Table 3. Percentage distribution of microscopically verified cases by histological type
Thyroid (C73) - Both sexes

	Follic.	Papil.	Carcinoma Medul.	Anapl.	Other	Unspec.	Sarcoma	Other	Unspec.	Number of cases MV	Total
Algeria, Algiers	25.6	46.3	5.3	0.9	5.3	16.7	-	-	-	227	244
Algeria, Batna	21.4	60.7	-	7.1	7.1	3.6	-	-	-	28	31
Algeria, Constantine	34.1	17.1	12.2	-	14.6	12.2	-	-	9.8	41	42
Algeria, Oran	10.6	24.2	-	1.5	13.6	45.5	1.5	-	3.0	66	69
Algeria, Setif	32.5	45.0	-	-	15.0	5.0	2.5	-	-	40	43
Burkina Faso, Ouagadougou	100.0	-	-	-	-	-	-	-	-	1	1
Congo, Brazzaville	20.0	40.0	-	-	20.0	20.0	-	-	-	5	7
France, La Reunion	22.2	51.1	6.7	2.2	13.3	-	-	-	4.4	45	45
The Gambia	50.0	50.0	-	-	-	-	-	-	-	2	4
Guinea, Conakry	16.7	66.7	-	-	8.3	8.3	-	-	-	12	23
Kenya, Eldoret	60.0	-	-	-	-	-	-	-	40.0	5	9
Malawi, Blantyre	75.0	25.0	-	-	-	-	-	-	-	4	7
Mali, Bamako	9.5	14.3	-	-	42.9	33.3	-	-	-	21	32
Namibia	31.8	38.6	9.1	2.3	6.8	6.8	2.3	-	2.3	44	46
Niger, Niamey	20.0	70.0	-	10.0	-	-	-	-	-	10	16
Nigeria, Ibadan	38.5	53.8	-	-	-	7.7	-	-	-	13	15
Rwanda, Butare	100.0	-	-	-	-	-	-	-	-	2	3
South Africa: Black	34.8	26.1	3.4	4.9	8.7	6.2	0.5	0.3	15.1	647	647
South Africa: White	18.7	59.3	3.7	2.4	9.4	4.6	0.3	0.1	1.5	737	737
South Africa: Indian	13.5	40.5	2.7	5.4	9.5	8.1	1.4	-	18.9	74	74
South Africa: Mixed race	40.4	45.6	3.5	5.3	1.8	3.5	-	-	-	57	57
South Africa, Elim	-	-	-	-	-	-	-	-	-	-	-
South Africa, Transkei, Umtata	50.0	50.0	-	-	-	-	-	-	-	2	2
South Africa, Transkei, 4 districts	-	33.3	-	-	33.3	33.3	-	-	-	3	3
Swaziland	61.5	15.4	15.4	-	7.7	-	-	-	-	13	26
Tanzania, Dar Es Salaam	28.6	14.3	-	14.3	14.3	28.6	-	-	-	7	7
Tanzania, Kilimanjaro	7.7	53.8	-	-	23.1	7.7	-	-	7.7	13	15
Tunisia, Centre, Sousse	11.8	76.5	-	8.8	2.9	-	-	-	-	34	34
Tunisia, North, Tunis	11.9	79.1	1.5	1.5	1.5	4.5	-	-	-	67	67
Tunisia, Sfax	12.5	75.0	-	-	-	-	-	-	12.5	8	8
Uganda, Mbarara	50.0	50.0	-	-	-	-	-	-	-	2	3
Uganda, Kyadondo County	56.8	9.1	2.3	-	9.1	18.2	-	-	4.5	44	53
Zimbabwe, Harare: African	58.3	16.7	-	8.3	8.3	6.3	-	-	2.1	48	75
Zimbabwe, Harare: European	16.7	66.7	-	-	-	16.7	-	-	-	6	8

5 Childhood cancer

Studies of the incidence of cancer in childhood in Africa are even more difficult than those of adults. Because of the relative rarity of cancer in this age group, population-based studies must involve rather large populations (or long time periods) in order that sufficient cases be assembled to permit calculation of valid rates. For this reason, most African studies have been of case series, with inevitable difficulties in interpretation.

The rather special nature of the tumours affecting children requires the use of a classification system other than the familiar ICD, which is based upon cancer site (and designed primarily for the study of epithelial neoplasms, which comprise only a small proportion of childhood cancers). Childhood cancers, in contrast, are histologically very diverse and some types can occur in many different sites. A classification based principally on histological type is therefore more appropriate. The current standard is the International Classification of Childhood Cancer (ICCC: Kramárová *et al.*, 1996) that was used for the IARC monograph *International Incidence of Childhood Cancer*, Volume II (IICC-2: Parkin *et al.*, 1998). An earlier version (Birch & Marsden, 1987) was used for the first volume of *International Incidence of Childhood Cancer* (IICC-1: Parkin *et al.*, 1988). There are 12 main diagnostic groups, as follows: leukaemia; lymphomas and reticuloendothelial neoplasms; central nervous system (CNS) and miscellaneous intracranial and intraspinal neoplasms; sympathetic nervous system tumours; retinoblastoma; renal tumours; hepatic tumours; malignant bone tumours; soft-tissue sarcomas; germ-cell, trophoblastic and other gonadal neoplasms; carcinomas and other malignant epithelial neoplasms; other and unspecified malignant neoplasms. All except retinoblastoma are divided into a number of subgroups. In this chapter, geographical and ethnic patterns of incidence will be considered for each major diagnostic group in turn. A series of tables summarizes the data on childhood cancers from the cancer registries contributing to this volume.

Leukaemia

In white populations of Europe, the Americas and Oceania, and also in much of eastern Asia, around a third of all childhood cancers are leukaemias, with age-standardized incidence rates (ASR) of 35–50 per million. Acute lymphoblastic leukaemia (ALL) comprises 75–80% of the total in these populations, with ASRs generally in the range 25–40 per million, and a marked peak in incidence at age 2–3 years. In black children in the United States, leukaemia accounts for about a quarter of all childhood cancer; the incidence of ALL is only half that among whites, largely because of a much reduced early childhood peak. In the United Kingdom, however, the incidence among children of West Indian origin is only slightly less than that among whites (Stiller *et al.*, 1991).

In North Africa, although data are relatively sparse, it appears that the incidence of leukaemia is not far below that in Europe, with a similar distribution by subtype, and a peak in incidence of ALL in young children. In a case series from the National Cancer Institute, Cairo, (El Bolkainy *et al.*, 1984), 87% of 123 childhood leukaemias were ALL, with a modest peak in frequency at ages 3–6 years.

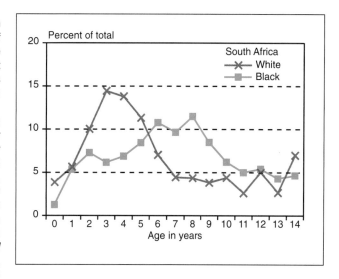

Figure 1. Age distribution of childhood lymphoid leukaemia

In sub-Saharan Africa, recorded incidence rates of leukaemia are considerably lower (Table 1). The incidence of ALL is especially low (Table 2), with little or no sign of a peak in the age–incidence curve (Figure 1).

This low incidence is partly a consequence of underdiagnosis and underreporting (Davies, 1973; Fleming, 1993). Cancer registries in Africa may have less efficient methods of detecting cases diagnosed by blood smears or cytology. Diagnosis may be missed because the common clinical presentation of childhood leukaemia—fever, lymphadenopathy and anaemia—is easy to confuse with other common conditions in paediatric practice in the tropics. The diagnosis may be missed on examination of blood smears, where blast cells may be mistaken for the activated lymphocytes common in children with malaria. Finally, children with the above symptoms (particularly the very young) may not be brought to medical attention before the rapid evolution of the disease has caused death.

An additional problem in interpreting epidemiological patterns of childhood leukaemia has been the reliance upon clinical series and relative proportions of cases of leukaemia of different cell types, and in different age groups, to infer differences in occurrence.

However, even taking these factors into account, all data are consistent in suggesting that incidence rates are low in African children (although this was disputed, on the basis of hospital admissions to paediatric wards in Kampala, Uganda in 1966, by Vanier & Pike, 1967).

Among cases of lymphoid leukaemia, the common ALL immunophenotype accounts for around 70% of classifiable cases among most white populations, including those in less developed countries, and the early childhood peak in the incidence of ALL is due to the even more marked peak for this subtype (Greaves, 1984). Common ALL accounts for only a minority of cases among

Table 1. Childhood cancer: age-standardized (world) incidence per million
Leukaemia

	MALE Cases ASR(W)		FEMALE Cases ASR(W)		TOTAL Cases	M/F	ASR(W)
Africa, North							
Algeria, 4 registries	108	25.6	63	16.0	171	1.7	20.9
*Egypt, Alexandria (1980-1989)	162	24.5	97	15.3	259	1.7	20.0
Tunisia, 3 registries	32	26.6	33	29.0	65	1.0	27.8
Africa, West							
The Gambia (1988-1998)	8	3.4	5	2.1	13	1.6	2.7
Guinea, Conakry (1993-1999)	7	4.4	4	2.5	11	1.8	3.5
Mali, Bamako (1988-1997)	1	0.6	5	2.8	6	0.2	1.8
Niger, Niamey (1993-1999)	4	5.1	6	6.9	10	0.7	6.0
Nigeria, Ibadan (1993-1999)	3	4.8	2	2.1	5	1.5	3.0
Africa, Central							
Congo, Brazzaville (1996-1999)	6	11.3	-	-	6	-	5.8
Africa, East							
France, La Reunion (1988-1994)	17	30.4	17	29.7	34	1.0	30.1
Kenya, Eldoret (1998-2000)	11	26.9	6	14.5	17	1.8	20.7
Malawi, Blantyre (1991-2001)	3	1.6	6	3.2	9	0.5	2.5
Uganda, Kyadondo County (1993-1997)	9	8.7	9	7.2	18	1.0	7.9
Zimbabwe, Harare: African (1990-1997)	41	24.4	34	19.0	75	1.2	21.6
Africa, South							
*Namibia (1983-1992)	17	6.3	16	6.0	33	1.1	6.2
South Africa: Black (1989-1992)	259	11.8	191	8.9	450	1.4	10.4
South Africa: Indian (1989-1992)	41	67.5	21	34.1	62	2.0	51.0
South Africa: Mixed race (1989-1992)	40	18.8	25	11.5	65	1.6	15.2
South Africa: White (1989-1992)	111	50.4	84	42.5	195	1.3	46.5
Swaziland (1996-1999)	6	6.7	5	6.5	11	1.2	6.6
Europe/USA							
USA, SEER: White (1993-1997)	492	49.3	402	42.4	894	1.2	45.9
USA, SEER: Black (1993-1997)	65	36.0	46	26.2	111	1.4	31.2
France, 8 registries (1993-1997)	122	45.7	86	33.4	208	1.4	39.7
The Netherlands (1993-1997)	342	49.2	231	34.8	573	1.5	42.2
UK, England (1993-1997)	1057	45.5	835	37.2	1892	1.3	41.4

International Incidence of Childhood Cancer Volume II

In italics: histopathology-based registries

South African blacks (MacDougall, 1985), in Nigeria (Williams, 1985) and Kenya (Dearden, 1985), so that T-cell ALL (the incidence of which is relatively constant throughout childhood) accounts for a correspondingly larger proportion.

The peak of ALL at age 2–3 years began to emerge in mortality data in England and Wales in the 1920s and it was well established among whites in the United States by the early l940s, the earliest period for which rates could be reliably calculated (Court Brown & Doll, 1961). The more moderate peak among American blacks emerged later (Miller, 1977). In the black population of South Africa, although the incidence of 'common' acute lymphocytic leukaemia (cALL) is low, this subtype still occurs with a peak incidence at around ages 2–5 years (Greaves et al., 1993). It has been suggested that the frequency of diagnosis of cALL in clinical series has increased in recent years, for example in Nigeria, South Africa, and Zimbabwe (Paul et al., 1992; Fleming, 1993).

A number of studies have found that residence in areas of higher socioeconomic status is associated with increased risk of childhood ALL (McWhirter, 1982, Alexander et al., 1990; Draper et al., 1991). In Ibadan, Williams (1985) observed that a higher percentage of childhood cases of ALL were of higher socioeconomic status (27%), compared with cases of acute myeloid leukaemia (AML) (6%) or Burkitt lymphoma (3.3%).

It seems likely that infection is an important factor in the etiology of childhood ALL, and several models have been proposed. According to the hypothesis of Greaves (1988), the association of high incidence of common ALL at age 2–3 years with higher levels of socioeconomic development may be explained by relatively late exposure to an infectious agent in more affluent societies. In these circumstances, a pre-malignant clone of B-cells in bone marrow will have had some time to proliferate in infancy, so that there are numerous cells in which a second mutation can occur under the promoting effect of antigenic challenge.

In the United States and Japan, improvements in public hygiene, as indicated by decreases in prevalence of hepatitis A infection, were followed by increases in childhood leukaemia incidence. This could have come about by an increase in the number of children susceptible to a putative leukaemia-inducing infectious agent also linked to public hygiene, consequent on an increase in the proportion of mothers who were seronegative for that agent (Smith et al., 1998b).

Williams et al. (1984), comparing admissions to University College Hospital, Ibadan, for childhood leukaemia in 1978–82 with those in 1958–68, suggested that there had been an increase in incidence rates. However, the estimated rates for the second period (5.5–19 per million), from Williams and Bamgboye (1983), seem no

Table 2. Childhood cancer: age-standardized (world) incidence per million
Acute lymphoid leukaemia

	MALE Cases	ASR(W)	FEMALE Cases	ASR(W)	TOTAL Cases	M/F	ASR(W)
Africa, North							
Algeria, 4 registries	71	17.0	40	10.3	111	1.8	13.7
*Egypt, Alexandria (1980-1989)	50	7.5	31	4.8	81	1.6	6.2
Tunisia, 3 registries	26	21.9	21	18.6	47	1.2	20.3
Africa, West							
The Gambia (1988-1998)	3	1.3	2	0.8	5	1.5	1.1
Guinea, Conakry (1993-1999)	3	1.9	3	1.7	6	1.0	1.8
Mali, Bamako (1988-1997)	-	-	-	-	-	-	-
Niger, Niamey (1993-1999)	4	5.1	2	2.4	6	2.0	3.7
Nigeria, Ibadan (1993-1999)	-	-	-	-	-	-	-
Africa, Central							
Congo, Brazzaville (1996-1999)	5	9.4	-	-	5	-	4.8
Africa, East							
France, La Reunion (1988-1994)	12	21.4	13	22.7	25	0.9	22.0
Kenya, Eldoret (1998-2000)	6	14.6	1	2.5	7	6.0	8.6
Malawi, Blantyre (1991-2001)	1	0.5	1	0.5	2	1.0	0.5
Uganda, Kyadondo County (1993-1997)	2	1.9	4	3.2	6	0.5	2.6
Zimbabwe, Harare: African (1990-1997)	26	15.3	15	8.4	41	1.7	11.8
Africa, South							
*Namibia (1983-1992)	11	4.2	13	4.9	24	0.8	4.5
South Africa: Black (1989-1992)	125	5.7	106	5.0	231	1.2	5.3
South Africa: Indian (1989-1992)	24	39.2	12	18.8	36	2.0	29.1
South Africa: Mixed race (1989-1992)	29	13.8	15	7.0	44	1.9	10.4
South Africa: White (1989-1992)	71	32.7	54	26.9	125	1.3	29.8
Swaziland (1996-1999)	1	1.2	2	2.6	3	0.5	1.9
Europe/USA							
USA, SEER: White (1993-1997)	408	41.1	328	34.7	736	1.2	38.0
USA, SEER: Black (1993-1997)	47	26.0	30	17.1	77	1.6	21.6
France, 8 registries (1993-1997)	92	34.8	66	25.8	158	1.4	30.4
The Netherlands (1993-1997)	268	38.6	193	29.1	461	1.4	34.0
UK, England (1993-1997)	827	35.8	650	29.0	1477	1.3	32.4

International Incidence of Childhood Cancer Volume II
In italics: histopathology-based registries

different from those recorded by the Ibadan Cancer Registry in 1960–69: 11.8 per million (Junaid & Babalola, 1988). In Kampala, Uganda, there is no evidence for an increase in incidence of childhood leukaemias: the incidence fell from 18.7 per million in 1960–71 to 8.6 per million in 1991–97 (Wabinga et al., 2000).

Apart from ALL, most childhood leukaemias are acute non-lymphocytic leukaemia (ANLL). In Europe and North America, the ASR is typically in the range 4–9 per million, with incidence highest in the first two years of life and relatively constant thereafter. ANLL (or acute myeloid leukaemia, AML) appears to be relatively common in series from Africa. However, this is most likely because of the deficit of cases of ALL, rather than a particularly high incidence of AML. Fleming (1993) considered that the incidence of AML in childhood may be increased in Africa, especially in boys aged 5–14 years. The basis for this speculation is not clear; although the rates estimated for Ibadan in 1978–82 were indeed high (Williams & Bamgboye, 1983), the numbers on which the calculation was based must have been small (and the population denominator very uncertain). None of the other reports from Ibadan have suggested a high incidence (Parkin et al., 1988, 1998), and in Cape Province, South Africa, the incidence in black children was no higher than in whites (Sayers et al., 1992).

Chloromas (solid leukaemic masses) have been reported to complicate about 10% of childhood cases of acute myeloid

leukaemia in Nigeria (Fleming & Peter, 1982; Williams et al., 1982) and an even higher proportion in Uganda (Davies & Owor, 1965; Barr et al., 1972; Owor, 1984) and South Africa (MacDougall et al., 1986).

Lymphoma
The epidemiology of lymphomas in Africa, including Burkitt lymphoma, has been described in Chapter 4.10. This section is confined to features specific to lymphoma in the childhood age range (Table 3).

Hodgkin disease
Stiller and Parkin (1990) observed that, although it was not possible to estimate incidence of childhood Hodgkin disease in Africa, most published series of childhood cancers contained "considerable numbers" of cases. Table 4 suggests that the incidence in sub-Saharan Africa is indeed similar to that in populations of the developed countries of Europe and North America, and that in North Africa, it may even be higher. The contrast between the pattern of incidence of childhood Hodgkin disease in western industrialized countries, where incidence rises steeply with age, and in some developing countries, where the increase in early adolescence is much gentler and there is sometimes even a modest peak at age 5–9 years, is described in Chapter 4.10. Figure 2 shows age-specific incidence in age groups 0–4, 5–9 and 10–14 years in

Table 3. Childhood cancer: age-standardized (world) incidence per million
Lymphoma

| | MALE | | FEMALE | | TOTAL | | |
	Cases	ASR(W)	Cases	ASR(W)	Cases	M/F	ASR(W)
Africa, North							
Algeria, 4 registries	124	**29.8**	57	**13.9**	181	2.2	**22.0**
*Egypt, Alexandria (1980-1989)	269	**40.9**	131	**20.7**	400	2.1	**30.8**
Tunisia, 3 registries	24	**18.7**	12	**10.4**	36	2.0	**14.7**
Africa, West							
The Gambia (1988-1998)	40	**16.8**	25	**10.6**	65	1.6	**13.7**
Guinea, Conakry (1993-1999)	34	**22.6**	30	**22.0**	64	1.1	**22.3**
Mali, Bamako (1988-1997)	22	**13.7**	10	**5.7**	32	2.2	**9.5**
Niger, Niamey (1993-1999)	20	**26.2**	12	**14.3**	32	1.7	**20.1**
Nigeria, Ibadan (1993-1999)	37	**62.9**	22	**20.1**	59	1.7	**34.7**
Africa, Central							
Congo, Brazzaville (1996-1999)	8	**15.2**	10	**20.2**	18	0.8	**17.6**
Africa, East							
France, La Reunion (1988-1994)	14	**22.7**	6	**10.6**	20	2.3	**16.7**
Kenya, Eldoret (1998-2000)	19	**46.4**	15	**37.1**	34	1.3	**41.7**
Malawi, Blantyre (1991-2001)	86	**47.9**	43	**23.2**	129	2.0	**35.2**
Uganda, Kyadondo County (1993-1997)	89	**79.1**	65	**52.8**	154	1.4	**65.3**
Zimbabwe, Harare: African (1990-1997)	33	**19.5**	15	**8.4**	48	2.2	**13.8**
Africa, South							
*Namibia (1983-1992)	22	**8.2**	9	**3.4**	31	2.4	**5.8**
South Africa: Black (1989-1992)	*198*	**9.0**	*90*	**4.1**	*288*	2.2	**6.6**
South Africa: Indian (1989-1992)	*10*	**15.5**	*6*	**9.6**	*16*	1.7	**12.6**
South Africa: Mixed race (1989-1992)	*29*	**13.0**	*10*	**4.7**	*39*	2.9	**8.9**
South Africa: White (1989-1992)	*67*	**28.6**	*34*	**15.5**	*101*	2.0	**22.2**
Swaziland (1996-1999)	12	**15.6**	10	**12.5**	22	1.2	**14.0**
Europe/USA							
USA, SEER: White (1993-1997)	187	**17.0**	117	**11.1**	304	1.6	**14.1**
USA, SEER: Black (1993-1997)	28	**14.8**	16	**8.5**	44	1.8	**11.7**
France, 8 registries (1993-1997)	84	**27.7**	42	**14.4**	126	2.0	**21.2**
The Netherlands (1993-1997)	154	**20.6**	84	**11.8**	238	1.8	**16.3**
UK, England (1993-1997)	446	**17.8**	193	**7.9**	639	2.3	**12.9**

International Incidence of Childhood Cancer Volume II

In italics: histopathology-based registries

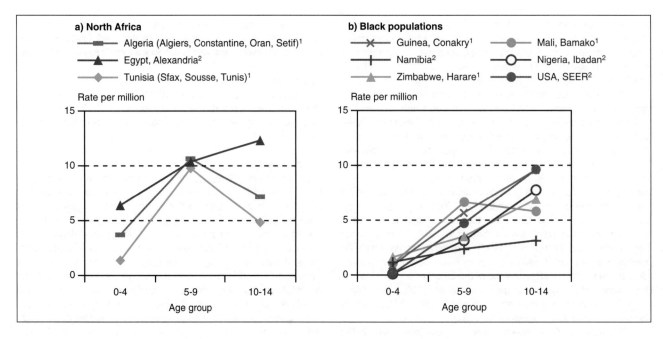

Figure 2. Hodgkin disease in children (Sources: 1 this volume; 2 *International Incidence of Childhood Cancer*, Vol. II)

Table 4. Childhood cancer: age-standardized (world) incidence per million
Hodgkin disease

	MALE		FEMALE		TOTAL		
	Cases	ASR(W)	Cases	ASR(W)	Cases	M/F	ASR(W)
Africa, North							
Algeria, 4 registries	39	**9.0**	19	**4.5**	58	2.1	**6.8**
*Egypt, Alexandria (1980-1989)	82	**12.5**	44	**6.7**	126	1.9	**9.5**
Tunisia, 3 registries	9	**6.7**	4	**3.4**	13	2.3	**5.1**
Africa, West							
The Gambia (1988-1998)	7	**2.9**	2	**0.9**	9	3.5	**1.9**
Guinea, Conakry (1993-1999)	11	**7.7**	3	**2.0**	14	3.7	**4.9**
Mali, Bamako (1988-1997)	11	**6.8**	3	**1.6**	14	3.7	**4.1**
Niger, Niamey (1993-1999)	4	**6.0**	-	**-**	4	-	**2.8**
Nigeria, Ibadan (1993-1999)	5	**7.9**	-	**-**	5	-	**2.7**
Africa, Central							
Congo, Brazzaville (1996-1999)	-	**-**	-	**-**	-	-	**-**
Africa, East							
France, La Reunion (1988-1994)	3	**5.4**	-	**-**	3	-	**2.7**
Kenya, Eldoret (1998-2000)	3	**7.2**	1	**2.5**	4	3.0	**4.9**
Malawi, Blantyre (1991-2001)	9	**5.0**	1	**0.5**	10	9.0	**2.7**
Uganda, Kyadondo County (1993-1997)	5	**4.4**	4	**3.2**	9	1.3	**3.8**
Zimbabwe, Harare: African (1990-1997)	9	**5.4**	4	**2.3**	13	2.3	**3.8**
Africa, South							
*Namibia (1983-1992)	8	**2.9**	3	**1.1**	11	2.7	**2.0**
South Africa: Black (1989-1992)	*86*	**3.9**	*24*	**1.1**	*110*	*3.6*	**2.5**
South Africa: Indian (1989-1992)	*3*	**4.5**	*1*	**1.5**	*4*	*3.0*	**3.1**
South Africa: Mixed race (1989-1992)	*17*	**7.4**	*2*	**0.9**	*19*	*8.5*	**4.1**
South Africa: White (1989-1992)	*18*	**7.5**	*6*	**2.4**	*24*	*3.0*	**5.0**
Swaziland (1996-1999)	4	**4.6**	1	**1.0**	5	4.0	**2.8**
Europe/USA							
USA, SEER: White (1993-1997)	60	**5.3**	61	**5.5**	121	1.0	**5.4**
USA, SEER: Black (1993-1997)	7	**3.5**	8	**4.1**	15	0.9	**3.8**
France, 8 registries (1993-1997)	26	**8.0**	16	**5.1**	42	1.6	**6.6**
The Netherlands (1993-1997)	37	**4.8**	32	**4.2**	69	1.2	**4.5**
UK, England (1993-1997)	169	**6.6**	87	**3.4**	256	1.9	**5.0**

International Incidence of Childhood Cancer Volume II
In italics: histopathology-based registries

selected populations. In several countries where Burkitt lymphoma is endemic, the incidence or relative frequency of Hodgkin disease is substantially higher at age 10–14 years than at 5–9 years, indicating an age–incidence pattern different from that which is typical of developing countries elsewhere.

The relative frequencies of histological subtypes of childhood Hodgkin disease vary considerably. Throughout North America and western Europe, nodular sclerosis is usually the most frequent, nearly always accounting for more than half the cases of known subtype. Lymphocyte predominance seldom accounts for more than 20% of cases, and lymphocyte-depleted Hodgkin disease is very rare. Case series from Africa with adequate detail on histological subtype are rather few (Levy, 1988; Wright, 1973; Edington et al., 1973; Cohen & Hamilton, 1980). African children have an excess of mixed cellularity (MC) subtype and a marked deficit of nodular sclerosing (NS) cases, while lymphocyte-depleted (LD) cases may comprise up to 30% in some series. Positivity for Epstein–Barr virus (EBV) in malignant cells is more common in childhood Hodgkin disease than in adults, in the MC subtype and in cases from developing countries (Glaser et al., 1997). There is a higher prevalence of EBV in Hodgkin disease cases from Kenya than in European countries, with almost all paediatric cases from Kenya being EBV-positive (Leoncini et al., 1996; Weinreb et al., 1996).

Non-Hodgkin lymphoma
Non-Hodgkin lymphoma in childhood is nearly always high-grade. The epidemiology of Burkitt lymphoma in Africa has been described in Chapter 4.10. Other types of non-Hodgkin lymphoma usually have a total ASR of 5–9 per million, though incidence rates may be a little higher than this in North Africa. In the United States, blacks have a lower rate than whites. Though these geographical patterns are assumed to be related to environmental exposures, the high incidence in young Jewish migrants to Israel from North Africa is retained in their Israeli-born offspring, indicating that genetic susceptibility may also be involved (Iscovich & Parkin, 1997).

Brain and spinal tumours
In developed countries, brain and spinal tumours typically account for 20–25% of all childhood cancer, with an ASR of 25–40 per million. The most common subgroup is astrocytoma, which covers a wide spectrum of histological types from the relatively benign juvenile astrocytoma (including optic nerve glioma) to the aggressive anaplastic astrocytoma and glioblastoma multiforme. The second most common category comprises primitive neuroectodermal tumours, most of which are cerebellar medulloblastoma. Ependymomas (including choroid plexus tumours) are relatively rare and, like astrocytomas, this category encompasses a wide range of degrees of malignancy.

Table 5. Childhood cancer: age-standardized (world) incidence per million
Brain and spinal neoplasms

	MALE Cases	MALE ASR(W)	FEMALE Cases	FEMALE ASR(W)	TOTAL Cases	TOTAL M/F	TOTAL ASR(W)
Africa, North							
Algeria, 4 registries	44	**10.2**	21	**5.2**	65	2.1	**7.7**
*Egypt, Alexandria (1980-1989)	136	**20.5**	115	**18.0**	251	1.2	**19.1**
Tunisia, 3 registries	11	**9.5**	12	**10.5**	23	0.9	**10.0**
Africa, West							
The Gambia (1988-1998)	1	**0.4**	-	**-**	1	-	**0.2**
Guinea, Conakry (1993-1999)	-	**-**	1	**0.8**	1	0.0	**0.4**
Mali, Bamako (1988-1997)	-	**-**	2	**1.2**	2	0.0	**0.6**
Niger, Niamey (1993-1999)	2	**2.1**	1	**1.4**	3	2.0	**1.8**
Nigeria, Ibadan (1993-1999)	13	**24.4**	5	**4.9**	18	2.6	**11.6**
Africa, Central							
Congo, Brazzaville (1996-1999)	-	**-**	-	**-**	-	-	**-**
Africa, East							
France, La Reunion (1988-1994)	8	**15.1**	6	**9.0**	14	1.3	**12.1**
Kenya, Eldoret (1998-2000)	6	**14.6**	5	**12.1**	11	1.2	**13.3**
Malawi, Blantyre (1991-2001)	-	**-**	1	**0.5**	1	0.0	**0.3**
Uganda, Kyadondo County (1993-1997)	3	**2.9**	1	**0.8**	4	3.0	**1.8**
Zimbabwe, Harare: African (1990-1997)	22	**13.3**	19	**10.7**	41	1.2	**11.9**
Africa, South							
*Namibia (1983-1992)	18	**6.8**	16	**6.0**	34	1.1	**6.4**
South Africa: Black (1989-1992)	*111*	**5.1**	*71*	**3.3**	*182*	*1.6*	**4.2**
South Africa: Indian (1989-1992)	*7*	**11.4**	*4*	**6.1**	*11*	*1.8*	**8.8**
South Africa: Mixed race (1989-1992)	*18*	**8.6**	*19*	**8.6**	*37*	*0.9*	**8.6**
South Africa: White (1989-1992)	*40*	**17.4**	*48*	**21.4**	*88*	*0.8*	**19.3**
Swaziland (1996-1999)	-	**-**	-	**-**	-	-	**-**
Europe/USA							
USA, SEER: White (1993-1997)	387	**37.6**	284	**28.7**	671	1.4	**33.2**
USA, SEER: Black (1993-1997)	46	**25.6**	43	**24.2**	89	1.1	**24.9**
France, 8 registries (1993-1997)	83	**29.0**	51	**19.0**	134	1.6	**24.1**
The Netherlands (1993-1997)	188	**26.0**	194	**28.4**	382	1.0	**27.2**
UK, England (1993-1997)	646	**27.0**	594	**25.5**	1240	1.1	**26.3**

International Incidence of Childhood Cancer Volume II

In italics: histopathology-based registries

In developing countries, brain and spinal tumours are usually outnumbered not only by leukaemias but also by lymphomas, and recorded incidence is lower than in developed countries. In Africa, rates are very variable, but in general very low, rarely exceeding 15 per million (Table 5). There is almost certainly considerable under-ascertainment, because of deficiencies in diagnostic facilities. The registries that collect cases mainly from pathology departments will also suffer a deficit if autopsies are rarely performed. There is some evidence, however, from comparisons of incidence rates within the same country that risk may vary between ethnic groups. Black children in the United States have a lower ASR than whites, while children of West Indian descent in the United Kingdom have a low frequency of brain tumours (Stiller et al., 1991). The lower recorded incidence in black children than in white in South Africa probably is largely related to differential biopsy rates.

Neuroblastoma

In the predominantly white populations of Europe, North America and Oceania, and also in Japan and Israel, the ASR is generally in the range 7–12 per million, and 6–10% of all childhood cancers are neuroblastomas (Stiller & Parkin, 1992). Rates are highest (25–50 per million) in the first year of life, when this is the commonest of all cancers. In the United States, blacks had a lower incidence than whites in infancy, but similar rates thereafter, whereas in the United

Kingdom, there is no sign of variation between ethnic groups (Stiller et al., 1991; Powell et al., 1994).

Although the highest recorded incidence rates for neuroblastoma have long been in industrialized countries with a high material standard of living, studies in Denmark and the United States found that it was more common among less affluent groups (Carlsen, 1986; Davis et al., 1987). This might be because children from families of lower socioeconomic status are generally more likely to be seen by doctors, giving greater opportunity for tumours to be detected. This explanation would not, however, account for the lower incidence among blacks in the United States, who are generally of lower socioeconomic status than whites. It seems likely that at least some of the deficit in developing countries compared with industrialized countries is due to underdiagnosis (Stiller & Parkin, 1992).

In North Africa, incidence rates of neuroblastoma are not much lower than in Europe and North America (Table 6). In southern Africa, there is some variability. Rates in black children in South Africa are considerably lower than rates in whites; since these data are histology-based, this may reflect different rates of investigation. In Zimbabwe, incidence in Harare is rather low, but the older series from Bulawayo (1963–77) did not suggest a particularly low incidence.

In West and East Africa, however, the rates are very low indeed, and neuroblastoma appears to be a rare cancer.

Table 6. Childhood cancer: age-standardized (world) incidence per million
Neuroblastoma

	MALE		FEMALE		TOTAL		
	Cases	ASR(W)	Cases	ASR(W)	Cases	M/F	ASR(W)
Africa, North							
Algeria, 4 registries	38	**9.7**	15	**4.0**	53	2.5	**6.9**
*Egypt, Alexandria (1980-1989)	42	**6.6**	24	**4.0**	66	1.8	**5.4**
Tunisia, 3 registries	9	**9.0**	11	**11.3**	20	0.8	**10.1**
Africa, West							
The Gambia (1988-1998)	1	**0.4**	1	**0.5**	2	1.0	**0.5**
Guinea, Conakry (1993-1999)	-	**-**	-	**-**	-	-	**-**
Mali, Bamako (1988-1997)	-	**-**	-	**-**	-	-	**-**
Niger, Niamey (1993-1999)	2	**2.6**	-	**-**	2	-	**1.2**
Nigeria, Ibadan (1993-1999)	2	**4.0**	1	**1.2**	3	2.0	**2.1**
Africa, Central							
Congo, Brazzaville (1996-1999)	-	**-**	-	**-**	-	-	**-**
Africa, East							
France, La Reunion (1988-1994)	2	**4.1**	5	**9.9**	7	0.4	**7.0**
Kenya, Eldoret (1998-2000)	-	**-**	-	**-**	-	-	**-**
Malawi, Blantyre (1991-2001)	1	**0.5**	-	**-**	1	-	**0.3**
Uganda, Kyadondo County (1993-1997)	-	**-**	-	**-**	-	-	**-**
Zimbabwe, Harare: African (1990-1997)	7	**4.1**	5	**2.8**	12	1.4	**3.4**
Africa, South							
*Namibia (1983-1992)	9	**3.6**	9	**3.6**	18	1.0	**3.6**
South Africa: Black (1989-1992)	*58*	**2.7**	*36*	**1.7**	*94*	*1.6*	**2.2**
South Africa: Indian (1989-1992)	*-*	**-**	*-*	**-**	*-*	*-*	**-**
South Africa: Mixed race (1989-1992)	*13*	**6.6**	*12*	**6.0**	*25*	*1.1*	**6.3**
South Africa: White (1989-1992)	*26*	**13.0**	*23*	**11.5**	*49*	*1.1*	**12.2**
Swaziland (1996-1999)	1	**1.4**	1	**1.4**	2	1.0	**1.4**
Europe/USA							
USA, SEER: White (1993-1997)	139	**14.9**	108	**12.1**	247	1.3	**13.5**
USA, SEER: Black (1993-1997)	25	**15.1**	17	**10.4**	42	1.5	**12.8**
France, 8 registries (1993-1997)	35	**14.0**	22	**9.5**	57	1.6	**11.8**
The Netherlands (1993-1997)	54	**8.2**	46	**7.3**	100	1.2	**7.8**
UK, England (1993-1997)	200	**9.2**	166	**7.8**	366	1.2	**8.5**

International Incidence of Childhood Cancer Volume II
In italics: histopathology-based registries

A low frequency of neuroblastoma has been reported in numerous other series from tropical Africa (O'Conor & Davies, 1960). Miller (1977) noted that neuroblastoma cases were infrequent in series from East Africa (Kenya, Tanzania, Malawi, Zambia); in the data from Uganda, and from West Africa (Dakar and Ibadan), the relative frequency was higher, but the ratio of neuroblastoma cases to Wilms tumour cases was less than half of that in blacks in the United States. In a series of 1522 histologically diagnosed solid tumours of children in Kenya, Kung'u (1984) observed only two cases of neuroblastoma (although there were many "unspecified small round-cell sarcomas" of young children in the series) and more recent series (Makata et al., 1996; Mwanda, 1999) have reported similarly low relative frequencies (0.5% and 0%, respectively). Miller(1989) drew upon relative frequency data cited above (Miller, 1977) and data in International Incidence of Childhood Cancer (Parkin et al., 1988) to draw attention to the very low frequency (<1% of childhood cancers) in Kenya, Malawi, Tanzania, Uganda, Zaire and Zambia. Figure 3 shows an updated version of the map of Miller (1989), drawing upon data in this volume, as well as the original series.

The low rates of neuroblastoma in Ibadan, Nigeria, reported in Table 6 echo the rather modest frequency of this cancer in series for the same centre in 1960–72 (2.6%) (Williams, 1975) and 1960–84 (4.3%) (Parkin et al., 1988).

Wessels and Hesseling (1996) calculated minimum incidence rates for the population of Namibia to be 7.6 per million for urban areas and 3.5 for rural dwellers.

Retinoblastoma
In most developed countries, retinoblastoma has an ASR of 3–5 per million and accounts for 2.5–4% of all childhood cancers. It is predominantly a tumour of early childhood, though the proportion of cases occurring among infants aged under one year is rather less than for neuroblastoma. In the United States, incidence among blacks (5.3 per million) is somewhat higher than among whites (4.9 per million) (Parkin et al., 1998).

The data from Africa (Table 7) suggest that, in many of the populations of sub-Saharan Africa, rates are rather higher than in Europe and the United States, with several countries having rates in the range 5–11. The explanation for the very low recorded rate in Alexandria (Egypt) is unknown.

High relative frequencies of retinoblastomas have been reported in several clinical or pathology series (although the latter are often restricted to solid tumours), e.g. from Nigeria (Kodilinye, 1967; Williams, 1975; Obioha et al., 1989), Sudan (Hussan et al., 1988;

Table 7a. Childhood cancer: age-standardized (world) incidence per million
Retinoblastoma

| | MALE | | FEMALE | | TOTAL | | |
	Cases	ASR(W)	Cases	ASR(W)	Cases	M/F	ASR(W)
Africa, North							
Algeria, 4 registries	22	5.9	18	5.2	40	1.2	5.5
*Egypt, Alexandria (1980-1989)	3	0.5	5	0.8	8	0.6	0.7
Tunisia, 3 registries	3	2.8	3	3.1	6	1.0	3.0
Africa, West							
The Gambia (1988-1998)	6	2.6	7	3.0	13	0.9	2.8
Guinea, Conakry (1993-1999)	21	11.6	10	5.6	31	2.1	8.6
Mali, Bamako (1988-1997)	13	7.8	13	7.6	26	1.0	7.7
Niger, Niamey (1993-1999)	6	6.4	4	4.3	10	1.5	5.3
Nigeria, Ibadan (1993-1999)	15	33.5	10	11.3	25	1.5	19.0
Africa, Central							
Congo, Brazzaville (1996-1999)	1	1.9	2	4.0	3	0.5	3.0
Africa, East							
France, La Reunion (1988-1994)	1	2.1	4	8.4	5	0.3	5.2
Kenya, Eldoret (1998-2000)	2	5.0	1	2.5	3	2.0	3.8
Malawi, Blantyre (1991-2001)	10	6.1	13	7.4	23	0.8	6.8
Uganda, Kyadondo County (1993-1997)	12	9.5	8	6.0	20	1.5	7.7
Zimbabwe, Harare: African (1990-1997)	24	14.0	13	7.3	37	1.8	10.6
Africa, South							
*Namibia (1983-1992)	10	4.1	12	4.9	22	0.8	4.5
South Africa: Black (1989-1992)	*66*	*3.2*	*56*	*2.8*	*122*	*1.2*	*3.0*
South Africa: Indian (1989-1992)	*4*	*7.4*	*1*	*1.6*	*5*	*4.0*	*4.5*
South Africa: Mixed race (1989-1992)	*8*	*4.1*	*9*	*4.6*	*17*	*0.9*	*4.4*
South Africa: White (1989-1992)	*6*	*3.1*	*6*	*3.4*	*12*	*1.0*	*3.3*
Swaziland (1996-1999)	1	1.4	2	2.6	3	0.5	2.0
Europe/USA							
USA, SEER: White (1993-1997)	43	4.6	41	4.6	84	1.0	4.6
USA, SEER: Black (1993-1997)	8	4.9	8	5.0	16	1.0	5.0
France, 8 registries (1993-1997)	13	5.5	3	1.3	16	4.3	3.5
The Netherlands (1993-1997)	33	5.0	35	5.6	68	0.9	5.3
UK, England (1993-1997)	92	4.3	92	4.4	184	1.0	4.4

International Incidence of Childhood Cancer Volume II

In italics: histopathology-based registries

Parkin *et al.*, 1988), Congo (Democratic Republic) (Massabi *et al.*, 1989) and Kenya (Kung'u 1984). However, care must be taken when interpreting comparisons of relative frequencies. It is likely that retinoblastoma—a relatively easily diagnosed cancer—will be more often correctly diagnosed in Africa than other deep-seated cancers.

It is generally considered that there is less variation in incidence between populations for bilateral tumours (all of which represent the heritable form of the disease, with a genetic etiology) than for unilateral cases, most of which are sporadic (Draper *et al.*, 1992). In Europe, the percentages of bilateral cases are 21% in France, 29% in Germany and 37% in England and Wales (Parkin *et al.*, 1998). In the United States SEER registries, the percentage of bilateral cases (1983–92) was 29% in whites and 44% in blacks. The numbers of cases in the individual series from Africa in this volume are generally too small (or laterality is not recorded) to allow any clear analysis of this feature. In the larger series in Table 7, for which laterality was recorded, bilateral cases were 0/27 cases in Ibadan and 4/22 in Namibia. In the national histopathology series from Malawi (1991–95), there were five bilateral tumours in a total of 32 registrations (Parkin *et al.*, 1998). The percentage of bilateral cases in a 20-year clinical series from Johannesburg was 18% (Freedman & Goldberg, 1976), while in a long case series from Congo (Democratic Republic), Kayembi-Lubeji (1990) reported 33% of cases to be bilateral. A deficit of bilateral tumours may represent a higher relative incidence of

Table 7(b) Retinoblastoma. Mean age at diagnosis

	Mean age (years)
Algeria, 4 registries (1993–97)	3.0
Tunisia, 3 registries (1993–97)	3.7
Guinea, Conakry (1996–98)	3.3
Mali, Bamako (1988–97)	3.4
Nigeria, Ibadan (1985–92)	3.4
Uganda, Kyadondo (1993–97)	3.1
South Africa: Black (1989–92)	2.8
South Africa: White (1989–92)	2.9
Zimbabwe, Harare: African (1990–97)	2.4
USA, SEER: White (1993–97)	1.3
USA, SEER: Black (1993–97)	0.9
France, 8 registries (1993–97)	1.3
The Netherlands (1993–97)	1.3
UK, England (1993–97)	1.3

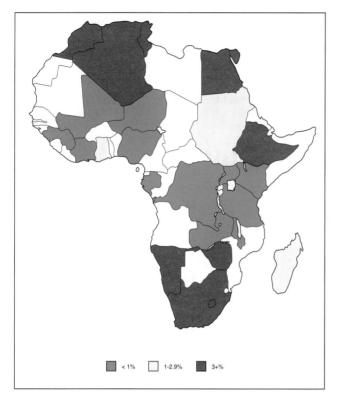

Figure 3. Frequency of neuroblastoma among childhood cancers (excluding Kaposi sarcoma and Burkitt lymphoma)

□ < 1% □ 1-2.9% ■ 3+%

sporadic, as opposed to heritable cases, but it could also be a consequence of poor survival from the first tumour, or simply failures of recording.

Most case series have noted the rather higher age at diagnosis of cases in Africa than in Europe or North America. The mean age of the cases in the registry series in Table 7 is shown in Table 7(b). The older age at diagnosis in African children relates to the lower frequency of bilateral tumours (which have an earlier age of onset than sporadic, unilateral cases) and probably also to the relatively advanced stage at which tumours present in clinical practice in Africa (Wessels & Hesseling, 1995).

Renal tumours

The great majority of childhood renal tumours are Wilms tumours. It has long been noted that, worldwide, the highest incidence rates of Wilms tumour are observed among black populations, both in Africa and in series from the United States (Stiller & Parkin, 1990). However, recent data from the SEER program (1983–92) do not suggest a higher incidence in black children (ASR 8.8 per million) than in white children (ASR 10.0 per million). In the United Kingdom, children of West Indian descent also have a relatively high frequency of Wilms tumour (Stiller *et al.*, 1991).

Among white populations, Wilms tumour usually has an ASR of 6–10 per million and accounts for 5–7% of all childhood cancers, though higher rates have been recorded in several Nordic countries, Estonia and New Zealand. The age distributions in white and black populations are similar, with the highest incidence occurring in the second year of life.

The results from the African registries in this volume are varied (Table 8). Several incidence rates in southern and eastern Africa (e.g., in Kenya, Reunion, Uganda and Zimbabwe) are relatively high; the registries in West Africa report moderate incidence (with the exception of Conakry, Guinea).

Since incidence of Wilms tumour apparently varies along ethnic rather than geographical lines, it is possible that there is a strong element of genetic predisposition in its etiology, despite the fact that very few cases can be identified as directly hereditary.

Liver tumours

Most malignant liver tumours of childhood are either hepatoblastomas or hepatocellular carcinomas.

Hepatoblastoma is one of the rarer embryonal tumours. Nearly all cases are diagnosed in the first few years of life and incidence is highest in infancy. There is apparently very little geographical variation, with ASRs around 1–2 per million worldwide.

Hepatocellular carcinoma shows much more geographical variation, though everywhere most cases are in older children (10–14 years). In Europe and North America, it is rare in childhood, occurring with well under half the frequency of hepatoblastoma. It is much more common, however, in regions of the world with high rates of adult liver cancer (sub-Saharan Africa, East and South-East Asia and Melanesia). Most childhood cases of liver cancer in these areas occur in chronic carriers of hepatitis B (Cameron & Warwick, 1977; Moore *et al.*, 1997).

Bone tumours

In most childhood cancer registries, bone tumours (Table 9) comprise about 5% of all childhood cancers, compared with less than 1% in adults. Almost all are either osteosarcoma or Ewing sarcoma, with fewer than 10% being of other types.

The risk of osteosarcoma shows a bimodal distribution throughout life, with the first peak at age 15–19 years, so that incidence within childhood increases with age and more than 70% occurs at age 10–14 years. In the United States, the incidence was formerly somewhat higher in the black population than among whites (Parkin *et al.*, 1988), but during the l980s rates were very similar for the two ethnic groups (Parkin *et al.*, 1998). A link between the risk of osteosarcoma and bone growth has long been suspected (Johnson, 1953). More than three quarters of tumours arise in the long bones of the legs and there is an excess in girls before age 13 years and in boys thereafter, corresponding to their relative rates of growth.

The data from Africa are very sparse, as many bone tumours do not have adequate histological examination. In *International Incidence of Childhood Cancer*, Vol. II (Parkin et al, 1998), incidence rates were presented for just two centres with more than five cases of osteosarcoma registered: Harare, Zimbabwe (ASR 4.3 per million, based on eight cases), and Namibia, 1983–92 (ASR 2.7 per million, histology-only cases).

There is considerably more variation in risk between populations for Ewing sarcoma, with particularly low incidence in black populations. This was first noted in comparisons between rates in black and white children in the United States (Fraumeni & Glass, 1970; Glass & Fraumeni, 1970). The ratio between osteosarcoma and Ewing sarcoma in childhood in African registries is around 10:1, compared with approximately equal numbers in white populations (Parkin *et al.*, 1993). This suggests that genetic factors are important in predisposition to (or protection against) Ewing sarcoma. Incidence increases with age, though less steeply than for osteosarcoma. Compared with osteosarcoma, Ewing sarcoma arises more frequently in the ribs, pelvis (especially in older children) and skull (in younger children) and correspondingly less frequently in the long bones.

Soft-tissue sarcomas

Among white populations, soft-tissue sarcomas account for 4–8% of all childhood cancers and have a combined ASR of 6–11 per million. Between two thirds and three quarters are rhabdomyosarcomas, 10–20% are fibrosarcomas (including malignant fibrous histiocytoma and neurofibrosarcoma) and the remainder are other rare types. Among blacks in the United States, rhabdomyosarcoma has a similar incidence whereas fibrosarcoma is somewhat more common.

Table 8. Childhood cancer: age-standardized (world) incidence per million
Wilms tumour

	MALE		FEMALE		TOTAL		
	Cases	ASR(W)	Cases	ASR(W)	Cases	M/F	ASR(W)
Africa, North							
Algeria, 4 registries	25	**6.6**	38	**10.1**	63	0.7	**8.3**
*Egypt, Alexandria (1980-1989)	31	**4.9**	19	**3.2**	50	1.6	**4.1**
Tunisia, 3 registries	7	**6.8**	5	**5.2**	12	1.4	**6.0**
Africa, West							
The Gambia (1988-1998)	10	**4.1**	7	**3.0**	17	1.4	**3.6**
Guinea, Conakry (1993-1999)	14	**9.3**	5	**3.2**	19	2.8	**6.3**
Mali, Bamako (1988-1997)	10	**6.1**	4	**2.3**	14	2.5	**4.2**
Niger, Niamey (1993-1999)	-	-	2	**2.1**	2	0.0	**1.1**
Nigeria, Ibadan (1993-1999)	2	**3.8**	3	**3.3**	5	0.7	**3.5**
Africa, Central							
Congo, Brazzaville (1996-1999)	3	**5.8**	3	**6.2**	6	1.0	**6.0**
Africa, East							
France, La Reunion (1988-1994)	3	**4.9**	9	**18.3**	12	0.3	**11.5**
Kenya, Eldoret (1998-2000)	8	**19.8**	6	**14.9**	14	1.3	**17.4**
Malawi, Blantyre (1991-2001)	12	**7.0**	8	**4.4**	20	1.5	**5.7**
Uganda, Kyadondo County (1993-1997)	12	**9.9**	6	**4.5**	18	2.0	**7.2**
Zimbabwe, Harare: African (1990-1997)	22	**12.8**	27	**15.2**	49	0.8	**14.0**
Africa, South							
*Namibia (1983-1992)	17	**6.8**	13	**5.2**	30	1.3	**6.0**
South Africa: Black (1989-1992)	*110*	**5.2**	*112*	**5.3**	*222*	*1.0*	**5.3**
South Africa: Indian (1989-1992)	*3*	**5.8**	*1*	**1.6**	*4*	*3.0*	**3.7**
South Africa: Mixed race (1989-1992)	*10*	**4.9**	*8*	**4.1**	*18*	*1.3*	**4.5**
South Africa: White (1989-1992)	*20*	**9.7**	*17*	**8.6**	*37*	*1.2*	**9.2**
Swaziland (1996-1999)	3	**4.3**	6	**8.4**	9	0.5	**6.4**
Europe/USA							
USA, SEER: White (1993-1997)	94	**9.9**	88	**9.6**	182	1.1	**9.8**
USA, SEER: Black (1993-1997)	16	**9.3**	28	**16.6**	44	0.6	**12.9**
France, 8 registries (1993-1997)	27	**10.6**	27	**11.6**	54	1.0	**11.1**
The Netherlands (1993-1997)	72	**10.7**	62	**9.7**	134	1.2	**10.2**
UK, England (1993-1997)	164	**7.4**	156	**7.2**	320	1.1	**7.3**

*International Incidence of Childhood Cancer Volume II

In italics: histopathology-based registries

In Africa, incidence rates of childhood soft-tissue sarcomas other than Kaposi sarcoma are unremarkable (Table 10).

In the 1970s, Kaposi sarcoma had an ASR of 2–2.5 per million in Kampala, Uganda, and Bulawayo, Zimbabwe, and in Bulawayo it was the most common childhood soft-tissue sarcoma (Parkin et al., 1988). These data from the period preceding the AIDS epidemic in sub-Saharan Africa give an indication of the incidence of childhood Kaposi sarcoma attributable to the endemic form of the disease. Since then, there have been very large increases in the incidence of Kaposi sarcoma among children in East and Central Africa. In Kampala during 1993–97, the ASR was 52.7 per million and among African residents of Harare, Zimbabwe, during 1990–97 it was 10.3 per million (Table 11). In these two series, Kaposi sarcoma accounted for 33% and 10% of all childhood cancers respectively. In Zambia over a similar period, the relative frequency was 19% (Chintu et al., 1995). It is clear that the great majority of the increase in incidence is related to the AIDS epidemic, which has been particularly severe in East and Central Africa. As very high rates of HIV infection are a more recent phenomenon in western and southern Africa, the peak incidence of childhood Kaposi sarcoma may also occur later in these countries. In Harare, however, while the incidence of Kaposi sarcoma at all ages combined doubled between 1990–92 and 1993–95, in children it rose by only around 15% (Bassett et al., 1995; Chokunonga et al., 2000).

Even before the onset of the AIDS epidemic, however, Kaposi sarcoma in childhood had very different clinical features from endemic Kaposi sarcoma of adults, and more resembled epidemic AIDS-related Kaposi sarcoma. Thus, it was often poly-lymphadenopathic, with either absent or sparse and anomalously sited skin lesions. Progression was rapid (Slavin et al., 1970; Olweny et al., 1976).

Germ-cell and gonadal tumours
Germ-cell tumours generally account for less than 4% of all childhood cancers. Testicular tumours are rare in black children in the United States (Miller, 1977); incidence rates for germ-cell tumours are about one third to one quarter those in white children (Parkin et al., 1998). These cancers are rare in all series of childhood cancers from Africa (Davies, 1973; Williams, 1975). Table 12 shows the rates from the series in this volume.

Epithelial tumours
By far the highest relative frequency of childhood nasopharyngeal carcinoma is in North Africa, a region of intermediate risk for adults, where it accounts for 7–15% of all childhood cancers; the ASR in Algeria was 2.6 per million. Among Israeli-born Jews, the highest incidence is among those whose parents were born in North Africa (Parkin & Iscovich, 1997). In the United States, black children had

Table 9. Childhood cancer: age-standardized (world) incidence per million
Bone tumours

	MALE Cases	MALE ASR(W)	FEMALE Cases	FEMALE ASR(W)	TOTAL Cases	TOTAL M/F	TOTAL ASR(W)
Africa, North							
Algeria, 4 registries	34	7.2	32	7.4	66	1.1	7.3
*Egypt, Alexandria (1980-1989)	54	8.4	47	6.9	101	1.1	7.6
Tunisia, 3 registries	5	3.6	5	3.6	10	1.0	3.6
Africa, West							
The Gambia (1988-1998)	3	1.4	5	2.3	8	0.6	1.9
Guinea, Conakry (1993-1999)	11	7.6	3	2.3	14	3.7	5.0
Mali, Bamako (1988-1997)	3	1.8	3	1.7	6	1.0	1.8
Niger, Niamey (1993-1999)	9	11.4	5	5.8	14	1.8	8.5
Nigeria, Ibadan (1993-1999)	3	5.5	1	0.8	4	3.0	2.4
Africa, Central							
Congo, Brazzaville (1996-1999)	1	1.9	-	-	1	-	1.0
Africa, East							
France, La Reunion (1988-1994)	4	6.0	2	2.8	6	2.0	4.5
Kenya, Eldoret (1998-2000)	2	4.9	1	2.3	3	2.0	3.6
Malawi, Blantyre (1991-2001)	3	1.8	3	1.7	6	1.0	1.7
Uganda, Kyadondo County (1993-1997)	5	4.6	5	3.8	10	1.0	4.3
Zimbabwe, Harare: African (1990-1997)	9	5.5	5	2.8	14	1.8	4.1
Africa, South							
*Namibia (1983-1992)	11	4.0	9	3.3	20	1.2	3.7
South Africa: Black (1989-1992)	52	2.3	55	2.5	107	0.9	2.4
South Africa: Indian (1989-1992)	5	7.9	3	4.6	8	1.7	6.3
South Africa: Mixed race (1989-1992)	2	0.9	4	1.7	6	0.5	1.3
South Africa: White (1989-1992)	15	6.1	31	12.9	46	0.5	9.4
Swaziland (1996-1999)	3	3.7	9	9.7	12	0.3	6.7
Europe/USA							
USA, SEER: White (1993-1997)	88	7.7	58	5.3	146	1.5	6.6
USA, SEER: Black (1993-1997)	11	5.5	7	3.6	18	1.6	4.5
France, 8 registries (1993-1997)	18	5.7	19	6.2	37	0.9	6.0
The Netherlands (1993-1997)	54	7.1	46	6.3	100	1.2	6.7
UK, England (1993-1997)	139	5.3	141	5.6	280	1.0	5.4

*International Incidence of Childhood Cancer Volume II

In italics: histopathology-based registries

an ASR of 0.8 per million, five times that in whites, and nasopharyngeal carcinoma was the most frequent epithelial neoplasm in the case series from Ibadan, Nigeria (Williams, 1975), Uganda (Davies, 1973) and Zambia (Chintu et al., 1995)

Ascertainment of skin carcinoma is probably incomplete in most registries but incidence is exceptionally high in Tunisia, where it accounts for 9% of all registrations in a series from the National Cancer Institute (Parkin et al., 1988). Among the 81 cases, 70% were squamous cell carcinoma and 30% were basal cell; 89% of cases were in children with xeroderma pigmentosum.

References

Alexander, F.E., Ricketts, T.J., McKinney, P.A. & Cartwright, R.A. (1990) Community lifestyle characteristics and risk of acute lymphoblastic leukaemia in children. Lancet, 336, 1461–1465

Barr, R.D., McCulloch, P.B., Mehta, S. & Kendall, A.G. (1972) Acute leukaemia in Kenya. Scot. Med. J., 17, 330–333

Bassett, M.T., Chokunonga, E., Mauchaza, B., Levy, L., Ferlay, J. & Parkin, D.M. (1995) Cancer in the African population of Harare, Zimbabwe, 1990-1992. Int. J. Cancer, 63, 29–36

Birch, J.M. & Marsden, H.E. (1987) A classification scheme for childhood cancers. Int. J. Cancer, 40, 620–624

Cameron, H.M. & Warwick, G.P. (1977) Primary cancer of the liver in Kenyan children. Br. J. Cancer, 36, 793–803

Carlsen, N.L. (1986) Epidemiological investigations on neuroblastomas in Denmark 1943-1980. Br. J. Cancer, 54, 977–988

Chintu, C., Athale, U.H. & Patil, P.S. (1995) Childhood cancers in Zambia before and after the HIV epidemic. Arch. Dis. Child., 73, 100–105

Chokunonga, E., Levy, L.M., Bassett, M.T., Mauchaza, B.G., Thomas, D.B. & Parkin, D.M. (2000) Cancer incidence in the African population of Harare, Zimbabwe: second results from the Cancer Registry 1993-1995. Int. J. Cancer, 85, 54–59

Cohen, C. & Hamilton, D.G. (1980) Epidemiologic and histologic patterns of Hodgkin's disease: comparison of the black and white populations of Johannesburg, South Africa. Cancer, 46, 186–189

Court Brown, W.M. & Doll, R. (1961) Leukaemia in childhood and young adult life. Trends in mortality in relation to aetiology. Br. Med. J., 1, 981–988

Davies, J.N.P. (1973) Childhood tumours. In: Templeton, A.C., ed., Tumours in a Tropical Country (Recent Results in Cancer Research No. 41), Berlin, Springer Verlag

Davis, J.N.P. & Owor, R. (1965) Chloromatous tumours in African children in Uganda. Br. Med. J., ii, 405–407

Davis, S., Rogers, M.A. & Pendergrass, T.W. (1987) The incidence and epidemiologic characteristics of neuroblastoma in the United States. Am. J. Epidemiol., 126, 1063–1074

Table 10. Childhood cancer: age-standardized (world) incidence per million
Soft tissue sarcomas

	MALE		FEMALE		TOTAL		
	Cases	ASR(W)	Cases	ASR(W)	Cases	M/F	ASR(W)
Africa, North							
Algeria, 4 registries	21	**5.0**	8	**1.9**	29	2.6	**3.5**
*Egypt, Alexandria (1980-1989)	24	**3.7**	9	**1.5**	33	2.7	**2.6**
Tunisia, 3 registries	3	**2.4**	4	**3.9**	7	0.8	**3.1**
Africa, West							
The Gambia (1988-1998)	1	**0.4**	4	**1.7**	5	0.3	**1.0**
Guinea, Conakry (1993-1999)	6	**4.3**	2	**1.4**	8	3.0	**2.9**
Mali, Bamako (1988-1997)	1	**0.6**	2	**1.2**	3	0.5	**0.9**
Niger, Niamey (1993-1999)	3	**4.1**	1	**1.0**	4	3.0	**2.5**
Nigeria, Ibadan (1993-1999)	4	**6.4**	5	**4.8**	9	0.8	**5.3**
Africa, Central							
Congo, Brazzaville (1996-1999)	4	**7.6**	1	**2.0**	5	4.0	**4.9**
Africa, East							
France, La Reunion (1988-1994)	1	**1.3**	2	**3.5**	3	0.5	**2.4**
Kenya, Eldoret (1998-2000)	5	**12.2**	2	**4.8**	7	2.5	**8.5**
Malawi, Blantyre (1991-2001)	28	**16.1**	18	**10.0**	46	1.6	**13.0**
Uganda, Kyadondo County (1993-1997)	88	**76.8**	53	**42.0**	141	1.7	**58.6**
Zimbabwe, Harare: African (1990-1997)	31	**18.1**	18	**10.1**	49	1.7	**14.0**
Africa, South							
*Namibia (1983-1992)	5	**1.9**	10	**3.7**	15	0.5	**2.8**
South Africa: Black (1989-1992)	76	**3.5**	69	**3.3**	145	1.1	**3.4**
South Africa: Indian (1989-1992)	7	**12.3**	2	**3.5**	9	3.5	**8.0**
South Africa: Mixed race (1989-1992)	7	**3.3**	7	**3.3**	14	1.0	**3.3**
South Africa: White (1989-1992)	16	**7.0**	8	**3.9**	24	2.0	**5.5**
Swaziland (1996-1999)	9	**10.9**	4	**5.4**	13	2.3	**8.1**
Europe/USA							
USA, SEER: White (1993-1997)	60	**5.8**	67	**6.6**	127	0.9	**6.2**
USA, SEER: Black (1993-1997)	12	**6.1**	6	**3.2**	18	2.0	**4.7**
France, 8 registries (1993-1997)	14	**4.8**	10	**3.9**	24	1.4	**4.3**
The Netherlands (1993-1997)	51	**7.2**	37	**5.4**	88	1.4	**6.3**
UK, England (1993-1997)	94	**3.9**	94	**4.1**	188	1.0	**4.0**

*International Incidence of Childhood Cancer Volume II

In italics: histopathology-based registries

Dearden, C.E. (1985) Preliminary communication on leukaemia cell markers in Kenya. *Leuk. Res.*, **9**, 753–754

Draper, G.J., Vincent, T.J., O'Conor, C.M. & Stiller, C.A. (1991) Socioeconomic factors and variation in incidence rates between county districts. In: Draper, G.J., ed., *The Geographical Epidemiology of Childhood Leukaemia and Non-Hodgin's Lymphoma in Great Britain 1966-83*, London, OPCS, pp. 47–56

Draper, G.J., Sanders, B.M., Brownbill, P.A. & Hawkins, M.M. (1992) Patterns of risk of hereditary retinoblastoma and applications to genetic counselling. *Br. J. Cancer*, **66**, 211–219

El Bolkainy, M.N., Gad-El-Mawla, N., Tawfik, H.N. & Aboul-Enein, M.I. (1984) Epidemiology of lymphoma and leukaemia in Egypt. In: Magrath, I., O'Conor, G.T. & Ramot, B., eds, *Pathogenesis of Leukemias and Lymphomas: Environmental Influences* (Progress in Cancer Research and Therapy, Vol. 27), New York, Raven Press, pp. 9–16

Edington, G.M., Osunkoya, B.O. & Hendrickse, M. (1973) Histologic classification of Hodgkin's disease in the western state of Nigeria. *J. Natl Cancer Inst.*, **50**, 1633–1637

Fleming, A.F. (1993) Leukaemias in Africa. *Leukemia*, **7** (suppl. 2), s138–s141

Fleming, A.F. & Peter, B. (1982) The epidemiology of leukaemias in the Guinea savannah region of Nigeria. *Nigerian Med. J.*, **12**, 223–233

Fraumeni, J.F., Jr & Glass, A.G. (1970) Rarity of Ewing's sarcoma among U.S. Negro children. *Lancet*, **i**, 366–367

Freedman, J. & Goldberg, L. (1976) Incidence of retinoblastoma in the Bantu of South Africa. *Br. J. Ophthalmol.*, **60**, 655–656

Glaser, S.L., Lin, R.J., Stewart, S.L., Ambinder, R.F., Jarrett, R.F., Brousset, P., Pallesen, G., Gulley, M.L., Khan, G., O'Grady, J., Hummel, M., Preciado, M.V., Knecht, H., Chan, J.K. & Claviez, A. (1997) Epstein-Barr virus-associated Hodgkin's disease: epidemiologic characteristics in international data. *Int. J. Cancer*, **70**, 375–382

Glass, A.G., & Fraumeni, J.F., Jr (1970) Epidemiology of bone cancer in children. *J. Natl Cancer Inst.*, **44**, 187–195

Greaves, M.F. (1984) Subtypes of acute lymphoblastic leukaemia: implications for the pathogenesis and epidemiology of leukaemia. In: Magrath, I., O'Conor, G.T. & Ramot, B., eds, *Pathogenesis of Leukemias and Lymphomas: Environmental Influences* (Progress in Cancer Research and Therapy, Vol. 27), New York, Raven Press, pp. 129–139

Greaves, M.F. (1988) Speculations on the cause of childhood acute lymphoblastic leukaemia. *Leukemia*, **2**, 424–429

Greaves, M.F, Colman, S.M., Beard, M.E.J., Bradstock, K., Cabrera, M.E., Chen, P.M., Jacobs, P., Lam-Po-Tang, P.R., MacDougall, L.G., Williams, C.K. & Alexander, F.E. (1993) Geographical distribution of acute lymphoblastic leukaemia

Table 11. Childhood cancer: age-standardized (world) incidence per million
Kaposi sarcoma

	MALE		FEMALE		TOTAL		
	Cases	ASR(W)	Cases	ASR(W)	Cases	M/F	ASR(W)
Africa, North							
Algeria, 4 registries	-	·	-	·	-	-	·
*Egypt, Alexandria (1980-1989)	-	·	-	·	-	-	·
Tunisia, 3 registries	-	·	-	·	-	-	·
Africa, West							
The Gambia (1988-1998)	1	**0.4**	1	**0.4**	2	1.0	**0.4**
Guinea, Conakry (1993-1999)	-	·	-	·	-	-	·
Mali, Bamako (1988-1997)	-	·	-	·	-	-	·
Niger, Niamey (1993-1999)	-	·	-	·	-	-	·
Nigeria, Ibadan (1993-1999)	-	·	-	·	-	-	·
Africa, Central							
Congo, Brazzaville (1996-1999)	1	**1.9**	-	·	1	-	**1.0**
Africa, East							
France, La Reunion (1988-1994)	-	·	-	·	-	-	·
Kenya, Eldoret (1998-2000)	3	**7.2**	-	·	3	-	**3.6**
Malawi, Blantyre (1991-2001)	26	**15.0**	16	**8.9**	42	1.6	**11.8**
Uganda, Kyadondo County (1993-1997)	81	**70.2**	46	**36.6**	127	1.8	**52.7**
Zimbabwe, Harare: African (1990-1997)	26	**15.2**	10	**5.6**	36	2.6	**10.3**
Africa, South							
*Namibia (1983-1992)	2	**0.8**	2	**0.7**	4	1.0	**0.7**
South Africa: Black (1989-1992)	*3*	**0.1**	*6*	**0.3**	*9*	*0.5*	**0.2**
South Africa: Indian (1989-1992)	-	·	-	·	-	-	·
South Africa: Mixed race (1989-1992)	*2*	**0.9**	-	·	*2*	-	**0.5**
South Africa: White (1989-1992)	*1*	**0.4**	-	·	*1*	-	**0.2**
Swaziland (1996-1999)	5	**6.1**	2	**2.8**	7	2.5	**4.4**
Europe/USA							
USA, SEER: White (1993-1997)	-	·	-	·	-	-	·
USA, SEER: Black (1993-1997)	-	·	-	·	-	-	·
France, 8 registries (1993-1997)	-	·	-	·	-	-	·
The Netherlands (1993-1997)	-	·	1	**0.1**	1	0.0	**0.1**
UK, England (1993-1997)	1	**0.0**	-	·	1	-	**0.0**

*International Incidence of Childhood Cancer Volume II

In italics: histopathology-based registries

subtype: second report of the Collaborative Group Study. *Leukemia*, **7**, 27–34

Hussan, M.A.M., Abass, F.E.M. & Ahmad, H.M. (1988) Malignanat disease in Sudanese children. *E. Afr. Med. J.*, **65**, 507–513

Iscovich, J. & Parkin, D.M. (1997) Risk of cancer in migrants and their descendants in Israel: I. Leukaemias and lymphomas. *Int. J. Cancer*, **70**, 649–653

Johnson, L.C. (1953) A general theory of bone tumours. *Bull. N.Y. Acad. Med.*, **29**, 164–171

Junaid, T.A. & Babalola, B.O. (1988) Nigeria: Ibadan Cancer Registry, 1960–1984. In: Parkin, D.M., Stiller, C.A., Draper, G.J., Bieber, C.A., Terracini, B. & Young, J.L., eds, *International Incidence of Childhood Cancer* (IARC Scientific Publications No. 87), Lyon, IARC, pp. 37–41

Kayembi-Lubeji, D. (1990) Retinoblastoma in Zaire. *Tropical Doctor*, **20**, 38

Kinlen, U. Epidemiological evidence for an infective basis in childhood leukaemia. *Br J Cancer 1995*, **71**, 1-5

Kodilinye, H.C. (1967) Retinoblasoma in Nigeria: problems of treatment. *Am. J. Ophthalmol.*, **63**, 469–481

Kramárová, E., Stiller, C.A., Ferlay, J., Parkin, D.M., Drtaper, G.J., Michaelis, J., Neglia, J. & Qureshi, S., eds (1996) *International Classification of Childhood Cancer* (IARC Technical Report No. 29), Lyon, IARC

Kung'u, A. (1984) Childhood cancers in Kenya: a histopathological and epidemiological study. *E. Afr. Med. J.*, **61**, 11–24

Leoncini, L., Spina, D., Nyong'o, A., Abinya, O., Minacci, C., Disanto, A., De Luca, F., De Vivo, A., Sabattini, E, Poggi, S., Pileri, S. & Tosi, P. (1996) Neoplastic cells of Hodgkin's disease show differences in EBV expression between Kenya and Italy. *Int. J. Cancer*, **65**, 781–784

Levy, L.M. (1988) Hodgkin's disease in black Zimbabweans. A study of epidemiologic, histologic, and clinical features. *Cancer*, **61**, 189–194

MacDougall, L.G. (1985) Acute childhood leukaemia in Johannesburg. *Leuk. Res.*, **9**, 765–767

MacDougall, L.G., Jankowitz, P., Cohn, R. & Bernstein, R. (1986) Acute childhood leukemia in Johannesburg. Ethnic differences in incidence, cell type, and survival. *Am. J. Pediatr. Hematol. Oncol.*, **8**, 43–51

Makata, A.M., Toriyama, K., Kamidigo, N.O., Eto, H. & Itakura, H. (1996) The pattern of pediatric solid malignant tumours in Western Kenya, East Africa, 1979-1994; an analysis based on histopathologic study (sic). *Am. J. Trop. Med. Hyg.*, **54**, 343–347

Massabi, M., Muaka, B.K. & Tamba, N. (1989) Epidemiology of childhood cancer in Zaire. *Lancet*, **ii**, 501

McWhirter, W.R. (1982) The relationship of incidence of childhood

Table 12. Childhood cancer: age-standardized (world) incidence per million
Germ cell tumours

	MALE		FEMALE		TOTAL		
	Cases	ASR(W)	Cases	ASR(W)	Cases	M/F	ASR(W)
Africa, North							
Algeria, 4 registries	6	1.7	7	1.9	13	0.9	1.8
*Egypt, Alexandria (1980-1989)	8	1.2	12	2.0	20	0.7	1.6
Tunisia, 3 registries	2	1.7	2	1.5	4	1.0	1.6
Africa, West							
The Gambia (1988-1998)	1	0.4	-	-	1	-	0.2
Guinea, Conakry (1993-1999)	1	0.5	1	0.6	2	1.0	0.5
Mali, Bamako (1988-1997)	-	-	-	-	-	-	-
Niger, Niamey (1993-1999)	1	1.1	-	-	1	-	0.5
Nigeria, Ibadan (1993-1999)	3	5.5	2	2.0	5	1.5	3.2
Africa, Central							
Congo, Brazzaville (1996-1999)	-	-	-	-	-	-	-
Africa, East							
France, La Reunion (1988-1994)	3	5.6	2	4.2	5	1.5	4.9
Kenya, Eldoret (1998-2000)	-	-	-	-	-	-	-
Malawi, Blantyre (1991-2001)	-	-	3	1.7	3	0.0	0.9
Uganda, Kyadondo County (1993-1997)	1	0.8	2	1.8	3	0.5	1.3
Zimbabwe, Harare: African (1990-1997)	1	0.6	6	3.3	7	0.2	2.0
Africa, South							
*Namibia (1983-1992)	-	-	6	2.3	6	0.0	1.1
South Africa: Black (1989-1992)	14	0.7	42	2.0	56	0.3	1.3
South Africa: Indian (1989-1992)	8	14.7	-	-	8	-	7.4
South Africa: Mixed race (1989-1992)	3	1.6	8	3.6	11	0.4	2.6
South Africa: White (1989-1992)	5	2.2	8	3.7	13	0.6	3.0
Swaziland (1996-1999)	-	-	2	2.5	2	0.0	1.2
Europe/USA							
USA, SEER: White (1993-1997)	54	5.3	48	4.7	102	1.1	5.0
USA, SEER: Black (1993-1997)	5	2.5	14	8.4	19	0.4	5.4
France, 8 registries (1993-1997)	12	4.4	6	2.6	18	2.0	3.5
The Netherlands (1993-1997)	30	4.2	48	7.0	78	0.6	5.6
UK, England (1993-1997)	67	2.9	100	4.2	167	0.7	3.5

International Incidence of Childhood Cancer Volume II
In italics: histopathology-based registries

lymphoblastic leukaemia to social class. Br. J. Cancer, **46**, 640–645

Miller, R.W. (1977) Ethnic differences in cancer occurrence: genetic and environmental influences with particular reference to neuroblastoma. In: Mulvihill, J.J., Miller, R.W. & Fraumeni, J.F., Jr, eds, Genetics of Human Cancer, New York, Raven Press, pp. 1–14

Miller, R.W. (1989) No neuroblastoma in Zaire. Lancet, **ii**, 978–979

Moore, S.W., Hesseling, P.B., Wessels, G. & Schneider, J.W. (1997) Hepatocellular carcinoma in children. Pediatr. Surg. Int., **12**, 266–270

Mwanda, O.W. (1999) Cancers in children younger than age 16 years in Kenya. E. Afr. Med. J., **76**, 3–9

O'Conor, G.T. & Davies, J.N.P. (1960) Malignant tumors in African children with special reference to malignant lymphomas. J. Pediatr., **56**, 526–535

Obioha, F.I., Kaine, W.N., Ikerionwu, S.E., Obi, G.O. & Ulasi, T.O. (1989) The pattern of childhood malignancy in eastern Nigeria. Ann. Trop. Pediatr., **9**, 261–265

Olweny, C.L.M., Kaddumukasa, L.A., Atine, I., Owor, R., Magrath, I. & Ziegler, J.L. (1976) Childhood Kaposi's sarcoma: clinical features and therapy. Br. J. Cancer, **33**, 555–560

Owor, R. (1984) Geographic distribution of malignant lymphomas and leukaemias in Uganda. In: Magrath, I., O'Conor, GT. &

Ramot, B., eds, Pathogenesis of Leukemias and Lymphomas: Environmental Influences (Progress in Cancer Research and Therapy, Vol. 27), New York, Raven Press, pp 29-33

Parkin, D.M. & Iscovich, J.A. (1997) The risk of cancer in migrants and their descendants in Israel: II Carcinomas and germ cell tumours. Int. J. Cancer, **70**, 654–660

Parkin, D.M., Stiller, C.A., Bieber, C.A., Draper, G.J., Terracini, B. & Young, J.L., eds (1988) International Incidence of Childhood Cancer (IARC Scientific Publications No. 87), Lyon, IARC

Parkin, D.M., Stiller, C.A. & Nectoux, J. (1993) International variations in the incidence of childhood bone tumours. Int. J. Cancer, **53**, 371–376

Parkin, D.M., Kramárová, E., Draper, G.J., Masuyer, E., Michaelis, J., Neglia, J, Qureshi, S. & Stiller, C.A., eds (1998) International Incidence of Childhood Cancer, vol. II (IARC Scientific Publications No. 144), Lyon, IARC

Paul, B., Mukiibi, J.M., Mandisodza, A., Levy, L. & Nkrumah, F.K. (1992) A three-year prospective study of 137 cases of acute leukaemia in Zimbabwe.Cent. Afr. J. Med. , **38**, 95–99

Powell, J.E., Parkes, S.E., Cameron, A.H. & Mann, J.R. (1994) Is the risk of cancer increased in Asians living in the UK? Arch. Dis. Child., **71**, 398–403

Sayers, G.M., Rip, M.R., Jacobs, P., Klopper, J.M.L., Karabus, C.D., Rosenstrauch, W.J., Hesseling, P., Hoffman, M. & Sayed, R.

Table 13. Childhood cancer: age-standardized (world) incidence per million
All cancers

	MALE Cases	ASR(W)	FEMALE Cases	ASR(W)	TOTAL Cases	M/F	ASR(W)
Africa, North							
Algeria, 4 registries	495	119.1	320	79.7	815	1.5	99.7
*Egypt, Alexandria (1980-1989)	799	121.8	516	81.1	1315	1.5	101.4
Tunisia, 3 registries	110	92.9	98	88.0	208	1.1	90.5
Africa, West							
The Gambia (1988-1998)	89	37.7	73	31.6	162	1.2	34.7
Guinea, Conakry (1993-1999)	119	76.9	74	50.9	193	1.6	64.0
Mali, Bamako (1988-1997)	74	45.5	59	33.6	133	1.3	39.4
Niger, Niamey (1993-1999)	61	76.5	58	67.1	119	1.1	71.7
Nigeria, Ibadan (1993-1999)	110	205.7	66	64.9	176	1.7	113.1
Africa, Central							
Congo, Brazzaville (1996-1999)	32	60.9	24	48.6	56	1.3	54.9
Africa, East							
France, La Reunion (1988-1994)	59	102.5	63	112.7	122	0.9	107.5
Kenya, Eldoret (1998-2000)	58	141.7	42	103.2	100	1.4	122.6
Malawi, Blantyre (1991-2001)	155	87.8	108	59.2	263	1.4	73.2
Uganda, Kyadondo County (1993-1997)	246	217.3	169	134.4	415	1.5	173.9
Zimbabwe, Harare: African (1990-1997)	215	127.4	171	96.0	386	1.3	111.3
Africa, South							
*Namibia (1983-1992)	128	48.8	107	40.7	235	1.2	44.8
South Africa: Black (1989-1992)	*1285*	*59.4*	*1010*	*47.5*	*2295*	*1.3*	*53.5*
South Africa: Indian (1989-1992)	*106*	*178.0*	*51*	*84.3*	*157*	*2.1*	*131.8*
South Africa: Mixed race (1989-1992)	*164*	*78.2*	*133*	*62.8*	*297*	*1.2*	*70.5*
South Africa: White (1989-1992)	*445*	*204.3*	*374*	*179.5*	*819*	*1.2*	*192.2*
Swaziland (1996-1999)	44	55.1	49	61.1	93	0.9	58.1
Europe/USA							
USA, SEER: White (1993-1997)	1660	163.2	1365	140.0	3025	1.2	151.9
USA, SEER: Black (1993-1997)	254	140.1	204	116.6	458	1.2	128.5
France, 8 registries (1993-1997)	456	163.9	309	116.8	765	1.5	140.9
The Netherlands (1993-1997)	1086	153.0	887	131.1	1973	1.2	142.3
UK, England (1993-1997)	3352	142.4	2724	118.9	6076	1.2	130.8

*International Incidence of Childhood Cancer Volume II

In italics: histopathology-based registries

(1992) Epidemiology of acute leukaemia in the Cape Province of South Africa. *Leuk. Res.*, **16**, 961–966

Slavin, G., Cameron, H.M., Forbes, C. & Morton Mitchell, R. (1970) Kaposi's sarcoma in East African children. A report of 51 cases. *J. Path. Bacteriol.*, **100**, 187–199

Smith, M.A., Simon, R., Strickler, H.D., McQuillan, G., Ries, L.A.G. & Linet, M.S. (1998b) Evidence that childhood acute lymphoblastic leukemia is associated with an infectious agent linked to hygiene conditions. *Cancer Causes Control*, **9**, 285–298

Stiller, C.A. & Parkin, D.M. (1990) International variations in the incidence of childhood lymphomas. *Paediat. Perinatal Epidemiol.*, **4**, 303–324

Stiller, C.A. & Parkin, D.M. (1992) International variations in the incidence of childhood renal tumours. *Br. J. Cancer*, **62**, 1026–1030

Stiller, C.A., McKinney, P.A., Bunch, K.J., Bailey, C.C. & Lewis, I.J. (1991) Childhood cancer and ethnic group in Britain: a United Kingdom Children's Cancer Study Group (UKCCSG) study. *Br. J. Cancer*, **64**, 543–548

Vanier, T.M. & Pike, M.C. (1967) Leukaemia incidence in tropical Africa. *Lancet*, **i**, 512–513

Wabinga, H.R., Parkin, D.M., Wabwire-Mangen, F. & Nambooze, S. (2000) Trends in cancer incidence in Kyadondo County, Uganda, 1960-1997. *Br. J. Cancer*, **82**, 1585–1592

Weinreb, M., Day, P.J., Niggli, F., Green, E.K., Nyong'o, A.O., Othieno-Abinya, N.A., Riyat, M.S., Raafat, F. & Mann, J.R. (1996) The consistent association between Epstein-Barr virus and Hodgkin's disease in children in Kenya. *Blood*, **87**, 3828–3836

Wessels, G. & Hesseling, P.B. (1995) Epidemiology of childhood cancer in Africa. *Int. J. Pediatr. Hematol. Oncol.*, **2**, 263–268

Wessels, G. & Hesseling, P.B. (1996) Unusual distribution of childhood cancer in Namibia. *Pediatr. Hematol. Oncol.*, **13**, 9–29

Williams, A.O. (1975) Tumors of childhood in Ibadan, Nigeria. *Cancer*, **36**, 370–378

Williams, C.K., Folami, A.O., Laditan, A.A. & Ukaejiofo, E.O. (1982) Childhood acute leukaemia in a tropical population. *Br. J. Cancer*, **46**, 89–94

Williams, C.K.O. & Bamgboye, E.A. (1983) Estimation of incidence of human leukaemia subtypes in an urban African population. *Oncology*, **40**, 381–386

Williams, C.K.O., Essien, E.M. & Bangboye, E.A. (1984) Trends in leukaemia incidence in Ibadan, Nigeria. In: Magrath, I., O'Conor, GT. & Ramot, B., eds, *Pathogenesis of Leukemias and Lymphomas: Environmental Influences* (Progress in Cancer Research and Therapy, Vol. 27), New York, Raven Press, pp 17–27

Williams, C.K.O. (1985) Influence of life style on the pattern of leukaemia and lymphoma subtypes among Nigerians, *Leuk. Res.*, **9**, 741–745

Wright, D.H. (1973) Epidemiology and histology of Hodgkin's disease in Uganda. *Natl Cancer Inst. Monogr.*, **36**, 25–30

6 AIDS and cancer in Africa

Introduction

The epidemic of the acquired immunodeficiency syndrome (AIDS) currently ravaging the world population was initially recognized in the early 1980s among the male homosexual community in the United States (CDC, 1981). An early manifestation, and one that was identified before the nature of the disease was recognized, was the occurrence of Kaposi sarcoma (KS)—normally an exceedingly rare cancer in the United States. This was the first signal that infection with the human immunodeficiency virus (HIV), later recognized as the etiological agent of AIDS, increases the risk of certain cancers. Subsequent observation has confirmed a greatly enhanced risk of not only KS, but also non-Hodgkin lymphoma (NHL), and these two diseases, along with cancer of the cervix, are now considered to be "AIDS-defining conditions"—that is, an HIV-positive subject with these cancers is considered to have AIDS (CDC, 1992). Subsequently, increased risks for several other cancers have been reported. The most convincing data come from follow-up of cohorts of HIV-positive subjects, comparing the occurrence of cancers with the number expected in the general population. Such studies suggest increased risks of several cancers, especially Hodgkin disease, anal cancer, seminoma, myeloma, and, less certainly, cancers of the lip, brain and lung (Goedert et al., 1998; Grulich et al., 1999; Frisch et al., 2001). This relationship between HIV/AIDS and cancer has led to a better understanding of the immunology and biology of HIV infection, and indirectly to increasing knowledge about the relationship between viruses and cancer. The knowledge that these cancers occur in association with a virus that targets the immune system has led to the supposition that immunosuppression may be a strong factor in their pathogenesis. Cancer risk is also high in primary immunodeficiency states and organ transplant patients, but HIV-immunosuppressed populations seem to have higher rates of virus-associated cancers.

However, immunosuppression may not necessarily be the direct causal factor in HIV-associated cancers. The virus is not known to be oncogenic, but the infection induces production of various cytokines and growth factors, which can act as growth promoters.

Although the vast majority of research into the link between AIDS and cancer has been carried out in 'western' populations (mainly in the United States, and to a lesser extent in Europe and Australia), these populations account for only a minority of the cases of AIDS occurring in the world today, or of the numbers of individuals who are carriers of HIV. As described below, sub-Saharan Africa accounted for about 70% of all such persons in the world at the beginning of the 21st century. This chapter reviews what is known of the impact of the epidemic of HIV/AIDS on cancer in the African continent, and what this has contributed to knowledge of the role of HIV in cancer etiology.

The AIDS epidemic in Africa

Table 1 shows estimates from the United Nations Programme on HIV/AIDS (UNAIDS) on the extent of the epidemic worldwide, and in the countries of the African continent, at the beginning of the 21st century.

In Africa, there were an estimated 29 million persons infected with HIV at the end of 2001 (72.5% of the world total), of whom 28.5 million were in sub-Saharan Africa. The regions most affected are southern and eastern Africa, where 21% and 10%, respectively, of the adult population are infected with HIV. The figures suggest a fairly brisk increase in sufferers (from 24.5 million at the end of 1999 to 28.5 million at the end of 2001), although the estimated number of deaths (2.2 million) was the same in 1999 and 2001. There are now 12 countries in which more than one tenth of the adult population aged 15–49 years is infected with HIV. In seven countries, all in the southern cone of the continent, at least one adult in five is living with the virus. In Botswana, 38.8% of adults are now infected with HIV, while in South Africa, 20.1% are infected, an increase from 12.9% at the end of 1997. With a total of five million infected people, South Africa has the largest number of people living with HIV/AIDS in the world. While West Africa is relatively less affected by HIV infection, the prevalence rates in some large countries are creeping up. Prevalence in Côte d'Ivoire is the highest in the region (around 10%) while Nigeria, by far the most populous country in sub-Saharan Africa, has over 5% of adults infected with HIV (2.7 million persons). The prevalence rates in other West African countries remain below 3%. Infection rates in East Africa, once the highest on the continent, hover above those in the West of the continent but have been exceeded by the rates now being seen in the southern cone.

In Africa, AIDS was first recognized in the Rakai district of south-west Uganda in 1982, where it was known locally as "slim disease" (Serwadda et al., 1985). It was characterized by fever, general malaise, itchy maculopapular rash, prolonged diarrhoea, oral candidiasis, occasional respiratory symptoms and profound wasting and weight loss.

Subsequently, descriptions of this disease were published in the international scientific literature, from Rwanda (Van de Perre et al., 1984), Congo/Zaire (Piot et al., 1984) and Zambia (Bayley, 1984). From this focus in East/Central Africa, the disease has spread to involve an increasingly wide area of the continent (Figure 1). The spread of this sexually transmitted disease has been aided and enhanced by the movement of troops and traders across borders. Though the main mode of transmission is sexual, particularly heterosexual sex in these areas, reuse of unsterilized injection needles and scarification marks are possible alternative routes that may have favoured the spread of the disease. In any event, as can be seen from the sex ratio of cases in Table 1, the disease is rather more common in women than in men in Africa, in contrast to other parts of the world, where homosexual intercourse or intravenous drug abuse are the major routes of transmission. The serious problem of HIV/AIDS in much of Africa is compounded by the lack of resources to manage the infection and its related issues. Unfortunately, various serious problems and determinants (e.g., wars, poverty) that fuel the spread of the epidemic abound in sub-Saharan Africa (Ateka, 2001). At the same time, it has been

Table 1. Estimates of HIV/AIDS in Africa

Region, Country	Estimated number of people living with HIV/AIDS, end 1999				Estimated AIDS deaths 1999: adults & children		Estimated number of people living with HIV/AIDS, end 2001			Estimated AIDS deaths 2001: adults & children	
	Adults and children	Sex ratio (M/F)	Prevalence adult (%)	Prevalence child (%)	Number	Rate per 1000	Adults and children	Prevalence adult (%)	Prevalence child (%)	Number	Rate per 1000
Northern Africa	...	...	**0.2**	...	...	...	**478 000**	**0.5**	**0.05**	**23 000**	**0.15**
Algeria	...	...	0.1	...	...	...	...	0.1*	...	...	...
Egypt	...	...	0.0	...	...	...	8000	<0.1	...	...	...
Libyan Arab Jamahiriya	...	...	0.1	...	...	...	7000	0.2	...	...	...
Morocco	...	...	0.0	...	...	...	13 000	0.1	...	...	...
Sudan	...	...	1.0	...	...	...	450 000	2.6	0.24	23 000	0.8
Tunisia	...	...	0.0	...	...	...	...	...	...	...	...
Western Africa	**4 788 600**	**0.84**	**4.6**	**0.22**	**463 410**	**2.4**	**5 672 400**	**4.9**	**0.49**	**363 200**	**1.74**
Benin	70 000	0.81	2.4	0.11	5600	1.0	120 000	3.6	0.40	8100	1.4
Burkina Faso	350 000	0.83	6.4	0.35	43 000	4.0	440 000	6.5	1.06	44 000	4.1
Cape Verde	...	...	...	...	...	...	...	...	...	...	...
Côte d'Ivoire	760 000	0.83	10.8	0.52	72 000	5.6	770 000	9.7	1.22	75 000	5.1
Gambia	13 000	0.82	2.0	0.10	1400	1.2	8400	1.6	0.09	400	0.3
Ghana	340 000	0.83	3.6	0.17	33 000	1.9	360 000	3.0	0.42	28 000	1.6
Guinea	55 000	0.79	1.5	0.08	5600	0.8	...	...	...	...	...
Guinea-Bissau	14 000	0.78	2.5	0.11	1300	1.2	17 000	2.8	0.28	1200	1.1
Liberia	39 000	0.76	2.8	0.16	4500	1.7	...	...	...	...	...
Mali	100 000	0.83	2.0	0.10	9900	1.0	110 000	1.7	0.24	11 000	1.0
Mauritania	6600	0.80	0.5	0.02	610	0.3	...	...	...	...	...
Niger	64 000	0.79	1.4	0.06	6500	0.7	...	...	...	...	...
Nigeria	2 700 000	0.86	5.1	0.24	250 000	2.5	3 500 000	5.8	0.51	170 000	1.6
Senegal	79 000	0.90	1.8	0.08	7800	0.9	27 000	0.5	0.07	2500	0.3
Sierra Leone	68 000	0.81	3.0	0.16	8200	1.9	170 000	7.0	0.79	11 000	2.7
Togo	130 000	0.82	6.0	0.32	14 000	3.5	150 000	6.0	0.73	12 000	2.8
Middle Africa	**2 242 100**	**0.81**	**5.4**	**0.23**	**205 720**	**2.4**	**3 085 900**	**6.5**	**0.72**	**244 370**	**2.76**
Angola	160 000	0.83	2.8	0.13	15 000	1.3	350 000	5.5	0.57	24 000	2.0
Cameroon	540 000	0.79	7.7	0.35	52 000	4.0	920 000	11.8	1.05	53 000	3.9
Central African Republic	240 000	0.77	13.8	0.58	23 000	7.2	250 000	12.9	1.54	22 000	6.6
Chad	92 000	0.80	2.7	0.12	10 000	1.5	150 000	3.6	0.48	14 000	1.9
Congo	86 000	0.82	6.4	0.30	8 600	3.3	110 000	7.2	1.04	11 000	3.9
Dem. Republic of the Congo	1 100 000	0.83	5.1	0.22	95 000	2.1	1 300 000	4.9	0.66	120 000	2.5

Table 1 (Cont.). Estimates of HIV/AIDS in Africa

Region, Country	Estimated number of people living with HIV/AIDS, end 1999				Estimated AIDS deaths 1999: adults & children		Estimated number of people living with HIV/AIDS, end 2001			Estimated AIDS deaths 2001: adults & children	
	Adults and children	Sex ratio (M/F)	Prevalence adult (%)	Prevalence child (%)	Number	Rate per 1000	Adults and children	Prevalence adult (%)	Prevalence child (%)	Number	Rate per 1000
Equatorial Guinea	1100	0.79	0.5	0.00	120	0.3	5900	3.4	0.20	370	0.9
Gabon	23 000	0.83	4.2	0.16	2000	2.0	…	…	…	…	…
Eastern Africa	**12 398 000**	**0.81**	**10.7**	**0.52**	**1 219 970**	**5.6**	**13 160 700**	**10.0**	**1.20**	**1 123 350**	**4.82**
Burundi	360 000	0.79	11.3	0.61	39 000	6.4	390 000	8.3	1.78	40 000	6.7
Comoros	…	…	0.1	…	…	…	…	…	…	…	…
Djibouti	37 000	0.84	11.8	0.55	3100	5.4	…	…	…	…	…
Eritrea	…	…	2.9	…	…	…	55 000	2.8	0.24	350	0.1
Ethiopia	3 000 000	0.81	10.6	0.54	280 000	5.1	2 100 000	6.4	0.79	160 000	2.8
Kenya	2 100 000	0.82	13.9	0.61	180 000	6.7	2 500 000	15.0	1.62	190 000	6.6
Madagascar	11 000	0.72	0.1	0.01	870	0.1	22 000	0.3	0.01	…	…
Malawi	800 000	0.81	16.0	0.81	70 000	7.2	850 000	15.0	1.21	80 000	7.6
Mauritius	…	…	0.1	…	…	…	700	0.1	…	<100	…
Mozambique	1 200 000	0.75	13.2	0.62	98 000	5.7	1 100 000	13.0	0.98	60 000	3.6
Réunion	…	…	…	…	…	…	…	…	…	…	…
Rwanda	400 000	0.76	11.2	0.69	40 000	6.1	500 000	8.9	1.85	49 000	6.7
Somalia	…	…	…	…	…	…	43 000	1.0	…	…	…
Uganda	820 000	0.83	8.3	0.51	110 000	5.6	600 000	5.0	0.93	84 000	3.8
United Republic of Tanzania	1 300 000	0.79	8.1	0.40	140 000	4.7	1 500 000	7.8	1.05	140 000	4.3
Zambia	870 000	0.84	19.9	0.96	99 000	11.9	1 200 000	21.5	3.03	120 000	12.4
Zimbabwe	1 500 000	0.75	25.1	1.08	160 000	14.6	2 300 000	33.7	4.13	200 000	17.0
Southern Africa	**5 020 000**	**0.79**	**20.7**	**0.76**	**315 100**	**7.9**	**6 090 000**	**21.3**	**1.99**	**436 000**	**9.86**
Botswana	290 000	0.87	35.8	1.49	24 000	16.6	330 000	38.8	4.28	26 000	18.4
Lesotho	240 000	0.85	23.6	0.99	16 000	8.8	360 000	31.0	3.34	25 000	14.0
Namibia	160 000	0.76	19.5	0.89	18 000	11.8	230 000	22.5	3.84	13 000	8.1
South Africa	4 200 000	0.78	19.9	0.70	250 000	7.3	5 000 000	20.1	1.68	360 000	9.3
Swaziland	130 000	0.79	25.2	0.93	7100	8.0	170 000	33.4	3.59	12 000	14.3
Sub-Saharan Africa	**24 500 000**	**0.81**	**8.6**	**0.38**	**2 200 000**	**4.1**	**28 500 000**	**9.0**	**0.92**	**2 200 000**	**3.8**
Global Total	**34 300 000**	**1.10**	**1.1**	**0.07**	**2 800 000**	**0.6**	**40 000 000**	**1.2**	**0.16**	**3 000 000**	**0.6**

Source: UNAIDS (http://www.unaids.org/epidemic_update/report/index.html)

estimated that close to 80% of resources earmarked for HIV/AIDS-related expenditure are utilized in regions accounting for less than 5% of the pandemic (Ateka, 2001).

According to UNAIDS, at the beginning of 2000, in most sub-Saharan countries adults and children were acquiring HIV at a higher rate than ever before: the number of new infections in the region during 1999 was 4.0 million. However, such rises are not inevitable. In Uganda, the prevalence of infection has decreased from around 14% in the early 1990s to about 5%. Studies of population-based cohorts have suggested that this is linked to changes in sexual behaviour (Mbulaiteye *et al.*, 2002). Similar observations have been made in Senegal (Meda *et al.*, 1999) and Zambia (Fylkesnes *et al.*, 2001).

In reviewing statistical data on HIV infection and AIDS, it is important to note that the clinical case definition for AIDS in Africa (WHO, 1986) relies on observed symptoms and signs, with almost no requirement for laboratory tests. The CDC/WHO definition for AIDS (CDC, 1987), which requires sophisticated laboratory support for diagnosis of opportunistic infections, estimation of CD4+ cell counts and exclusion of other known causes of immunodeficiency, is not a practical option in Africa and therefore not applied. Apart from the expense, the results of sero-diagnosis and confirmatory tests for HIV/AIDS in Africa are often complicated by the presence of cross-reacting antibodies from other common infections (Biggar, 1986). The clinical case definition, which was developed for the AIDS surveillance in Africa, lacks sensitivity and specificity. In addition, most of the data from sub-Saharan Africa relate to patients attending health centres, often the accessible and convenient study population, who unfortunately do not represent the general population, as usually only the sick attend health facilities and often only at late stages.

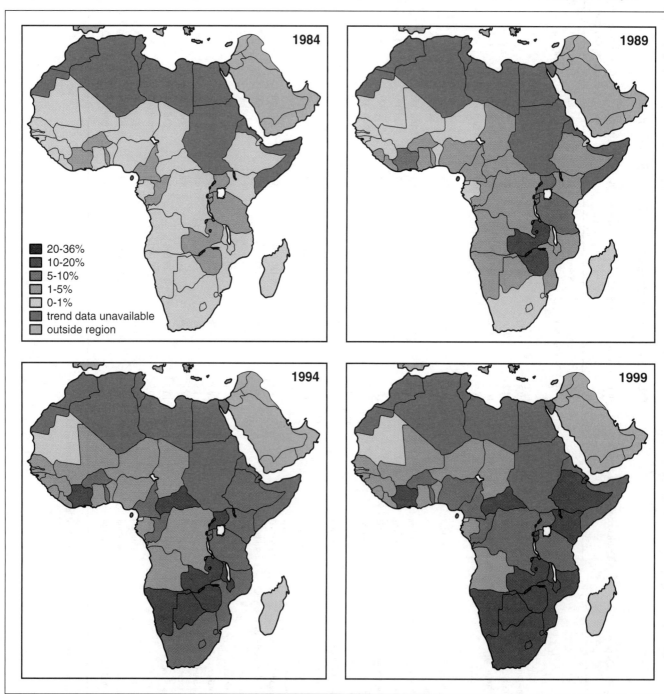

Figure 1. The spread of the AIDS epidemic in Africa, 1984–99
Source: UNAIDS (http://www.unaids.org/epidemic_update/report/index.html)

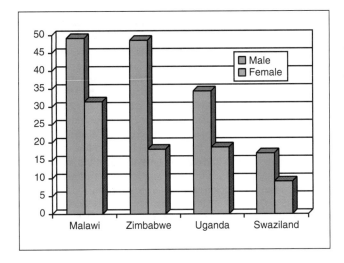

Figure 2. Incidence of Kaposi sarcoma in South and East Africa

As noted earlier, perinatal and heterosexual transmission predominate in Africa. The spectrum of associated diseases is rather different from the patterns in Europe and North America, with tuberculosis the main infectious complication (Lucas et al., 1991; Berkley et al., 1989). Several studies have suggested that the progression of HIV infection to clinical AIDS is more rapid in Africa than elsewhere (N'Galy et al., 1988; Whittle et al., 1992). However, there are few observations based upon incident infections (sero-converters). In the longitudinal, prospective population cohort study of people infected with HIV-1 and randomly selected subjects negative for HIV-1 antibodies in Uganda, the median time from seroconversion to death was 9.8 years, similar to that in developed countries before the use of anti-retroviral therapy. The median time from seroconversion to AIDS was 9.4 years and from AIDS to death was 9.2 months (Morgan et al., 2002a). It was also observed that most of the clinical conditions and symptoms used to define the disease and its progression, although more frequent in HIV-positive individuals than in controls, were also common in the latter (Morgan et al., 2002b), an observation similar to findings in Rwanda (Leroy et al., 1995). Herpes zoster, oral candidiasis and pulmonary tuberculosis were, however, found to be more predictive of HIV infection. The high background levels of these defining conditions in the population, as a result of poverty, malnutrition, endemic malaria, infections, poor sanitation and inadequate health care, make it seem that the progression of HIV infection is more rapid in Africa.

Evidence for associations between HIV/AIDS and cancer in Africa

Routine surveillance of cancer incidence in high-risk populations was a valuable tool in identifying the increased risks of KS and NHL in populations at high risk of AIDS in the United States (Biggar et al., 1984, 1985; Casabona et al., 1993). In Africa, cancer registries face many difficulties in complete enumeration of cases (due to lack of access to limited health-care facilities and poor medical records), consistent recording and coding of diagnosis, and definition and enumeration of populations at risk (ill-defined place of residence, infrequent population censuses, and rural–urban migration). Nevertheless, some data are available from cancer registries in various countries on trends in incidence of different cancers in relation to the advancing epidemic of AIDS.

In theory, linkage studies between cohorts of AIDS patients and cancer registries (in areas where they exist) are feasible in Africa, but none have been performed. In contrast, several case–control studies have been reported, comparing prevalence of HIV infection in cancer cases and control populations. Some care is needed in

interpreting the results. First, the cases are not always well defined, and may include 'cancers' diagnosed on clinical grounds only, without histological confirmation. The potential for bias due to inclusion of diseases related to HIV as cancer cases (for example, tuberculosis or HIV-related lymphadenopathy) should be considered. Secondly, as in all case–control studies, the nature of the control group must be carefully scrutinized—is it likely to represent the population from which the cases came, with respect to prevalence of HIV infection, or are persons included who are more, or less, likely to be infected?

Kaposi sarcoma

Before the onset of the HIV/AIDS epidemic, cumulative incidence of KS in the United States and Europe was ≤ 0.5 per 100 000, comprising about 0.3% of male and 0.1% of female cancers. Though the incidence was higher in East and Central Africa (comprising 3–10% of all cancers), it was rare in the western, northern and southern parts, where it accounted for ≤ 1% of cancers. The epidemiology of this 'endemic KS' in Africa is described in Chapter 4.6.

In the United States and Europe, KS is the most frequently reported AIDS-associated cancer, its incidence being 1000–5000 times higher in some high-risk population groups with HIV infection than in the general population (Serraino et al., 1997). In Africa, KS was reported to occur in 18% of AIDS cases in Rwanda (Van de Perre et al., 1984), 16% and 10% of cases in Kinshasa, Congo (Democratic Republic) (Piot et al., 1984; Nelson et al., 1993) and 4% in Uganda (Berkley et al., 1989).

Surveillance data from cancer registries have shown a large increase in incidence in many countries since the onset of the AIDS epidemic, and KS has become the most common cancer of men in Kampala, Uganda (Wabinga et al., 2000), Harare, Zimbabwe (Chokunonga et al., 1999), Blantyre, Malawi and Swaziland (this volume). Incidence is rather lower in women (Figure 2), but in these four countries, KS is second in frequency, behind cancer of the cervix.

In Bulawayo, Zimbabwe, the earlier (1963–72) estimated age-adjusted incidence rates in males and females were 2.3 and 0.3 per 100 000, respectively, but the recent rates from Harare (1993–95) are as high as 48.0 and 17.9 per 100 000 (Chokunonga et al., 1999), with median ages of 35 and 32 years in males and females. In Kampala, Uganda, the age-standardized incidence of KS in 1960–71 was 3.6 per 100 000 in men and around 0.2 per 100 000 in women; these rates had increased to 39.3 and 21.8 per 100 000, respectively, in 1995–97 (Parkin et al., 1999). Although the incidence of KS was low among the black population in South Africa until 1992, it approximately trebled between 1993 and 1995 (Sitas et al., 1998).

In parallel with these increases in incidence, there have been a narrowing of the sex ratio to less than 2:1 (Figure 2) and a change in the age distribution, with, in the 1990s, a slight peak in childhood at ages 0–4 years, a decline until age 15 years and the main peak at 35–39 years in males and 25–29 years for females (see Figure 3 of Chapter 4.6)

The four case–control studies in Africa which have estimated relative risk are summarized in Chapter 4.6. They suggest moderately elevated risks of 35 in Rwanda (Newton et al., 1995), 54 in Uganda (Newton et al., 2001), and 62 and 22 in two studies in Johannesburg, South Africa (Sitas et al., 1997, 2000). These risks are much lower than those reported in developed countries. Probably this relates to the much higher background incidence (non-HIV-related) in these populations, so that with similar levels of absolute risk in AIDS cases, relative risk is much lower in the African setting.

The relationship of KS to the associated oncovirus HHV-8 and the role that the epidemiology of this virus may have in the distribution of AIDS-related KS in Africa is reviewed in Chapter 4.6.

Lymphoma

The increased frequency of NHL in AIDS was noted in 1982 (Ziegler et al., 1982) Since then, the elevated risk has been confirmed in studies in the United States and Europe (Beral et al., 1991; Casabona et al., 1991). About 3% of AIDS cases present with a lymphoma, but lymphomas may occur in up to 10% of AIDS cases at some point. Almost all lymphomas in AIDS cases are of B-cell type. The cohort study of Coté et al. (1997) provides the most accurate estimate of excess risk in AIDS—about 160 times that in HIV-negative subjects. Risk is highest for high-grade lymphomas, especially diffuse immunoblastic (x 630) and undifferentiated Burkitt lymphoma (BL) (x 220). Extranodal lymphomas are more common in AIDS than usual (Beral et al., 1991), although this is probably because of the great excess of central nervous system lymphomas (15-fold increase); other extranodal lymphomas are not in excess (Coté et al., 1997). Immunoblastic and central nervous system lymphomas occur later in the course of AIDS (with more profound immunosuppression) than do Burkitt-type lymphomas (Roithmann et al., 1991). Males are more commonly affected, but this might be simply because of risk-group differences. Thus, the risk in females is 1.2 times that in males in heterosexually acquired cases of AIDS (Serraino et al., 1992). Risk is higher in white (compared with black) patients, and in those of higher socioeconomic status (Beral et al., 1991; Biggar & Rabkin, 1992; Franceschi et al., 1999).

Chromosomal translocations have been found in AIDS-associated lymphomas. They include t(8;14)(q24;q32), t(8;22)(q24;q11) and t(2;8) (p12;q24) involving the c-myc locus, and rearrangements of the switch region of the heavy chains of immunoglobulins (chromosome 14) or light chains (chromosome 22 for λ, chromosome 2 for κ), especially for BL, but also in certain immunoblastic lymphomas with plasmocytic differentiation (Delecluse et al., 1993). Rearrangements of bcl 6 situated in 3q27 were reported in 20% of diffuse large-cell lymphomas, but not small-cell types (Gaidano et al., 1994). Mutations in TP53 and n-ras are reported in a high proportion of AIDS-related BL and immunoblastic lymphomas (Ballerini et al., 1993).

Epstein–Barr virus (EBV) is present in two thirds of AIDS-related lymphomas (Hamilton-Dutoit et al., 1993) and may play an important role in lymphomagenesis (IARC, 1996, 1997). Its frequency varies by lymphoma type: it is found in almost all central nervous system lymphomas, 70–80% of immunoblastic lymphomas and 30–40% of small-cell/BL-type lymphomas.

– Non-Hodgkin lymphoma and AIDS in African adults

Relatively little is known concerning the effects of the AIDS epidemic on the occurrence of lymphomas in Africa, despite the very high seroprevalence of HIV in some countries. Particular care is needed in characterizing lymphomas when studying the possible link with HIV, since lymphadenopathy and lymphoid proliferation are common features of AIDS and the AIDS-related complex (Ioachim et al., 1990; Baroni & Uccini, 1993), and a high percentage of persons undergoing lymph node biopsy in Africa now are therefore likely to be HIV-positive (Bem et al., 1996).

Autopsy studies in Africa have found a very low prevalence of lymphomas in HIV-positive subjects. Abouya et al. (1992) found no cases among 53 subjects in Côte d'Ivoire, and Nelson et al. (1993) no cases among 63 subjects in Kinshasa, Congo (Democratic Republic). Lucas et al. (1994) detected seven cases of lymphoma among 247 autopsies (2.8%) in Côte d'Ivoire. Clinical descriptions of AIDS cases rarely mention lymphoma (Standaert et al., 1988; Gilks et al., 1992; Reeve, 1989; Karstaedt, 1992; Hira, 1990).

In Zimbabwe, Bassett et al. (1995) did not observe a very high incidence of NHL in the black population of Harare in 1990–92, although they did note that NHL comprised a rather higher percentage of lymphoreticular neoplasms than in an earlier series in 1979–84 (Levy, 1988). There are indications that incidence increased in the period 1991–95, at least in adult females (Chokunonga et al., 1999).

In Uganda, the most recent data from the cancer registry in Kampala suggest that the incidence of NHL increased significantly between 1991–94 and 1995–97, especially in children and young adults (Parkin et al., 1999).

To date, three studies have estimated the risk of NHL (all histological subtypes) in HIV-positive compared with HIV-negative subjects. Newton et al. (1995) found an odds ratio of 12.6 (95% CI 2.2–54.4) based on 19 cases tested for HIV in Rwanda, although some of these cases had been diagnosed on clinical suspicion only. In South Africa, Sitas et al. (1997, 2000) compared NHL cases with hospital 'controls', who had cancers unrelated to HIV or (in women) vascular disease. The most recent analysis (Sitas et al., 2000) of 105 NHL cases (all histologically confirmed) gave an odds ratio (OR) of 5.0 (95% CI 2.7–9.5). In a similar study of 31 adult cases of histologically confirmed NHL in Uganda (Parkin et al., 2000), the OR was 2.1 (95% CI 0.3–6.7); 12 of the cases (39%) were BL, of whom 3/7 (43%) were HIV-positive. Otieno et al. (2001) identified 29 cases of adult (age 16+) cases of BL from hospitals throughout Kenya in the period 1992–96. The number of cases identified in the main teaching hospital in Nairobi (19) was considered to be three times greater than in earlier years. Nineteen of the cases (66%) were HIV-positive, with ages typical of AIDS patients in Kenya (median 35 years) and a clinical presentation (diffuse lymph node involvement) differing from the HIV-negative cases, who were younger (16–25 years) and had a clinical picture reminiscent of typical endemic BL, with complete sparing of peripheral lymph nodes.

These are very low excess risks compared with those observed in Europe and the United States. Probably this relates to the poor prognosis of AIDS cases in Africa. The degree of immune dysfunction at AIDS diagnosis, as measured by CD4+ counts, is less in Africa than in industrial countries and median survival times are much shorter (Boerma et al., 1998). Since the risk of NHL in AIDS (and other immunodeficiency states) is related to the degree of immune dysregulation, it could be that the apparently low risk of lymphoma in HIV-positive subjects in Africa is a result of competing mortality—particularly from infectious diseases—in AIDS patients with relatively low levels of immunosuppression. In the study in Uganda (Parkin et al., 2000), the CD4+ cell count at diagnosis in HIV-positive lymphomas was higher than generally observed in Europe and North America (Roithmann et al., 1991; Roithmann & Andrieu, 1992). Lucas et al. (1994) found that NHL was present undiagnosed at autopsy in 2.8% of HIV-positive subjects in Côte d'Ivoire (4% of subjects with AIDS), a figure not very different from the cumulative probability of developing a lymphoma observed in cohorts of AIDS patients in the USA (Coté et al., 1997).

– Non-Hodgkin lymphoma of childhood

In the United States and Europe, NHLs are the most common malignancy in paediatric AIDS patients (Arico et al., 1991; Serraino & Franceschi, 1996) and about one third are BL (Mueller, 1998). This form of BL is clinically and cytogenetically similar to BL as it is observed in non-AIDS cases (sporadic BL) in North America and Europe, and the proportion of cases with detectable EBV genome is similar (around 30%). It is thus quite distinct from the endemic form of BL that was common in equatorial Africa long before the AIDS epidemic. Endemic BL in some areas comprised more than 90% of NHL in children and its relationship with EBV and malaria is well documented (see Chapter 4.10). The effect of the AIDS epidemic on the occurrence of BL in these areas is therefore of considerable interest.

Hospital and autopsy series do not provide any evidence for an increased frequency of childhood BL cases since the onset of the AIDS epidemic. The autopsy series of Lucas et al. (1994) in Côte d'Ivoire found no NHL in 78 HIV-positive children, while in Zambia, there was a decrease in the number of histological diagnoses of BL in the main teaching hospital between 1980–82 (pre-HIV epidemic) and 1990–92 (during the HIV epidemic) (Chintu et al., 1995).

However, in Uganda, one of the first countries in Africa to be affected by the AIDS epidemic in the early 1980s, registry data show a three-fold increase in the incidence in children (0–14 years) between the 1960s and 1995–97 (Parkin et al., 1999).

In studies of childhood BL since the onset of the AIDS epidemic, it seems that cases remain predominantly of the endemic type, which is not associated with HIV. Among 56 childhood BL cases from Uganda (Parkin et al., 2000), all were EBV-positive, and the median age of seven years, the predominance of males and the localization in facial and abdominal sites were characteristic of endemic BL. There was no association with HIV (OR = 1.0, 95% CI 0.3–3.9). In a previous study in Uganda, Mbidde et al. (1990) reported the absence of HIV infection among 50 children with BL studied early in the AIDS epidemic. All 17 cases of childhood BL in a series from the Nairobi Hospital, diagnosed in 1995–96, were HIV-negative (Lazzi et al., 1998). In a larger series from Kenya, Otieno et al. (2001) reported that only 5/767 (0.65%) childhood cases of BL were HIV-positive—the sex ratio (2.5:1) and peak age at 5–7 years was typical of endemic BL. It is possible that the lack of an association between HIV and BL relates to the poor survival of children infected perinatally with HIV—only 34% of HIV-infected children in Uganda survived to the age of three years (Marum et al., 1997).

It seems unlikely that the increased incidence of BL in Kampala, Uganda, is the consequence of the epidemic of HIV, and other factors, such as malaria infection, may be responsible.

– Hodgkin disease
Hodgkin disease represents one of the common tumours occurring in a context of immunodeficiency, including in HIV-infected populations, in whom 10-fold increases in risk have been observed (Dal Maso et al., 2001). HIV-associated Hodgkin disease has been reported more often in European countries and to a lesser extent the United States. All series have documented unusually aggressive disease, including a higher frequency of the unfavourable histological subtypes (mixed cellularity and lymphocyte-depleted), advanced stages and poor therapeutic response compared with the behaviour of Hodgkin disease outside the HIV setting. Such increases have not been reported from sub-Saharan Africa and there is no change in the age-specific incidence pattern.

HPV-associated cancers and HIV/AIDS
Human papillomavirus (HPV)-associated malignancies occur frequently in patients with HIV infection and AIDS (Frisch et al., 2000). In part, this may simply reflect the lifestyle factors associated with both infections; HIV-positive individuals are more likely to be infected with HPV. On the other hand, HIV may alter the natural history of HPV-associated oncogenesis through loss of immune control, facilitating infection with HPV or enhancing its persistence in cells and therefore increasing the development of squamous intraepithelial lesions (SIL).

– Cervical cancer
The Centers for Disease Control (CDC) designated high-grade SIL (HSIL) (moderate or severe dysplasia) as a category B defining condition, and invasive cervical cancer a category C defining condition of AIDS in 1993 (CDC, 1992). Although studies in the United States and Europe have reported 5–15-fold increases in risk of invasive cervical carcinoma in women who develop AIDS (Chapter 4.3), similar risks have not been demonstrated in sub-Saharan Africa. Numerous studies have investigated whether there is an increased risk of pre-invasive disease (cervical intraepithelial neoplasia (CIN) or SIL) in the presence of HIV infection.

Prevalence of CIN in relation to HIV status. In 4058 women attending two family planning clinics in Nairobi, Kenya, Maggwa et al. (1993) found a higher prevalence of cytologically diagnosed

CIN in women who were HIV-positive compared with those who were negative (4.9% versus 1.9%). The OR was little affected by adjustment for reported sexual behaviour or prior history of sexually transmitted diseases (OR = 2.78, 95% CI 1.32–5.85). In a similar study in Abidjan, Côte d'Ivoire (La Ruche et al., 1998a), the 2198 women were attending gynaecology clinics for various symptoms and hence had a relatively high prevalence of abnormal Pap smears (11.7% with low-grade SIL (LSIL) or worse). The prevalence of SIL was significantly higher in women who were HIV-positive (OR = 3.6 for LSIL and 5.8 for HSIL) and risk of LSIL (only) increased with increasing immunosuppression, as measured by CD4+ count. Kapiga et al. (1999) found that the risk of SIL among 691 HIV-positive women in Dar es Salaam, Tanzania, was increased among those with a CD4+ cell count below 200/μL. Leroy et al. (1999) tested pregnant women in antenatal clinics in Kigali, Rwanda, for HIV, in 1992–93. Among 103 HIV-positive and 107 HIV-negative women tested by Pap smears; the prevalence of SIL was significantly higher in the HIV-positive group (OR = 4.6, 95% CI 1.8–12.3), but, within this group, was not associated with immunosuppression.

CIN in relation to HPV and HIV infection. Studies in which HPV infection can be assessed as well as HIV are likely to be more informative concerning the contribution of HIV to cervical neoplasia. Most of these studies show that HPV infection is significantly more prevalent in women who are HIV-positive than in HIV-negative women (Laga et al., 1992; Ter Meulen et al., 1992; Seck et al., 1994; Langley et al., 1996; Miotti et al., 1996; La Ruche et al., 1998b; Piper et al., 1999; Serwadda et al., 1999; Temmerman et al., 1999; Womack et al., 2000). However, in other studies, there was no apparent association between the two infections. In their study of Nairobi prostitutes, Kreiss et al. (1992) found that HIV infection was associated with only a modest increase in HPV infection (37% versus 24%, OR = 1.7, not significant). In women attending an antenatal clinic in Mwanza, Tanzania, the OR of HPV infection in association with HIV was 1.02 (95% c.i. 0.6-1.6) (Mayaud et al., 2001).

Because of the close association of HPV and HIV infection, it is not surprising that, in most studies, CIN/SIL is more prevalent in HIV-positive than in HIV-negative women. Laga et al. (1992), in a group of 95 prostitutes from Kinshasa, Zaire, observed a significantly higher prevalence of CIN in women positive for HIV (27%) than in those negative (3%) (OR = 14.7). Seck et al (1994) reported on 35 HIV-positive women (18 with HIV-1; 17 with HIV-2) and 58 HIV-negative women attending an infectious disease service in Dakar, Senegal; HIV infection was associated with the presence of dysplastic smears (OR = 5.5, 95% CI 1.02–29.7). Miotti et al. (1996) studied 268 post-partum women in Malawi; cytologically diagnosed SIL was significantly related to HIV status (OR = 2.2). Langley et al. (1996) found that SIL was associated with HIV-2 infection (the association with HIV-1 was not statistically significant) among 759 prostitutes in Dakar, Senegal. In a later study in Dakar, Vernon et al. (1999) observed a strong association between SIL and both HIV-1 and HIV-2 in women participating in a study of mother–child transmission of HIV, but there was no association in a group of 278 prostitutes. HSIL was strongly associated with HIV positivity (OR = 4.5, 95% CI 1.8–12.4) in family-planning attenders in Kenya (Temmerman et al., 1999). However, in the studies in which HPV infection was not associated with HIV-positivity (Kreiss et al., 1992; Mayaud et al., 2001), there was no difference in CIN prevalence between women positive or negative for HIV, and in their series of gynaecology inpatients in Dar es Salaam, Tanzania, Ter Meulen et al. (1992) found that the prevalence of abnormal Pap smears did not differ between HIV-positive and -negative women.

The results of some of these studies allow the independent effects of HPV and HIV to be evaluated (Table 2). In the studies by Kreiss et al. (1992) and Mayaud et al. (2001), there was no

Table 2. Case–control studies of CIN and infection with HIV in women positive or negative for HPV infection

Reference	Location	Source of subjects	Measure of exposure	No. of cases/ no. of controls		Cases/controls HIV+ (%)	Odds ratio	95% CI
Kreiss et al. (1992)	Nairobi, Kenya	Prostitutes	Cytological CIN (all grades)	HPV–	3/34	66.7/61.7	1.24	0.06–78.6
				HPV+	13/13	69.2/76.9	0.68	0.08–5.34
Miotti et al. (1996)	Malawi	Women one year post-partum	Cytological SIL	HPV–	6/145	50/33.1	2.02	0.26–15.6
				HPV+	19/59	63.2/59.3	1.18	0.36–3.90
La Ruche et al. (1998b)	Abidjan Cote d'Ivoire	Gynaecology Outpatients	Cytological LSIL Biopsy/colposcopy HSIL	HPV–	57/292	19.3/14.7	1.38	0.62–3.03
				HPV+	151/95	53.6/31.6	2.51	1.42–4.46
Temmerman et al. (1999)	Nairobi Kenya	Family planning clinic attenders	HSIL on cytology	HPV–	11/421	27.3/6.9	5.07[a]	0.82–22.5
				HPV+	22/59	37.5/22.0	1.33[a]	0.35–4.55
Womack et al. (2000)	Chitungwiza Zimbabwe	Primary care attenders	SIL on biopsy or colposcopy	HPV–	29/217	41.4/35.5	1.28	0.54–3.01
				HPV+	87/133	83.9/65.4	2.76	1.34–5.73
Mayaud et al. (2001)	Mwanza Tanzania	Antenatal clinic attenders	SIL on cytology	HPV–	16/354	18.8/15.8	1.23	0.22–4.67
				HPV+	25/162	24.0/13.6	2.01	0.59–5.99

[a] OR for HSIL vs lesser abnormality and normal cytology

independent effect of HIV on risk of CIN—HIV did not influence risk of SIL, independent of HPV. A similar result is evident in the data presented by Miotti et al. (1996); however, at a follow-up visit, one year later, HPV infection in HIV-positive women was significantly more persistent (75% still positive) than in those women who were HIV-negative (23%).In the subset of subjects in the Abidjan study (described above) who were tested for the presence of HPV by polymerase chain reaction (PCR) analysis (La Ruche et al., 1998b), HIV did not have a significant effect on the risk of SIL in women negative for HPV (OR for all grades of SIL combined = 1.38; 95% CI 0.62–3.03), although, in the presence of HPV, there was an additional effect of HIV on the risk (OR for all grades of SIL combined = 2.51; 95% CI 1.42–4.46)). HIV-infected women with abnormal cytology were not highly immunosuppressed (median CD4+ count 450/µL). A subset of 461 of the women from the screening study in Chitungwiza, Zimbabwe, were tested for HIV, as well as being examined for CIN (by colposcopy and/or biopsy); cells obtained by cytobrush were tested for HPV by hybrid capture II test (HC II) (Womack et al., 2000). The prevalence of HSIL was almost three times higher in HIV-positive women than in HIV-negative (17.3% versus 5.9%,   p < 0.001), but, in women negative for HPV, HIV did not have a significant effect on the risk of SIL (OR for all grades of SIL combined = 1.28; 95% CI 0.54–3.01). However, in the presence of HPV, there was an additional effect on the risk (OR for all grades of SIL combined = 2.76; 95% CI 1.34–5.73). HIV infection was associated with a seven-fold increase in HPV viral burden in women who were colposcopically normal.

The mechanism underlying the role played by HIV in the pathogenesis of cervical precancer has been the subject of much speculation. The most likely explanation seems to be that HIV infection leads to enhanced persistence of infection with HPV, as has been observed in various prospective studies, and that this may be related to immunosuppression (Jay & Moscicki, 2000). Studies so far performed in Africa suggest that immunosuppression (as measured by CD4 cell counts) is associated with a higher prevalence of HPV infection in seropositive women (Miotti et al., 1996; Vernon et al., 1999).

Invasive cancer of the cervix. With respect to invasive cervix cancer, the close association between HIV and HPV infection, as shown in these studies, should imply an increased risk in HIV-positive women, if only because of this confounding. However, in early studies, both Rogo & Kavoo-Linge (1990) and Ter Meulen et al. (1992) found prevalence of HIV in cancer patients to be lower than in the normal population. In 18 cervix cancer cases among gynaecology outpatients, the prevalence of HIV (22%) was the same as in subjects with normal Pap smears (La Ruche et al., 1998a). Prevalence of HIV among 1323 cases of cervix cancer (almost all histologically confirmed) in Johannesburg was higher (12.6%) than in the comparison group of hospital patients with a mixture of non-HIV-related cancers or vascular disease (9.0%), yielding an OR of 1.6 (95% CI 1.1–2.3) (Sitas et al., 2000). Newton et al. (2001) found a similar slight excess of HIV infection (32%) in 65 women diagnosed as having cervix cancer in Kampala, Uganda, compared with 21% in 'controls' with non-infection-related cancer or non-cancerous conditions (OR = 1.6; 95% CI 0.7–3.6).

The lack of a clear effect of HIV on the risk of invasive cancer may result from competing causes of mortality in HIV-infected women in Africa (mainly tuberculosis or other infections) during the long progression from HPV infection through CIN to invasive cancer. In a setting where an organized screening programme is not normally available, the suggestion that active screening among HIV-positive women may have prevented progression to invasive cancer is not a plausible explanation.

The observation of younger age of cases of cervix cancer who were HIV-positive, compared with those who were HIV-negative (Lomalisa et al., 2000) has no etiological significance, merely reflecting the very different age structures of the respective populations at risk.

– Anal cancer

Various studies have indicated an association between HIV infection and anal cancer (Palefsky et al., 1990), with the risk being higher in men than women in the United States (Frisch et al., 2000) and in homosexual males compared with non-homosexual men (Melbye et al., 1994). No change in incidence has been noted in Africa since the onset of the AIDS epidemic.

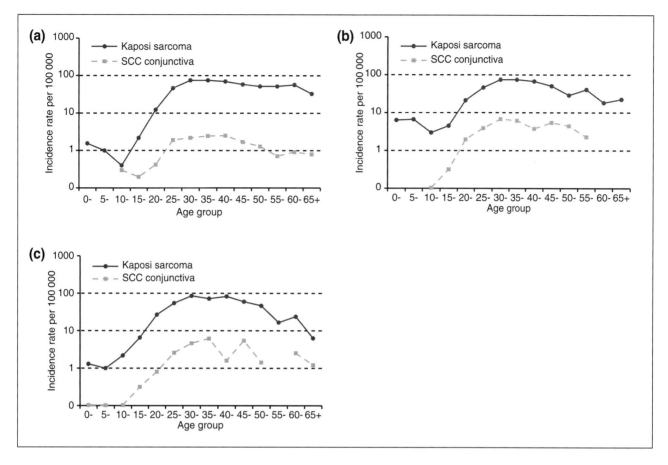

Figure 3. Incidence of Kaposi sarcoma and squamous cell carcinoma of the conjunctiva (both sexes) in (a) Harare, Zimbabwe, (b) Kampala, Uganda, and (c) Blantyre, Malawi

Ocular tumours

HIV infection is associated with a number of ocular manifestations. Ocular involvement by KS occurs and 20% of patients with systemic KS may develop the lesions on the eyelids, conjunctiva and rarely in the orbit. Although orbital lymphoma occurs in Africa, from observation, it is not common even in HIV-related cases.

HIV infection was suspected to be a risk factor for the development of squamous-cell dysplasia and neoplasia of the conjunctiva when striking increases in the number of patients with conjunctival neoplasms were noticed in Malawi, Rwanda and Uganda (Kestelyn *et al.*, 1990; Ateenyi-Agaba, 1995; Waddell *et al.*, 1996). In the pathology department at Moshi, Tanzania, about 10 cases of conjunctival squamous-cell cancer (SCC) were observed between 1976 and 1984, increasing to 40 cases by 1997 (Poole, 1999). The tumours occur at a relatively young age, mostly arising in the limbus of the eye, with duration of symptoms less than six months and an aggressive course. The Kampala cancer registry recorded a ten-fold increase in the incidence of conjunctival SCC between 1960–71 and 1995–97 (Parkin *et al.*, 1999). The high age-standardized rates of SCC of the conjunctiva now observed in registry data from Kampala, Uganda (2.0 per 100 000 in males and 2.3 in females) are also found in Blantyre, Malawi (2.1 per 100 000 in males and 2.8 in females) and Harare, Zimbabwe (1.5 per 100 000 in males and 2.5 in females). The close association with HIV infection is suggested by the age-specific incidence curve, which shows maximum rates at ages 30–39 years, very similar to the peak for age-specific incidence of Kaposi sarcoma (Figure 3) and reflecting the peak ages for HIV infection in these populations.

Five case–control studies have been completed in Africa, comparing prevalence of HIV infection in cases of SCC of the conjunctiva with that in control subjects (Table 3). All suggest a strong association, with an estimated OR between 8 and 13. The association has been confirmed in follow-up of cohorts of HIV-positive subjects in the United States (Goedert & Coté, 1995; Frisch *et al.*, 2001).

Since HPV (particularly type 16 and sometimes 6, 11, 18) has been found in some lesions (Newton, 1996), there is speculation that HIV plays a permissive role in enhancing the persistence of HPV and allowing its oncogenic potential to be expressed. HPV 16 was isolated in 7 out of 20 cases (35%) of conjunctival carcinoma samples from Uganda and Malawi (Waddell *et al.*, 1996). However, in the case–control study in Uganda (Newton *et al.*, 2002), no association was found with infection by HPV 16, 18 or 45 (as measured by serology), although the prevalence of infection by the latter two types was very low, and the estimates of risk were correspondingly imprecise.

Conjunctival SCC has always been comparatively more common in Africa than in Europe and America, as a result of the effects of ultraviolet light, the probable prime risk factor (Newton *et al.*, 1996b). High ambient solar ultraviolet radiation may act synergistically with HIV or potentiate the effects of the virus in promoting neoplastic transformation.

Other cancers

Leiomyosarcoma has been associated with HIV/AIDS, particularly in children, but there has been no evidence of an increase in this tumour in sub-Saharan Africa.

Incidence of liver cancer remains high in most regions in Africa, but there has been no significant increase associated with HIV/AIDS, in spite of the viral etiological basis. Nasopharyngeal cancer, associated with EBV, has also shown no increase.

Table 3. Case–control studies of infection with HIV and conjunctival cancers

Reference	Location	Cases	Controls	No. of cases/ no. of controls	Cases/controls HIV positive (%)	Odds ratio	95% CI
Kestelyn *et al.* (1990)	Kigali, Rwanda	Conjunctival squamous-cell neoplasms: 5 intraepithelial 6 invasive	Other eye clinic patients, age- and sex-matched	11/22	82/27	13.0	2.2–76.9
Ateeni-Agaba (1995)	Kampala, Uganda	Histologically confirmed SCC of conjunctiva	Other patients from same clinic, age- and sex-matched	48/48	75/19	13.0	4.5–39.4
Newton *et al.* (1995)	Kigali Rwanda	Eye cancer excl melanoma and KS	Other cancers excl. KS and NHL	8/200	25/4	8.4	0.8–96.9
Waddell *et al.* (1996)	Kampala, Uganda	Conjunctival squamous-cell neoplasms: 11 intraepithelial 27 invasive	Other eye clinic patients, age- and sex-matched	38/76	71/16	13.1	4.7–37.6
Newton *et al.* (2002)	Kampala, Uganda	Conjunctival tumours, 60% confirmed SCC	Other cancers (excl. cancers related to HIV, HPV, KSHV or sunlight)	60/1214	70/14.5	10.1[a]	5.2–19.4

[a]Adjusted for age and sex

References

Abouya, Y.L., Beaumel, A., Lucas, S., Dago-Akribi, A., Coulibaly, G., N'Dhatz, M., Konan, J.B., Yapi, A. & De Cock, K.M. (1992) Pneumocystis carinii pneumonia. An uncommon cause of death in African patients with acquired immunodeficiency syndrome. *Am. Rev. Respir. Dis.*, **145**, 617–620

Arico, M., Caselli, D., D'Argenio, P., Del Mistro, A.R., DeMartino, M., Livadiotti, S., Santoro, N., Terragna, A. (1991) Malignancies in children with human immunodeficiency virus type 1 infection. The Italian Multicenter Study on Human Immunodeficiency Virus Infection in Children. *Cancer*, **68**, 2473–2477

Ateenyi-Agaba, C. (1995) Conjunctival squamous cell carinoma associated with HIV infection in Kampala, Uganda. *Lancet*, **345**, 695–696

Ateka, G.K. (2001) Factors in HIV/AIDS transmission in sub-Saharan Africa. *Bull. WHO*, **79**, 1168

Ballerini, P., Gaidano, G., Gong, J.Z., Tassi, V., Saglio, G., Knowles, D.M., Dalla Favera, R. (1993) Multiple genetic lesions in acquired immunodeficiency syndrome-related non-Hodgkin's lymphoma. *Blood*, **81**, 166–176

Baroni, C.D. & Uccini, S. (1993) The lymphadenopathy of HIV infection. *Am. J. Clin. Pathol.*, **99**, 397–401

Bassett, M.T., Chokunonga, E., Mauchaza, B., Levy, L., Ferlay, J. & Parkin, D.M. (1996) Cancer in the African population of Harare, Zimbabwe, 1990-1992. *Int. J. Cancer*, **63**, 29–36

Bayley, A.C. (1984) Aggressive Kaposi's sarcoma in Zambia, 1983. *Lancet*, **i**, 1318–1320

Bem, C., Patil, P.S., Bharucha, H., Namaambo, K. & Luo, N. (1996) Importance of human immunodeficiency virus-associated lymphadenopathy and tuberculous lymphadenitis in patients undergoing lymph node biopsy in Zambia. *Br. J. Surg.*, **83**, 75–78

Beral, V., Peterman, T., Berkelman, R. & Jaffe, H. (1991) AIDS-associated non-Hodgkin lymphoma. *Lancet*, **337**, 805–809

Berkley, S., Okware, S. & Naamara, W. (1989) Surveillance for AIDS in Uganda. *AIDS*, **3**, 79–85

Biggar, R.J. (1986) Possible nonspecific association between malaria and HTLV-III/LAV. *New Engl. J. Med.*, **315**, 457–458

Biggar, R.J. & Rabkin, C.S. (1992) The epidemiology of acquired immunodeficiency syndrome-related lymphomas. *Curr. Opin. Oncol.*, **4**, 883–893

Biggar, R.J., Melbye, M., Kestems, L., Sarngadharan, M.G., de Feyter, M., Blattner, W.A., Gallo, R.C. & Gigase, P.L. (1984) Kaposi's sarcoma in Zaire is not associated with HTLV-III infections. *New Engl. J. Med.*, **311**, 1051–1052

Biggar, R.J., Horm, J.W., Lubin, J.H., Goedert, J.J., Greene, M.H. & Fraumeni, J.F., Jr (1985) Cancer trends in a population at risk of acquired HIV immunodeficiency syndrome. *J. Natl Cancer Inst.*, **74**, 793–797

Boerma, J.T., Nunn, A.J. & Whitworth, J.A. (1998) Mortality impact of the AIDS epidemic: evidence from community studies in less developed countries. *AIDS*, **12 suppl. 1**, S3–14

Casabona, J., Melbye, M., Biggar, R.J. and the AIDS Registry Contributors (1991) Kaposi's sarcoma and non-Hodgkin's lymphoma in European AIDS cases. *Int. J. Cancer*, **47**, 49–53

Casabona, J., Salas, T. & Salinas, R. (1993) Trends and survival in AIDS-associated malignancies. *Eur. J. Cancer*, **29A**, 877–881

CDC (Centers for Disease Control) (1981) Kaposi's sarcoma and Pneumocystis pneumonia among homosexual men – New York City and California. *Morb. Mortal. Wkly Rep.*, **30**, 305–308

CDC (Centers for Disease Control) (1987) Revision of the CDC surveillance case definition for acquired immunodeficiency syndrome. *Morb. Mortal. Wkly Rep.*, **36 (Suppl. 15)**, 15–155

CDC (Centers for Disease Control) (1992) 1993 revised classification system for HIV infection and expanded surveillance case definition for AIDS among adolescents and adults. *Morb. Mortal. Wkly Rep.*, **41**, 1–19

Chintu, C., Athala, U.H. & Patil, P.S. (1995) Childhood cancers in Zambia before and after the AIDS epidemic. *Arch. Dis. Child.*, **73**, 100–105

Chokunonga, E., Levy, L.M., Basset, M.T., Borok, M.Z., Mauchaza, B.G., Chirenje, M.Z. & Parkin, D.M. (1999) AIDS and cancer in Africa: the evolving epidemic in Zimbabwe. *AIDS*, **13**, 2583–2588

Coté, T.R., Biggar, R.J., Rosenberg, P.S., Devesa, S.S., Percy, C., Yellin, F.J., Lemp, G., Hardy, C., Goedert, J.J. & Blattner, W.A. (1997) Non-Hodgkin's lymphoma among people with AIDS: incidence, presentation and public health burden. AIDS/Cancer Study Group. *Int. J. Cancer*, **73**, 645–650

Dal Maso, L., Serraino, D. & Franceschi, S. (2001) Epidemiology of AIDS-related tumours in developed and developing countries. *Eur. J. Cancer*, **37**, 1188–1201

Delecluse, H.J., Raphael, M., Magaud, J.P., Felman, P., Alsamad, I.A., Bornkamm, G.W. & Lenoir, G.M. (1993) Variable morphology of human immunodeficiency virus-associated lymphomas with c-myc rearrangements. The French Study Group of Pathology for Human Immunodeficiency Virus-Associated Tumours, I. *Blood*, **82**, 552–563

Franceschi, S., Dal Maso, I. & La Vecchia, C. (1999) Advances in the epidemiology of HIV-associated non-Hodgkin's lymphoma and other lymphoid neoplasms. *Int. J. Cancer*, **83**, 481–485

Frisch, M., Biggar, R.J. & Goedert, J.J. (2000) Human papillomavirus associated cancers in patients with human immunodeficiency virus infection and acquired immunodeficiency syndrome. *J. Natl Cancer Inst.*, **92**, 1500–1510

Frisch, M., Biggar, R.J., Engels, E.A. & Goedert, J.J. (2001) AIDS-Cancer Match Registry Study Group. Association of cancer with AIDS-related immunosuppression in adults. *JAMA*, **285**, 1736–1745

Fylkesnes, K., Musonda, R.M., Sichone, M., Ndhlovu, Z., Tembo, F. & Monze M. (2001) Declining HIV prevalence and risk behaviours in Zambia: evidence from surveillance and population-based surveys. *AIDS*, **15**, 907–916

Gaidano, G., Lo Coco, F., Ye, B.H., Shibata, D., Levine, A.M., Knowles, D.M. & Dalla-Favera, R. (1994) Rearrangements of the BCL-6 gene in acquired immunodeficiency syndrome-associated non-Hodgkin's lymphoma: association with diffuse large-cell subtype. *Blood*, **84**, 397–402

Gilks, C.F., Otieno, L.S., Brindle, R.J., Newnham, R.S., Lule, G.N., Were, J.B., Simani, P.M., Bhatt, S.M., Okelo, G.B., Waiyaki, P.G. *et al.* (1992) The presentation and outcome of HIV-related disease in Nairobi. *Q. J. Med.*, **82**, 25–32

Goedert, J.J. & Coté, T.R. (1995) Conjunctival malignant disease with AIDS in USA. *Lancet*, **2**, 257–258

Goedert, J.J., Coté, T.R., Virgo, P., Scoppa, S.M., Kingma, D.W., Gail, M.H., Jaffe, E.S. & Biggar, R.J. (1998) Spectrum of AIDS-associated malignant disorders. *Lancet*, **351**, 1833–1839

Grulich, A.E., Wan, X., Law, M.G., Coates, M. & Kaldor, J.M. (1999) Risk of cancer in people with AIDS. *AIDS*, **13**, 839–843

Hamilton-Dutoit, S.J., Raphael, M., Audouin, J., Diebold, J., Lisse, I., Pedersen, C., Oksenhendler, E., Marelle, L. & Pallesen, G. (1993) In situ demonstration of Epstein-Barr virus small RNAs (EBER 1) in acquired immunodeficiency syndrome-related lymphomas: correlation with tumor morphology and primary site. *Blood*, **82**, 619–624

Hira, S.K., Ngandu, N., Wadhawan, D., Nkowne, B., Baboo, K.S., Macuacua, R., Kamanga, J., Mpoko, B., Heiba, I.M. & Perine, P.L. (1990) Clinical and epidemiological features of HIV infection at a referral clinic in Zambia. *J. Acquir. Immune Defic. Syndr.*, **3**, 87–91

Ioachim, H.L., Cronin, W., Roy, M. & Maya, M. (1990) Persistent lymphadenopathies in people at high risk for HIV infection. Clinicopathologic correlations and long-term follow-up in 79 cases. *Am. J. Clin. Pathol.*, **93**, 208–218

IARC (1996) *IARC Monographs on the Evaluation of Carcinogenic Risks to Humans*. Vol. 67, *Human Immunodeficiency Viruses and Human T-cell Lymphotropic Viruses*, Lyon, IARC

IARC (1997) *IARC Monographs on the Evaluation of Carcinogenic Risks to Humans*. Vol. 70, *Epstein-Barr Virus and Kaposi's Sarcoma Herpesvirus/Human Herpesvirus 8*, Lyon, IARC

Jay, N. & Moscicki, A.B. (2000) Human papillomavirus infections in women with HIV disease: prevalence, risk, and management. *AIDS Read.*, **10**, 659–668

Kapiga, S.H., Msamanga, G.I., Spiegelman, D., Mwakyoma, H., Fawzi, W.W. & Hunter, D.J. (1999) Risk factors for squamous intraepithelial lesions among HIV seropositive women in Dar es Salaam, Tanzania. *Int. J. Gynaecol. Obstet.*, **67**, 87–94

Karstaedt, A.S. (1992) AIDS—the Baragwanath experience. Part III. HIV infection in adults at Baragwanath Hospital. *S. Afr. Med. J.*, **82**, 95–97

Kestelyn, P., Stevens, A.M., Ndayambage, A., Hansens, M. & van de Perre, P. (1990) HIV and conjunctival malignancies. *Lancet*, **336**, 51–59

Kreiss, J.K., Kiviat, N.B., Plummer, F.A., Roberts, P.L., Waiyaki, P., Ngugi, E. & Holmes, K.K. (1992) Human immunodeficiency virus, human papillomavirus and cervical intraepithelial neoplasia in Nairobi prostitutes. *Sex. Trans. Dis.*, **19**, 54–59

Laga, M., Icenogle, J.P., Marsella, R., Manoka, A.T., Nzila, N., Ryder, R.W., Vermund, S.H., Heyward, W.L., Nelson, A. & Reeves, W.C. (1992) Genital papillomavirus infection and cervical dysplasia – opportunistic complications of HIV infection. *Int. J. Cancer*, **50**, 45–48

Langley, C.L., Benga-De, E., Critchlow, C.W., Ndoye, I., Mbengue-Ly, M.D., Kuypers, J., Woto-Gaye, G., Mboup, S., Bergeron C., Holmes K.K. & Kiviat, N.B. (1996) HIV-1, HIV-2, human papillomavirus infection and cervical neoplasia in high-risk African women. *AIDS*, **10**, 413–417

La Ruche, G., Ramon, R., Mensah-Ado, I., Bergeron, C., Diomande, M., Sylla-Koko, F., Ehouman, A., Toure-Coulibaly, K., Wellfens-Ekra, C. & Dabis, F. (1998a) Squamous intraepithelial lesions of the cervix, invasive cervical carcinoma and immunosuppression induced by human immunodeficiency virus in Africa. *Cancer*, **82**, 2410–2408

La Ruche, G., You, B., Mensah-Ado, I., Bergeron, C., Montcho, C., Ramon, R., Toure-Coulibaly, K., Wellfens-Ekra, C., Dabis, F. & Orth, G. (1998b) Human papillomavirus, and human immunodeficiency virus infections: relation with cervical dysplasia-neoplasia in African women. *Int. J. Cancer*, **76**, 480–486

Lazzi, S., Ferrari, F., Nyongo, A., Palummo, N., de Milito, A., Zazzi, M., Leoncini, L., Luzi, P. & Tosi, P. (1998) HIV-associated malignant lymphomas in Kenya (equatorial Africa). *Hum. Pathol.*, **29**, 1285–1289

Leroy, V., Msellati, P., Lepage, P., Batungwanayo, J., Hitimana, D.G., Taelman, H., Bogaerts, J., Boineau, F., Van de Perre, P., Simonon, A., *et al.* (1995) Four years of natural history of HIV-1 infection in African women: a prospective cohort study in Kigali (Rwanda), 1988-1993. *J. Acquir. Immune Defic. Syndr. Hum. Retrovirol.*, **9**, 415–421

Leroy, V., Ladner, J., De Clercq, A., Meheus, A., Nyiraziraje, M., Karita, E. & Dabis, F. (1999) Cervical dysplasia and HIV type 1 infection in African pregnant women: a cross sectional study, Kigali, Rwanda. The Pregnancy and HIV Study Group (EGE). *Sex. Trans. Infect.*, **75**, 103–106

Levy, L.M. (1988) The pattern of haematological and lymphoreticular malignancy in Zimbabwe. *Trop. Geogr. Med.*, **40**, 109–114

Lomalisa, P., Smith, T. & Guidozzi, F. (2000) Human immunodeficiency virus infection and invasive cervical cancer in South Africa. *Gynecol. Oncol.*, **77**, 460–463

Lucas, S.B., Odida, M. & Wabinga, H. (1991) The pathology of severe morbidity and mortality caused by HIV infection in Africa. *AIDS*, **5 (suppl. 1)**, S143–S148

Lucas, S.B., Diomande, M., Hounnou, A., Beaumel, A., Giordano, C., Kadio, A., Peacock, C.S., Honde, M. & de Cock, K.M. (1994) HIV associated lymphoma in Africa: an autopsy study in Cote d'Ivoire. *Int. J. Cancer*, **59**, 20–24

Maggwa, B.N., Hunter, D.J., Mbugua, S., Tukei, P. & Mati, J.K. (1993) The relationship between HIV infection and cervical intraepithelial neoplasia among women attending two family planning clinics in Nairobi, Kenya. *AIDS*, **7**, 733–738

Marum, L.H., Tindyebwa, D. & Gibb, B. (1997) Care of children with HIV infection and AIDS in Africa. *AIDS*, **11 suppl. B**, S125–134

Mayaud, P., Gill, D.K., Weiss, H.A., Uledi, E., Kopwe, L., Todd, J., ka-Gina, G., Grosskurth, H., Hayes, R.J., Mabey, D.C. m& Lacey, C.J. (2001) The interrelation of HIV, cervical human papillomavirus, and neoplasia among antenatal clinic attenders in Tanzania. *Sex. Transm. Infect.*, **77**, 248–254

Mbidde, E.K., Banura, C., Kazura, J., Desmond-Hellman, S.D., Kizito, A. & Hellmann, N. (1990) NHL and HIV infection in Uganda. *5th International Conference on AIDS in Africa*, abstract FPB1

Mbulaiteye, S.M., Mahe, C., Whitwoth, J.A.G., Ruberantwari, A., Nakiyingi, J.S., Ojwiya, A. & Kamali, A. (2002) Declining HIV-1 incidence and associated prevalence over 10 years in a rural population in south-west Uganda: a cohort study. *Lancet*, **360**, 41–46

Meda, N., Ndoye, I., M'Boup, S., Wade, A., Ndiaye, S., Niang, C., Sarr, F., Diop, I. & Carael, M. (1999) Low and stable HIV infection rates in Senegal: natural course of the epidemic or evidence for success of prevention? *AIDS*, **13**, 1397-405.

Melbye, M., Coté, T.R., Kessler, L., Gail, M. & Biggar, R.J. (1994) High incidence of anal cancer among AIDS patients. *Lancet*, **343**, 636–639

Miotti, P.G., Dallabetta, G.A., Daniel, R.W., Canner, J.K., Chiphangwi, J.D., Liomba, G., Yang, L.-P. & Shah, K.V. (1996) Cervical abnormalities, human papillomavirus, and human immunodeficiency virus infections in women in Malawi. *J. Infect. Dis.*, **173**, 714–717

Morgan, D., Mahe, C., Mayanja, B., Okongo, J.M., Iubega, R. & Whitworth, J.A. (2002a) HIV-I infection in rural Africa: is there is difference in median time to AIDS and survival compared with that in industrialized countries? *AIDS*, **16**, 597–603

Morgan, D., Mahe, C., Mayanja, B. & Whitworth, J.A.G. (2002b) Progression to symptomatic disease in people infected with HIV-I in rural Uganda: prospective cohort study. *Br. Med. J.*, **324**, 193–196

Mueller, B.U. (1998) Cancers in human immunodeficiency virus-infected children. *J. Natl Cancer Inst. Monogr.*, **23**, 31–35

Nelson, A.M., Perriens, J.H., Kapita, B., Okonda, L., Lusamuno, N., Kalengayi, M.R., Angritt, P., Quinn, T.C. & Mullick, F.G. (1993) A clinical and pathological comparison of the WHO and CDC case definitions for AIDS in Kinshasa, Zaire: is passive surveillance valid? *AIDS*, **7**, 1241–1245

Newton, R. (1996) A review of the aetiology of squamous cell carcinoma of the conjunctiva. *Br. J. Cancer*, **74**, 1511–1513

Newton, R., Grulich, A., Beral, V., Sindikubwabo, B., Ngilimana, P.J., Nganyira, A. & Parkin, D.M. (1995) Cancer and HIV infection in Rwanda. *Lancet*, **345**, 1378–1379

Newton, R., Ferlay, J., Reeves, G., Beral, V. & Parkin, D.M. (1996) Effect of ambient ultraviolet radiation on incidence of squamous cell carcinoma of the eye. *Lancet*, **347**, 1450–1451

Newton, R., Ziegler, J., Beral, V., Mbidde, E., Carpenter, L., Wabinga, H., Mbuletieye, Appleby, P., Reeves, G., Jaffe, H. & Uganda Kaposi's sarcoma Study Group (2001) A case-control study of HIV infection and cancer in adults and children in Kampala Uganda. *Int. J. Cancer*, **91**, 622–627

Newton, R., Ziegler, J., Ateenyi-Agaba, C., Bousarghin, L., Casabonne, D., Beral, V., Mbidde, E., Carpenter, L., Reeves, G., Parkin, D.M., Wabinga, H., Mbulaiteye, S., Jaffe, H., Bourboulia, D., Boshoff, C., Touze, A. & Coursaget, P. (2002) The epidemiology of conjunctival squamous cell carcinoma in Uganda. *Br. J. Cancer*, **87**, 301–308

N'Galy, B., Ryder, R.W., Bila, K., Mwandagalirwa, K., Colebunders, R.L., Francis, H., Mann, J.M. & Quinn, T.C. (1988) Human immunodeficiency virus infection among employees in an African hospital. *New Engl. J. Med.*, **319**, 1123–1127

Otieno, M.W., Remick, S.C. & Whelan, C. (2001) Adult Burkitt's lymphoma in patients with and without human immunodeficiency virus infection in Kenya. *Int. J. Cancer*, **92**, 687–691

Palefsky, J.M., Gonzales, J., Greenbalt, R.M., Ahn, D.K. & Hollander, H. (1990) Anal intraepithelial neoplasm and anal papilloma virus infection among homosexual males with group IV HIV disease. *JAMA*, **263**, 2911–2916

Parkin, D.M., Wabinga, H., Nambooze, S. & Wabwire-Mangen, F. (1999) AIDS-related cancers in Africa: maturation of the epidemic in Uganda. *AIDS*, **13**, 2563–2570

Parkin, D.M., Garcia-Giannoli, H., Raphael, M., Martin, A., Katangole-Mbidde, E., Wabinga, H. & Ziegler, J. (2000) Non-Hodgkin's lymphoma in Uganda: a case-control study. *AIDS*, **14**, 2929–2936

Piot, P., Quinn, T.C., Taelman, H., Feinsod, F.M., Minlangu, K.B., Wobin, O., Mbendi, N., Mazebo, P., Ndangi, K., Stevens, W., Kalambayi, K., Mitchell, S., Bridts, C. & McCormick, J.B. (1984) Acquired immunodeficiency syndrome in a heterosexual population in Zaire. *Lancet*, **ii**, 65–69

Piper, M.A., Severin, S.T., Wiktor, S.Z., Unger, E.R., Ghys, P.D., Miller, D.L., Horowitz, I.R., Greenberg, A.E., Reeves, W.C. & Vernon, S.D. (1999) Association of human papillomavirus with HIV and CD4 cell count in women with high or low numbers of sex partners.*Sex Transm. Infect.*, **75**, 253–257

Poole, T.R. (1999) Conjunctival squamous cell carcinoma in Tanzania. *Br. J. Opthalmol.*, **83**, 177–179

Reeve, P.A. (1989) HIV infection in patients admitted to a general hospital in Malawi. *Br. Med. J.*, **298**, 1567–1568

Rogo, K.O. & Kavoo-Linge (1990) Human immunodeficiency virus seroprevalence among cervical cancer patients. *Gynecol. Oncol.*, **37**, 87–92

Roithmann, S. & Andrieu, J.-M. (1992) Clinical and biological characteristics of malignant lymphomas in HIV-infected patients. *Eur. J. Cancer*, **28A**, 1501–1508

Roithmann, S., Toledano, M., Tourani, J.M., Raphael, M., Gentilini, M., Gastaut, J.A., Armengaud, M., Morlat, P., Tilly, H., Dupont, B., Taillan, B., Theodore, C., Doniado, D. & Andrieu, J.M. (1991) HIV-associated non-Hodgkin's lymphomas: clinical characteristics and outcome. The experience of the French Registry of HIV-associated tumors. *Ann. Oncol.*, **2**, 289–295

Seck, A.C., Faye, M.A., Critchlow, C.W., Mbaye, A.D., Kuypers, J., Woto-Gaye, G., Langley, C., De, E.B., Holmes, K.K. & Kiviat, N.B. (1994) Cervical intraepithelial neoplasia and human papillomavirus infection among Senegalese women seropositive for HIV-1 or HIV-2 or seronegative for HIV. *Int. J. STD AIDS*, **5**, 189–193

Serraino, D. & Franceschi, S. (1996) Kaposi's sarcoma and non-Hodgkin's lymphomas in children and adolescents with AIDS. *AIDS*, **10**, 643–647

Serraino, D., Francheschi, S., Tirelli, U. & Monfardini, S. (1992) Epidemiology of acquired immunodeficiency syndrome and associated tumours in Europe. *Ann. Oncol.*, **3**, 595–603

Serraino, D., Pezzotti, P., Dorrucci, M., Alliegro, M.B., Sinicco, A. & Rezza, G. (1997) Cancer incidence in a cohort of human immunodeficiency virus seroconverters: HIV Italian seroconvertion study group. *Cancer*, **79**, 1004–1008

Serwadda, D., Sewankambo, N.K., Carswell, J.W., Bayley, A.C., Tedder, R.S., Weiss, R.A., Mugerwa, R.D., Lwegaba, A., Kirya, G.B., Downing, R.G., Clayden, S.A. & Dalgleish, A.G. (1985) Slim disease: a new disease in Uganda and its association with HTLV-II infection. *Lancet*, **ii**, 849–852

Sitas, F., Bezwoda, W.R., Levin, V., Ruff, P., Kew, M.C., Hale, M.J., Carrera, H., Beral, V., Fleming, G., Odes, R. & Weaving, A. (1997) Association between human immunodeficiency virus type 1 infection and cancer in the black population of Johannesburg and Soweto. South Africa. *Br. J. Cancer*, **75**, 1704–1707

Sitas, F., Madhoo, J. & Wessie, J. (1998) Incidence of Histologically Diagnosed Cancer in South Africa, 1993-1995. Johannesburg, National Cancer Registry of South Africa, South African Institute of Medical Research

Sitas, F., Pacella-Norman, R., Carrara, H., Patel, M., Ruff, P., Sur, R., Jentsch, U., Hale, M., Rowji, P., Saffer, D., Connor, M., Bull, D., Newton, R. & Beral, V. (2000) The spectrum of HIV-1 related cancers in South Africa. *Int. J. Cancer*, **88**, 489–492

Standaert, B., Kocheleff, P., Kadende, P., Nitunga, N., Guerna, T., Laroche, R. & Piot, P. (1988) Acquired immunodeficiency syndrome and human immunodeficiency virus infection in Bujumbura, Burundi. Trans. R. Soc. Trop. Med. Hyg., 82, 902–904

Temmerman, M., Tyndall, M.W., Kidula, N., Claeys, P., Muchiri, L. & Quint, W. (1999) Risk factors for human papillomavirus and cervical precancerous lesions, and the role of concurrent HIV-1 infection. *Int. J. Gynaecol. .Obstet.*, **65**, 171–181

Ter Meulen, J., Eberhardt, H.C., Luande, J., Mgaya, H.N., Chang-Claude, J., Mtiro, H., Mhina, M., Kashaija, P., Ockert, S., Yu, X., Meinhardt, G., Gissman, L. & Pawlita, M. (1992) Human papillomavirus (HPV) infection, HIV infection and cervical cancer in Tanzania, East Africa. *Int. J. Cancer*, **52**, 515–521

Van de Perre, P., Rouvroy, D., Lepage, P., Bogaerts, J., Kestelyn, P., Kayihigi, J., Hekker, A.C., Butzler, J.P. & Clumeck, N. (1984) Acquired immunodeficiency syndrome in Rwanda. *Lancet*, **ii**, 62–65

Vernon, S.D., Unger, E.R., Piper, M.A., Severin, S.T., Wiktor, S.Z., Ghys, P.D., Miller, D.L., Horowitz, I.R., Greenberg, A.E. & Reeves, W.C. (1999) HIV and human papillomavirus as independent risk factors for cervical neoplasia in women with high or low numbers of sex partners. *Sex. Transm. Infect.*, **75**, 258–260

Wabinga, H.R., Parkin, D.M., Wabwire-Mangen, F. & Nambooze, S. (2000) Trends in cancer incidence in Kyandondo County, Uganda, 1969-1977. *Br. J. Cancer*, **82**, 1585–1592

Waddell, K., Lewallen, S., Lucas, S., Ateenyi, C., Herrington, C.S. & Liomba, G. (1996) Carcinoma of the conjunctiva and HIV infection in Uganda and Malawi. *Br. J. Ophthalmol.*, **80**, 503–508

Whittle, H., Egboga, A., Todd, J., Corrah, T., Wilkins, A., Demba, E., Morgan, G., Rolfe, M., Berry, N., Tedder, R. (1992) Clinical and laboratory predictors of survival in Gambian patients with symptomatic HIV-1 or HIV-2 infection. *AIDS*, **6**, 685–689

WHO (World Health Organization) (1986) Acquired immunodeficiency syndrome (AIDS): WHO/CDC case definition for AIDS. *Wkly Epidemiol. Rec.*, **61**, 69–73

Womack, S.D., Chirenje, Z.M., Gaffikin, L., Blumenthal, P.D., McGrath, J.A., Chipato, T., Ngwalle, E., Munjoma, M. & Shah, K.V. (2000) HPV-based cervical cancer screening in a population at high risk for HIV infection. *Int. J. Cancer*, **85**, 206–210

Ziegler, J.L., Drew, W.L., Miner, R.C., Mintz, L., Rosenbaum, E., Gershow, J., Lennette, E.T., Greenspan, J., Shillitoe, E., Beckstead, J., Casavant, C. & Yamamoto, K. (1982) Outbreak of Burkitt's-like lymphoma in homosexual men. *Lancet*, **2**, 631–633

Index

Achevé d'imprimer sur les presses
de l'Imprimerie Darantiere
à Dijon-Quetigny en
juin 2003

N° d'impression : 23-0818
Dépôt légal : juin 2003

Imprimé en France